HOMŒOPATHIC
DRUG PICTURES

HOMŒOPATHIC DRUG PICTURES

By

M. L. TYLER

M.D.Brux., L.R.C.P., L.R.C.S.Edin.,
L.R.F.P.S.Glas.

HEALTH   SCIENCE   PRESS
Rustington,   Sussex,   England

First Published 1942
Reprinted (with Supplement) 1944
Revised Edition 1952
Reprinted 1970

SBN 85032 021 6

MADE AND PRINTED IN GREAT BRITAIN BY
MORRISON AND GIBB LIMITED, LONDON AND EDINBURGH

CONTENTS

CONTENTS

CONTENTS

FOREWORD TO THE SECOND EDITION

THE second edition of " Homœopathic Drug Pictures " from the pen of the late Dr. Tyler is probably the most valuable contribution to the homœopathic Materia Medica that has been written in our day.

The early compilations of drug provings were an unorganised collection of symptoms produced by drugs on the healthy together with clinical observations gathered from the experiences of physicians using the drugs.

In recent years many Materia Medicas have been composed to assist the practitioner to sort out this indiscriminate mass of drug symptoms and to bring to his help an apprehension of the nuances of each drug.

To this task, Dr. Tyler has brought a lifetime of experience and has put on record a Materia Medica which fulfils this need to a high degree. Her drug studies are terse and exact.

This magnum opus was written in under ten years ; a remarkable tribute to her industry and to her gift of presenting the insight she had acquired into the essence of each drug's activity on the sick.

It is not surprising that such an intrepid homœopathic physician as Dr. Tyler should have interpolated into her book various theories which were in vogue in her time in support of the homœopathic principle ; for instance the applicability of the Arndt-Schulz law to the doctrine *Similia Similibus Curentur*. But the real and enduring value of her work lies in that her genius enabled her to give a pattern to each drug which can be readily equated with the pattern of the patient's symptoms ; his reactions, environmental, physical and emotional. The similarity between the configuration of the sick patient's symptoms and that of the drug is an approach especially congenial to the British School of Homœopathy of to-day.

We are fortunate to have Dr. Tyler's vast knowledge set down in this book which will remain of abiding value to every practitioner of our art.

Once again, we salute the memory of a great lady and a great homœopathic physician.

J. D. KENYON.

February, 1952.

ENUNCIATION

HOMŒOPATHY arrived a full hundred years before its time. It was then completely revolutionary and met with fierce opposition. But its unanswerable appeal was to results, and those who had once witnessed its amazing powers of relief in sickness and pain, had perforce to adopt it in their practice. Homœopathy, being POWER, has survived. But it is only in our day that science is demonstrating its absolute reasonableness, and showing that it is not only up to date, but has always been before-date.

* * * *

Its name proclaims it—the *pathy of " like sickness "*, because its medicines are used to cure only the exact conditions they can produce in the healthy. " Drugs are sick-making, and sick-curing, and the sickness is the same."

* * * *

Apart from what is common to both schools of medicine, Homœopathy concerns itself solely with *Materia Medica* : with the discovery of medicines, the testing or " proving " of medicines, the preparation of medicines, the exhibition of medicines ; and in all these it is entirely heterodox.

* * * *

The medicine of the schools has been mainly based on *physiological action* : therefore its dosage is material. " So much of this hypnotic will compel sleep and not prove lethal."

Homœopathy is the medicine of *vital stimulation* : its aim, not physiological action, but *vital reaction*. And the amount of stimulus required to provoke reaction, in an organism rendered hypersensitive by disease, is seldom material.

* * * *

In order to make such therapy possible, it was imperative that innumerable drugs should be fully tested as to their subversive powers, and their pathogeneses registered. Such "Provings ", carefully conducted and faithfully recorded, form the *Materia Medica Pura* of HAHNEMANN ; who thus made the Law *similia similibus curentur* practical and, in long years of patient investigation, established also its corollaries.

Time has added, and adds, invaluable drugs to our wealth of available data. But not one jot or tittle has had to be superseded, for this reason : that Hahnemann dealt with, and taught us to deal with FACTS—" facts simply expressed in the changeless language of nature "—and FACTS ARE FOR ALL TIME.

PREFACE

On Adam, we are told, was laid the task of naming all things living : a tremendous opportunity and responsibility : since things nameless are lost to any wide use, while things misnamed are hurtfully mislaid.

The choice of a name for his epoch-making discovery in Medicine devolved on Hahnemann, who, being a man of erudition, was able to express, for all time and for all the world, in happy Greek phrase, at once its powers and its possibilities. It was the Medicine of LIKES, the Medicine of the cure of LIKES BY LIKES— HOMŒOPATHY. Perfect name ! Perfect description !

That was the first stage—incontrovertible, yet incomplete, as he was to discover ; when remedies, in certain individual cases, after first apparently curing, presently failed. WHY ? . . . Success spells FINIS : partial failure goads to fresh effort. So it was here. And eleven years of intense work and verifications enabled him to further reveal *The Origin and Nature of Chronic Diseases, and the Manner of their Cure.*

But the times were not ripe for such teachings, and his followers have, more or less, failed to follow. Essentials have been whittled down. Even the Law of Healing is, for some, a mere Rule. And the power he envisaged for the healing of the nations has been, to some extent, neglected—even called in question.

As to the initial part of his revelation, which concerns the Medicine of Likes, that goes without saying.

The merest tyro must grasp the fact that you cannot, for instance, cure chronic constipation with purgatives : this the centuries have demonstrated, and—the chemists still flourish.

In the same way that you cannot cure constipation by purgatives, you cannot cure sleeplessness by hypnotics,—except, perhaps, where it is merely the question of breaking a habit ; nor pain by analgesics. To cure, you must not merely deaden sensation, but cut at the root, at the cause of the pain. This is self-evident when we reflect that a thing CURED, IS cured, and does not demand ever-readjusted dosage to keep up the fiction.

On the other hand you *can* cure simple constipation by the agent capable of causing just that kind of constipation ; sleeplessness by the very same subversive agent that can cause that kind of inability to sleep, and so on. One recalls the story of the miserable insomniac, huddled away behind closed shutters

and heavy curtains, lest his remorseless enemy, NOISE—even
the slightest noise, should penetrate to reawake consciousness,
irritability—despair.   To whom came a wise man of not only
medicine but psychology, who ordered him away to spend his
nights in a dockyard ; where heavy hammerings never ceased,
and where his terrors, perforce, had to give it up ; when he
was cured.   And again, recently, a treatment for shell-shock is to
employ gramophone records reproducing all the horrific noises
associated with modern warfare, in order to restore, by the
familiarity which breeds contempt, the shattered nerves of war
victims.   If this is not pure Homœopathy, what is ?

Great satisfaction lies in the knowledge that it is possible to
discover curative agents for each curable case, by means of the
testing (" proving ") of drugs, as we have been taught to test them.
But not on animals, which cannot supply the symptom-picture we
need ; and not on the sick of diverse diseases, who can, at best,
yield only a medley of drug-plus-disease symptoms, impossible to
disentangle and inscribe for the permanent use of humanity.   But
Homœopathy investigates and records the effect of drugs on
healthy, sensitive humans, who can supply the exact information
desired.

One feels regret for the enthusiastic expectation that seeks
otherwise to discover the effects of medicines, with no law as to
their application, in order that it may, some day, somehow, be
able to employ them with a reasonable prospect of success. . . .
for is it not thus that Medicine has painfully evolved itself ?—now
dogmatizing ; now doubting ; now discarding in favour of a new hope ;
till Hahnemann came on the scene to upset every preconceived
opinion, tradition or teaching contrary to FACTS.   Till his day it
seems never to have occurred to " science " to test remedies on
healthy persons, and thus discover their precise effects on human
organs, tissues and mentalities, before prescribing them for the
sick.   Is it not self-evident that knowledge of diseases and
knowledge of drug-action are of little value, lacking the essential
fore-knowledge, how to apply the one for the relief of the other.

But, while considering the cure of curable sickness by the
Therapy of Likes, there are incurable cases of disease, or results of
disease.   You cannot put back lung tissue that has ulcerated out,
any more than you can readjust an amputated limb, so that it
shall survive and functionate normally.   But, for the most
incurable conditions, the Medicine of Likes still holds good.   It
may, and does, palliate, and indefinitely prolong life.   What is left
of the ulcerated lung may heal and suffice to carry on with—even
for years.   Besides which, who shall dogmatize as to what is

incurable ?   Homœopathy in the hands of courageous, enthusiastic and imaginative physicians, can narrow down the range of incurability : can even work seeming miracles of healing.

Homœopathy has been described under different names, some of them the reverse of complimentary, since Hahnemann fitted it with that name of perfect expression, in order that no one should ever mistake its nature, or pervert its purpose.

Burnett hit the mark when he styled Homœopathy " Scientific Medicine ". It is all that. It is medicine based on ascertained facts and abundantly proved deductions. And our experience is, that the wider our knowledge and the more conscientiously applied, the better results we get. Knowledge in any department is not necessarily all knowledge : everywhere it is just a question of degrees. If we knew all, even in regard to our own corner of medicine, who shall set the bounds to our great deeds of healing ? But because the goal is not attained—is not attainable—it is something to keep it steadily in view and, by pursuing it, to be nearing, daily, more light and power . . . .   Aye, POWER. For that is the new name we would propose for the system of Hahnemann.

HOMŒOPATHY, THE MEDICINE OF POWER.

After all, what is POWER ? Is it not the most intangible, yet most compelling of conceivable agents ? As Robert Louis Stevenson has it :

> *I only saw the things you did,*
> *But always you yourself you hid.*

Power is not peculiar to earth, nor to any of the solar systems it holds together and rules. For its recognition it needs neither bulk, quantity, texture, colour, odour. It may be constant, or instantaneous in action : evidenced, here, by apparent immovable stability in a torrent of orderly motion, there, by the vivid flash, more devastating, often, than the most fiendish explosive. And yet, since *He giveth them a law which shall not be broken*, His powers may be drawn upon for humanity's puny uses by studying and mastering their modes and limitations, and the correct manner of their application.

" *Potencies* "—powers—as Hahnemann came to know them, are the strange " infinitesimals " latent in things—perhaps in all things of substance, and only to be disclosed and rendered serviceable by "dynamization" : and that in inverse ratio to their concentration. He found that by the addition of a first non-lethal dose of such a " like " as *Belladonna* to a " like " such as *scarlet fever*, you will be adding fire to consuming fire ; therefore he attempted, in his orderly way, by dilution—one part of medicine in 99 parts of some medicinally inert substance ; ensuring the perfect diffusion of the former throughout the latter by a series of succussions, or triturations, in order to decrease activity, that he was really more and more liberating curative power.

In one of his writings where he discusses Potentization, he emphasizes his claim to its discovery. " I was apparently the first who made this great, this °extraordinary *discovery*, that the properties of crude medicinal substances gain, when they are fluid by repeated *succussion* with unmedicinal substances, and when they are dry by frequent continued *tritivration* with unmedicinal powders, such an increase of medicinal power, that when these processes are carried very far, even substances in which for centuries no medicinal power has been observed in their crude state, display under this manipulation a power of acting on the health of man that is quite astonishing."

Moreover he demonstrated that, while the inherent latent powers of medicinal, or apparently non-medicinal substances were modified by being thus developed into " a series of degrees of potency, many of which were never known before ", that, besides this alteration in their *medicinal* properties, the homœopathic method of preparation produces an alteration in their *chemical* properties. Those which in crude form are insoluble, become entirely soluble in both water and alcohol, by means of this homœopathic transformation. " This discovery is invaluable to the healing art."

And again, " The medicinal chemical substances which have been thus prepared, are no longer subject to chemical laws."

" A dose of phosphorus of the highest potency may remain for years enclosed in its paper in a desk, without losing its medicinal properties, or even changing them to those of phosphoric acid.

" A remedy which has been elevated to the highest potency, and by this means has become almost spiritualized, is no longer subject to the laws of neutralization. . . ." And Hahnemann, accounted one of the greatest analytical chemists of his day, knew what he was writing about.

In regard to *Chronic Diseases*, absolutely convinced of the truth of his discoveries, and having reached his seventy-third year, to avoid the danger of their loss to mankind, he disclosed them, as he says, " to two of his most deserving disciples . . . lest he should be called into eternity before having completed his work ". As a matter of fact, it was left unfinished. He had grouped all the chronic non-venereal diseases under one name—*Psora* ; but as he says, " in the subsequent list of anti-psoric remedies no ISOPATHIC remedies are mentioned, for the reason that their effects upon the healthy organism have not sufficiently been ascertained ". By *isopathic remedies* he evidently means, or includes, disease products—our " *nosodes* ", one of which, his *Psorinum*, made from the muco-purulent matter of a scabies vesicle, " he pronounces homœopathic and *not isopathic*, since the homœopathic preparation, by which it is sterilized, and potentized, has changed its nature and properties, till they are no longer *identical*, but ' *like* ' ; not *isopathy*, but *Homœopathy*".

This has needed some hundred years before obtaining anything like recognition ; indeed, his greatest work, the successful treatment of chronic non-venereal diseases, is only beginning its triumphal march into that territory of despair—*Chronic Disease.*

*   *   *   *

Moreover that Homœopathy can successfully combat a disease never seen, but whose symptoms are known, was abundantly proved by statistics, which poured in from all parts of the world when CHOLERA, described by Hahnemann as " that mysterious and murdrous pest " was " rushing on Europe in 1830 ". He prepared his followers to deal with it, with what success the following statistics, among many others, exemplify.   His chief remedies were CAMPHOR, for the early stages ; very frequently repeated, " till consciousness, rest, and sleep return, and he is saved ".

Camphor poisoning displays all the symptoms of early cholera. " In the second and more difficult stage of clonic spasmodic character, with vomiting, purging and excessively painful cramp in calves, etc., if *Camphor* has not helped in fifteen minutes give *Cuprum*, in potency, every hour or half-hour ; or, where there are excessive vomiting, excessive purging, *excessive cold sweats*, the remedy is *Veratrum alb.*"

We read, *inter alia*, " Cholera, came first by way of .*Russia*. The Russian Consul General reported results from Homœopathic treatment in Russia in 1830-1.   Of 70 cases treated in two places, all were cured.   And of 1,270 cases, 1,162 were cured and only 108 died.   (The allopathic mortality in Russia was 60 to 70 per cent.)"[1]

Dr. Wilde, an allopathic surgeon (Ed. *Dublin Quarterly Journal of Medicine*), in his *Austria, its Literary, Scientific and Medical Treatments*, wrote : " Upon comparing the report made of the treatment of cholera in the Homœopathic Hospital at Vienna with that of the other hospitals at the same time, it appears that while two-thirds of those treated homœopathically were *cured*, two-thirds of those treated by the other hospitals *died*. This extraordinary result led Count Kolowrat, Minister of the Interior, to repeal the law relative to the practice of Homœopathy."[1]

A Dr. Perrussel (South of France) attended the poor villagers who have been suffering from sweating sickness and from cholera. His mortality under (homœopathic) treatment was 5 to 7 per cent. ; the allopathic mortality there was 90 per cent.[2]

In Guatemala in 1854, a Baptist missionary was given ten days' imprisonment by a coroner. His real offence was curing, by gratuitous administration of homœopathic medicines, a large proportion of cholera patients, when the hospital treatment did not cure one.

In 1854 Cholera broke out violently round our, then, London Hospital, whose 25 beds were devoted to the treatment of cholera and choleraic diarrhœa. Returns give 61 cases of cholera with 10 deaths, and 341 cases of choleraic diarrhœa with 1 death. While, besides the cases treated in hospital over 1,200 bottles of *Camphor* were given to the poor who flocked in crowds to get them.

Detailed returns had to be made by all hospitals and practitioners as to treatment and results in cholera. When these were presented to Parliament the homœopathic statistics were missing ; were demanded, and had to be produced. The excuse was embodied in the following resolution of the Medical body concerned :

" Resolved that by introducing the returns of homœopathic practitioners, they would not only compromise the value and utility of their average of cure, as deduced from the operation of known remedies, but they would give an unjustifiable sanction to an empirical practice alike opposed to the maintenance of truth and to the progress of science."—*British Journal of Homœopathy*, xiii., p. 466.

But the most brilliant cholera work was done by Dr. Rubini in the Naples epidemic of 1854-5. With camphor alone he treated in the R. Albergo dei Poveri 225 cases of cholera without a single death, and 166 soldiers of the 3rd Swiss Regiment with the same success. " Spirits of Camphor", in consequence, for many years—probably still—has borne his name.

Bradford, *Logic of Figures*, states, p. 137, " The aggregate statistics of results of allopathic treatment of cholera in Europe and America show a mortality of over 40 per cent. ; statistics of homœopathic treatment a mortality of less than 9 per cent."

---

[1] Bradford's *Logic of Figures* (1900).
[2] *British Journal of Homœopathy* 1854, pp. 521, 686.

ABROTANUM

(Southernwood)

Artemesia Abrotanum : Old Man Tree : Boy's Love : Lad's Love

In *Abrotanum* we have a valuable remedy of marasmic children. It has many symptoms in common with *Aethusa cynapium*, and many others that sharply differentiate the two drugs. In both we find extreme weakness; inability to stand, or even to hold the head erect. But the *Abrotanum* child, instead of being unable to take milk, craves bread boiled in milk, to satisfy its gnawing hunger. Both drugs have, "Thinking difficult ; loss of comprehension.

But the mental symptoms of *Aethusa* and *Abrotanum* help to distinguish between them. In *Aethusa*, " Fools' Parsley ", there is confusion, inability to think, almost idiocy. *Abrotanum* has also incapacity for thought ; but may be extremely irritable, cross, ill-natured : even violent and inhuman : would like to do something cruel. No humanity.

Our idea of *Abrotanum*, " Lad's Love ", is a greyish-green shrubby plant, growing just inside the garden gate of country cottages. In passing in or out one instinctively crushes what Culpepper describes as " its numerous leaves divided into many fine bristly segments, of a fine pale green colour ", in order to retain on one's fingers its charming scent. This, no doubt, gained it the name of Lad's Love : for in all the centuries it must have been plucked by our lads for shy presentation to the maidens of their choice ; doubtless to be pressed and sacredly preserved in many an ancient Bible, after the manner of our country-folk, to rekindle, throughout life, its sweet memories of youth and courtship.

Abrotanum is one of our old English herbal remedies. In CULPEPPER'S *English Physician* (its Preface is dated 1653), we read in regard to *Abrotanum*,

" The seed bruised, heated in warm water, and drank, helps those that are troubled with cramps or convulsions of the sinews, and sciatica, and bringing down women's courses. The same taken in wine is an antidote against all poisons. The backbone anointed with the oil cures the ague, it removes inflammations in the eyes, if part of a roasted quince and a few crumbs of bread be boiled and added. Boiled with barley-meal, it removes pimples and wheals from the face, or other parts of the body.

The seed and the dried herb kills worms in children; the herb bruised and applied draws out splinters and thorns from the flesh. The ashes mingled with old salad oil, helps those that are bald, causing the hair to grow again on the head or beard. A strong decoction of the leaves is a good worm medicine, but is disagreeable and nauseous. The leaves are a good ingredient in fomentations for easing pain, dispersing swellings, or stopping the progress of gangrenes." He speaks of its fine pale green colour, and pleasant smell.

Black Letter Symptoms

Great weakness and prostration with a kind of hectic fever : with children, after influenza.

Itching chilblains (compare Nux, Agaricus).

Painful, inflammatory rheumatism before the swelling commences.

Gout. Painful and inflamed wrists and ankle joints.

And Some Notable Symptoms

Sensation of creeping chills along convolutions of brain.

Appetite very great ; ravenous, while emaciating.

(Or, loss of appetite.)

Sensation as if stomach were hanging, or swimming in water, with a peculiar feeling of coldness and dullness to all irritants.

After sudden checking of diarrhœa, rheumatism.

Piles appeared and became worse as rheumatic pains abated.

Frequent desire for stool, but little but blood passed.

Destroys worms, especially ascarides.

Twitching, ovarian regions ; pains extend to back.

Suppressed menses.

In pleurisy (after *Acon.* and *Bry.*) when a pressing sensation remains in affected side, impeding free breathing.

Hectic fever, very weakening (marasmus).

Contraction of the limbs from cramps, or following colic.

In marasmus, the skin is flabby and hangs loose.

*   *   *

Nash mentions *Abrotanum* six times in his *Leaders*. Its chief uses, for him, are summed up as :

Marasmus, most pronounced in lower extremities, from malnutrition.

Diarrhœa.

Diarrhœa alternating with rheumatism.

We will quote these passages because they give very definite indications as regards the uses of the remedy, and what is so important, his useful comparisons with other remedies of like conditions or symptoms.

In regard to marasmus, he points out that, whereas *Sanicula, Natrum mur.* and *Lycopodium* emaciate from above downwards, *Abrotanum* emaciates from below, upwards.

Of *Nat. mur.* he says, No remedy is more hungry, yet he loses flesh while eating well (*Acet. a., Abrotanum, Iodine, Sanicula* and *Tuberculinum*).

In *Nat. mur.* emaciation is most noticeable in the neck : *Abrotanum* in the legs. . . .

In the marasmus of children we have to choose among remedies such as *Bar. carb., Silica, Abrotanum, Nat. m., Sulphur, Calc.* and *Iod.* Under all these remedies we may find emaciation of the rest of the body, while the abdomen is greatly enlarged. Again, under every one of them, the child may have a voracious appetite ; eat enough, but grow poor all the time. It is a defective assimilation.

Certain remedies alternate symptoms, as *Kali bi.* where rheumatic and dysenteric symptoms alternate. Also *Abrotanum.*

Abrotanum has ravenous hunger : losing flesh while eating well (*Iod., Nat. m., Sanic., Tub.*).

Marasmus of the lower limbs only.

* * *

Abrotanum is also a remedy of boils, of rheumatism : of gout ; especially of wrists and ankle joints (*Ruta*).

It has a reputation for hydrocele in children : this we have rapidly cured, before now, with *Rhododendron.*

By far the best picture of *Abrotanum* is to be found in Allen's *Keynotes.*

ACONITUM

"My heart is disquieted within me: and the fear of death is fallen upon me.

" Fearfulness and trembling are come upon me : and an horrible dread hath overwhelmed me."

THE Sweet Psalmist of Israel, the Warrior King, who nearly three thousand years ago swept the strings of all human emotions and experiences: who has inspired a hundred generations with courage, reliance, confidence—repentance : who reached the sublimest heights, and fathomed the depths of suffering, bereavement, and remorse,. even he had his *Aconite* moment of *solid, unreasoning* FEAR.

His words, above, are practically those of the provings of *Aconite*.

KENT says, " *Aconite* is like a great storm ; it comes, and sweeps over, and passes away." . . . " It is a short-acting remedy : a violent poison in large doses, either destroying life, or passing away in its effects quite soon, so that if the patient recovers, recovery is not delayed. There are no chronic diseases following it."

The very face of *Aconite* expresses FEAR, and *Aconite* is curative in ailments from fright, mental, or physical, even to jaundice ; just as *Chamomilla* is curative of ailments, even to jaundice, caused by rage and anger, or *Staphisagria* of ailments caused by real, or imaginary, insults and grievances.

But the fears of *Aconite* are more or less intangible. The known, the definite, has no terrors for *Aconite*. It has not the fear of poverty of BRYONIA, the fear of thunder of PHOSPHORUS, the fear of dogs of BELLADONNA, the fear of approach of ARNICA, the fear when alone of *Arsenicum, Argentum nit.* But *Aconite* has the FEAR OF DEATH, the fear of darkness, the fear of bed, the fear of ghosts. *Aconite* has not only the fear of death, but it predicts the very hour of death. As Kent puts it, " If a clock is in the room, he will say that when the hands reach a certain point, he will be a corpse." It is *Aconite* who calls his friends around, and takes leave of them. *Aconite* has thoughts of death, the presentiment of death, predicts the time of death. And such a mental state, occurring in the course of any illness, or after any shock, fright or operation, calls for *Aconite*.

Aconite is a quick-acting, superficial remedy, for acute and most distressing conditions, when the patient, getting *Aconite*, lies down, relaxes, and sleeps. The storm has passed.

It is homœopathy that can administer to intangible, but torturing distress. And remember, *Aconite* is no dope, it is merely promptly *curative* of the conditions it has actually produced in poisonings and in provings.

Dr. Clarke once said, " If ever you come across a book by Henry N. Guernsey, buy it." And GUERNSEY has an illuminating article on *Aconite*. He says :

" The genius of this highly useful remedy is through the mental sphere, and it is always important to consider the mental symptoms. Almost certainly this remedy should never be given in cases where the sickness is borne with calmness and patience. If *Aconite* is even to be thought of, we will find mental uneasiness, worry, or fear, accompanying a most trifling ailment, such as inflammation of the eyelids .   .   .   Great and uncontrollable anguish, anxiety, and great fear, are characteristic of the *Aconite* disease.   .   .   .

" *Complaints caused by fright, and the fear remains. (Opium.)*

" Predicts the expected day of his death, is very characteristic.

" In the delirium is unhappiness, worry, despair, raving, with expression of fear upon the countenance, but there is rarely unconsciousness.   .   .   .

" Easy bleeding, of bright, pure, red blood, attended by a great fear of death.   .   .   .

" Active hæmorrhages from any part of the body, uterine or other, accompanied with fear of death and nervous excitability."

Fear of death may be so great, that people have actually killed themselves for fear of dying !   (I myself knew one such case.)

Shakespeare says that " *There is nothing either good or bad, but thinking makes it so.*" And with *Aconite*, it is largely the thinking that makes it so.

It is the unreal, the intangible, that strike terror into *Aconite*, and failing *Aconite*, you may almost have to fake the clock, in order to save life.

Kent says, " The patients most in need of *Aconite* are the strong, robust people.

" The patient seems threatened with sudden, violent death, but recovery is quick.   A great storm, and soon over."

Aconite is the remedy of *cold, dry weather*, like *Hepar, Nux* and a few others ;   while *cold, wet weather* affects such people as need *Dulcamara, Rhus*, etc.

NASH gives *Aconite* as one of the greatest PAIN remedies : his trio here being *Aconite, Chamomilla* and *Coffea*.

But the pains of *Chamomilla* are accompanied by intense irritability, those of *Coffea* by excitement, by " a sensitiveness of the skin beyond comprehension ", and are curiously aggravated by noise, while those of *Aconite*, as said, are intolerable and accompanied by anguish and FEAR.

As Kent puts it, *Aconite* " *screams with pain.* Pains like knives. . . . Some awful thing must be upon him, or he could not have such dreadful sufferings. Predicts the day of his death, as a result of the awfulness that seems to be overwhelming him. And this mental picture is always present, in pneumonia, in inflammations of the kidneys, of the liver, of the bowels, in any part of the body where *Aconite* is useful."

Nash says, " *Aconite* has great distress in the heart and chest, while with *Belladonna* everything seems to centre in the head."

And he quotes Hering as to the *Aconite* fever. " Heat, with thirst ; hard, full and frequent pulse, anxious impatience, inappeasable, beside himself, tossing about with agony."

Aconite has been, perhaps, rather neglected in our day. The old homœopaths knew how to use it. But someone gave vent to the unfortunate platitude, which has been passed on, " By the time you see the case, it is already too late for *Aconite*." Rubbish ! The *Aconite* condition may come on at any moment, in any illness, after surgical interference, when *Aconite* will restore speedy peace, and leave no after-effects.

Aconite has been styled the Homœopathic Lancet : for it was *Aconite*, that finished " bloodletting ", by the signal relief it gave in the onset of most inflammatory conditions (pleurisy, pneumonia, etc.) where, *not to bleed* was actually regarded as tantamount to murder.

Aconite is an example of the uselessness of getting your knowledge of drugs from their effects on animals. Clarke records an attempt to destroy an elephant, where a carrot was scraped out, and enough *aconitine* to poison 2,000 men was put in. The elephant ate it readily, but nothing happened, and three hours later a large dose of prussic acid had to be administered, which soon proved fatal.

As Clarke says, " *Aconite* is one of the deadliest and most rapidly acting of poisons, yet, through Hahnemann's discoveries, it has been transformed into the best friend of the nursery."

" *Aconite* is the remedy of the rosy, chubby, plethoric baby," says Kent. And one visualizes a scene—a small, healthy baby girl, with high fever, crying out and throwing herself about in her mother's arms ; anguished and unable to express her trouble except by bursts of crying : her mother almost frantic:—"I don't want to lose her ! " And then, just a wee dose of sweet sugar medicated with *Aconite*, the potency immaterial, and the storm soon over.

For *Aconite* is at its most indispensable in households and in the nursery, for sudden, severe effects, following *chills* and *frights*, with restlessness, anxiety, fear, and exalted sensibility.

And this is what HAHNEMANN says. " *Aconite* is the first and main remedy, in minute doses, in inflammations of the windpipe (croup, membraneous laryngitis), in various kinds of inflammations of the throat and fauces, as also in the local acute inflammations of all other parts, particularly where, in addition to thirst and quick pulse, there are present *anxious impatience, an inappeasable mental agitation, and agonizing tossing about.* . . . In the selection of *Aconite* as a homœopathic remedy particular attention should be paid to the symptoms of the disposition, so that they should be very similar." He points out that it is also "an indispensable accessory remedy even in the most obstinate chronic affections, when the system requires a diminution of the so-called *tension of the blood vessels*".

Elsewhere, in Sir John Weir's paper, " *Homœopathy, an Explanation of its Principles,*" will be found a case, which is worth repeating here. " At 10.30 p.m. one night, I was called to see a man suffering from urticaria—anaphylactic—after anti-tetanus serum. He was almost beside himself with fear and anxiety: very restless, couldn't keep still: certain he was going to die. Thirsty, felt hot, great fear of being alone. Very apprehensive. Everything had to be done at once. Rheumatic pains intolerable: said they were driving him crazy.

" Here *Aconite*, in the 30th potency, gave almost instant relief, and in fifteen minutes the patient was quite himself again. This was one of the most dramatic things I have ever seen."

One could run on indefinitely with *Aconite*, its wonderful soothing effect in *heart disease*, where an acute condition has supervened, with palpitation, anguish, and great distress. Such as with a Belgian refugee during the early days of War ; a bad heart case, with condition dangerously, almost fatally aggravated, while waiting for days for embarkation, exposed on the quay to cold, exhaustion, and fear ; in Kidney disease, as with a boy in hospital, with general dropsy, better every time for *Aconite*, then permanently benefited by *Sulphur*—which is the " chronic " of *Aconite*. It is well to remember that, where *Aconite* is too superficial for what has already become chronic, *Sulphur*, its " chronic" is generally the remedy, in the same way that *Calcarea* is the chronic of *Belladonna*. Then, again, in inflammation of the bladder, in suppressed urine, or menses ; and endless other conditions resulting from, or accompanied by, *chill, shock, fright, fear.*

Aconite, remember, is a very great FEVER remedy : but is only the fever remedy of *Aconite* fevers. Kent says, " Never give *Aconite* in blood-poisoning, such as we find in scarlet fever, typhoid, etc. We find nothing of the violent symptoms of *Aconite* in such conditions. The nervous irritability of *Aconite* is never present, but the opposite ; the stupor, the laziness, the purple skin : whereas *Aconite* is bright-red. *Aconite* has no symptoms like the slow types of continued fevers. The *Aconite* fever is generally one short, sharp attack. Some remedies have periodicities, or waves : *Aconite* has no such thing. The most violent attack of fever will subside in a night if *Aconite* is the remedy."

The sensations of the various drugs are suggestive and helpful, as, for instance, *Aconite* tingles, *Lachesis* hammers, *Arsenicum* may stitch with hot needles, *Bryonia, Kali carb.*, and *Spigelia stitch and stab*, the first and the last on movement especially ; *Kali carb. independently of movement* also, and so on.

We will conclude with extracts from the actual provings of *Aconite*, given in black type by Hahnemann, in Allen's *Encyclopedia* and in Hering's *Guiding Symptoms* ; that is to say, symptoms again and again brought out in healthy provers, and again and again found curative in the sick *of a like sickness.*

BLACK LETTER SYMPTOMS (*Hahnemann and Allen*)

Nightly raging delirium.
Variable humour, gay, then dejected.
He did all things hurriedly.
Great vexation about trifles.
Great anxiety : great internal anxiety.
Inconsolable anxiety.
Extremely disposed to be cross.
Fear of approaching death.
Lamentable fears of approaching death.
Apprehension : sadness : solicitude.
Fear of some misfortune happening to him.
Inconsolable anxiety and piteous howling, with complaints and reproaches about (often trivial) evils.
Excessive restlessness and tossing about for hours.

Very restless nights.   Restless tossings in bed.

Palpitation of the heart and great anxiety, increased heat of body, especially in the face.   She is as if stupified from flying redness in the face.

Unsteadiness of ideas : if she wants to pursue a train of thought a second chases this away, and a third again displaces this, until she becomes quite confused.

Want of memory, as if what he had just done were a dream, and he can scarcely recall what it was.

Weakness of memory.

HEAD *in front as if nailed up.*

Pain is intolerable, drives him crazy.

Fullness and heaviness in forehead, as if an out-pressing weight lay there, and as if all would be forced out at the forehead.

Heat in head.   Burning headache as if brain were agitated by boiling water.

Fullness in head.   Semilateral drawing in head.

Throbbing left side forehead : while strong beats occur in the right side by fits.

Vertigo : staggers especially to the right.

Vertigo with nausea, especially rising from sitting.

Vertigo worse shaking head, whereby complete darkness comes before the eyes.

Dilated pupils.   Photophobia.

Inflammation EYES *with lachrymation, which causes so much pain and fright that he wishes for death.*

Inflammation of eyes, extremely painful.

Great sensitiveness to NOISE.

EPISTAXIS.

Great sensibility of olfactory nerve.

Creeping pain in CHEEKS.

Sensation of the face growing large.

Penetrating fine stitches in tip of TONGUE.

Tongue swollen.

Dryness of mouth.

Burning in THROAT.

Great thirst.

Empty eructations.   Nausea.

Vomits lumbrici.

Inclination to vomit, as if had eaten something disgustingly sweet or greasy.

Violent vomiting.

Pressive pain, STOMACH, like a weight.

Tensive pressing pain like a weight in stomach and hypochondria.

Swollen, distended ABDOMEN, like ascites.

Flatulent colic in hypogastrium as if he had taken a flatus-producing purgative.

Burning in umbilical region.

Sensitiveness of abdomen to touch, as from slight peritoneal inflammation. Burning in abdomen.

Cutting in intestines.

Great swelling of abdomen which is painful to touch.

White STOOL.

Pain in rectum. Shooting and aching in anus.

Anxious desire to urinate.

URINE hot, dark-coloured.

Fetid breath.

Sensitiveness of LARYNX to touch.

Hoarseness. Hoarse, dry, loud cough.

Expectoration of bright red blood. Hæmoptysis.

Difficult respiration.

Squeezing pain in chest.

Creeping pain in chest. Stitches in chest with cough.

Anxiety about HEART. Palpitation and anxiety.

Pulse contracted, full, powerful, febrile, exceeding 100 beats to minute.

Rheumatic pain nape of NECK : only on moving.

Violent, shooting, digging pain left of spine.

Bruised pain in articulation of lowest lumbar vertebra with sacrum : sacrum feels hacked off.

Cool sweat on PALMS.

Creeping pain in fingers.

Coldness of feet.

Weakness and laxity of the ligaments of all joints.

Yawns often without being sleepy.

Light SLEEP.

Very restless nights : tossing in bed. Excessive restlessness.
Anxious dreams : wakes with a start.

Chill of whole body, with hot forehead : hot ear lobe, and internal
dry heat.
Slight perspiration all over body.
Very fine stinging, or stinging burning pain in many parts, skin.

Redness and heat of one, coldness and paleness of the other cheek.
Towards evening, burning heat in head and face, redness of
cheeks and out-pressing headache.
Towards evening, dry heat in face with anxiety.

NOTABLE, OR QUEER SYMPTOMS AND INDICATIONS

Constriction at throat. Scratching and constriction. Dryness,
as if something had struck in throat.

He frequently pulled at the throat.

The abdomen seemed as if full of water.

Burning feeling from stomach up through œsophagus to mouth.

White fæces and red urine.

Slight sensation of splashing in bladder when urinating.

Numb sensation, small of back into legs.

Whole body sensitive to touch : child will not allow itself to
be moved : it whines.

Most of the symptoms are accompanied by shivering and
anxiety.

Fine pricking, as from needles here and there on body.

Convulsions of teething children : heat, startings, twitching of
single muscles. Child gnaws its fists : frets ; cries.

Violent chills, dry heat.

After a violent chill, dry heat with difficult breathing, lancinating pain through chest.

Inflammatory fevers and inflammations, with heat, dry skin,
violent thirst, red face, or alternate red and pale face ; groaning
and tossing about ; shortness of breath ; congestion to head.

Bad effects from suppressed sweats, etc.

Pains intolerable. Numbness : tinglings ; formications.

Measles ; dry barking cough ; painful hoarseness ; cannot
bear light.

Tongue red.

Local congestions and inflammations.

Neuritis with tingling. Gastric catarrh from chilling stomach
with ice water when heated. (*Ars.*)

AESCULUS HIPPOCASTANUM

(Horse Chestnut)

As NASH says, " this is one of the remedies that is not so remarkable for its wide range of action, as it is for positiveness within its range ".

Its sensations are, *heaviness and lameness*, especially in the sacro-iliac regions. *Fullness to bursting* in fauces, stomach, bowels, rectum and chest : fullness in various parts, as if they contained an undue amount of blood—heart, lungs, stomach, brain, skin. And, as Kent emphasizes, *purpleness* of congested parts. He says: " *Aesculus* is a venous remedy, engorged and full, sometimes to bursting. Now there is another feature I want to bring out. You will notice that where congestion takes place it is *purple*, or blue in colour. . . . The remedy is not active in its inflammatory state, it is sluggish and passive . . . the heart is labouring and the veins are congested. . . . It is one of the most frequently indicated remedies in the *hæmorrhoidal constitution*, as it used to be called."

While GUERNSEY (*Keynotes*) lays his finger, as usual, on the spot when he says : " *The guiding thread directing the use of this remedy is found in the rectum, hæmorrhoidal vessels, sacrum and back.*"

Popular use and observations, as so often, point to its remedial uses : as when Hering tells us" that it causes prolapsus ani in cattle which feed on it "—and we learn that " the nuts are carried in the pocket to avoid, or to cure piles ".

The *black letter symptoms* of a drug, i.e. the symptoms outstandingly caused and cured by it, are pretty strong pointers to its most frequent and brilliant exploits of healing. Glance down them : " Rectum feels full : sore with burning and itching ; full of small sticks " (a great characteristic of the drug). Then the usually " blind " hæmorrhoids, protruding, aching, burning, purplish, with shooting pains to sacrum and back. And then the dull backache that makes walking almost impossible, and is agony, if one stoops, or rises from stooping. Even the headache appears to affect the sacrum and hips ; again worse by walking, and by stooping forwards.

For such backache, one has also to consider (*inter alia*) *Agaricus*. In the Repertory both have sacral pain in black type : *Agar.* when sitting, *Aesc.* when rising from sitting, when stooping, when walking, and extending to hips. And *Aesc.* takes also the sacro-iliac articulations. But—don't be caught out by a sacro-iliac subluxation, after a fall, a twist, an awkward lift, a confinement, an operation. Here *Aesculus*, or whatever the drug of the symptoms may be, will palliate, but *it will not cure*. Don't lose your faith in the remedy of like symptoms, because it cannot release the catch, and let the joint snap home. Hahnemann warned us one hundred years ago that mechanical lesions must be mechanically treated. They are not the province of medicine. By mechanical readjustments of pelvis a large number of cases of sciatica may be cured ; till one is apt to think *all* cases ; and then one comes along, where manipulation fails, and some other operative procedure is indicated, or some simple remedy in which you had lost faith because it did not cure what had been beyond its province, comes in brilliantly. Sciatica may have many causes : one remembers well one hospital case where a bulge on the femur in its upper third was discovered and which X-ray diagnosed as probable sarcoma, but which practically disappeared with— of all things !—*Ferrum*. This was prescribed, not on account of the bone condition, not because of the probable diagnosis, but because of some silly little symptoms, peculiar to that patient with, whatever might be the matter with him ! The hospital case books still contain the apparently significant pictures : while the man so far recovered that he was called up for war, and only exempted on the strength of those X-ray pictures : but he remained well, to our knowledge, years after.

But we must get back to *Aesculus*, and here one remembers in war days a very suffering nurse, who had attended a cold and humid funeral, with the result that she did not know how she was to go on duty, because of the awful pain in the lower part of her back ; a pain that would not let her stoop, or rise from stooping. The Repertory was asked for the remedy—*Aesculus*, and she was given a dose and sent to lie down. In a couple of hours she reappeared happy and ready for work, and one heard no more of the backache. There are people who have an idea that Homœopathy is slow. *Is it !* In simple acute sickness nothing can be quicker ; only it must be *Homœopathy* ; i.e. the symptoms in patient and drug must correspond. The worst of working by law is, *that it won't work when it isn't law !* Give it a fair chance if you want to pull it off. But one must allow that it *is* sometimes difficult. But you will find that " the more you put into it, the more you get out "

By the way, one should contrast *Aesculus* with *Nitric acid*. Both afflict woefully, and marvellously comfort rectum and anus.

Aesculus has his rectum *full of sharp sticks* (*Collinsonia* also) ; *Nitric acid* has a splinter there, pricking sharply during the passage of stool. *Nitric acid* endures agonies during stool, and for hours after stool : with *Aesc.* the pain seems to come on some hours after stool. *Nit. ac.* has fissures and bleeding piles. *Aesc.* the large, purple protruding piles, with perhaps the sawing knife-pain that will not permit of standing, sitting or lying, but only *kneeling*. Curious " personalities " these remedies of ours ! with their very definite and peculiar characteristics, and where no one will do for another : a very complicated lock, which only the one key of many fine wards will fit. They make Homœopathy very easy, and very difficult, and very interesting.

But in *Aesc.* not only the sacral regions, but the whole spine is weak ; aches dully, and is worse from motion.

And not only the rectum but the whole digestive tube, with liver (even to jaundice), has burning distress, with sensations of fullness, flatulency and colicky pain ; but probably associated with rectal and hæmorrhoidal symptoms.

And with the characteristic backache there may be leucorrhœa, dark yellow, thick and sticky ; and *Aesc.* has caused and cured misplacements, enlargements, and induration of the womb, with great tenderness, heat, and throbbing. But all this with *lameness in the lower back, which gives out when walking.*

*   *   *

HALE (*New Remedies*) writes of *Aesculus.*—" A veritable polycrest, having a wide range of action, but like some other polycrests it has a central point of action, from which radiate a series of reflex symptoms.

" This central point of action is the *liver and portal system*, and nine out of every ten of its symptoms are due to this action. I have found it analogous in its effects to *Aloe, Collinsonia, Nux vom., Sulphur* and *Podophyllum.* . . .

" I have been most successful with it in *congestion of the liver*, when accompanied by *piles*. Indicated by the symptoms—aching, pinching pains in the right hypochondrium, aggravated by walking. The pain extends up between the shoulders.

" *Constipation*, with hard, dry, knotty stools, which are *white*.

" *Hæmorrhoids*, if the following symptoms are present, are promptly removed by *Aesc.* . . . The tumours are protruding, or, internal, are usually purple, hard and very sore (not *raw* as in *Aloes*, but a bruised feeling), with aching, burning, rarely bleeding. . . . The rectal symptoms are characteristic—very disagreeable sensations of dryness, soreness, constriction, fullness, and a feeling as if sticks, splinters, gravel or other foreign substances had become lodged in the rectum . . . fullness—protrusion, with a desire to strain . . . with, usually, *absence of actual constipation*. . . .

" *The pains in the back* which attend its rectal symptoms are quite notable . . . sometimes shooting or cutting, but usually consist of a lameness as if strained, extending to hips or legs, or an aching and weakness aggravated by walking, stooping, or any movement." Dr. Hale adds, " Like *Rhus* its pain and stiffness often go off after continued motion. . . . "

He says also, " Dr. Hart claims to have discovered a keynote in a symptom not found in its pathogenesis—*Throbbing in abdominal and pelvic cavities* ; especially the latter."

* * *

And in *Aesc.* not only the piles, but the varices and ulcers are purple, or rather their surroundings; dusky and purple.

Even heart and chest are not exempt from the attentions of *Aesculus*, and probably its real range is wider than we usually realize : for Hering gives it in black type for the " *chest complaints of horses* ",—hence its name, supposedly, *horse-chest-nut*. The provings show its action on the lungs—while Nash has found it a second *Arsenicum* in coryza. This is what he writes :

" I have used *Aesculus* with very good results in coryza and sore throat. The coryza is very like the *Arsenic* coryza, thin, watery and burning ; but what characterizes *Aesc.* here is sensation of rawness ; *sensitive to inhaled cold air*. In the throat it has the same sensation of rawness, both in the acute form and also in chronic follicular pharyngitis, for which it is often a good remedy."

This again the provings suggest, dryness of posterior nares and throat, with sneezing, followed by severe coryza. Stinging and burning in posterior nares and soft palate. Pricking, formication, burning and stinging in fauces ; shooting in left side. Violent burning in throat, with raw feeling. Dryness and roughness of throat, as from taking cold. Dry, constricted fauces. *Dark congested fauces*, with full feeling and irritation. Catarrhal laryngitis ; larynx dry and stiff.

But everywhere it will show its peculiar characteristics— fullness to bursting—dull aching back, etc. prohibits movement— and everywhere congestion and *purpleness*, and dryness, and burning.

By the way, Kent tells us that *Aesc.* " is a wonderful eye remedy, especially when the eyes have ' hæmorrhoids ' : i.e.

enlarged blood vessels. Redness, burning, lachrymation, with enlarged blood vessels. Increased determination of blood to the eyes also ". And he points out that in common with all the remedies of venous plethora, *Pulsatilla*, etc., the *Aesculus* patient feels better " when surrounded by cold air ".

BLACK LETTER SYMPTOMS

RECTUM *feels full : dryness and itching.*
Rectum feels full of small sticks (characteristic). (*Coll.*)
Hard dry stool passed with difficulty, with dryness of rectum and heat.
Stool followed by rectal fullness.
Hæmorrhoids, blind and painful, rarely bleeding.
Hæmorrhoids painful, burning, purplish ; generally " blind ".
Pain in hæmorrhoids like a knife, sawing up and down : could not sit, stand or lie ; only kneel.
" *Some carry the nuts in their breeches pockets as a preventive.*"

LEUCORRHŒA *with lameness in back across sacro-iliac articulations, with great fatigue walking : that part of the back gives out when walking even a little way.*

" CHEST *complaints of horses.*"

Constant dull BACKACHE ; *walking almost impossible : scarcely able to stoop, or to rise after sitting.*
Constant headache affecting the sacrum and hips, much worse by walking, or stooping forwards.

Paralytic feeling in arms, legs and spine.

Heaviness and lameness.
Fullness in various parts.
Mucous membranes dry, swollen ; burn and feel raw.
Glandular swellings of bone (whatever that may mean !).

By the way, people carry a horse chestnut about in their clothing " to cure rheumatism ".

AETHUSA CYNAPIUM
(Fools' Parsley)

ONE of our minor, but very precious remedies. Generally thought of as a remedy of childhood : of babies who cannot tolerate milk : of sudden vomiting : of water, copious ; of greenish phlegm : of weakness and drowsiness after vomiting—after " fearful vomiting ", with or without diarrhœa and extreme colic. Also a remedy of " idiotic children ".

But its virtues extend beyond the times of childhood. It was Dr. Clarke's great remedy for a form of examination funk, as will be seen later, in a quotation from his *Dictionary*. The " funk " that *Aethusa* banishes is portrayed in its provings :—" unable to read anything, after over-taxation of the mental faculties " ; " incapacity to think : confused " ; " cannot retain any idea " ; " great anxiety " ; " Head confused : brain feels bound up ". In other words, the condition—we have all been through it—when working to our limit for an exam., we find it is useless to attempt further study ; a condition of mental repletion with non-assimilation, when the greatest efforts to wrestle with things that *may* be demanded are a mere waste of time :—they refuse to go in : and when the only hope is to lay aside books and chance it, or—*Aethusa*. Another form of examination funk asks for *Argentum nitricum*. Here the condition is not that of " stalemate ", but of acute anxiety, worry, and premonition of failure. The victim is hurried ; tormented with anxiety, and with nerves unstrung. Intense apprehension—even to diarrhœa, before the mildest ordeal (*Gels.*). *Argentum nitricum* is a remedy of great mental strain and apprehension : *Aethusa* of simple sense of incapacity, . . . that is as we see it. *Aethusa* more violently upsets the stomach—with its extreme vomiting : while *Argentum nitricum* bloats the stomach with flatulent dyspepsia : as if it would burst with wind. Both have diarrhœa, with green mucus. *Argentum nitricum* is the remedy of craving for sweets and sugar, which disagree. Kent gives a case where a nursing infant got green diarrhœa because its mother ate candy. He had prescribed *Chamomilla*, *Mercurius*, and *Ars.*, with no relief, till he found out about the candy. Asked, at last, if she ate sweet things, sugar, etc., she said, no. " Why, yes, you do," said her husband. " I bring you home a pound of candy every day. What do you do with it ? " " Oh, that's nothing," she said. " But," says Kent, " the baby did not get well until it got *Argentum nitricum* and the mother stopped eating candy." He tells us that quite a number of medicines have a craving for sweets, but many of them can eat sweets with impunity. *Aethusa* is worse from coffee, and has a desire for wine, but the mental symptoms are increased after taking it.

Aethusa should also be remembered as one of the remedies of epilepsy. With this drug, in convulsions, the eyes are turned down, thumbs clenched, face red, pupils dilated ; foam at mouth ; jaws locked, etc.

And a thing to be remembered in regard to the children it can help is their great weakness ; and their inability to hold up the head (*Abrot.*). All its symptoms are apt to be worse at 3 to 4 a.m.

" *Aethusa cynapium* in infants that are fed every time they cry. Draws up the knees when carried, in the same general position that the *Medorrhinum* assumes, but *Aethusa* patients do not sleep in the knee-chest posture, as far as I know. I came across one eighteen-year-old girl who slept in the knee-chest posture and for whom *Medorrhinum* was the indicated remedy. This is the only time in an adult that I have found this particular symptom. It interested me so much that I asked her why she slept in that position. She said at times she had a feeling in the abdomen as if there were ten thousand worms twisting around in there and when she took the knee-chest position, the feeling immediately ceased."—Dr. UNDERHILL, from a discussion quoted in an old *Homœopathic Recorder* (U.S.A.).

ALLEN (*Keynotes*), draws attention to complete absence of thirst. And, not only the intolerance of milk, but the great weakness of children ; even to idiocy.

*   *   *

NASH points out that : " AETHUSA is one of our best remedies for vomiting in children. The milk comes up as soon as swallowed, by great effort, after which the child becomes greatly relaxed and drowsy ; or if the milk stays down longer, it finally comes up in *very sour curds, so large that it would seem almost impossible the child could have ejected them.* If this condition of stomach is not cured, the case will go on to cholera infantum, with green watery or slimy stools, colic and convulsions. The convulsions are peculiar, in that the eyes turn downwards, instead of up or sideways. . . . He says the sunken face with *linea nasalis*, a surface of pearly whiteness on upper lip bounded by a distinct line from outer nasal orifice to angles of mouth. This symptom is more characteristic of *Aethusa than of any other remedy.* . . . The absence of thirst rules for *Aethusa* instead of *Arsenicum*."

*   *   *

CLARKE (*Dictionary*) gives cases illustrating the action of *Aethusa*, which has not received its name, " Fools' parsley " for nothing. He calls it indeed a medicine for "fools". There is great weakness of mind or body. One very characteristic symptom is : *Inability to think or fix the attention.* Guided by this symptom I once gave it to an undergraduate preparing for an examination, with complete success. He had been compelled to give up his studies, but was able to resume them, and passed a brilliant examination. To a little waif in an orphan home who suffered with severe headaches and inability to fix his attention on his lessons, I sent single doses of *Aethusa*, at rare intervals, with very great relief. The little boy asked for the medicine himself subsequently on a return of the old symptoms.

He says, the symptoms of *Aethusa* are particularly clearly defined, in fact *violence* is one of the notes of its action—violent vomiting, violent convulsions, violent pains, violent delirium. Then, idiocy ; in some cases alternating with furor. . . . He notices the intolerance of milk. The great weakness and exhaustion after vomiting ; the child is so exhausted *it falls asleep at once.* "Hungry after vomiting", is a keynote here. . . . Adults complain of a sensation, as if the stomach was turned upside down. . . .

*   *   *

And a couple of peculiar symptoms, we seem to have missed. Tongue feels too long.

Swelling of glands round neck like a string of beads. In fever, there is complete absence of thirst, though there is great heat.

BLACK LETTER SYMPTOMS

A drawn condition, beginning at the ala nasi, and extending to the angle of the mouth, gave the face an expression of great anxiety and pain.

Intolerance of milk : the children throw up their milk almost as soon as swallowed, curdled or not curdled, in from ten to fifteen minutes, by a sudden and violent vomiting ; then weakness makes them drowsy for some minutes.

Vomiting curdled milk.

NOTABLE SYMPTOMS, ITALICIZED, OR STRANGE

Liable to transports of rage. Fury : frenzy.
Imagined she saw rats run across the room.
Imagines he sees dogs and cats.
Great anxiety and restlessness.
Fretful and cross in open air : better in room.

Awkwardness : discontent.

Stupefaction, as if of a barrier between his organs of sense and external objects.

Lies stretched out without consciousness.

Vertigo with sleepiness.   He cannot keep upright.

Moist tongue, white-coated after milk.

Or, tongue feels too dry.   Or, copious salivation.

Aphthae : pungent heat in mouth and throat.   Difficulty in swallowing.

Taste : sweet ; insipid ; bitter ; salt ; of onions ; of cheese.

Slow speech : speech almost prevented.

Inflamed aphthae and pustules in throat : condition almost desperate.

Itching and scraping in œsophagus.

Inability to swallow.

Horrible vomiting.

Copious greenish vomiting.

Vomits bloody mucus.

Tearing pain, pit of stomach, extending into œsophagus.

Coldness of abdomen, objective and subjective : with coldness in lower extremities.

Sensation of pressure as of a band round chest.

Swelling of mammary gland.

Violent palpitations of heart ; resounds in head.

Distressing pain, occiput and nape of neck, extending down spine.

A feeling as if pain in back would be ameliorated by straightening and bending stiffly backwards, as in opisthotonos.

Numbness of arms ; heaviness ; weakness ; cramps : contraction of fingers.

Formication referred to bones of lower limb.

Bloating : whole body becomes swollen and livid.

Violent epileptic spasms, with clenched thumbs, red face, eyeballs turned down, pupils dilated, insensible, milky foam from mouth, clenched teeth, small hard, frequent pulse.

Spasms : delirium ; stupor.

Stiffness of whole body.

Inability to hold head erect, or to sit up.

Whole body bluish-black.

He cannot bear to be uncovered during the sweat.

AGARICUS MUSCARIUS

Agaricus—Amanita (the name under which its symptoms appear in Hering's *Guiding Symptoms*)—the Fly Agaric (or fungus) —the Bug Agaric—the " fou " fungus of the French, has its own peculiar place and very distinctive symptoms in homœopathic Materia Medica. Its proving by Hahnemann appeared in *Stapf's Archives*, a contemporary periodical, with his provings of some other drugs—notably *Psorinum*, of which we have, I believe, no translation. But that of *Agaricus* is to be found in Vol. II of his *Chronic Diseases*.

Here Hahnemann describes the fungus as " surmounted by a scarlet-coloured top, which is studded with whitish excrescences, and white leaflets ". He says it is to be first triturated, then dynamized in the usual way to, as he suggests, the 30*th* potency.

One associates *Agaricus* especially with chorea : but its notable twitchings and jerkings are only a small part of its drug-picture. One remembers Dr. Blackley of old in the London Homœopathic Hospital, who used *Agaricus* for things where, to one's profound ignorance, it seemed strangely inappropriate : but he probably knew its uses better than most of us !—For instance, it seemed a curious drug to give for pneumonia !—and yet, this is what KENT says about it :—

" *Agaricus* is a great medicine in *chest* troubles, though seldom thought of. It has cured what seemed to be consumption. Catarrhal condition of the chest, with night sweats and history of nervous symptoms. Violent cough in isolated attacks ending in sneezing. Convulsive cough, with sweats toward evening, with frequent pulse, expectoration of pus-like mucus, worse in the mornings and when lying on back. Add to this the symptoms of *Agaricus* as described, and *Agaricus* will take hold of that case. Cases of incipient phthisis. It closely relates to the tubercular diathesis.

" I remember starting out to prove *Tuberculinum* on an individual I suspected would be sensitive to it from his history and symptoms. The first dose almost killed him, and, considering the use that that substance is put to in diagnosing the disease in cattle, it seemed to stir him up. He became emaciated and looked as if he would die. I let it alone, and watched and waited patiently and the symptoms of *Agaricus* came up and established the relationship between these two remedies, and confirmed Hering's observation of the relationship of *Agaricus* to the tubercular diathesis. *Agaricus* cured him and fattened him up."

Among HERING'S symptoms are, " Chest feels too narrow. Oppression, constriction of chest. Convulsive cough with anxious sweat. After each cough violent sneezing ; sometimes so rapidly that he does not know if he coughs or sneezes. Inflammation of the lungs. Tuberculous consumption."

This poisonous fungus affects the digestive organs. Turmoil in abdomen—full of colic : everything ferments. Horribly offensive flatus. Tympanitic abdomen. Violent urging to stool. Sensation as if the rectum would burst—even after stool. Straining after stool (*Merc. cor.*).

Agaricus has its own severe backache, especially sacral, and especially worse when sitting. (But here look out for a possible mechanical cause—sacro-iliac subluxation.) One has seen it curative in a difficult case of rheumatism where the indication was " *diagonal pains*, as left forearm and right thigh, or right knee and left hand". And here *Agaricus* is worse at rest and sitting, and better moving about.

But much of its malignancy and its beneficence centre round the spine and the nervous system. As Kent says, " the most striking things running through this medicine are twitchings and tremblings. Jerking of the muscles and trembling of the limbs. The twitching of the muscles becomes so extensive that it is a well developed case of chorea. . . . Difficulty in co-ordinating the movements of the muscles of the body. Inco-ordination of brain and spinal cord. Clumsy motions. Drops things. Fingers fly spasmodically open while holding things." Kent says " you may sometimes cure Bridget in the kitchen, when the trouble is that she is continually breaking dishes by letting them fall, with *Agaricus* or *Apis*." And he adds this distinction between the two drugs, that whereas *Agaricus* hugs the fire, *Apis* wants to get out of the kitchen !

One remembers the classical description of the onset of chorea. " The child gets scolded for making faces : then it gets smacked for dropping and breaking the cups and saucers " ; then at last it dawns on the most unobservant that it is no case of original sin, but St. Vitus' Dance, and the victim is hurried away to the doctor who takes the temperature, listens to the heart, and orders " Bed ! "—and, if a homœopath, prescribes *Agaricus*, or whichever of these jerky medicines most resembles, in its drug-picture, the individual symptoms of this particular patient.

As Kent says, " *All remedies are full of freaks, and it is the figuring out of these peculiarities that enables us to do good prescribing."*

Agaricus affects the heart also, with stitching pains; with oppression of heart, as well as lungs; with shock and palpitation : but several other remedies, *Hyos.—Stram.—Mygale—Ignatia*, and so on, cause even greater (choreaic) distortion of the face.

GUERNSEY (*Key Notes*) says of *Agaricus*, " This remedy is exceedingly rich in symptoms on almost every organ and function of the body . . . I am always well rewarded in its study and use when I find cropping out, *itching, redness and burning, on any part of the body, as if frost-bitten; or burning and itching of internal parts.*" While NASH, who does not have a great deal to say about *Agaricus*, while recording the tenderness of spinal column, extending into lower limbs, and the twitchings of eyelids, face and extremities which cease during sleep, is more obsessed with the skin symptoms. " Ears, face, nose and skin, red and itch as if from chilblains." He says this itching, redness and burning, as if from being frozen, " may lead to the choice of this drug in many different diseases ".

And of course most people know *Agaricus*, if for nothing else, as a remedy for chilblains. *Agaricus* suffers intensely from the cold, and its chilblains are terribly painful when the hands, or feet, are cold. *Pulsatilla* chilblains, on the contrary, " terrify " (as they say of cattle when the flies are at them in the hot sunshine) when they get warm. The chilblains of *Agaricus* are dreadfully sore when cold ; those of *Pulsatilla* itch and burn to distraction when hot. These are the remedies that especially occur to one for chilblains . . . *and Rue !* One remembers well the days of rue ointment for a nephew, whose chilblains were so bad as to confine him to bed from time to time during his schooldays. His mother, finding that nothing but rue ointment helped, used to post off her annual appeals for fresh supplies.

But there is rue ointment, *and* rue ointment. It was one of our gardeners who supplied the pharmacology:—he always grew rue in the garden in order to make an ointment for the cows when their udders were sore. And we still grow rue, that ancient " Mithridate"; only one is often too lazy to turn it into ointment— and misses it accordingly. *Rue* should be prepared from the fresh plant—always ; and this is the way of it. Heat lard till liquid (a tall soup bottle is excellent for the purpose) and plunge into this a good bunch of fresh rue with its flowering tops at their best. Leave it to extract for some hours in a warm place, till the rue is pale and the lard green and smelly ; then lift up the bunch, and let it drain.   Cover the pot when the ointment is cold and solid. It is a useful application for bunions, for synovitis of knee—but here *Ruta* in potency will act as well, and is not greasy—for sores, for chilblains, for broken chilblains.   But in those days one had not made the acquaintance of *Agaricus* and *Pulsatilla* in this connection, whose action is longer-lasting and far more curative.

But the " Mad Fungus " of course affects the brain and senses : —in its milder stages with ill-humour, indifference, does not want to work, or to answer questions : when in full blast with delirium—which knows nobody—throws things at people—sings and talks but won't answer.   It is one of the medicines of delirium—even raving delirium.   " It is used by tribes of Asiatic savages in the form of a real intoxicating drink."   It is so like alcoholism that it has taken its place as one of our remedies for *delirium tremens*.   And certainly Boger's terse description of *Agaricus* suggests not only chorea but intoxication,—" *Agaricus has irregular, uncertain and exaggerated motions : he reaches too far—steps too high—drops things . . . with indistinct and jerky speech.*"

Black Letter Symptoms

Delirium tremens.

Delirium with constant raving.

Dull, drawing HEADACHE *in morning, extending into root of nose, with nosebleed or thick mucous discharge.*

Headaches of those who are subject to chorea ; or who readily become delirious in fever or with pain ; twitchings or grimaces.

Redness, burning itching of EARS, *as if they had been frozen.*

TONGUE *dry.*

Very drowsy after dinner, quite unusual ; he SLEEPS *very deeply and gets awake with pains in all limbs.*

Sudden convulsive COUGHS, *< forenoons, or during day.*

Pain in LUMBAR REGION AND SACRUM ; *and while sitting ; pain, sore aching ; back not sensitive to touch.*

Burning itching on both HANDS, *as if frozen ; parts hot, swollen, red.*

Trembling of hands.

Stiffness in fingers from gout.

Twitching of gluteal muscles.

Pain in bones of lower LEGS, *sometimes as if in the periosteum.*

Pain and inflammation of frost-bitten toes.

Chilblains.

Tearing in limbs < in rest or sitting, > moving.

Pains in limbs with lameness and numbness.

Uncertainty in walking, tumbling over everything in the way.

Twitchings; of eyelids and eyeballs; of cheeks; in chest posteriorly; in abdomen.

Involuntary movements (especially with children) while awake; ceasing during sleep.

Spasmodic motions, from simple involuntary motions and jerks of single muscles, to a dancing of whole body. Chorea.

Paralysis of upper and lower limbs. Incipient softening of spinal marrow.

During sleep, one does not notice any motion of eyes whatever in clonic spasms of eyes.

Chilblains, frost-bite, and all consequences of exposure to cold, particularly in face.

Shiverings over body, run from above downward.

Shudders; with bitter vomiting after supper.

Sweat when walking, or with slightest exertion.

Profuse sweat.

Burning, itching, redness and swelling, as from frost-bites.

Drunkards, especially for their headaches.

SOME PECULIAR OR ITALIC SYMPTOMS

Agaricus is one of the few remedies of diagonal symptoms : they may appear at the same time on opposite sides of the body —but diagonally.

Cold sensations : icy cold feeling on a small place, left chest near shoulder-blade.

Formication and burning in gluteal muscles.

Neuralgic pains as though sharp pieces of ice touched the parts or as if cold needles ran through the nerves. (*Ars.* hot needles.) It seems as if the whole body would dwindle to nothing.

Itching and burning all over with great distress.

AILANTHUS GLANDULOSA :

Tree of Heaven

IN our old garden at Wyvenhoe, years ago, there were two magnificent Ailanthus trees, whose memory has helped to rivet attention to this little-known, but invaluable remedy.

Its dramatic history, as a medicine, is only recorded, so far as we have been able to discover, by Dr. Hughes, but since this serves to impress on the mind what *Ailanthus* is good for, and its peculiarities of malevolence, i.e. its magnificent curative power in some desperate cases of acute disease, it is worth repeating.

Dr. Hughes tells us that one of our most accomplished physicians " supplies the first chapter ". His own child was seized with all the symptoms of early malignant scarlet fever : vomiting, severe headache, intolerance of light, dizziness, hot red face, inability to sit up, rapid small pulse ; drowsiness, yet great restlessness ; much anxiety. Two hours later the drowsiness had become insensibility, with constant, muttering delirium, and the child did not recognize the members of her family. She was now covered, in patches, with an eruption of miliary rash, with efflorescence between its points, all of a dark, almost livid colour ; the eruption more profuse on forehead and face than elsewhere. The father gave his child up for lost. But in a few hours a change came about which gave a new aspect to the case. Enquiry ascertained that she had largely sucked the juice of the stalks of the Ailanthus. The doctor ends his tale by suggesting that we have here a possible aid in those frightful cases of scarlet fever which prove fatal in the first stage, with symptoms of cerebral intoxication.

This was written in 1864 : but, published in a journal little known, seemed to have made no impression. Later, our Dr. Pope, realizing the significance and value of these facts, called attention to them, and his remarks soon bore fruit :—for Dr. Chalmers, in 1868, found himself in the midst of an epidemic of malignant scarlatina. New, at that time, to the use of homœopathic remedies, he was disappointed at their action here. His attention was called to *Ailanthus*, and he procured some, and at once found he had the agent he needed. The fever was characterized by a dark-coloured and partial eruption, and the constant effects of the medicine were shown in the change to a rash more bright-hued and general, with marked diminution in the frequency of the pulse, with more regularity and firmness, and with restoration to consciousness. Other doctors, later, who had had large experience with the drug in scarlatina, corroborated the favourable reports of its use. But an Australian doctor said that he found it necessary to discontinue it when the eruption began to fade, or it might cause a pemphigoid rash during and after desquamation. It has also been suggested in cases of cerebral and spinal congestion. Its effect on head and mental faculties being very like the dull heavy head with confusion and incapacity for labour, from brain fag or over worry ; while the pains in the back, all up the spine, and the contractive feeling in chest and abdomen, with numbness and tingling in upper and lower extremities are the symptoms of spinal congestion.

Ailanthus is also suggested, says Hughes, in bad cases of measles where the rash fails to come out, or recedes suddenly, or is livid ; in diphtheritic and other low forms of sore throat ; and in epidemic cerebrospinal meningitis.

We have quoted at some length, though endeavouring to condense. because of the importance of the drug, and the little that one can learn in regard to its fascinating history elsewhere.

Allen's *Encyclopedia* gives a few provings, besides those of the dramatic symptoms of poisoning case which emphasize its place in acute, malignant, deadly and rapid cases of disease. The lividity of the scanty eruption, that fails to appear as it should, the drowsiness and, soon, muttering delirium, with vomiting, headache, intolerance of light, hot red face, rapid, small pulse ; great restlessness and anxiety . . . let us see how the provings bear out what we in a lesser degree learn from the poisoning.

Mentals. Great anxiety. Inability to concentrate : cannot add up a row of figures correctly. Loss of memory : mental alienation. Stupor, delirium, insensibility, after suppressed scarlatina.

Tottering gait ; staggering ; giddy, with nausea, retching and some vomiting. The figures on the ledger began to dance up and down on the column. Apoplectic fullness of head. Electrical thrill starts from brain and goes to extremities. Tingling left arm and hand with dull headache.

Pupils widely dilated. Photophobia.

Face and forehead dark mahogany, in suppressed scarlatina.

Tongue dry, parched, cracked. Covered with whitish coat, brown in centre ; or moist and covered with white fur ; tip and edges livid.

Thick, œdematous, and dry choky feeling in throat : may become chronic.

Constant efforts to raise lumps of mucus. Throat tender and sore on swallowing, and on admission of air. Parotid and thyroid glands tender and enlarged. Throat livid and swollen with deep, angry-looking ulcerations. Tonsils studded with ulcerated points.

Nausea similar to that of pregnancy.

Tenderness over liver : tympanites. Burning in stomach and bowels. Feeling of insecurity, as if he would be attacked by diarrhœa any minute. Frequent watery dejections, expelled with great force. Dysentery ; frequent painful stool ; little fœcal matter : much bloody mucus.

Deep exhausing cough, with asthmatic expansion of lungs ; excessive soreness and tenderness of lungs.

The eruption is described above : dark, almost livid ; more profuse on forehead and face. .Intolerable pain in the back of neck, in upper part of back, and right hip-joint.

If odour gives any indication, *Ailanthus* should prove a good remedy in malignant puerpural fever.

BOGER has some black-type symptoms that emphasize points : Rapid prostration. Advancing malignancy and stupor. Fœtor and stupor. Face and throat dark and swelled. Deep ulcers stud the tonsils. Eruption in dark sparse patches. Scarlatina suppressed. Affects especially Blood, Throat, Skin, Mind.

KENT says : This remedy is especially suitable in low, zymotic forms of fever—diphtheria, scarlet fever, blood poisoning ; typhoids, especially where characterized by capillary congestions in spots—red, mottled spots. Malignant scarlet fever ; where the regular rash does not come out, but red spots appear ; bleeding from gums and nose, and dreadful tumefaction of throat. Face is purple, besotted ; eyes congested—even bleeding from eyes. Stupefaction : stupid and bemused. Throat œdematous with purple patches. Blood decomposing rapidly. Biisters may form at finger-tips and other parts of body. Fœtid odours from mouth and nose. . . . When a case suddenly assumes this prostration, with rapid heart, fœtid, purple or blue patches, blood poisoning is going on. A remittent or a diphtheria may suddenly take on this form. . . .

Cannot concentrate ; cannot answer correctly ; semi-conscious with great anxiety ; finally, complete unconsciousness. In quite a number of such cases in Brooklyn, many patients were saved by it. It seemed able to change the character of the malignant form of scarlet fever into a mild kind.

It has been observed in addition, that hair falls out ; flashes of light play before the eyes on closing lids at night . . . countenance indicates much distress. Face dark as mahogany ; purple, puffed, besotted. . . . This remedy corresponds to most malignant types. . . . With these zymotic states there is pain at the back of the neck and head, no matter what the name of the disease is.

Feeling of a rat running up the leg occurred in one of my provers.

Kent says again : " When you go to the bed of scarlet fever, you should not call to mind the names of the medicines you have heard recommended for scarlet fever. Let the appearance of the patient bring to mind such remedies as appear like this patient, regardless of whether they have been associated with scarlet fever or not.

" You may see what looks like an *Aconite* rash, but there is such scanty zymosis in the nature of *Aconite*, that it is no longer thought of. *Belladonna* is not suitable, for the *Bell.* rash is shiny and smooth. . . . *Pulsatilla* has a measly rash with often a low form of fever, but not so low as the typhoid state. In the prostration, worse after sleep, general stupor and delirium, almost at a glance you see *Lachesis* ; the type of such forms of disease. Or in scarlet fever where the child keeps picking the skin from lips and nose, lies pale and exhausted, no rash to speak of, and urine nearly suppressed,—and in a moment you think of *Arum triph.* Or, purple appearance, horrible fœtor, sore throat, and the child cannot get water enough, wants a stream running down its throat all the time, and you may safely trust to *Phosphorus.* . . . There is always something to tell the story, if you will only listen, study and wait long enough."

(We make no apology for repetitions. They serve to impress unusual facts and symptoms on the mind, and make prescribing easier.)

ALLIUM CEPA (Onion)

WE all know what happens when we cut a raw onion and experience its emanations, or when one happens to rub ones eyes with a hand that has been in contact with its cut surface. Nose tingles : eyes water profusely, and all the symptoms of an acute catarrh instantly appear.

Therefore *Allium cepa* is one of our very best and most frequently indicated remedies for an early, more or less superficial, cold. Get it in while symptoms agree, and you will have saved yourself.

* * *

KENT gives us the PARTICULARS OF THE CORYZA. . . . " Sneezing which comes with increasing frequency. Watery discharge drips from the nose constantly ; burns like fire, and excoriates upper lip and wings of the nose, till there is redness and rawness. Notice (he says) that the fluid from the nose is excoriating, and the fluid from the eyes bland. But when we come to study *Euphrasia*, we will find just the opposite—just such a watery discharge from the nose, and just such copious lachrymation : but the lachrymation here is acrid, and the discharge from the nose bland. The nasal discharge of *Cepa* fairly eats the hair off the upper lip. There is so much congestion that the patient has a sensation of fullness in the nose, with throbbing and burning, sometimes nosebleed. Pain through jaws, in face, extending into the head. Frontal and occipital headaches—so severe that the eyes cannot stand light. . . .

He gives another phase of the medicine : " Why it begins on the left side and goes over to the right, I do not know, but it usually does this. Stuffing up of the side of the nose; watery, acrid discharge from left side of nose—in another twenty-four hours the right side is invaded. Profuse nasal discharge. Colds after damp cold winds. Fluent coryza with headache ; tears from eyes ; want of appetite, cough and trembling of hands ; feels hot and thirsty ; worse evenings and indoors ; better in open air. Every year in August, morning coryza with violent sneezing ; very sensitive to the odour of flowers and skin of peaches. This is one form of hay fever cured by *Allium cepa*. It will wipe out an attack of hay fever in a few days when symptoms agree."

Of hay fever he says further, " It is really an explosion of chronic disease. It may be wiped out in one season by a short-acting remedy, only to return the next just the same, and perhaps another remedy will be required. As soon as the hay fever is stopped you must begin with constitutional treatment. There will be symptoms, if you know how to hunt for them, that differ altogether from the acute attack. . . . It is difficult to find a constitutional remedy when the hay fever is at its height.

" The inflammation soon spreads to ears, throat and larynx. The old mother used to put onions on the baby's ear when it had earache. . . . In households where a medicine case is kept, *Pulsatilla* is the standard remedy for earache, and only occasionally has a doctor to be sent for. *Pulsatilla* will cure earache in almost all sensitive children who cry pitifully. But those who are snappish, who are never suited, who will throw away something they have asked for and slap the nurse in the face, must have *Chamomilla*. With *Pulsatilla*, *Chamomilla* and *Allium cepa* you can cure the majority of earaches in children."

He also says, " We all know what a flatulent vegetable the onion is, it is a wonderful medicine for babies with colic. Cutting, tearing pains draw the poor little thing almost double. It screams with the violent cutting pains in the lower abdomen. . . ." Again " A wonderful remedy for whooping cough, with indigestion, vomiting and flatulence. Flatus offensive ; doubled up with the colic . . . it also cures a ragged, sensitive anus, with bleeding, in infants."

" Violent, rapid inflammations of larynx. Sensation as if something were torn loose, or as if a hook were dragging up through larynx with every cough. In whooping cough the child shakes and shudders, and you can see it dreads the cough because of the tearing pain in larynx. . . . *Cepa* has a reputation for croupy cough. The old lady binds onion on the throat of the child with croup. . . . Another affection over which this remedy has marvellous power is traumatic neuritis in a stump after amputation. Pains almost unbearable, rapidly exhausting the strength of the patient."

* * *

H. C. ALLEN in his invaluable *Keynotes of Leading Remedies*, gives a few more valuable hints, as to the scientific uses of *Allium cepa*—homœopathically prepared and potentized *onion*. " It is a great eye medicine, where eyes burn, smart as from smoke, are watery and suffused, capillaries injected and excessive lachrymation." He says, " Useful for nasal polypus ; for catarrhal laryngitis, where cough compels patient to *grasp larynx* ; seems as if *cough would tear it*. Neuralgic pains like a long thread, in face, neck, chest, head.

" Panaritis ; with red streaks up arm ; pains drive to despair —in child-bed."

" Sore and raw spots on feet, especially heel, from friction." He quotes Dioscorides, " *Efficacious when feet are rubbed sore* ".

CLARKE used to say, " Whenever you find a book by H. N. GUERNSEY, buy it." He had the greatest respect for his knowledge and acumen as regards our Materia Medica. So we will turn up for possible further valuable hints in regard to the onion as a remedy, to Guernsey. We will not repeat, only attempt to add more to the curious and characteristic symptoms.

He starts, " *Catarrhal conditions* most decidedly lead the way to the useful employment of this remedy. All catarrhal symptoms and pains are, as a rule, worse in the evening. Lachrymation and running from the nose, worse in a warm room. Coughs are worse in cold air.

" Fear that the pains will become unbearable . . . pain in temples, aggravated by winking. *Eyes.* Very much lachrymation and coryza. Paralysis left-half of face ; also of limbs of the same side : copious flow of urine.

" Hawking of lumpy mucus from posterior nares, sometimes tough and difficult to detach. Pain in throat as if one had swallowed too large a substance, the pain extends into the right ear.

" Strong craving for raw onions. Cannot take any other nourishment. Nausea from stomach up into throat. Belching and rumbling and puffing up of abdomen.

" Pains liver region. Violent pains left hypogastrium, with urging to urinate, urine scalding.

" Patient inflates the lungs, raises up, gives a *hearty sneeze.*

" Chilly crawls run down the back ; especially at night, with frequent urination."

Old CULPEPPER, some 300 years ago, wrote of onions : " They are wholly flatulent, or windy, and provoke appetite, increase thirst, ease the bowels, provoke the courses, help the bites of mad dogs and of other venomous creatures, used with honey and rue . . . kill worms in children. . . . Roasted under the embers, and eaten with honey, or sugar and oil, they much conduce to help an inveterate cough, and expectorate tough phlegm." (And here comes a little bit of Homœopathy.) " The juice, snuffed up the nostrils, purges the head, and helps the lethargy : yet often eaten is said to procure pains in the head." He tells us that the juice is good for scalds and burns. " Used with vinegar it takes away all blemishes, spots and marks on the skin ; and dropped into the ears, eases the pains and noise in them. Applied also with figs beaten together, helps to ripen and break imposthumes (boils) and other sores. . . . Onion bruised, with the addition of a little salt, and laid on fresh burns, draws out the fire and prevents them blistering."

ALUMINA

(Pure Aluminium Oxide)

WE have been asked for a drug picture of *Alumina*. People are much interested in this metal and its compounds, because of its extensive use, now that it can be cheaply produced, as a strong, light, heat-defying material for domestic cooking pots. In fact, we are told that it is almost impossible, in these days, to procure anything else. A great controversy has been raging intermittently in regard to these useful cooking utensils. The public has even been officially reassured in regard to their harmlessness :— by those who have not our exact knowledge of the symptoms of any poisoning, or the smallness of the dose that may, in sensitives, give rise to symptoms. Occasional ingestions of any deleterious substance may be practically harmless—easily dealt with by the organism and overcome, whereas constant small poisonings must tell on health :—in the way that, as we are told, the smallest quantity of lead in drinking water may produce a profound anæmia. As a matter of fact, if there were no danger in the use of aluminium for cooking purposes, why should purchasers be warned that soda must not be used in cleansing them ? and why should we be assured that there is far less danger in the employment of the more expensive aluminium saucepans, made of purer material. If there were *no* danger, could there be *less*.

Well, anyway, aluminium becomes interesting to us all now that we are absorbing it, most of us, all day long and every day. It is not needed in our make-up, and is, at best, a foreign body. If we have been wise, and discarded aluminium for any cooking purpose in our homes, yet in places away from home, where London's millions get at least coffee and light foods at mid-day and in the tea hour, they are exposed to the danger of milk boiled in aluminium saucepans and to eggs contaminated in the same way. Curiously enough, cases have been reported where persons have declared that they could not eat eggs; that they found eggs absolutely poisonous : and yet, when induced to " venture on an egg " cooked in iron or enamel, it has proved to be perfectly digestible.

One had an idea that aluminophobia was just a fad about which tiresome persons were always writing and making a fuss. But one's scepticism was first shaken a couple of years ago, when a very level-headed doctor described the curious condition of her precious puppy, dying at three-and-a-half months old of what no one, even a very eminent " vet.", could diagnose. She had been doing his cooking herself in the best aluminium saucepan procurable, and in a few days he began to vomit p.c. After a month of incessant vomiting, he was emaciated, and after six weeks he could not stand. He was "a dreadful sight", and vomited even after a drink of water. She was going to have him " put to sleep " when the post brought a pamphlet on aluminium poisoning in dogs. She got an enamel saucepan, and the dog at once improved and never looked back. A friend's dog was suffering in the same ways, and her dog—and husband—both improved in health when aluminium was banished from the kitchen.

But all persons do not seem to suffer equally from aluminium. Why ? Doubtless because what we call idiosyncrasy, for want of wider or more particular knowledge, comes in here. One man is poisoned by strawberries—by mushrooms—by dates : a thousand are not. " *One man's meat is another man's poison*" :—is it not in proverbs that the collective experience of mankind is embodied ? Probably it is an individual question of certain conditions of blood, of secretions—of food or drink ingested, that make for poisonous compounds of aluminium in certain persons.

A rather alarming case of supposed aluminium poisoning is given in an American medical journal—mislaid at the moment, but doubly interesting because of a similar case just now in one's private practice. It was malignant disease of œsophagus, which cleared up when aluminium cooking vessels were discarded ! Is there, in the provings of *Alumina*, anything suggestive here ? We will quote from Allen's *Encyclopedia of Pure Materia Medica :* " *Sense of constriction from the œsophagus down to the stomach every time he swallows a morsel of food. . . . Contraction of the œsophagus. . . . Violent, pressive pain, as if a portion of the œsophagus were contracted or compressed in the middle of the chest, especially during deglutition, but also when not swallowing, with oppression of the chest. . . . Spasmodically pressive pain in middle of chest, on swallowing food and drink.*" One would point out that in these cases it is the lower end of the œsophagus that is the site of the mass, and therefore constriction—" the middle of the chest ".

Again to quote *Allen*, a compound of *Alumina*, *Alum* (a double sulphate of aluminium and potassium) is responsible for the following, quoted from *Hufeland :*
" *Alum* causes induration and scirrhus uteri, if continually used for copious menstruation and hæmorrhages."

Evidently *Alum* may be one of the irritants of tissues on which cancer grafts itself.

Alumina, of course, is one of our greatest remedies in constipation,—that is, of the peculiar form of constipation it induces : " *no desire for stool ; and—no power to strain at stool, however soft* ". Here one has used it from time to time with great success. And from what one has observed of the effects of *Alumina*, one opines that the almost universal use of aluminium cooking vessels must be worth thousands a year to the chemists who sell laxatives and purgatives galore to the public. As said, idiosyncrasy no doubt comes in : but whatever else the aluminium salts may do in the way of vitiating health, interference with the normal bowel function is certainly one. No power to strain even for a soft stool ; and no desire for stool—for a week or two, even : and as one has observed, the hold-up seems to be in the neighbourhood of the splenic flexure, or the upper part of the descending colon.

But not only here, but in many parts of the body, *Alumina* is a remedy of paresis and paralysis. In its ptosis of eyelids, one thinks of *Causticum*. Again in its paralytic effects on intestines, one thinks of *Plumbum*, to which, by its similarity of symptoms, it stands in the relation of antidote. But its pitiful, increasing, and chronic condition of weakness and heaviness of the lower limbs especially, make the drug very interesting. It weakens alike mentally and physically. In these days when national fitness is the ideal of the moment, a possible constant source of deterioration, mental and physical, does not appeal to one as particularly helpful.

* * *

Apparently, as usual, the crude poison is antidoted, by its potencies (200, etc.).

* * *

In regard to its appetites : *Alumina* is down as one of the drugs that craves indigestible things : slate pencils, earth, chalk, clay, white rags, charcoal, cloves, acids, coffee and tea-grounds, dry rice. Besides its aversion to potatoes, which greatly disagree, it has aversion to meat, which has no taste ; to beer ; and a longing for fruits and vegetables—barring potatoes. It is worse also from all irritating things, like salt, vinegar, pepper ; gets a sore throat from eating onions ; gets easily drunken from the weakest spirituous drinks ; and is worse from tobacco smoke. Considering its dryness and irritation of mucous membranes, one can understand some of these things.

Black Letter Symptoms

Eyes inflamed ; itching at inner canthus ; agglutination at night, lachrymation by day. Burning ; dryness ; smarting.
Yellow halo round the candle.
Eyelids thickened, dry, burning.

Redness of nose.
Point of nose cracked.

Involuntary spasmodic twitching of lower jaw : with hæmorrhage of bowels, and dark offensive stools.

In evening, dryness of throat, which induces frequent clearing of throat.

Worse from eating potatoes.

Painter's colic.

Inactivity of rectum ; even the soft stool needs great straining.
Rectum seems paralysed.
No desire for, and no ability to pass stool till there is a large accumulation.
Stools : hard, knotty, covered with mucus ; like sheep's dung, with cutting in anus, followed by blood ; like pipe-stems.
Soft and thin stool, passing with difficulty.
Severe hæmorrhage from bowels, with flow of urine.
Diarrhœa whenever she urinates.
Evacuation of a small quantity of hard fæces, with pressure and a sensation of excoriation in the rectum.

Urine voided when straining at stool ; or cannot pass urine without straining.
Constipation of sucklings.

Continual . dry, hacking cough, with vomiting and arrest of breathing ; with frequent sneezing.
Every morning a long attack of dry cough, ends with difficult raising of a little white mucus.

Great heaviness in lower limbs ; he can scarcely drag them.
When walking he staggers and has to sit down.
Great weariness of the legs when sitting.

Faint and tired ; must sit down.

Some Italic and Curious Symptoms

Seeing blood on a knife, has horrid ideas of killing herself, though she abhors the idea. (Comp. *Ars., Nat. sulph., Thuja.*)

Great dread of death, with thoughts of suicide.

Fear of losing his reason.

Uneasiness, evening, as if evil impending.

Weeps constantly, without wishing it.

Sneers at everything. Peevishness. Grumbles.

Intolerable ennui : no disposition for any kind of work.

Headache ; violent stitches in brain ; stabs : as with a knife.

Headache, as if hair pulled.

Vertigo.

Inability to walk, except with eyes open and in daytime.

Cloudiness and drunken feeling, alternating with pain in kidneys.

Easily made drunk, by weakest spirituous drink.

Sees fiery spots ; white stars.

Objects appear yellow.

As if looking through a fog, or feathers.

Itching, corners of eyes, and of lids.

Upper lids seem to hang down, as if paralysed, especially the left. (*Caust., Sep.,* etc.)

Ears hot and red : especially evenings.

It seems as if, in right ear, he had an entirely different voice.

Skin of face tense, even round eyes, as if the white of an egg had dried upon it.

Stitches in throat on swallowing ; something pointed seems to stick in throat.

Sense of constriction, œsophagus down to stomach, every time he swallows a morsel of food.

Violent pressive pain, as if part of œsophagus were contracted or compressed in middle of chest.

Rabid hunger ; or, aversion to food ; no desire to eat.

No taste in food ; or everything tastes like straw or shavings.

Rancid eructations ; pyrosis ; waterbrash.

Worse after potatoes ; a loathing which makes him shiver.

Crawling at pit of stomach, as from a worm.

Crawling in rectum as from worms.

Dropping of blood, or a stream of blood during, or after evacuation.

(*Alumina's* characteristic constipation is given elsewhere.)

And, can only urinate when straining for stool. Can only pass stool when standing, is one of its curious symptoms.

Oppression, chest : constriction round chest.

Twitching and involuntary movements of limbs and fingers.

Heaviness of legs, can hardly lift them.

Heaviness in feet, with great lassitude of legs.

Pain in sole of foot, on stepping on it, as if it were too soft and swollen.

Lassitude : great ; of whole body ; slow, tottering gait ; excessively faint and tired ; great fatigue, especially upon talking.

* * *

Different teachers emphasize one point, or another, in regard to a drug, and in accordance with their own experience of its utility : we endeavour to cull the experience of many.

HUGHES says : " In mucous membranes, the characteristic feature seems to be *dryness* with more or less irritation : . . . in morbid sensitiveness of nasal mucous membrane to cold ; in chronic dry catarrh of conjunctivæ, even when granular ; in chronic pharyngitis, where membrane looks dry, red, glazed ; in dry, hacking coughs from pharyngeal or laryngeal irritàtion ; in dyspepsia from deficiency of gastric juice ; in constipation from lack of intestinal secretion. Has also cured a frequent desire to urinate during the night. Chronic affections of old people, or dry, thin persons." He says, Dunham recommends it for violent cough excited by an elongated uvula.

* * *

GUERNSEY : " Peculiarities about rectum and stool afford hints to the use of this remedy. . . . *Inactivity* of the rectum, requiring great straining to evacuate even a soft stool. No desire for stool for days, sometimes a week, until there is a large accumulation, and even then evacuation seems only after great effort. Even if the accumulated stool be very soft, the same effort is required to pass it. One must strain at stool in order to urinate. We see this in dysentery, typhus, and in many other disorders, when *Alumina* will be very likely the remedy.

* * *

FARRINGTON says : " *Alumina* has been used in *nervous affections* of a very grave character. Bœninghausen used the metal *Aluminium* for the following symptoms in that dreaded disease, locomotor ataxia : frequent dizziness ; objects turn in a circle ; ptosis ; diplopia or strabismus ; inability to walk in the dark or with the eyes closed without staggering ; feels as if walking on cushions. Formication, or sensation of creeping as from ants in the back and legs. The nates go to sleep when sitting. The heels become numb when walking. A feeling in face as though it was covered with cobwebs, or as if white of egg had dried upon it. Pain in the back, as though a hot iron were thrust into the spine. These are the symptons indicating *Alumina*, and these are the symptoms which led Bœninghausen to *Alumina*, and enabled him to cure four cases of the disease."

" Hypochondriacal men, with lassitude and indifference to labour or to work. An hour seems to them half a day. Peevish and fretful, here rivalling *Nux* and *Bry*. . . .

" *Alumina* acts on *skin* just as it does on mucous membranes; produces dryness and harshness ; indicated in rough dry eruptions which crack, and *may* bleed, but not often—but which itch and burn intolerably, and are worse in the warmth of the bed. . . .

" Feeling of constriction along œsophagus when swallowing food. Always worse from potatoes is a good indication for *Alum*. There is aversion to meat, and a craving for indigestible substances.

" There are diseases of the blood to which it is applicable. Anæmia, chlorosis, especially in young girls at puberty. Menses pale and scanty. Abnormal craving for indigestible articles, such as slate pencils, chalk, whitewash. Leucorrhœa may be profuse, even running down to the feet (*Luet*.)."

Farrington also says, " *Alumina* acts best in spare aged persons, rather wrinkled and dried-up looking ; and in girls at puberty, especially if chlorotic. Also in delicate children, especially those who have been artificially fed, i.e. nourished by the many varieties of baby foods with which the market is glutted. Such children are weak and wrinkled ; nutrition is decidedly defective. Bowels inactive—(with the characteristic constipation as described). The child too may suffer, when teething, from strabismus ; from weakness of internal rectus of affected eye."

* * *

As so frequently, we must ask KENT to make *Alumina* live for us, in his graphic manner. From him we best get its mental symptoms. . . . " It affects intellect; confuses intelligence; so that patient is unable to make a decision. Judgment is disturbed. Unable to realize ; things he knows seem to him to be unreal " (for unreality, compare *Med.*). Kent quotes Hahnemann, in *Chronic Diseases*, as giving the best expression of *Alumina* mentality that occurs anywhere. . . . "When he says anything, he feels as if another person had said it ; when he sees anything, as if another person had seen it, or as if he could transfer himself into another and only then could see. . . ." The consciousness of personal identity is confused. He 'is dazed ; makes mistakes in writing and speaking ; uses words not intended.

"Then, another phase : gets into a hurry. Nothing moves fast enough ; time seems slow, everything delayed.

"Then, *impulses :* when he sees sharp instruments or blood, impulses rise within him, and he shudders because of these impulses. An instrument that could be used for murder or for killing causes these impulses. Impulse to kill herself.

"Thinks surely he is going to lose his reason. Thinks about this frenzy and hurry and confusion of mind ; how he hardly knows his own name, and how fretful he is, and finally thinks he is going crazy."

*   *   *

EFFECTS ON SENSITIVES OF ALUMINIUM EMANATIONS.

Practical, anyway, this radiator !—light, bright, and gave out unusual heat. . . . Yet, after a bit, the room did not feel good ; one was glad to turn it off. WHY ? Aluminium pots were taboo : but the aluminium or aluminium plated radiator was not suspect.

Next—what was happening ? A curious vertigo ; when eyes suddenly went out of focus, and one had to halt, at risk of falling ; or, when typing, one had to wait for normal vision, and the abrupt end of what one called " *visual vertigo* " ; or when, seeing oddly, one would discover a yellow-grey cloud across right-eye vision coupled with alarming instability. An umbrella for a prop, was a god-send ; while just to touch objects in a room, was reassuring.

At last, it dawned !—perhaps aluminium symptoms ?—and Materia Medica answered, " Yes "—soon confirmed by the fact that, the radiators savagely smashed, the trouble rapidly disappeared. And when a once-time nurse came to ask help because she was becoming paralysed, the symptoms she detailed were with curious exactitude those one had spotted as symptoms of aluminium emanations. *Was she using one of those radiators ? Well, the housemaid where she was nursing had been leaving one of these radiators on in her bedroom all day during this bitter weather.* . . . And so the poor soul departed reprieved and happy.

One yearns to say to the many one meets, walking warily with the help of an umbrella, " Pardon me, but have you got one of those splendid aluminium radiators? "

AMMONIUM CARBONICUM

It was one of Dr. Younan's " Hints " especially applicable to-day in the somewhat trying conditions in which we exist, which drew one's attention to *Ammonium carb.* for the cough that may be left by Influenza; which should yield to *Bryonia,* but may fail to do so.

He says, " Since my own experience with *Ammonium-carbonicum* I have used it in many cases, especially those of children, with much success. It has cured the cough of Influenza when everything else has failed, and I have more than once not found it necessary to give a second dose."

Ammon. carb. is a remedy of severe, if not desperate, conditions ; one of very great value, but where, having no personal experience, we shall call upon some of our best prescribers to paint its Drug picture for us. On first trying to envisage it, it seemed a bit vague and colourless : but as one persevered, it grew in luminosity, till it assumed definite and unmistakable proportions: while its very vagueness and want of definition as regards symptoms, seem to have led to its successful prescribing. Its salient features are : want of energy, power, strength, tone. Typical *Ammon. carb.* is weak, tired, played out, mind and body : sometimes without a single apparent ailment or disease to account for the condition : or it may come in at the end of serious and (without its stimulus) fatal illnesses.

When one studies a little-regarded drug, it is astonishing how often the very patient who needs it, appears on the scene ; or how one remembers just the very patient, of long ago, who might have benefited by it. For instance somebody, ill for months, generally in bed, with what is diagnosed (so her people say) " heart failure "—" degenerated heart "—a healthy and energetic middle-aged woman, puts up the *Ammonium carb.* condition, and ought to cure rapidly. She is " absolutely in despair and cannot go on like this ! "—and is, as is so often the case, coming to see whether Homœopathy can again score one of its triumphs. It should !

*   *   *

Ammonium carb. is one of Hahnemann's remedies ; see his *Chronic Diseases.* He found it useful where the mental condition was one of fearfulness, disobedience, want of docility, loathing of life : uneasiness, anxiety, weakness.

Chronic headache, as if something would get out at the forehead ; hammering headache.

Burning or coldness in eyes.   One of the remedies of cataract.

Itching in ear, in nose.   Pustules and boils on nose, and nose-bleed especially on washing, in a.m. (all the authorities make a point of this symptom).

Looseness of teeth.   Sore, raw throat.

Rawness and burning, œsophagus, after a meal; headache and nausea after a meal.   Giddiness during a meal, unconquerable desire to eat sugar.   .   .   .   Plenty of stomach symptoms include pain, heartburn, pain in stomach when stretching oneself.

Shortness of breath :   asthma, cough—with hoarseness, the body being warm.   Cough from tickling in throat : by day : by night ;   stitches in small of back when coughing.   Burning in chest : stitches in chest.

Goitre.

Pain in wrist joint where sprained long ago.   Warts.   Burning stitches and tearing in corns.

Drowsy by day : sleepless by night.   Heat in head with cold feet.

These are merely Hahnemannian extracts, showing to some extent the range of drug action of *Ammon. carb.*   By the way, the salt is triturated, and then the potencies are run up.   Hahnemann also says :

" This drug is especially suitable to *adynamic, weak, nervous, venous or lymphatic constitutions :* to individuals of a *torpid phlegmatic, melancholy temperament*, to people leading *a sedentary life*, and to *the female organism* ; in persons who are easily impressed, but react slightly and for a short time ; when there is laxity of fibre, disposition to lymphatic accumulation, accumulation of mucus and fat ; and to nervous affections.   .   .   .

"·It is remarkable that *ammonium* should be useful against a tendency to gangrene, and that cancerous and mortifying ulcers should evolve a large quantity of ammonium : that ammonium should play an important part in the affections of the sexual organs of the female and that a considerable quantity of ammonium should be evolved through the skin during menstruation ; and, lastly, that ammonium should relieve the symptoms of poisoning by fungi, and that ammonium should be a characteristic constituent of these growths.   It is well known that a similar relation exists between the itch and sulphur : that the itch vesicle smells of sulphur, and that sulphur is a specific against the itch."

*   *   *

One notices that many of the symptoms of *Ammon. carb.* are worse while, or after eating : " the stomach feels over-loaded for hours after eating." It is worse for cold, wet weather : for washing (*Sulph.*) ; during menses. It is better in dry weather ; when lying on the painful side, or on the abdomen.

Among other trials, it has itching at anus, and hæmorrhoids which bleed and protrude.

It affects especially the right side : and its bad hour is 3 a.m.

All the rest one gets, emphasized, in the following extracts and quotations.

Black Letter Symptoms

Sense of oppressive fullness, pushing as if FOREHEAD *would burst.*

Nosebleed : when washing hands or face in a.m. NOSE *bleeds from left nostril.*

Stoppage, nose, mostly at night : must breathe through mouth.

A good deal of hunger and appetite. Rabid HUNGER : *yet she is immediately satiated after having eaten little.*

Heat in the face, during and after dinner.

Qualmishness.

One of the best remedies in emphysema.

Cough at night : every morning at 3 a.m. ; dry cough from tickling of throat, as of dust.

Angina pectoris.

Right ARM *appeared to weigh a hundredweight, and to be without strength.*

Spasm in right arm, which drew it backwards.

Panaritium : finger inflamed ; deep-seated periosteal pain.

Better for external pressure : headache better : constrictive pain in stomach better : pain in bowels better.

Body red, as if covered with scarlatina
Malignant scarlatina with somnolence, etc.

Body feels bruised.

* * *

NASH, quoting Guernsey, says : Delicate women who faint easily and want smelling salts around them most of the time. Weak ; with deficient reaction ; generally of the lymphatic temperament. Want stimulants, especially such as act through olfactory nerves—Ammonia, Camphor, Musk, Alcohol, etc. A good remedy to excite reaction in the first onset of such a suddenly prostrating disease as cerebro-spinal meningitis. Good for dry, stuffed coryza, acute or chronic ; patient is worse at night, has to breathe with mouth open. . . . Very useful in scarlatina, body very red, almost bluish red, and the throat seems the centre where the force of the disease seems to be expended in malignant intensity. The eruption is faintly developed, from inability, owing to weakness, of vitality to keep it on the surface (Zinc). *Ailanthus* is also comparable here.

*   *   *

We will cull also from FARRINGTON—sketchily.

Vital powers are weakened. Hæmorrhages of a dark fluid blood appear. There is degeneration of blood tissue. Muscles become soft and flabby, teeth loosen and decay, and gums recede and ulcerate.

Its symptoms in uræmia are very important, and are not only characteristic in uræmia, but in any other disease in which this remedy may be indicated : as in scarlatina, also in heart disease. They are : somnolence or drowsiness with rattling of large bubbles in lungs ; grasping at flocks ; bluish or purplish hue of lips from lack of oxygen in blood, and brownish colour of tongue. Its nearest analogue here is *Antimonium tart.* (*Arnica* also, in typhoid states.)

With such symptoms remember *Ammon. carb.* for œdema of lungs and emphysema.

To be remembered also for poisoning by charcoal fumes.

It is useful in the beginning of cerebro-spinal meningitis : when patient is stricken by the violence of the poison, and falls into a stupid, non-reactive state. He is cold, and the body surface is cyanotic. Pulse weak. In just such cases *Ammonium carb.* will bring about reaction.

Useful again in dilatation of heart. Patient suffers going up stairs, or up hill : suffers intolerably in a hot room. There is often a cough with bloody sputum. Palpitation, dyspnœa and retraction of epigastrium. Perhaps cyanosis.

In pneumonia with great debility, with symptoms pointing to a heart clot.

Indicated in chronic bronchitis, with atony of bronchial tubes, favouring emphysema. Copious accumulation of mucus in lungs, dilatation of bronchial tubes, and œdema pulmonum. He is weak, sluggish in movements, coughs continually, raises with difficulty or not at all. May be drowsy, delirious, muttering.

Then, scarlatina (all the authors speak of this). It is rather a malignant type. Throat swollen internally and externally, glands enlarged, bluish or dark red swelling of tonsils. In addition to swelling of cervical lymphatics, inflammation of the cellular tissues.

Then the characteristic obstructed nose, particularly at night. The child starts from sleep as if smothering ; or has to lie with its mouth wide open, to breathe. Enlargement often of the right parotid gland. Like *Apis* : but *Apis* has more œdema, for instance, of the uvula.

* * *

Lastly, to epitomize KENT. " If we were practising in the old-fashioned way and considered the wonderfully volatile nature of *Ammonium carb.* in some of its forms, we would only look upon it as an agent to relieve faintness . . . and use it in the form of hartshorn to comfort old maids and some other women. But it is a deep-acting, constitutional medicine, an antipsoric. It effects rapid blood changes : it disturbs the whole economy. Its fluids are all acrid. The acrid saliva excoriates the lips, so that they crack in corners and middle, and become raw, dry, scabby.

Eyelids fester and become dry and cracked from the excoriating fluids. The stool is acrid and excoriates. There is rawness from acrid menstrual discharge and leucorrhœa. Wherever there is an ulcer the fluids that ooze excoriate the parts around.

It bleeds black blood, often fluid, that will not coagulate. Skin mottled, intermingled with great pallor.

It has violent action on the heart : there is violent, audible pulsation, worse for every motion. Strange that the ancients knew that *Ammon. carb.* would overcome difficult breathing from cardiac attacks. (When indicated, the single dose, very high, is enough.) He says, the ancients used *Ammon. carb.* in the low form of pneumonia : it had a homœopathic relation to some of the cases. Once in a while they would cure the awful stage of prostration with heart failure at the end of pneumonia, and because they relieved such a one, it was established as a remedy for all future use.

It has a state analogous to blood poisoning (as in erysipelas, and malignant scarlet fever), with prostration and great dyspnœa, as if heart were giving out : with patchy surface, dusky and puffy face.

Enfeebled weak heart : absence of symptoms: lack of response to remedies. Patient has to lie in bed and do nothing, for palpitation and difficult breathing on motion.

Such a case, he says, furnished me much amusement for a year and a half. There was a woman, who answered this description. Her state was one of peculiar weakness with dyspnœa and palpitation on motion. I had been treating her, but had not fully studied the case, and as she did not progress, she was put under an able neurologist for a " rest cure ". She was to be well in six weeks, but as, then, she was worse than ever, a heart specialist was called in to examine her. The heart was not vigorous, but there was no organic affection. Then a lung specialist, and all kinds of other specialists, to investigate fully all her organs : but there was nothing the matter with them ; yet the poor woman could not walk because of her sufferings and palpitating heart. . . . After three months, steadily failing, Dr. Kent was called to see her again. The case was extremely vague, with nothing but those few symptoms. " Finally I settled on *Ammon. carb.*, and she has been on this remedy for eighteen months : one dose helping her from six weeks to two months. She now climbs mountains, and does everything she wants to do. This shows how deeply this remedy acts."

Exhaustion, every M.P. An attack like cholera coming the first day of each M.P. There may be exhaustion with vomiting, coldness, blueness, sinking dyspnœa. (*Verat.*)

Its asthma has this peculiarity, worse in a warm room, till suffocates ; as if he would die for want of breath. Yet the headache and bodily complaints are worse from cold.

Bones ache : ache as if they would break. Teeth ache violently from change of weather, or of temperature in the mouth. Hair falls out ; nails become yellowish ; gums receded from teeth and bleed : scorbutic, or scrofulous constitution.

Hysteria : nervous women carry a bottle of ammonia hanging to their chain. A great similarity between the symptoms of this drug and snake poisonings—where it has a great reputation.

Many complaints from bathing.

In diphtheria and chest troubles, worse after sleep. (Very like *Lach.* in many of its symptoms.)

Seems as if all her inner parts were raw and sore.

Full of catarrhal symptoms and cough ; rattling of mucus all through chest. Oppression of breathing. A catarrhal dyspnœa. Hypostatic congestion of lungs : chest filling up with mucus difficult to expel. Coldness, prostration and weakness of chest.

Worse 3 a.m. ; wakes with cold sweat and difficult breathing. Almost pulseless. Face pale and cold.

" Heart failure. Patient got on well, then the heart failed." Here *Ammon. carb.*, given in time, would save life.

ANACARDIUM ORIENTALE
(Marking Nut)

THE indications for *Anacardium* are so striking and so definite that it seems hardly necessary to Drug picture it.

But, a word of warning. We once complained to a very wise and learned homœopathic chemist that *Anacardium*, in some digestive troubles, had failed to work. Of course there may have been one of two reasons for this : the drug may have been wrongly prescribed, or it may not have been a good preparation. The old man was too polite to suggest any but the second alternative, and he proceeded to explain. He said, the dark juice from which it derives its name is not in the nut but in the husk. Whereas ignorant persons put tinctures on the market made from the nut itself ; useless for medicinal purposes. A successor of that same chemist with whom we were discussing the point the other day, sent us two samples of *Anacardium* ø which lie before us as we write : the potent preparation nearly black : the reputed *Anacardium*, a pale brown. So once again we reiterate the warning :—Get your homœopathic remedies from homœopathic chemists who know what they are selling, and do not pick up cheap, ill-prepared, perhaps vitiated drugs, just anywhere. To get results, remedies must be made from the medicinal parts of a plant, grown in its own habitat, culled at its best, and prepared and preserved without contamination. We are absolutely at the mercy of our chemists ; and we are very grateful to them.

Anacardium is best known for its peculiar and extreme mental symptoms : its loss of memory : its senses of duality and unreality (the latter makes one think of *Medorrhinum*) ; its perversions, blasphemous and cruel : its illusions, delusions, and fears : its peculiar sensations—bursting, binding, plugging. We will call on various outstanding prescribers to describe the manner in which they have found it useful, and the indications on which they have come to rely.

But, first, *Anacardium*, one of Hahnemann's drugs, is to be found in Vol. ii of his *Chronic Diseases*. Here we read, that " Caspar Hoffman has called the *Confectio anacardina seu sapientium* (celebrated as a distinguished remedy against weakness of mind, memory and the senses) a *Confection of fools* : because many had lost their memory and had become mad on account of using it *too often and inconsiderately*." " Hence it was only the improper and too frequent use of *Anacardium* that made it hurtful," **as**

Hahnemann points out. "If applied correctly it became curative." In other words, just another illustration of his discovery :—" That which can cause, can cure ; and, in order to cure, seek out that which can cause."

Hahnemann tells us that this is one of the drugs that come from the Arabs. He says : " This powerful drug, together with others of which the ancients availed themselves with great benefit, had been completely forgotten for the last thousand years." And he identifies and describes it thus : " Between the external black, shining, *heart-shaped*, hard shell, and the sweet kernel which is covered with a brown reddish thin skin, there is a thickly, blackish juice contained in a cellular tissue with which the Indians mark their linen in an indelible manner, and which is so sharp that moles may be etched away by means of it. A wrong *Anacardium* ' *occidentale* ' is kidney-shaped," he says.

Black Letter Symptoms

Great weakness of MEMORY.
Loss of memory.
Irresistible desire to curse and swear.
Hypochondriasis.
When walking he felt anxious, as if someone were pursuing him :
he suspected everything around him.
He is separated from the whole world : has no confidence in himself ; despairs of being able to do that which is required of him.
Weakness of all the senses.

Pain HEAD, *relieved entirely when eating : worse during motion and work.*
Gastric and nervous headaches.
Dull pressure as from a plug, left vertex.

VISION *indistinct.*
Dull pressure as from a plug, upper border right orbit.

Flat, offensive taste in MOUTH.

Symptoms disappear during dinner, but begin anew after two hours.
Pain about NAVEL *as if a blunt plug were squeezed into intestines.*
Great and urgent desire for stool, passes without evacuation.
Rectum powerless, with sensation as if plugged up.

Dull pressure as from a plug in right side CHEST.

Cramp calves when walking.

Sensation as of a hoop or band round the part.

SOME CURIOUS OR ITALIC SYMPTOMS OF *Anacardium*

Recollections only come after the time he is in need of them.

Has a devil in his ear, whispering blasphemous words.

Everything perceived has no reality.

Thinks he is double : that mind and body are separated : that a stranger is at his side : that strange forms accompany him.

Her husband is not her husband : her child not her child.

Screams loudly : swears : thinks himself a demon.

Contradiction between reason and will : has two wills, one commanding to do what the other forbids.

In one ear a devil, in the other an angel prompts him to do murder, or acts of benevolence.

Cowardice.

Takes everything in bad part and becomes violent.

Sensation of obstruction as from a plug in ear.

Abdomen feels as if it would burst when coughing.

Dull pressure like a plug in right chest.

Two quickly succeeding stitches, pierce through and through the heart at night.

Sleepiness after coughing.

Legs stiff, as if bandaged : tense, as if too short.

Wave-like twitches here and there in legs.

Pressing or pentrating pain as from a plug in different parts.

Frequent tenesmus during the day for many days, without his ever being able to expel anything.

Any part which he leaves unmoved, immediately goes to sleep.

*   *   *

GUERNSEY says :—" There are few remedies in the entire Materia Medica having ' impaired memory ' as so marked a characteristic. In restoring the memory, it often cures the patient of all other troubles."

Forgets everything : consciousness of this takes away the appetite.

Feels blasphemous words constantly suggested, with desire to curse and swear.

Fixed ideas : that he is double : that there is no reality in anything : all a dream : mind and body separated : a stranger at his side, one to the right, the other to the left : her husband is not her husband, or her child her child . . . is being pursued : suspects everyone : constantly expecting trouble.

Two different influences exerted on him at the same time, the one to do murder, the other to do good. . . .

Frequently screams loudly, as if to call someone.

3

Objects appear too far off.

All the symptoms disappear while eating, returning afterwards.

(Then the ubiquitous plug sensations, and the sensations of a hoop or band round parts.)

*   *   *

KENT emphasizes the following points :—Full of strange notions and ideas. Feeble mind, to complete imbecility. Disturbed by everything : cursing. In continuous controversy with himself : controversy between two wills, two impulses. Hallucinations : a demon sits on one shoulder an angel on the other. Contradiction between will and reason.

" I have learned much from *Anac.*, *Aurum* and *Argentum*, of the strange action of medicines on the human mind. By this means we can get at facts and lay aside many hypotheses."

Nothing real : all seems in a dream. Fixed ideas : that he is double : that a stranger is by his side. One moment he sees a thing and understands it and another moment he does not understand it. One moment sees it is her child and another that it is not. . . . One moment thinks it is so, and next moment has enough reason left to know that it is not so. Delusion is an advanced stage of illusion. In the repertory we have the same remedies, often, for illusion and delusion ; it is a matter of grade. . . . He sees demons, and at first he knows from his intelligence that a demon is not there, but later he wants you to drive him out.

Fears everything and everybody : he is pursued : expects enemies : internal anxiety : no peace. . . . All moral feeling is taken out of him. He feels cruel. Can do bodily injury without feeling. Cruel, malicious, wicked. Suitable in religious mania when the conflict between the external and internal will is kept up. " Skins " like *Rhus*. Tetanus. Epilepsy.

*   *

NASH says :—*Anacardium orientale* is a very valuable remedy, not generally appreciated by our school. It ought often to be used in that hydra-headed complaint called dyspepsia, for which *Nux* is so indiscriminately used. And he stresses that *Anac.* has a pain in stomach *only* when the stomach is empty, and is *relieved by eating*, while *Nux* is relieved after the process of digestion is over. *Nux* is at its worst two or three hours after meals, but only till digestion is accomplished, then comes relief : whereas with *Anac.* this is the time when the *suffering* is worst. Nash found almost as many *Anac.* as *Nux* cases : and found the 200th here more efficacious than the lower potencies. " The potency here as well as elsewhere and with all remedies has more to do with success in curing than some imagine."

In regard to stool, he says, *Nux* has the desire, but with irregular or overaction. *Anac.* has the desire, with not sufficient action to carry it out. Then *Anac.* has a sense of lump or plug in anus which ought to come away ; which does not appear in *Nux*.

* * *

Anacardium, marking nut,
Plugged sensations, eyes to gut.
Anacardium, here's your guide,
Plug within, tight band outside.
Mentally two wills oppose,
Which to obey he never knows.
Think of *Anacardium* where
Patient wants to curse and swear :
Should he never cease to pray,
Give *Stramonium* right away.

Marking nut will potent be,
To restore lost memory.
Anacardium vies with *Nux*
In dyspepsia : here's the crux
Pain till food's digested, see ?
Spells *Tinct. Nucis vomicæ* :
Pain when stomach's empty—tut !—
Cure him with the marking nut.

ANTIMONIUM CRUDUM

" Stibium Sulphuratum nigrum. "—HAHNEMANN.

HAHNEMANN says it is found in nature, in the shape of black parallel needles, having a metallic lustre ; is composed of twenty-eight parts of sulphur and one hundred parts of antimony. The different triturations are prepared according to the method which has been already pointed out. The smallest dose, he says, is sufficient to produce the desired effect, in chronic diseases. . . . He says :—

Antimony is useful when the following symptoms are indicated : A child cannot bear to be touched or looked at.

Rush of blood to the head ; troublesome itching on head : with falling off of hair.

Redness and inflammation of the eyelids. Sore nostrils : heat and itching of cheek. *Pain in hollow teeth.*

Chronic loss of appetite : *eructations tasting of ingesta.*

Nausea, loathing, disposition to vomit consequent upon a spoiled stomach, etc., etc. . . .

One has, perhaps unfortunately, a certain limited number of remedies that have become such friends that they are always at hand, tendering their services ; while a host of others remain mere names and need to be laboriously looked up. *Ant. crud.* has, with us, remained more or less in the latter category. Indeed, one's ideas of the *Ant. crud.* personality resolve themselves into this :—*Greedy, fat, sentimental, with sore corners to mouth, and crippled feet.*

But the drug ought to be considered in cases of " rheumatic inflammation of muscles. In arthritic affections, with swelling and nodosities. In rheumatic contraction of muscles, with curvature of limbs " (JAHR). Then, together with its sentimentality, it has the irresistible desire to talk in rhymes, or to repeat verses : and with its " ecstatic love ", it is said to be useful for the bad effects of disappointed affections (*Nat. mur., Calc. phos.*). Allen's *Keynotes* tell us that its symptoms change locality, or go from one side of the body to the other. (Compare *Lach.*, from left to right : *Lyc.*, from right to left : or *Lac. can.* when they cross and then go back. One has verified this in the diphtheria of a *Lyc.* case : and (again curatively) with *Lac. can.* in ovarian pain.)

BLACK LETTER SYMPTOMS

Allen, Hering ; also Hahnemann's stressed symptoms in his *Chronic Diseases*, where no black type is given.

Peevish. Sulky. Loathing of life.
Child fretful and peevish, turns away and cries when touched.

HEADACHE : *after bathing; from deranging stomach; alcoholic drinks ; after a chill ; suppressed eruptions ; from a cold.*

EYES : *soreness of outer canthi.*
Redness and inflammation of eyelids.
Chronic blepharophthalmia of children.
Sore, cracked and crusty NOSTRILS.
Suppurating and long lasting eruption on CHEEKS.

Toothache, in hollow TEETH : *pain sometimes penetrates into head. Worse at night, after eating and from cold water: touching tooth with tongue causes pain as if nerve were torn : better walking in open air.*
Gnawing pain in carious teeth ; after every meal.

TONGUE *coated ; thick white ; milky white, yellow.*
White tongue.
Lips dry. Cracks in the corners of mouth, painful like sores.
Gums detach from teeth and bleed easily.

STOMACH : *violent thirst, with dryness of lips.*
Thirst in the evening with desire to drink.
Gulping up of food, tasting of the ingesta.
Vomiting after sour wine.
After vinegar or acid wine, loose stools.
Constant discharge of wind, up and down, immediately reproduced, for years; (cured case).
Belching with taste of what has been eaten.
Loathing, nausea and desire to vomit.
Gastric symptoms predominate : disgust for drink and food, bitter mouth and vomit.
Vomiting.
Stomach weak. Easily disturbed digestion.
Gastric catarrh : white tongue : nausea and vomiting. . . .

Very liquid STOOLS.
Diarrhœa: watery with undigested food: watery with little hard lumps. Worse from vinegar—acids—sour wine ; overheating ; after cold bathing ; at night and early morning.

Diarrhœa of old people.
Alternate diarrhœa and constipation of old people.
Difficult, hard stool : faeces too large.
Elderly people with diarrhœa, all at once get costive.
Mucous piles, pricking, burning ; continuous mucous discharge, staining yellow. Sometimes ichor oozes out.

COUGH : *first attack is always most severe, subsequent ones weaker and weaker ; (whooping cough).*
Pain in chest with heat.
Blenorrhœa pulmonum, or phthisis mucosa.
Severe continual itching on chest the whole day.
Violent itching on BACK.
Arthritic pain in FINGERS.
Drawing pains in fingers and their joints.
Drawing pain in the left hip-joint.
Large horny places on soles, close to toes.
Great sensitiveness of soles when walking.

Great SLEEPINESS *during the day, mostly forenoon.*

Exhausted in warm weather.
Cannot bear HEAT *of sun.*
Worse overheating near the fire.
After overheating, diarrhœa.
Sensitive to COLD : *to inhaling cold air : after taking cold.*
Pertussis, worse cold washing.
Cold bathing : causes violent headache ; cold in head ; gastric catarrh ; diarrhœa ; suppressed menses.

FEVER : *heat attended by sweat.*
Violent chill without thirst ; heat with thirst followed by sweat.
After the sweat is over, heat and thirst return.
Gastric fevers.

Mucous membranes generally affected.
Horny excrescences.
Measles-like eruptions : or measles delayed : vomiting during measles.

ITALIC, OR NOTABLE, OR QUEER SYMPTOMS

Decided disposition to shoot himself, to no other kind of suicide. This forced him to leave his bed, otherwise he was unable to get rid of it.

Continual condition of ideal love and ecstatic longing for some ideal being, which filled his fancy ; more when walking in the pure open air than when in a room.

Irritated state of mind : feeling of grief. The sound of bells, or the sight of that which surrounds him, moves him to tears.

Feeling of emptiness in the head, or headache as if forehead would burst : felt intoxicated.

Small, flat, tender tubercles on scalp, with crawling sensation.

Roaring in ears. Violent din in ears, as if someone were beating against the door of the house.

A kind of deafness in right ear, as if a leaflet were placed before the tympanum.

Coryza with sore crusty nostrils. Both nostrils chapped and covered with crusts.

Nosebleed.

Nose painful, as from inspiring cold air or acrid vapours.

Cracks in corners of mouth, painful like sores.

Burning, stinging, as from a red-hot spark on chin and upper lip. On touching it, hand seems to move over sore places.

Dryness of mouth : rawness of palate.

Much saltish saliva in mouth.

Violent thirst with dryness of lips.

Hiccough. Nausea with vertigo.

Violent vomiting, with attacks of anxiety.

Terrible vomiting which nothing can stop.

Fearful vomiting with convulsions.

Violent vomiting and diarrhœa, with excessive anguish.

Pain in stomach, as from excessive fullness, without fullness.

Pain in stomach as after too much eating, with distended, but not hard, abdomen.

Burning at pit of stomach like heartburn, with good appetite.

Burning, spasmodic pain, pit of stomach, drove him to despair, and to the resolution of drowning himself.

Loud rumbling in abdomen, which is much distended.

Protrusion of rectum during stool. Expulsion of black blood.

Stool first natural, then several small loose evacuations, then a small but hard evacuation with violent straining.

Violent spasms in larynx and pharynx, as if throat were filled with a plug, which becomes alternately thicker and thinner, with a feeling of soreness.

Suffocating catarrh. (Death from suffocating catarrh, from a few grains of antimony.)

Feeling as if limbs were enlarged.

Finger-nails did not grow as formerly : painfully sensitive beneath the nails.

Bluish spots on thighs.   Bluish spots on tibiæ.

Mortification of foot : it is quite black.   Intolerable burning, lancinating pain in a mortifying foot, it being insensible to touch or the prick of a pin.

Her foot so heavy she cannot lift it.

Icy cold feet.

Large horny places on skin of soles of feet, with pain like corns which returned after having been cut out.

Great sensitiveness of soles of feet.

Immense swelling of whole body.   Dropsical swelling of body.

Getting fat : or, Emaciation and exhaustion.

Apoplexy with such a profuse flow of saliva, that he expelled a large quantity of watery foam from nose and mouth.

Great sleepiness by day.   At 7 p.m. overwhelmed with sleep.

*   *   *

NASH draws attention to the thick, milky-white coating on the tongue which may occur in many complaints :—

To the derangements from overloading the stomach, especially with fat food : nausea.

To the crushed finger-nails, which grow in splits like warts and with horny spots :

To the corns and callosities on soles, with excessive tenderness, so that he can only walk with pain and suffering :

To the alternate constipation and diarrhœa in old people, especially with the characteristic (white) tongue.

Child cannot bear to be touched or looked at : fretful, cross.

He says many remedies have white tongue, but this one leads them all : thickly coated, white, white as milk tongue.   (We have once seen a tongue not coated, but quite white.   So far as memory serves, it was *Ant. crud.* that quickly cured.)

It is a great stomach remedy . . .   disorders that arise from overeating . . .   gastric derangements of recent date.   The sufferer feels he must throw up before there will be any relief. A few pellets of *Ant. crud.* on the tongue will often settle the business, save the loss of a meal and all further suffering.

Then the peculiar stools, partly solid and partly fluid.   And the form of diarrhœa oftenest with old people, which alternates with constipation, where *Antimonium crud.* is the only remedy. The peculiar mental symptoms—the greatest sadness and woeful mood : the sentimental mood in the moonlight; ecstatic love.

" *Child cannot bear to be touched or looked at—a gem !* "   Nash says that often in cases of gastric or remittent fever he has been led to the use of *Ant. crud.* by this condition of the mind. The cross child, not like *Cham.* which wants to be carried and soothed, but which will scream and cry and show temper at every little attention. Here the fever is apt to run higher at night, and the white tongue is almost always present.

He notices the finger-nails growing in splits, with horny spots : and the toe-nails that grow out of shape, or shrivel up and do not grow at all. And the very tender corns and callosities. (Here one remembers a case cured by *Ant. crud.*) He says some of the worst cases of chronic rheumatism have been cured by *Ant. crud.*, guided by the extreme tenderness of the soles of the feet. Horny excrescences anywhere on the skin make one think of *Ant. crud.*

This remedy is most often needed in the extremes of life, in children and old people.

He draws attention to its aggravations from heat of sun : also from radiate heat of fire ; and also to its aggravations from cold bathing. He says that, when a case of long standing comes, dating the beginning of the trouble from swimming or falling into the water, we think of *Ant. crud.*, and examine for further indications. (N.B.—Burnett's great remedy here was *Bellis per.*)

*　　*　　*

HUGHES, *Pharmacodynamics*, gives a very brief account of this drug : but he quotes Dr. Clotar Muller in regard to its extraordinary efficacy in affections of the skin : " I have reason to think that *Antimonium crudum* is an invaluable remedy where pimples, pustules, pocks or furuncular elevations arise primarily or secondarily, especially when at the same time there is severe continued pricking itching of the skin, and after rubbing tenderness and soreness. Especially when such phenomena occur on the face or genitals."

In regard to its " horny places on the skin of the soles of the feet ", he quotes a recorded case where one of twenty years standing involving the entire sole, and very sensitive, was soon cured by the drug.

*　　*　　*

KENT points out that all the symptoms seem to centre about the stomach. No matter what the complaint, the stomach takes part in it.

It produces a very serious state of mind, an absence of the desire to live. " When I hear a patient say, ' Oh, doctor, if I could only die ! ' I do not like such a case." The prostration is similar to *Arsenicum*, but *Ars.* has overwhelming fear of death, while this medicine has loathing of life. . . . These over-excitable, intense, nervous, hysterical young girls and women are overcome by mellow lights such as flow through stained glass windows, or by the mellow light from the moon in the evening : that is what is meant by " Sentimental mood in the moonlight ".

Worse cold, damp weather : cold bathing. Yet many of the symptoms come on in the sun's rays, and from the heat of an open grate. . . . A child with whooping cough will cough more after looking into the fire. . . . Constant nausea : stomach feels too full, as if he had eaten too much, when he has not eaten at all : feels distended when the abdomen is flat. Gouty persons where the nodules on fingers and joints become painless and the stomach and intestines become distended and painful.

Skin ulcerated : a tendency to grow warts, callosites, bad nails and bad hair. The thickened skin on soles of feet are very sore to walk upon, because of their numerous centres of little corns. Warts on hands : nails brittle, black, can hardly be cut.

P.S.—Dr. Schwartz of California writes me that *Antimonium crud.* is " an almost specific in Rheumatoid Arthritis ".

ANTIMONIUM TARTARICUM

(" Tartar emetic ")

HERING says of this drug, " An invention of the alchemists, very popular with them, forbidden by the French Academy, finally introduced and much used and much abused by the Old School."

Old School, Farrington says, does not make much play in these days with *Tartar emetic* : and he is borne out by its present day teachings, for we are told (Hale White) that " many years ago an ointment of *Tartar emetic* was applied as a counter irritant : but it causes too much pain and is now seldom used ". That *Tartar emetic* " cannot be recommended as an emetic, its action is slow and its general depression great. It should never be given to produce purgation ". It is also pronounced " an undesirable expectorant ". But this is qualified. . . . " The only cases in which it is permissible are those in which an emetic is required for laryngitis, bronchitis, or some other acute inflammatory condition of the respiratory tract, for then its depressant action on the circulation may perhaps be beneficial, but usually *Ipecacuanha* is preferable."

For its uses in the nervous and muscular systems, " it has now been abandoned " : and " it is much less used in medicine than formerly ".

Thus Old School, with its crude methods and crude dosage, fails to realize the precious life-savers at its command, and leaves practical and curative medicine to the disciples of Hahnemann.

*   *   *

" *Ant. tart.*" was proved by Hahnemann and some of his students: but his provings were only published in Stapf's Archives: —in our Hospital Library : but one does not joyfully grub in the old German books, when one can get the desired matter in other, later, English works. His proving of course appears in Allen, Hering, etc.

Hering (*Guiding Symptoms*) " makes use " also " of the masterly monograph of Dr. R. Hencke (1874) who collected all poisonings, provings and cures ".

In the hands of homœopaths *Antimonium tartaricum* is a very precious and indispensable remedy and has saved innumerable lives : the lives of infants and small children especially, dying of bronchitis and broncho-pneumonia, cyanosed and almost moribund ; and, at the other end of life, of old people, with chest full of rattles and wheezes, with lungs filling up, and no power to raise the phlegm. One of our early recollections was of a baby brother gasping, with blue lips and nails : a mother's distress ; how she took the matter out of the doctor's hands, and slipped into the baby's mouth a few of the little sweet things—so power-less, seemingly !—and yet so powerful where they fill the picture : and then the allopathic doctor's surprise at his next visit! after which he only looked on, while she prescribed.

Knowing the Law of Healing, one could do quite good curative work, if put to it, with an allopathic materia medica : going, however, by the rule of contraries when it comes to its deductions and teachings, and leaving its suggestions and warnings severely alone. They do not apply !

Old School calls Tartar emetic *a powerful irritant of the skin* . . . We use that action, and give the drug internally for just such powerful irritations of the skin as it can excite. One has seen over and over again, for instance, how a dose or two of *Ant. tart. cm* has cured impetigo contagiosa in a few days, without any external application whatever, except a little plain starch powder to " slop it up ". One remembers a grown-up brother and two little sisters who appeared at "out-patients" with exten-sive patches of that infection, even extending, in one case, to the neck. *Ant. tart. cm*, as usual, sufficed. *Pustular eruptions—* here, of course, it is one of our most useful remedies in small-pox. Among our great remedies in pustular eruptions are *Ant. tart.*, *Cicuta, Rhus, Thuja*, and especially *Variolinum*—Burnett's great remedy in herpes, by the way!—but, each and all, only according as the rest of the symptoms agree. We shall see, again and again emphasized, how *Ant. tart.* comes in for gastric and intestinal conditions, and its magnificent use in chest troubles, and most especially in the broncho-pneumonias and pneumonias of little children. Here, with us, the large mortality of the old school is almost obliterated.

*　　*　　*

HUGHES says,* " The best known action of *Tartar emetic*—that to which it owes its name—is its power of producing nausea and vomiting. The nausea which it causes is very intense and long lasting " : and he reproduces a useful little drug-picture :

" ' The face is pale, the skin cool, moist and relaxed, the pulse feeble, frequent and often irregular, the saliva flows copiously, and feelings are usually experienced of gastric uneasiness, languor, and unusual weakness, which are, sometimes, in the highest degree distressing ; so much so as, if long continued, to render the patient

---

* " *Pharmacodynamics.*"

utterly prostrate in body and mind, and indifferent to all things around him, even to life itself.' To these should be added universal muscular relaxation."

Hughes quotes (in dogs poisoned by *Ant. tart.*) " the lungs were always more or less affected : orange-red or violet throughout : destitute of crepitation, gorged with blood, and in some parts hepatized. . . . Lepelletier independently confirmed these observations and naïvely remarked, ' One would imagine that, admitting its action in man to be similar, far from being useful, its administration would be particularly pernicious in pneumonia ; but it is not so, for, instead of favouring engorgement of the lung, it promotes its resolution.' "

FARRINGTON points the characteristics, and gives valuable tips in regard to this drug. . . .

" Head confused : warmth of forehead and confused feeling, as if the patient ought to sleep (in passive congestion of brain). If the patient is a child we notice an unwillingness to be looked at or touched. If you persist in your unwelcome attention, it will have a convulsion.

" On awaking from sleep the child seems stupid, and is so excessively irritable that he howls if one simply looks at him.

" Suppressed eruptions with these head symptoms . . . and great difficulty in breathing. Face bluish or purple, the child becomes more drowsy and twitches. There is rattling breathing. . . . These symptoms that I have mentioned accompany two grand sets of phenomena for which *Ant. tart.* may be useful, namely pulmonary and gastro-enteric affections.

" For children, invaluable in diseases of the chest, when the cough is provoked whenever the child gets angry, which is very often. Eating brings on the cough, which culminates in vomiting of mucus and food.

" A nursing infant suddenly lets go of the nipple and cries as if out of breath, and seems better when held upright and carried about. Now, this is the beginning of capillary bronchitis. There are fine crepitant râles all through the chest. *Ant. tart.* here nips the whole disease in the bud and saves the child much suffering. Another form of cough . . . marked wheezing when child breathes. The cough sounds loose, and yet the child raises no phlegm. This increases till the child grows drowsy. Its head is hot and bathed in sweat. The cough grows less and less frequent. The pulse is weak. Symptoms of cyanosis appear. The quicker, in these cases, you give *Ant. tart.*, the better for your patient.

"*Ant. tart.* is also indicated in the affections of old people and particularly in orthopnœa, or threatening paralysis of the lungs in the aged. You hear loud rattling of phlegm in the chest yet the patient cannot get up the phlegm. (Here *Baryta carb.* is complementary, and may suffice when the other only partly relieves.)

" In this threatening paralysis of the lungs you must compare *Antimonium tartaricum* with several other drugs : with *Lachesis*, which has aggravation when arousing from sleep ; with *Kali hydriodicum*, especially where there is œdema pulmonum and a great deal of rattling of mucus in the chest. What little sputum is raised is frothy and greenish, and looks like soapsuds.

" *Carbo veg.* also suits these cases, but here the rattling is accompanied by cold breath and by coldness of the lower extremities from the feet to the knees.

" *Moschus* in paralysis of the lungs, when there is loud rattling of mucus and the patient is restless. Especially after typhoid fever. The pulse grows less and less strong and finally the patient goes into a syncope. (*Ant. carb.*)

" *Ant. tart.* produces a perfect picture of pleuro-pneumonia. Portions of the lungs are paralysed. Fine râles are heard, even over the hepatized portions. Great oppression of breathing, especially towards morning. The patient must sit up in order to breathe. . . .

" Pustules very nearly identical with those of small-pox.

" Diseases of intestinal tract. . . . Very like *Veratrum* : only here *Veratrum* has more cold sweat on forehead, *Ant. tart.* more drowsiness."

NASH, as usual, sums up the action of *Ant. tart.* in a few words of vital import.

" Great accumulation of mucus in air passages, with coarse rattling and inability to expectorate; impending paralysis of lungs.

" Face very pale or cyanotic from unoxidized blood.

" Great coma or sleepiness in most complaints.

" Vomiting; intense nausea, with prostration; general coldness, cold sweats and sleepiness.

" Trembling : internal ; head and hands.

" Thick eruptions like pocks, often pustular ; as large as a pea.

" Relief from expectoration.

" Both ends of life, childhood and old age.

" Child clings to those around ; wants to be carried ; cries and whines if anyone touches it ; will not let you feel the pulse.

" Nausea as intense as that of *Ipecac.*, but less persistent, and with *Ant. tart.* there is relief after vomiting."

And Nash says, " If *Antimonium tart.* possessed only the one power of curing, that it does upon the respiratory organs, it would be indispensable. No matter what the name of the trouble, whether it be bronchitis, pneumonia, whooping cough or asthma, if there is a great accumulation of mucus with *coarse rattling*, or filling up with it, but, at the same time, there seems to be in-ability to raise it, *Tartar emetic* is the first remedy to be thought of. This is true in all ages and constitutions, but particularly so in children and old people.".

" There is one symptom that is very apt to be present in these cases, i.e. great drowsiness, sometimes amounting to coma. . . ."

" In pneumonia, both *Tartar emetic* and *Opium* may have great sleepiness, but there is no need for any confusion here as to choice for in *Opium* the face is dark red or purple, and there may be sighing or stertorous respiration. With *Tartar emetic* the face is always pale, or cyanotic, with no redness, and the breathing is not stertorous."

He also says, " *Antimonium tart.* is also one of our best remedies for hepatization of lungs remaining after pneumonia. There is dullness on percussion, and lack, or absence of respiratory mur-murs, and the patient continues pale, weak, and sleepy."

KENT gives a wonderful picture of *Ant. tart.* We will quote, condensing. He says, " About the first thing we SEE in an *Ant. tart.* patient is expressed in *the face*. The face is pale and sickly— the nose drawn and sunken—the eyes are sunken with dark rings around them—the lips are pale and shrivelled—the nostrils dilated and flapping, with a dark sooty appearance inside them. The expression is that of suffering. The atmosphere in the room is pungent . . . it makes you feel that death is there."

He says, " We find this state and appearance in catarrhal patients, in broken down constitutions, in feeble children, in old people : in catarrhal conditions of trachea and bronchial tubes. And we HEAR *coarse rattling* and bubblings in the chest—coarse, like the ' death rattle '. The chest is steadily filling up with mucus. At first he may be able to throw it out, but finally he is suffocating from the filling up of mucus and the inability of chest and lungs to throw it out. It is a paralytic condition of the lungs. . . . The first few days of the sickness will not point to *Ant. tart.* So long as reaction is good and strength holds up you will not see this hippocratic countenance—sinking—and cold-ness, and cold sweat. You will not hear this rattling in the chest, because these symptoms are symptoms that indicate a passive condition. *Antimonium tart.* has weakness and lack of reaction."

He contrasts it with *Ipecac.* which may come in for the first period. He says, " *Ipecac.* has some of this coarse rattling, but it is attended with great expulsive power of the lungs. *Ant. tart.* has the coarse rattling that comes after many days. . . . It has, like *Ipecac.*, the coughing and gagging and retching, but only in the later stage of great relaxation, prostration and coldness. When you hear him cough you are impressed with the idea that there must be some profound weakness in his lung power. The lungs have lost the power to produce an expulsive action with deep inspiration. Here the chest is full of mucus and it rattles : the cough is a rattling cough, but the mucus does not come up, or only in such quantity as does not relieve. His chest is full of mucus, and he is really passing away, dying from carbonic acid poisoning due to lack of expulsive power."

He says, " Unlike *Aconite, Bell.* and *Bry.*, which come down with violence, the very opposite is present in *Ant. tart.*, where you have little fever, cold sweat, coldness, relaxation, hippocratic aspect. . . . Most of these severe cases of bronchitis and pneumonia die in the *Ant. tart.* state. . . . In very old people who have had catarrh of the chest for years, where every sharp cold spell brings on catarrh of the chest with thick white mucus— dyspnœa—must sit up and be fanned—cannot lie down because of the difficult breathing and filling up of the chest, *Ant. tart.* will ease him over a number of these attacks before he dies. . . . ' When the expectoration is yellow, *Ammoniacum* will pull him through, and *Ant. tart.* when it is white, and attended with prostration, sweat, coldness, pallor and blueness of the face.' "

Kent says further, " He does not want to be meddled with or disturbed. Everything is a burden. The child when sick doesn't want to be touched, or talked to, or looked at. Wants to be let alone. The infant is always keeping up a pitiful whining and moaning. Always in a bad humour, that is, extremely irritable when disturbed."

Note that with *Ant. Tart.* the sputum is WHITE.

" In most complaints this remedy is *thirstless*. Generally in these attacks of dyspnœa the friends of the patient will stand around with a very strong desire to do something, if it is only to hand a glass of water. This patient is irritated by being offered a swallow of water. He is disturbed and shows his annoyance. The child will make an offended grunt when offered water. Thirst-lessness with all these bronchial troubles, with copious discharge of mucus and great rattling in the chest. . . .

" Desire for acids and sour fruit, and they make him sick. Stomach troubles from vinegar, sour things, sour wine, sour fruit. Aversion to milk and every other kind of nourishment, but milk especially makes the patient sick, causing nausea and vomiting.

" With the stomach symptoms and bowel symptoms there is this *constant nausea*, but it is more than a nausea, it is a deadly loathing of every kind of food and nourishment, a nausea with the feeling that if he took anything into the stomach he would die ; not merely an aversion to food, not merely a common nausea that precedes vomiting, but a deadly loathing of food. Kind-hearted people very often want him to take something, for perhaps he has not taken any food all day, or all night ; but the thought of food only makes him breathe worse, increases the dyspnœa, increases his nausea, his loathing and his suffering."

In the same way that expectoration is difficult with *Ant. tart.* vomiting " is not an easy matter with this remedy. It is not merely to open the mouth and empty the stomach of its contents. The vomiting is more or less spasmodic. ' Violent retching. Gagging and retching and straining to vomit. Suffocation, gagging, through great torture.' The stomach seems to take on a convulsive action, and it is with the greatest difficulty, after many of these great efforts, that a little comes up, and then a little more, and this is kept up. ' Vomiting of anything that has been taken into the stomach, with quantities of mucus.' Thick, white, ropy mucus, sometimes with blood. . . . Old gouty patients, old drunkards, old broken-down constitutions. In children also that have broken-down constitutions, as if they had grown old. These take cold in the chest, with great rattling of mucus, and require this remedy. . . . All the forms of *Antimony* have that dropsical tendency, relaxation and weakness. *Ant. tart.* is full of it."

PECULIAR AND CHARACTERISTIC SYMPTOMS

from Guernsey's *Keynotes*, etc. etc. :

Pitiful whining and crying before and during the attacks, or paroxysms, whatever they may be. Despair of recovery.

A child coughs when angry. (Important symptom in whooping cough, etc.) Coughs and yawns alternately.

In pneumonia, when the edges of eyelids are covered with mucus : also, eyes inflamed, staring, dull, half-open, or one closed. Sees only as through a thick veil.

Nostrils flap (*Lyc.*).

Face a perfect picture of anxiety and despair. Cold, distorted, pale, with bluish spots, bathed in cold sweat, livid. Face-muscles twitch.

Sickly, sunken pale bluish or twitching face, covered with cold sweat.

Tongue covered with a thick, white, pasty coat ; open, parched upper lip drawn up; or tongue very red ; in streaks ; or dry down middle ; brown, dry.

Craves apples, fruits, acids, cold drinks, refreshing things. Aversion to milk. Thirstlessness, or intense thirst. Continuous anxious nausea with great effort to vomit, and sweat on forehead. The smallest quantity of drink is vomited, with eager desire for more. Nausea with great faintness.

Waves of nausea with weakness and cold sweat.

Violent pain in abdomen ; seems stuffed full of stones, but it does not feel hard.

Child at birth pale, breathless, gasping, although the cord feebly pulsates.

Rapid, short, difficult and anxious respiration ; seems as if he would suffocate without sitting erect the whole night ; spell may come on at 3 a.m. (or 4 a.m.) and has to sit up. *Great rattling of mucus in the bronchia, especially just below the larynx, like a little cupful about to run over, but very little is expectorated.*

Very drowsy, great shortness of breath, bronchial tubes over-loaded with mucus.

Somnolency : waning consciousness on closing eyes.

Weak, drowsy, lacking in reaction.

Respiration very unequal, now shorter, now longer, worse lying, lessened when carried about in an upright position . . . gasping for breath at the beginning of every coughing spell. Noisy, whistling, purring, bellowing, or sawing respiration ; with great rattling of mucus as if the child would suffocate, always relieved by spitting or vomiting the mucus. Cough excited by eating.

In the difficulty of breathing, face may be pale, dark red, blue lips, hot and sweaty head, muscular twitching.

Cough: compels one to sit up: it seems loose and rattling, but no expectoration : with great pain in chest or larynx, cries for help and grasps at larynx.

Sputa blood-streaked, rust coloured, adhering like glue.

Œdema of lungs. Impending paralysis of lungs. Emphysema.

Much palpitation : with uncomfortable warm, or hot feeling proceeding from heart.

In croup, often we find neck stretched out, and head bent back.

A chief characteristic of this remedy on the skin is to produce pustular eruption.

BLACK LETTER SYMPTOMS (*Hering and Allen*)

BAD HUMOUR.

The child wants to be carried (Cham.), cries if anyone touches it ; will not let you feel the pulse.

Dim, swimming eyes.

Pallor. Pale, sunken face.

Rheumatic toothache of intermitting type.

During dentition, catarrhal hyperæmia.

Tongue very red, dry in the middle.

Tongue red in streaks.

Tongue covered with thick, white, pasty coat.

Much mucus in throat with short breathing.

Disgust for food, frequent nausea and relief by vomiting.

Belching which relieves.

Nausea causes great anxiety.

Continuous anxious nausea, straining to vomit, with sweat on the forehead.

Nausea, vomiting and loss of appetite. Vomits with great effort.

Absence of thirst.

Absence of thirst the whole day.

Vomiting, followed by great languor, drowsiness, loathing, and desire for cooling things.

Great precordial anxiety with vomiting of mucus and bile.

Sharp cutting colic before stool.

Child at birth pale, breathless, gasping, though the cord still pulsates.

The mucus rattles in the chest.

Rattling of mucus when coughing or breathing.

Rattling originates in the upper bronchi and can be heard at a great distance.

Much rattling of mucus in trachea ; cannot get it up.

Shortness of breath from suppressed expectoration, especially if drowsy.

Unequal breath, now shorter, then longer, much more frequent when lying. Better when child is carried upright.

Respiration with great rattling of mucus.

Suffocated and oppressed about 3 a.m., must sit up to get air ; better after cough and expectoration.

Cough compels the patient to sit up, is moist and rattling, but without expectoration.

When the child coughs there appears to be a large collection of mucus in the bronchial tubes, and it seems as if much would be expectorated, but nothing comes up.

Coughing and gaping consecutively, particularly children, with crying or dozing, and twitching of the face.

Profuse mucus with feeble expulsive power (bronchitis in infants and old people).

Profuse mucus sputa, easily expectorated.

Cough grows less frequent, patient shows signs of " carbonized blood "

Rattling of phlegm on chest, better when carried in an upright position, worse lying down ; with oppression.

Inflammation of respiratory mucous membrane.

Sputa blood-streaked, rust coloured, adhering like glue to the vessel.

Atalectasis, with symptoms of asphyxia belonging to the remedy ; with œdema of unhepatized portions of the lungs ; breathing laboured, orthopnœa, mucous râles.

Œdema of lungs. Emphysema. Impending paralysis of lungs.

Grippe : acute pneumonia : broncho-pneumonia : pleuro-pneumonia.

Pulse hard, full, strong ; sometimes trembling ; very much accelerated with every motion.

Pulse rapid, weak, trembling.

Great restlessness. Tosses with anxiety.

Prostration and collapse.

Violent pain in lumbo-sacral region ; the slightest effort to move causes retching and cold clammy sweat.

Trembling of hands.

Great sleepiness : irresistible inclination to sleep, with nearly all affections.

Coma.

Or, great sleeplessness.

Worse at night and sleepless.

Warmth aggravates ; even getting warm in bed.

Skin covered with a running, sticky sweat.

The tissues it affects . . .

Collection of synovia in joints.

Mucous membranes : catarrhal inflammations ; conjunctivitis ; gastritis, enteritis ; laryngitis, trachitis, bronchitis, extending even into the air-cells ; cystitis.

Pustular eruptions ; on conjunctivae, face, mouth and fauces, œsophagus, stomach, jejunum, genitals.

Variola : backache, headache, cough and crushing weight on chest before or at the beginning of the eruptive stage ; diarrhœa, etc. Also when the eruption fails.

Chest, anterior surface of upper arms, wrists, abdomen and inner side thighs covered with closely set, bright-red, small, conic, hard pustules, with an inflamed, tetter-like base, itching intolerably.

Pustular eruption leaves bluish-red marks on face, etc.

Thick eruption like pocks, often pustular, as large as a pea.

Some of the Notable or Peculiar Symptoms, which appear in Italics

Furious delirium.

The child will not allow itself to be touched without whining and crying. Howls if looked at.

Flickering before eyes :—*sparks before eyes.

Convulsive twitchings in almost every muscle of face.

Swallowing almost impossible.

Great desire for apples.

Vomits till he becomes faint.

Nausea, then yawning and profuse lachrymation, followed by vomiting.

Abdomen seems to be stuffed full of stones, though he has eaten nothing and it does not feel hard.

Violent pressure in abdomen, as from stones, as if full ; much worse sitting and stooping. (*Coloc.* is > stooping and pressure.)

Seems as if he would suffocate, in bed. Cannot get air. Obliged to sit up the whole night.

About 3 a.m. suffocated and oppressed, had to sit up to get air ; only after cough and expectoration she became better.

Dyspnœa : had to be supported in a sitting position in bed.

Cold hands : icy-cold finger tips.

Feet go to sleep immediately after sitting down each time.

Had scarcely fallen asleep when seized with electric shocks and jerks (which came from abdomen).

Cold sweat all over body.

---

* *A lady, very ill with bronchitis (as one remembers well from long ago), was given Ant. tart., several doses, low, which she proceeded to prove with curious, most distressing flashes of light, " What's that ? What's that ? There, again ! " They, in her weak and suffering state, absolutely terrified her. The drug was discontinued, and no more was heard of the flashes.*

Effects of vaccination, when *Thuja* fails, and *Silica* is not indicated.

If the use of *Ant. tart.* was continued after it had produced an eruption like small-pox, the pustules got large, full of pus, deepened in the centre and became confluent : with great pain ; crusts were formed, leaving deep scars.

In prescribing *Ant. tart.*, then, look for drowsiness—nausea—irritability that hates to be touched or looked at : usually thirst-lessness : and in " chests ", breathing, expectorating, lying down, almost impossible. One sees how invaluable it is for desperate conditions, and how with *Carbo veg.*, it is one of the " last gasp " remedies.

APIS

(It was coming across the following that determined the choice of *Apis* for our present drug picture.)

" In 1847, the attention of the writer was first directed to *Apis mellifica* as a remedial agent by the following unique cure.

" A lad, aged about 12 years, had been afflicted for several months with ascites and hydrothorax. He had been treated for some three months by allopathic physicians first for dysentery, followed by ascites, and afterwards for several months by a homœopathic physician. No permanent benefit resulted from either mode of medication, and the symptoms finally became so urgent that I was called in consultation, and tapping was at once resorted to in order to save the patient from imminent danger. Appropriate homœopathic remedies were again prescribed, but without arresting the onward course of the malady. The patient commenced to fill up again with great rapidity. The secretion of urine was nearly suspended, the skin was dry and hot, pulse rapid and weak, respiration short and difficult, great tenderness of the abdomen, dryness of the mouth and throat, thirst, excessive restlessness and anxiety, short irritating cough, and an almost entire inability to sleep.

" At this stage of the case a strolling Indian woman—one of the few survivors of the Narragansett tribe, suggested to the family the use of a honey bee every night and morning. She enclosed the bees in a covered tin pail, and placed them in a heated oven until they were killed, and then after powdering them, administered one in syrup every night and morning. After the lapse of about twenty-four hours the skin became less hot and softer, the respiration less difficult and more free, the pulse slower and more developed, and there was a decided increase in the quantity of urine. From this time the symptoms continued steadily to improve, the dropsical effusion diminished day by day, until at the expiration of a few weeks, the patient was entirely cured.

" This was the first cure of dropsy by *Apis* which was ever reported. From this empirical fact—this *usu in morbis*, I perceived that the profession was as yet unacquainted with a powerful remedial agent, and accordingly commenced a series of provings and clinical trials with it. . . ."

Dr. E. E. Marcy and others: *Elements of a New Materia Medica*, p. 442.

And Kent says, " It is queer how old women knew, long before *Apis* was proved, that when the little new-born baby did not pass its water they could find a cure by going out to the bee-hive and catching a few bees, over which they poured hot water, and of which they gave the baby a teaspoonful. Some domestic things like that have been known among families and among nurses, and it is consistent, because it is just like what we give *Apis* for."

Some of our most valuable medicines have come from domestic use, from herbalistic lore, from accidental poisonings, from observing the effects of bites and stings of poisonous reptiles and insects, from traditions of country-folk and savages.

But Homœopathy leaps at knowledge in any form, and by testing or " proving " the poisonous material (for it must be remembered that all medicines are poisons, and all poisons can be used as remedial agents) it makes them, one by one, scientific, by disclosing their true uses, and the exact symptoms on which they can be prescribed with confidence.

There are different preparations of *Apis*, " there is but one right one ", says Hering. It is " the pure poison obtained by grasping the bee with a small forceps, and catching the minute drop of virus suspended from the point of the sting in a vial or watch glass. This is potentized "—according to directions. He says there is no object in drying and powdering the whole bee, with all the foreign matter and impurities.

It is Guernsey, Kent and Nash who give valuable pictures of *Apis*.

GUERNSEY says, " The PAINS are like *bee-stings*, with the *thirst* and the *burning* following. Scanty urine. Shrill, sudden piercing screams while sleeping or waking, form invaluable key-notes to the use of this remedy."

HERING'S description is, " redness and swelling, with stinging and burning pains—in eyes—eyelids—ears—face—lips—tongue—throat—anus—testicles ", with relief from cold, and aggravation from heat.

Apis has very definite symptoms, and is very definite in the tissues it affects, and in the way in which it affects them.

It affects, as KENT points out, the coverings of the body : not only the skin and the mucous membranes, but also the coverings of organs—the meninges of the brain—the pericardium : and always in the same way, with swellings, dropsical conditions, and its own peculiar stinging and burning pains. These sharp stinging pains often extort a shriek, as the *crie cerebrale* of meningitis. And everywhere where there is the *Apis* swelling, œdema, stinging and burning, there is the *Apis aggravation from heat*: aggravation from a hot room, aggravation from the heat of the fire, aggravation from a hot bath. Kent says, " in brain troubles, if you put an *Apis* patient with congestion of the brain into a hot bath he will go into convulsions, and consequently you see that warm bathing is not always ' good for fits '. It is taught in Old School text-books so much that the old women and nurses know that a hot bath is good for fits, and before you get there just as like as not you will have a dead baby. This congestion of the brain, with little twitchings and threatening convulsions, makes them put the baby in a hot bath, and it is in an awful state when you get there. If the baby needs *Opium* or *Apis* in congestion of the brain the fits become worse by bathing in hot water. If the nurse has been doing that kind of business you have learned the remedy as soon as you enter the house, for she will say the child has been worse ever since the warm bath, has become pale as a ghost and she was afraid he was going to die. There you have convulsions far worse from heat, pointing especially to *Opium* and *Apis*."

Kent says, " *Apis* is full of dropsy, red rash, eruptions, urticaria, erysipelas . . . in all these there is stinging and burning : burning like coals of fire, at times, and stinging as if needles or small splinters were sticking in."

" The complaints of *Apis* are attended with more or less violence and rapidity." And Kent describes the " effect of a bee sting on a sensitive ". Many people are stung with small effect : but a sensitive " comes down with nausea and anxiety that make him feel that he is dying, and in about ten minutes he is covered with urticaria from head to foot. He stings and burns and wants to be bathed in cold water : he fears that he will die if something is not done to mitigate his dreadful sufferings ; rolls and tosses as if he would tear himself to pieces. I have seen all that come on after *Apis*. The antidote for that is *Carbolic acid* no matter how high you have the potency. I have seen Carbolic acid administered in that state, and the patient described the sensation of the Carbolic acid going down his throat as a cooling comfort. He says, ' Why doctor, I can feel that dose go to the ends of my fingers.' " (Of course Kent here speaks of *potentized Carbolic acid!* the crude acid would be " a remedy worse than the disease ")

Apis is THIRSTLESS, especially in dropsy and *fever*.

Here is a recent instance of how *Apis* acts in skin troubles.

W.S., invalided home some time ago, after 13 years in the tropics with much malaria and much quinine (60 grs. a day). Came in September last for an eruption all over for the last three weeks. Excessive itching : worse at night : worse from warmth : "it itches and stings as if lying in a bed of nettles". He got *Apis cm.*

He wrote later, " The outer skin came off wherever it was affected in white powdery form. The new skin is quite clear. In fact the cure is practically complete. It took a definite turn after the *Apis* doses."

Apis is a great throat medicine. A medicine for diphtheria. But, always, with the *Apis* swelling, œdema, aggravation from heat, and burning and stinging pains: (or, Nash says, *painlessness*).

Nash describes the *Apis* throat : " In those intensely violent and rapid cases of diphtheria in which the whole throat fills right up with œdematous swelling, the uvula hanging down like a transparent sac filled with water, and the patient is in imminent danger of death· by suffocation from actual closure of throat and larynx, there is no remedy like *Apis*." And he gives a case from his early experiences.

" A number of years ago I was called to Watkins Glen, N.Y. in consultation in a very bad case of diphtheria. One had already died in the family and four lay dead in the place that day. Over forty cases had died in the place and there was an exodus going on for fear. Her attending physician, a noble, white-haired old man, and withal a good and able man, said, when I looked up to him and remarked I was rather young to counsel him: ' Doctor, I am on my knees to anybody, for every case has died that has been attacked.' The patient was two rooms away from us,.but I could hear her difficult breathing even then. *Apis* was comparatively a new remedy then for that disease, but as I looked into her throat I saw *Apis* in a moment, and a few questions confirmed it. I told the doctor what I thought and asked him if he had tried it. He said, ' No, he had not thought of it, but it was a *powerful blood poison ;* try it.' It cured the case, and not one case that took this remedy from the beginning and persistently, died. It was the remedy for the *genus epidemicus*."

But *Apis* affects the mind also. The *Apis* patient is sad, tearful. Depressed, with constant weeping. No sleep from worrying. Very irritable; and (with *Lachesis*, and *Nux*) suspicious and jealous. Wholly joyless and indifferent. But in all this, is *worse from heat—hot rooms—hot bath.* Fear of death. Fear of apoplexy.

Then *Apis* has hyperæsthesia among its peculiarities : " worse from touch—even the hair ", says Nash.

And here is a tip of Nash's : In inflammations and fevers, when there is alternate dry heat, then sweating, think of *Apis*.

Homœopathy is " slow " say people of little understanding. Slow ?—surely only to be expected in some chronic cases, with years of inefficient, or wrong treatment behind them. Such cases, even for Hahnemann, might need a couple of years in order to cure ; or might have become incurable :—when the utmost to be hoped for, so far as our present knowledge goes, must be palliation. But in acute work what about *this*—recently to hand ? We all know that one of the plagues of Egypt, in our day, is ophthalmia. Go there, if you want to study the destruction of eyes, and the various causes that contribute. Well, a year ago, a once-missionary (now third-year student of medicine) went back to Egypt in the pause in school-work which occurs in late summer and early autumn. One of her eyes got infected, and to the terror of the medical missionaries developed *trachoma*. They scraped the inside of the lids and, with the aid of a competent ophthalmologist " treated " the condition, and it slowly yielded, leaving the eye undamaged. But she was told to expect recurrences—which duly kept their appointment. When attack No. 3 started, she happened to be in the house of a homœopathic doctor who was not concerned with treatment, but cure ; and accordingly the Repertory was asked for the drug that met the symptoms. It worked out to APIS, and she got *Apis cm* that evening. Next morning she was jubilant ; the terror had practically subsided : and by night the eye was well. At that time she was just starting again for Egypt, and was provided with plenty of *Apis cm* for the eyes she might find there. Result ?—simple amazement !—and she, the not yet qualified, was allowed to treat all the eyes in one Dispensary—real bad eyes !—because, *after one dose of the Apis, again and again they cleared up in twenty-four hours.*

Other curious symptoms that belong to *Apis* are, anus wide open, with involuntary diarrhœa. (*Phos.* also has, anus open, from which oozes thin stool.) In *Apis*, " *the stools occur with every motion of the body, as if the anus were constantly open.*"

Then its curious sensations of tension, or tightness :—afraid to cough, because something will burst, or be torn away. Afraid to strain at stool, because something will break.

Here are Allen's black type symptoms:
Vertigo and headache.
Eyelids much swollen, red and œdematous.
No thirst, with heat.
Sensation of rawness in anus, with diarrhœa.
The stools occur with every motion of the body, as if the anus were constantly open.
Sensation in the toes and foot as if too large, swollen and stiff.
Most extreme sleepiness.
Closed rooms are perfectly intolerable.
Headache in warm room.
Enough has been said to suggest that whenever and wherever you have *swelling—œdema—relief from cold—aggravation from heat—burning and stinging pains*, consider APIS.

Honey-bee—APIS—its virtues we sing
For all manner of pains that *burn* and *sting*,
With bad aggravations from all kinds of heat,
With puffings and swellings and tension :—repeat,
Till you've got it by heart, that the *Bee* is the thing,
For all manner of pains that BURN and STING.

Then the *Bee* for effusions !—the *Bee* stands first
For dropsies and fevers with *absence of thirst* :—
Œdema of limbs, or of trunk, or of throat ;
Effusions, œdema of membranes :—you'll note
That its action on kidneys is great, and you'll see
That you've scored when the urine's increased by the *Bee*.

Then the " crie cerebrale ! "—at the thrill of that " crie "
You'll instantly hurry in quest of the *Bee* :
Or, when swellings and tensions and stiffnesses rule,
Says *she'll* " *burst!* " when she coughs, or when straining at stool.
By the way, you'll find *Apis* a wonderful thing
In ovarian diseases, where pains burn and *sting*.

ARGENTUM NITRICUM

DRUGS elicit queer and characteristic symptoms, mental and physical, from their provers : and when these match the queer and characteristic symptoms, mental and physical, of sick persons, they cure. The nearer the correspondence, the more certain the cure.

Argentum nitricum—silver nitrate—is the " devil's stone " or " hell-stone " of Old School, which has not much use for it, except as Lunar Caustic; because in allopathic doses, or when accidentally swallowed during the process of cauterizing the throat, it has turned people permanently blue—a condition known as " argyria." With us it is a most precious remedy, and no other can take its place.

The earlier provings of *Argentum nitricum*, given in Allen's *Encyclopedia* are, as we shall see, chiefly concerned with its physical symptoms, which are very definite and suggestive, and have led to splendid curative work in stomach conditions, etc. But other provings, given in Hering's *Guiding Symptoms*, bring out its interesting and unique mental peculiarities; and these are our most precious indications for its use.

Remedies, as we Homœopaths learn to realize them, step forth as *personalities*. They haunt us in 'bus and tram, and confront us in our patients. They become creatures of temperaments— mental and physical. They have likes and dislikes, cravings and aversions : sensitiveness to meteoric conditions, as well as to human intercourse and environment. We realize their terrors, real or imaginary—their strange obsessions. And in measure as this is so, we are able to apply them with success for the relief of persons of like idiosyncrasies and distresses.

Silver nitrate is a remedy of very vivid personality, quite unlike all others. It has such strange weaknesses and self-tormentings !—and knowing it so well, and having experienced its splendid power to help, it may seem a strange thing to say, but one regards it with something like affection.

Old School has no conception of the wonderful power to strengthen and to comfort, of this remedy. Its mental and intellectual distresses are great.

Let KENT, in his vivid way, detail for us some of the mental inwardness of *Arg. nit.* which we must condense. He describes,

" disturbances in memory—disturbances in reason." He says, " *Arg. nit.* is irrational : does strange things, and comes to strange conclusions : does foolish things.

" He is tormented by the inflowing of troublesome thoughts, which torment him till he is in a hurry and fidget, and he goes out and walks and walks, and the faster he walks the faster he thinks he must walk, and he walks till fatigued. He has an impulse that he is going to have a fit—or that he is going to have a sickness. A strange thought comes into his mind that if he goes past a certain corner of the street he will create a sensation— perhaps fall down in a fit : and to avoid that he will go round the block. He avoids going round that corner, for fear he will do something strange.

" There is an inflowing of strange thoughts into his mind. In crossing a bridge, or high place—the thought that he might kill himself—or jump off, or what if he should jump off : and sometimes the actual impulse comes to jump off that bridge into the water. When looking out of a high window, the thought comes into his head, what an awful thing it would be to jump out of that window ; and sometimes the impulse comes to actually jump out.

" There is a fear of death—the over-anxious state that death is near (*Acon.*). When looking forward to something he has to do, or has promised to do, or in expectation of things, he is anxious. When about to meet an engagement, he is anxious. Breaks into a sweat with anxiety . . . when going to a wedding—to the opera—to church, the anxiety is attended with fear—even to diarrhœa (*Gels.*).

" So we have a wonderfully queer medicine.

" Mental exhaustion, headaches, nervous excitement and trembling, and organic troubles of heart and liver ; in business men, students, brain workers, in those subject to long excitement, in actors who have kept up a long time the excitement of appearing well in public. . . .

" Like *Pulsatilla*, *Arg. nit.* wants cold air, cold drinks, cold things. Suffocates in a warm room. Cannot go to church or the opera, must stay at home. Dreads a crowd, dreads certain places.

" And then the *physical* side. . . . Full of ulceration— especially on internal parts, and mucous membranes. Kent says this tendency to ulcerate seems rather strange ; peculiar that it should have in its pathogenesis such a tendency, when the Old School has been using it to cauterize ulcers, and yet it heals them up. . . . It has cured prolonged and almost inveterate ulceration of the stomach, when there has been vomiting of blood.

" Do not forget that this medicine is one of the most flatulent medicines in the books. He is distended to bursting ; gets scarcely any relief from passing flatus or eructations.

" Desires sugar : feels he must have it and it makes him sick. He cannot digest it ; it acts like physic and brings on diarrhœa. So marked is the aggravation from sugar that the nursing infant will get a green diarrhœa if the mother eats candy." Kent gives a case where nothing helped the baby " till he found out that the mother ate candy—her husband brought her home a pound of candy every day. The baby did not get well ' till it got *Arg. nit.*, and the mother stopped eating candy.'

" *Arg. nit.* has the most intense eye symptoms : catarrhal, ulcerative ; to opacities of cornea. But all, worse for heat and relieved by cold. Profuse purulent discharge from lids."

NASH quotes Allen and Norton, in regard to eyes. " The greatest service that *Argentum nitricum* performs is in purulent ophthalmia. With a large experience in both hospital and private practice, we have not lost a single eye from this disease, and every one has been treated with *internal remedies*, most of them with *Argentum nitricum* of a high potency, 30th or 200th. We have witnessed the most intense chemosis, with strangulated vessels, most profuse purulent discharge, even the cornea beginning to get hazy and looking as though it would slough, subside rapidly under *Argentum nitricum* internally. The subjective symptoms are almost none. Their very absence, with the *profuse purulent* discharge, and the swollen lids from a collection of pus in the eye, or swelling of the sub-conjunctival tissue of the lids them-selves, indicates the drug." (One may say that such a case, in a child, during the 1914-18 War, with *Arg. nit.* 200 and bathing the eye with normal saline, was amazingly better the next day, and soon well. This was impressed on one's memory, since eye cases have seldom come one's way.)

Arg. nit. has some peculiar physical symptoms : Stick in the throat sensation (*Hepar*, etc.), simultaneous vomiting and purging —" gushing both ways " like *Arsenicum*.

All these things, *Argentum nitricum* has caused, and can (and has) cured.

Now for more of the physical symptoms, extracted from Allen's *Encyclopedia*.

" Anxiety which makes him walk rapidly.

Vertigo.

Vertigo, *general debility of limbs and trembling.*

Headache relieved by binding something tightly round head.

Ophthalmia : better cool open air, intolerable in warm room.

Ophthalmia with intense pains.

Grey spots and *bodies in shape of serpents move before vision.*

The canthi are red as blood : the caruncula lachrimalis is swollen. Stands out of the corner of the eye like a lump of red flesh : clusters of intensely red vessels extend from the inner canthus to the cornea.

The conjunctiva is puckered and interstitially distended. Vanishing of sight.   Must constantly wipe off the mucus which obstructs vision.

Sickly appearance.   Appearance of old age.

Pain in teeth :   worse when chewing—eating sour things—cold things.

Painful red tip to tongue.

Rawness throat.   *Rawness and soreness.*

Thick tenacious mucus in throat.

Sensation as if a splinter were lodged in throat when swallowing.

Uvula and fauces dark red.

Irresistible desire for sugar.

Violent belchings.

Nausea after eating.

Constant nausea, and frequent efforts to vomit.

Vomiting and diarrhœa with violent colicky pain.

Desire to vomit, *with sensation as if head were in a vice.*

Violent cardialgia.

After yawning, sensation as if stomach would burst.   Wind presses upwards.

Painful swelling in pit of stomach with great anxiety.

Abdomen swollen and distended, with much flatulence.

A slight colic wakes him from uneasy slumbers, and he has sixteen evacuations of greenish, very fœtid mucus, with a quantity of noisy flatus.

Four evacuations of green mucus, with retching, vomiting of mucus.

(After having eaten sugar greedily in the evening, he was attacked with) *scanty, watery diarrhœa about midnight, accompanied with flatulent colic, and much noisy flatulence during the evacuation.*

Violent diarrhœa, *like spinach flakes.*

Palpitation and irregular action of heart.

Staggering and paralytic heaviness of lower limbs.

Rigidity in calves :   great debility and weariness in calves, can scarcely walk.

Tremulous weakness.   Trembling and tremulous sensation.
Convulsions.
Peculiar discoloration of skin, from grey-blue,. violet or
bronze-coloured tinges to the real black.
Skin brown, tense, hard."

As said, *Arg. nit.* is one of the great remedies for the terrors
of *anticipation.* It has Examination funk. Its nervousness in
anticipation of a coming ordeal will go as far as diarrhœa—
(*Gelsemium*). One of our doctors makes great play with his
" Funk Pills "—*Arg. nit.* The Anticipation remedies are rather
scattered through Kent's repertory, but we have collected the
following, which should be inserted as a rubric.   .   .   .
ARG. NIT., *Ars., Carbo veg.,* GELS., *Lyc., Med., Pb., Phos. a.,*
SIL.
Arg. nit. has also *claustrophobia.* Wants the end seat in a
pew : to be near the door in church or theatre : needs an easy
escape. " Even in the street the sight of high houses always made
him giddy and caused him to stagger : it seemed as if the houses
on both sides would approach and crush him." *Arg. nit.* cannot
look down—and cannot look up.
Here are some cured symptoms.   .   .   .   " When walking
becomes faint with anxiety, which makes him walk faster."
.   .   .   " Often wakes his wife or child, to have someone to talk
to."   .   .   .   " Fears to be alone, because he thinks he will die."
.   .   .   " When walking becomes faint with anxiety, which makes
him walk the faster."   .   .   .   " When walking, fears he will have
a fit, or die, which makes him walk faster."   .   .   .   " Distressing
idea that all his undertakings must and would fail."   .   .   .
" Does not work, thinking it will do him harm, or that he is not
able to stand it."   .   .   .   " Fears, if passing a certain corner or
building that he will drop down and create a sensation ; is relieved
by going in another direction.   .   .   ."

                    *   *   *

A poor little schoolgirl of six, in such terrors of anticipation
that, when the school bell rang, she put her head in her hands,
and vomited. *Argentum nit.* finished that trouble promptly and
entirely, and sent her happily to school, to do well there.
A wee boy of $4\frac{3}{4}$ was curiously ill—mentally. The history
was : Measles before he was two : then double pneumonia and
(?) meningitis. He " rolled his head " and had evidently marked
opisthotonos (" was bent like a bow, backwards, between head and
heels "). " When he began to walk, walked backwards." Now

4

had " terrible nights, with much screaming," and " mad " attacks by day. Was in terror of his father, by night—" Daddy might look at me ! " He said of people, " They make me bleed, and I 'll make them bleed." He said the next house was " going to fall on him " ; that " the clouds were coming down on him." Great fear of noise.

The first* medicine did not help much. But, after a couple of doses of *Arg. nit.*, the next report was, " Very much better. Lost the things coming down on him. Fears all gone." Later he needed a few doses of *Belladonna*, and then its " chronic " *Calcarea* ; and in a few months he was well and normal. But for a wee boy to put up such a plea for *Argentum nitricum*, by such very peculiar and characteristic symptoms, was curious.

Homœopathy can do wonderful things in making children happy and normal.

A youthful dyspeptic, with almost daily severe flatulence and bursting sensations, worse for afternoon tea and long into the night, relieved pro tem by either *Pulsatilla* or *Carbo veg.*, but always recurring, took *Arg. nit.* in potency. Result, the gastric symptoms ceased to trouble, in fact, never again did trouble to the same extent. *Puls.* and *Carbo v.* had been palliative only— *Arg. nit.* had proved curative.

But, the *Arg. nit.* having proved such a boon, was continued for some time, till a new, most distressing symptom appeared— *numbness in the forearms at night.* The wristbands of the night-dress had to be cut, everything pulled away from arms ; nothing must touch or press them. This was only a proving of *Argentum nitricum*, and, when this was discontinued, was soon forgotten, never to recur. . . . Since when, when patients have, from time to time, complained of such numbness in the arms at night, *Arg. nit.* has cured them.

The symptom is found in Clarke's *Dictionary.* He says, " In a proving by myself, one of the most marked symptoms was a kind of numb sensitiveness of the skin of the arms—a hyper-æsthetic—anæsthetic state ; increased sensitiveness to touch, but diminished power of distinguishing sensations."

Symptom-groups often lead one to a particular remedy. *Desire for sweets, desire for salt, can't stand heat,* makes one think of *Argentum nit.* And if you find the patient *cannot look down from a height*, you may be sure. No other remedy has just that symptom complex.

One may note here, that Dr. Clarke's remedy for Examination funk was *Aethusa cynapium*, " fool's parsley "—well named ! One of its characteristic symptoms is " Inability to think, or fix the attention." He says, " guided by this symptom I gave it to an undergraduate preparing for an examination, with complete success. He had been compelled to give up his studies, but was able to resume them, and passed a brilliant examination. To a little waif in an orphan home who suffered from severe headaches and inability to fix his attention on his lessons, I sent a single dose of *Aethusa*, at rare intervals, with very great relief. The little boy asked for the medicine himself subsequently on a return of the old symptoms."

With *Argentum nit.* the condition is apprehension :—ill with anxiety in regard to what is before him :—fear of failure. With *Aethusa*, it is simply inability to fix the attention, or to think.

Homœopathy is very definite : and one remedy, even if you label both " Funk pills ", will not do for the other !

ARNICA MONTANA

MOUNTAIN ARNICA—" fall-kraut " (" fall-herb ")—" Panacea lapsorum "—should be in every house, and everybody should know of its uses.

Arnica grows all the world over in mountainous regions. A great-grandson of Nelson, hailing from the Andes, seen once only, years ago, is still remembered because he told the tale of *Arnica*. He told of the terrible falls in those mountains, and how the people there gather *Arnica*, pour boiling water on the plant, and give the infusion to drink to the injured men, with astonishing results.

In the scheme of the Almighty, wherever healing is needed, there it is to be found, whether in plant or venom—always at hand.

This wonderful remedy comes by hoary tradition from domestic practice. But Hahnemann has made its use scientific, and demonstrated how it falls into line with all the rest, by its power of *causing* what it can cure. That is to say, he " proved " it, by administering it to nine persons (mostly doctors) besides himself, and then faithfully recording what it can do in the way of altering health and giving rise to abnormal conditions and sensations in healthy provers.

Let us glance down the provings of *Arnica*, and find what they have to tell us in regard to its uses : remembering that *what a drug can cause, that it can cure.*

Felt as if *bruised* over the whole body.

General weakness, weariness, sensation of being *bruised*.

Pain in the back, *as after a violent fall.*

Pain in the heart, as if squeezed, or *as if it had got a shock.*

All the joints, bones and cartilages of chest painful, as if *bruised*, during motion and breathing.

Stitches in chest. Short panting breath. Tightness.

Bloody expectoration.

Cough, with feeling in ribs, as if they were all *bruised*.

Small of the back painful, as if it had *been beaten.*

Pain in limbs, as if joints *bruised* ; pain in all limbs, as if they had been *bruised*.

Pain in arms, *as from bruises* ; arms weary, *as if bruised*, by blows.

Pain as if from a *sprain* in wrist-joint. Pain in balls of thumbs, as if they had *knocked against something hard*.

Pain as from *a sprain* in hips.

Then some *typhoid symptoms* with involuntary stool during
sleep ; foul taste ; foul breath ; distention of abdomen,
etc., and its typical mental state.

Then some *peculiar symptoms*, mental and physical.

Cold nose.

Head burning hot, with cold body.

Forgetfulness ; absentmindedness.

Sudden horror of instant death.

Fear of being touched. . . .

HAHNEMANN says of *Arnica*, " Hence it is very beneficial " (not
only in " injuries caused by severe contusions and lacerations of
fibres ") " but also in the most severe wounds by bullets and *blunt
weapons* : in the pains and other ailments consequent on *extracting
the teeth*, and other *surgical operations*, whereby sensitive parts have
been violently stretched : as also *after dislocations* of joints, *after
setting fractures* of bones, etc. . . . And in some kinds of
false pleurisy it is very efficacious, where the symptoms correspond."

For internal use he recommends the 30th potency. For
external use, the parts are to be kept moistened for twenty-four
hours with wine, or brandy and water, in which five to ten drops
of *Arnica* (not the " φ " but the " 1c ") has been well mixed (five
to ten drops to the pint).

Of course, a few doses of *Arnica* internally, after tooth extraction, is the common practice of us all.

KENT (" Materia Medica ") gives some striking little pictures of
the action of *Arnica*. " After railway (or road) accident," " horror
of instant death, with cardiac symptoms at night. He goes off
into a sleep of terror, jumps up again with this sudden fear of
death, and says, ' Send for a doctor at once.' And this may happen
night after night."

Or, on the other hand, an *Arnica* case, in desperate sickness,
may say, " I am not ill. I do not need a doctor."

(We had such a case in our hospital during the 1914-18 War—a
Frenchwoman, with a very bad form of typhoid, contracted in
France during a virulant epidemic. She relapsed and relapsed. It
was a very anxious case. But, at her worse, she began to profess
herself as " so well ! "—" Ca va si bien—si bien, Mademoiselle ! "
So she got *Arnica*, and made a rapid recovery.)

Kent gives another little picture of the *Arnica* condition in old
cases of gout. The old grandfather, sitting away in a corner, in
terror of touch or approach. He feels that anything coming
towards him is going to hurt him, because he is so sore and tender.
If he sees little Johnnie running towards him, he says, " Oh, do

keep away !—keep away ! " " Give him a dose of *Arnica*," says Kent, " and he will let Johnnie run all over him ".

Then the *hard bed sensation*. That is such a splendid appeal for *Arnica*, in all sorts of sicknesses. The patient is restless, but only because the bed feels so hard and lumpy, that he is forced to try for a new position. (It is not the *anxious* restlessness of *Aconite* or *Arsenicum*, or the *pains* of *Rhus*, that seem as if movement would help—which it may not.)

Another great use for *Arnica* is in cerebral hæmorrhage ; generally the first thing to use. This is also foreshadowed in the provings, " Pain *as if the head were being distended from within outwards*, . . . as if brain were rolled up in a lump. Stitches in l. frontal eminence, accompanied by the sensation *as if an extravasation of blood had taken place*."

Illustrative cases in the ken of some of us.

(1) She was taken ill one night with *stitching pains in the chest* that made breathing a proposition. Her husband tried to help her with various remedies, probably *Aconite*, certainly *Bryonia*, but in vain. Then, in a " Domestic Homœopathy," he discovered " bastard pleurisy " with its remedy, *Arnica* ; and he gave her a few globules. They were scarcely swallowed when, with a long sigh, and " That's the first breath I've been able to draw tonight ! " she was fast asleep in a moment.

(2) He was a doctor who wrote that for more than a month he had had *distressing difficulty in breathing, since running eighty yards*. He would wake at night " with oppression in chest, anxiety and fear ". " Heart weakness suggests early death," he said, yet he was " calm and not anxious". " Legs heavy ; head fuzzy ; couldn't run upstairs. Heart sounds weak, but no disease." *Arnica* was suggested and he wrote back, " *Arnica* had the desired effect ! All symptoms went within forty-eight hours. I'm all right now."

(3) She was carrying awkward things downstairs, slipped and *sprained her ankle* badly, and put on an *Arnica* compress, probably rather strong. Ankle was well next day, but there was a brilliant eruption all over the foot, which died away when the *Arnica* was discontinued.

Here, N.B.—*Arnica* can bring out a very nasty dermatitis, when used externally too long or too strong—even a cellulitis when applied to wounds where the skin is broken ; and here it is better always to use *Hypericum*. Probably Hahnemann's " 1st centesimal potency " (the " 1c "), would be an improvement, always, on the " mother tincture " (" φ ") commonly in use.

(4) Another doctor, *overfatigued mentally and physically*, lost all interest in his work. His usual self-confidence disappeared, so that he began to doubt his prescriptions and wonder whether he had prescribed too much of this, or even the wrong medicine. He was never sure whether he had shut the door, or turned off the lights: had to go back and see. He was naturally keenly alert, and this change of mentality worried him. *Arnica* 1,000 put him right in a few days, restoring perfectly his memory and self-confidence.

(5) A person who tired very easily, and was knocked up by a day's shopping in London. Over fatigue always meant a bad night, unless she took *Arnica*. On one occasion she had been *vaccinated*, and her arm was swollen and sore, with painful glands in the armpit; on the top of which she had a dragging day in Town; so at night, she took *Arnica*. To her surprise she had no further discomfort from the vaccination ! (*Arnica* is capable of producing cellulitis and septic conditions, and here. it relieved promptly.) Some of us prescribe it always, with relief to the patient, after a vaccination. Unlike *Thuja*, which aborts the process entirely, *Arnica* simply relieves the discomfort, leaving the pustules to take their usual course.

(6) Two small girls, of nine and five, brought into hospital by the police after having been *knocked down by taxis*. Both comatose and limp. Both were seen by surgeons within a few hours of admission, and in both cases the surgeons pronounced them hopeless. Both were given *Arnica* internally, and both sat up to eat a hearty breakfast next morning.

(7) A patient writes from abroad. " My wife has been very ill here, . . . but I am happy to say that all has gone supremely well, and Strasbourg echoes amazement at the effect of *Arnica* 1,000 taken six hours after a *double ovariotomy with complications*. *Phosphorus* prevented all nausea and shock, and the *Arnica* made morphia entirely unnecessary. A wonderful piece of work."

(8) A very severely sprained ankle on the stairs late one night. The sufferer was too cute to try to walk on it ; she sat and wriggled it in every direction, crawled up somehow to bed, and took *Arnica*. Next day, again, *Arnica* and wriggling, feeling that bone after bone slipped back into place. . It was well in about twenty-four hours.

And here, a tip ! Don't go walking on a foot whose jig-saw puzzle of instep joints may be slightly disturbed. They will pinch nerves, and you will get pain and swelling and inflammation, and be laid up, more or less, for weeks. Shake the jig-saw bits home. Bend your knee ; hold on to something ; and with your toes on the ground, roll your foot backwards and forwards and round and round, while the parts slip home. *Arnica* will look after the rest.

Arnica is a short-acting remedy : but PROMPT.

INSECT STINGS

We forgot to mention the role of *Arnica* in insect stings. The strong tincture applied to a *wasp* sting, prevents the pain and swelling, and in a couple of hours the sting is forgotten.

Urtica is said to do likewise for bee stings.

And *Cantharis* 200, given internally, quickly cures the inflamed and horrible swellings that may follow gnat bites.—ED.

BLACK LETTER SYMPTOMS

Stupor, with involuntary discharge of fæces.

Forgetful ; what he reads quickly escapes his memory, even the word he is about to speak.

Says there is nothing the matter with him.

Delirium tremens.

Hopelessness ; indifference. (*After concussion.*)

Fears being struck by those coming towards him ; fears even the possibility of being touched (*in gout*).

Violent attacks of anguish. (*Angina pectoris.*)

Vertigo when shutting eyes.

Pressive headache as if head was being distended from within outward ; pain seems to arise from something soft in vertex, with drawing in vertex and occiput, and tearing towards temples.

Mechanical injuries ; especially with stupor from concussion ; fractures of skull, or even compression (apply externally warm cloths saturated with dilute tincture from the root ; give also internally).

Meningitis after mechanical or traumatic injuries, such as concussions, bruises, falling, concussion of brain, etc., when suspecting exudation of blood, fibrine or pus. In such cases we find great sopor and partial paralysis of tongue, oculmotors, iris or limbs.

Meningitis after lesion or concussion, provided there is no complete want of reaction.

Apoplexia sanguinea.

Head feels too large.

Inflammation of eyes, with suggillations after mechanical injuries.

Retinal hæmorrhage ; expedites absorption of clots.

A variety of eye troubles resulting from blows and various injuries ; sometimes applied locally (*tincture diluted with water*) *and sometimes given internally.*

Hard hearing from concussions.

Epistaxis.

Nosebleed ; preceded by tingling ; from mechanical causes ; whooping cough ; typhus.

Toothache after operation, plugging, etc.

Putrid smell from mouth.

Eructations ; frequent ; empty ; bitter.

Vomiting of dark red coagula, mouth bitter ; general soreness. After injuries.

Foul belching.

Dyspepsia. Prolapsus ani.

Offensive flatus ; smelling like rotten eggs.

Stool involuntary during sleep (also urine). Fevers. Apoplexy, etc.

Dysentery with ischuria, or tenesmus of neck of bladder with fruitless urging.

Most marked indication is long intervals between stools, namely from four to six hours.

Bladder affections after mechanical injuries.

Tenesmus from spasms of neck of bladder.

Constant urging while urine passes involuntarily in drops.

Frequent attempts to urinate.

Has to wait a long time for urine to pass.

Retention of urine from exertion.

Ischuria with dysentery.

Involuntary urination at night during sleep. Apoplexy. Typhus, etc.

Urine brown with lateritious sediment.

Hæmaturia from mechanical causes.

Urine thick, with much pus and some blood globules, but no tubes. Nephritis.

Urine very acid, with increase of specific gravity.

Penis and testes swollen purple-red ; after injuries.

Phymosis from friction ; parts bruised and much swollen.

Threatened abortion from falls, shocks, etc. ; nervous, excited ; feel bruised.

Soreness of parts after labour ; prevents hæmorrhage.

Sore nipples.

Asthma from fatty degeneration of heart.

Whooping cough ; child cries before paroxysm as though in fear of soreness it will cause, cough cause bloodshot eyes, nosebleed, expectoration of foaming blood, or clots of blood.

Hæmorrhage after mechanical injuries ; slight spitting of black, thick, viscid blood, or bright red, frothy blood, mixed with mucus and coagula.

Hæmoptysis.

Pleurisy after mechanical injuries; must continually change position, bed feels so hard.

Pneumothorax from external injuries.

" Strain of the heart " from violent running.

Fatty degeneration of heart.

Pulse, in rest, below 60, *after moving, above* 120. *Nephritis.*

Articulations and cartilaginous connections of chest feel as if beaten, when moving, breathing, or coughing.

Hygroma patellæ.

A splinter ran deep into sole a month ago, producing a great deal of proud flesh, came out after inner and outer use.

Paralytic pains in all joints during motion, as if bruised.

Complaints from exertion ; hoarse, overusing voice ; palpitation ; formication, lame ; paralysis ; bruised feeling ; sciatica ; weary, faint ; retained urine ; nosebleed.

Head feels too hot for him, body feels chilly and cold, between frequent attacks of violent convulsions. After Acon.

General sinking of strength ; he can scarcely move a limb. Typhus.

While answering, falls into a deep sleep before finishing. Typhus.

Frequent violent attacks of chill. Nephritis.

Chilly, with heat and redness of one cheek.

Head feels too hot to him, body chilly and cold ; < between frequent attacks of convulsions.

Malaria intermittents.

Traumatic fevers.

Typhoid conditions.

Putrid fevers.

Heat in oft-repeated short attacks.

Concussions and contusions.

Burrowing pus, not painful.

Prevents suppuration.

Hyperinosis is rather a contra-indication for Arnica.

Septicæmia ; tendency to typhoid forms.

Myalgia ; particularly after over-exertion.

Gout and rheumatism.

Inflammation of skin and cellular tissue ; tender on pressure.

Everything on which he lies seems too hard.

Sprains, with much swelling, bluish redness, intense soreness.

After bruises with blunt instruments. Iritis.

Concussions ; falls ; mechanical injuries.

Contusions with lacerations.

Stings of bees or wasps ; splinters.

Compound fractures, and their profuse suppuration.

Pressure ; aching in epigastrium < ; liver, sensitive ; spleen sore ; stitches in chest > .

Mechanical injuries ; concussion of brain while there are unconsciousness, pallor or drowsiness ; weak, intermitting pulse ; cold surface, and other indications of depressed vitality from shock ; threatened abortion ; ovarian troubles ; orchitis ; mastitis, etc.

Many small boils painful, one after another ; extremely sore.

Acon., Ipec., Veratr. ; *after* Apis *in hydrocephalus.*

Complementary to Acon.

ARSENICUM

Arsenicum is another of the *very* important homœopathic remedies : that is to say, when it is given in homœopathic potencies for its own striking and characteristic symptoms, previously brought out in provings and in poisonings.

One remembers a man, brought dying into our hospital, poisoned : and one knew from the symptoms that the poison was *Arsenic* or *Phosphorus*. Dr. (now Sir) Bernard Spilsbury when a few hours later, he carried away organs for examination, said " probably *Arsenic*, as more common ", and he proved to be correct.

The man lay there, deeply jaundiced, convulsed from time to time, quite unconscious, and gulping up mouthfuls of dark blood. *Arsenic* is a terrible poison : it is almost incredible that persons should deal such death to themselves or others : but they do ! Poisoner and suicide are not discriminating. In slow *Arsenic* poisonings the symptoms are also unbelievably cruel : the deadly nausea, vomiting and purging : the appalling anguish, fear and restlessness, combined with weakness and collapse . . . and it is just in terrible cases of similar suffering and prostration, that *Arsenic* does its most rapid and brilliant curative work. *Arsenicum* for ptomaine poisoning years ago, gave us a homœopathic doctor : and we have watched *its absolute magic* in other ptomaine poisonings.

These are the ghastly sufferings and symptoms for which we homœopaths prescribe *Arsenic* with confidence and joy . . . Restlessness—despair—intolerable anguish—fear : a restlessness that will not suffer the patient to stay in one room—in one bed : and withal prostration out of all proportion to the apparent condition. Such cases are of bad prognosis in any disease, unless *Arsenic*, in homœopathic potency, is given.

Of the symptom, " He can find rest in no place, continually changes his position in bed, will get out of one bed into another, and lie now here now there," Hahnemann says in a footnote, " *It scarcely occurs so markedly in any other medicine.*"

And here one remembers the effect of a Zeppelin raid on one of the patients in the hospital in the early days of the Great War. She was frantic for hours, and could not be appeased. She could not stay here ! But, where was she to go ? If she went into the country, they might come there ! And so on : till a dose of *Arsenicum*, and she became quiet and composed, and sank to the level of the other patients—so far as Zeppelins were concerned.

Of the symptoms, " Violent vertigo, complete exhaustion, continual vomiting, hæmaturia, and rapid extinction of life," Hahnemann says in a footnote, " Gehlen died thus from inhalation of arseniureted hydrogen."

And even in regard to its more trivial symptoms, such as " On account of nausea and sickness he must lie down in the forenoon " ; " drawing pain between the scapulæ, which compels him to lie down,"—" the perspiration exhausts him as he lies in bed, almost to the production of syncope," etc., Hahnemann gives us a very important footnote. . . . " *That symptoms of a not very important character and, otherwise, trivial affections induce a sudden and complete sinking of the strength, is a very important and characteristic peculiarity of Arsenicum.*"

Of the symptom, " Nocturnal stuffed catarrh, threatening suffocation," Hahnemann says in a footnote, " I cured myself rapidly with *Arsenic* of a similar suffocative catarrh that always came on more severely every evening after lying down, which brought me near to death : the dose I used was of a minuteness that passes all belief. The other symptoms of my malady were certainly also met with among the symptoms of *Arsenic.*"

Arsenicum is one of our great asthma remedies and asthmatic symptoms are very manifest in the provings. . . . " Constrictive sensation in the chest : painful respiration : oppression of the chest : difficult breathing : piteous lamentation that an intolerable anxiety and a very oppressive sensation in the abdomen hinders respiration : frequently recurring tightness of the chest, etc." Of these Hahnemann also says, " As the symptoms are not observed in the mass from any other known medicine, it is evident how *Arsenic* is homœopathic to inflammation of the chest, and that it can, and does cure it specifically."

In regard to the symptoms " sadness and restlessness and tossing about in bed, with unquenchable thirst ", he says, " This was from external application (of arsenic) on the head in two children. Death ensued after two days, and revealed *inflammation of the lungs* and *great inflammation in the stomach and small intestines.*"

And when he is scourging the malpraxis of his day, he describes the suffering—even to death, of persons who had had Arsenic applied to ulcers.

He says of one patient, " *Arsenic* worn in a bag on the bare chest for four days, produced anxiety so that he frequently fainted, besides a violent pain in the place, and black pocks on the spot."

Arsenic is not only acrid to mentality, eating into rest—hope—security : but all its secretions and discharges are acrid and corrosive. Acrid tears and eye-discharges:—acrid nasal discharges :

acrid leucorrhœa :—acrid, burning, corrosive discharges from
ulcers, which constantly extend in circumference rather than in
depth.

Then its characteristic BURNING pains—relieved by heat.
Burning pains in head—in eyes—in nostrils—in mouth—in throat
—in stomach—in bowels—in hæmorrhoids—in bladder—in
urethra—in ovaries—in genitalia generally—in breasts—in chest
—about the heart—in spine—in back—in veins—in ulcers—in
skin—in cancer—in anthrax—carbuncle, etc. Veins burn like
fire, especially at night.

Arsenic has very marked time-aggravations. Periodicity.
Different symptoms and sufferings at different hours or seasons.
But its special time of suffering is midnight and *after midnight* :—
all night, but after midnight : and 1 a.m. especially.

Arsenic has a very wide range of action, from more or less
trivial and ordinary complaints, up to, as we have seen, the most
terrible. It has its place in the nursery medicine chest, as well
as in the treatment of the most serious diseases, and in assuaging
the pain and suffering, mental and physical, of hopeless diseases.
It is one of our great remedies for shingles : it has produced and
is valuable in the treatment of œdema and ascites, earning the name
of " the homœopathic trocar " Only, always, the cardinal symptoms of *Arsenic* must be present : the *anguish—restlessness—prostration :—the burning pains relieved by heat.*

Hahnemann says, " A sensible homœopathic physician will not
give this remedy even in such a minute dose, unless he is convinced
that its peculiar symptoms have the greatest possible resemblance
to those of the disease to be cured. When this is the case it is
certain to be efficacious. . . .

" Such employment of *Arsenic* has shown its curative power in
countless diseased states ; among the rest, in several kinds of
quotidian fevers and agues of a peculiar kind ; in varicose veins ;
in stitches in the sternum ; vomiting after almost every kind of
food ; excessive loss of blood at the menstrual period, and other
disorders in connection with that function ; in constipation ; in
acrid leucorrhœa and excoriation caused thereby ; in indurations
of the liver ; oppression of the chest when going up hill ; fetid
smell from the mouth ; bleeding of the gums ; hæmoptysis ;
aching in the sternum ; gastralgia ; drawing, shooting here and
there in the face ; drowsiness in the evening ; shivering in the
evening and stretching of limbs, with timorous restlessness ;
difficulty of falling asleep, and waking up at night ; weariness in
the feet ; bruised pain in the knee joint ; itching tetters on the
knee ; pain in the ball of the big toe ; tearing shooting in the hip,

groin and thigh : nocturnal drawing tearing from the elbow to the shoulder ; painful swelling of the inguinal glands, etc."

(Mat. Med. Pura.)

One can personally recall striking cases where, with typical *Arsenic* symptoms, *Arsenic* has cured constantly recurring ague— vomiting after every kind of food—ptomaine poisonings— asthmatic conditions—gastralgia—facial neuritis, following herpes : and such neuritis elsewhere : and so on. *Arsenic*, in homœopathic preparation acts rapidly and curatively in all sorts of diseases and conditions *where the symptoms point to Arsenic* : even assuaging pain, and prolonging life, indefinitely and astonishingly, in some inoperable cases of carcinoma.

* * *

GUERNSEY says, of *Arsenicum*. " We find a great amount of anguish in the patient, and the greater the suffering the greater the anguish. Very great restlessness, which is exhibited in an anxious tossing and jerking about, every movement being followed by exhaustion. Exhaustion is not felt by the patient when lying still, but as soon as he moves, he is surprised to find himself so weak. Intense burning sensations, as if from coals of fire—usually found in the abdominal cavity. Fear of death. This is not the *Aconite* fear, but it is an anxiety, and a feeling that it is *useless to take any medicine*, as they are surely going to die. . . ."

It will be observed that homœopathy treats disease-conditions rather than named diseases. There is no disease, mild or urgent, in which *Arsenicum* may not be curative, provided drug symptoms and disease symptoms agree.

* * *

KENT says, "From the time of Hahnemann to the present day this has been one of the polychrests, one of the most frequently indi- cated medicines, and one of the most extensively used. In the old School it is most extensively abused, in the form of Fowler's solution.

" *Arsenic* affects every part of man : it seems to exaggerate or depress almost all his faculties, to excite or disturb all his functions . . . it has certain prevailing and striking features. *Anxiety, restlessness, prostration, burning* and *cadaveric odours* are prominent characteristics. The surface of the body is pale, cold, clammy and sweating, and the aspect cadaveric.

" The *Arsenicum* patient with this mental state is *always freezing*, hovers around the fire, cannot get clothing enough to keep warm, a great sufferer from the cold.

" *Arsenic* produces a tendency to *bleeding*. The patient bleeds easily and may bleed from any place. . . . Anywhere that mucous membranes exist there may be hæmorrhage (*Phos.*).

" Many of the mental troubles, as well as the physical troubles, come on and are increased at certain times . . . most of the sufferings of *Arsenicum* are worse from 1-2 p.m. and *from 1-2 a.m.* After midnight, very soon after midnight sometimes, his sufferings begin, and from 1-2 o'clock they are intensified. . . .

" Sensitiveness is a feature of *Arsenic :* sensitiveness to smell and touch, and every other circumstance ; oversensitiveness of all the senses . . . oversensitiveness to the circumstances and surroundings of the room. The *Arsenicum* patient is an extremely fastidious patient. Hering once described him as ' the gold-headed cane patient '. If this is carried out in a woman who is sick in bed she is in great distress if every picture on the wall does not hang perfectly straight. . . . A morbid fastidiousness has its simillimum in *Arsenic.*" (*Nux.*)

Arsenic has " Rigors and chills of a very violent character, and at such times he describes a feeling as if the blood flowing through the vessels were ice water. He feels a rushing through the body of ice-cold waves. When the fever comes on and he is intensely hot from head to foot, before the sweat has appeared, he feels that boiling water is going through the blood vessels."

Kent points a peculiar feature of the *Ars.* thirst. " During the chill, there is no thirst, except for hot drinks : during the heat there is thirst, little and often, for enough water to moisten the mouth, which is almost no thirst ; and during the sweat there is thirst for large drinks. . . . He will say, ' I can drink the well dry.' "

*　　　*　　　*

NASH gives the characteristic symptoms of *Arsenic* thus—
" Great anguish and restlessness, driving from place to place.
Great and sudden prostration : sinking of vital force.
Intense burning pains.
Intense thirst : drinks often, but little. Cold water disagrees.
Vomiting and stool simultaneously : worse for eating and
　　drinking. . . .
Dyspnœa worse on motion ; especially ascending.
Worse in cold air (except the head pains)—from cold things—
　　cold applications :—1 to 3 a.m. From movement.
Better by warm air or room, or hot applications : relieved by
　　sweat."

Arsenicum is pre-eminently one of the remedies that cures by bringing back—to cure—old suppressed skin troubles. Even asthma is seen to cure up, *with the return of an old eruption,* under *Arsenicum.* Nash gives such a case. . . .

He once had a case of severe gastralgia, and prescribed *Arsenicum* because the pains came on at midnight, lasting till 3 a.m., during which time the patient had to walk the floor in agony, and there was *great burning* in the stomach. She had but one slight attack after taking *Arsenicum*, but when he saw her next she asked whether that medicine would send out " salt rheum ? " And then he discovered that she had had eczema of the hands cured by ointment ; and he told her that she could have back the pain in her stomach any time she wanted it, by again suppressing the eruption. " She did not want it."

He says, " The pains of the stomach are terrible, and aggravated by the least food or drink, especially if *cold*. Abdominal pains are also intense, causing the patient to turn and twist in all possible shapes and directions. Diarrhœa of all kinds of stools, from simple watery to black, bloody and horribly offensive . . . finally, hæmorrhoids. But in all these affections, of the whole alimentary tract, we are apt to find the characteristic *burning* of this remedy . . . and the not less characteristic *amelioration from heat :* with usually the *midnight aggravation.*"

He says *Arsenicum* is particularly efficacious in lung troubles, where breathing is very much oppressed. Wheezing and frothy expectoration. Patient cannot lie down ; must sit up to breathe, can't move without being greatly put out of breath. The air passages seem greatly constricted. " It is especially useful," he says, " in asthmatic affections caused or aggravated by suppressed eruptions, or pneumonia from retrocedent measles—even chronic lung troubles from suppressed eczema."

He says the symptom, " *Acute, sharp, fixed or darting pain in apex and through upper third of right lung* " is a gem. (Burnett also emphasizes this somewhere.)

Of the *Arsenicum* WEAKNESS . . . he says, You may say it is common for sick people to be weak. True, but the *Arsenicum* patient is weak *out of all proportion* to the rest of his trouble, or apparently so : and it is a general prostration, not local.

Arsenicum affects, as he points out, all the tissues . . .

Attacks the blood, causing septic changes, exanthemata, ecchymoses, petechiæ, etc.

Attacks the veins ; varices burn like fire, especially at night.

Attacks serous membranes, causing copious serous effusions.

Attacks glands, which indurate and suppurate.

Causes inflammatory swellings, with burning lancinating pains. Attacks the periosteum.

Attacks joints causing pale swellings, burning pains, etc.

Causes general anasarca ; skin pale, waxy, or earth coloured ; here great thirst (*Apis* none).

Causes rapid emaciation ; atrophy in children.

Causes ulcerations, constantly extending in breadth. They *burn* like fire, pain even in sleep ; discharge may be copious or scanty, the base blue, black or lardaceous.

Anthrax burning like fire (*Anthracinum*), cold blue skin dry as parchment, peeling off in large flakes.

Gangrene, better from heat (worse *Secale*).

(Indeed one of Hahnemann's " polychrests ! ")

Nash adds, " Notwithstanding this, *Arsenicum* is not a panacea. Like every other remedy it must be indicated by its similar symptoms, or failure is the outcome.

" Its great keynotes are RESTLESSNESS—BURNING—PROSTRATION—and MIDNIGHT AGGRAVATION."

Black Letter Symptoms

Very violent delirium, especially at night, with great restlessness.

Her desire exceeds her need (eats and drinks more than is good for her ; walks further than she needs to do).

Despairs and weeps : imagines no one can help him, that he must die ; is cold and chilly, and afterwards generally weak.

Anguish. Excessive anguish.

Anguish and despair driving from one place to another, for relief.

With great anguish he turns and tosses to and fro in his bed.

Anxiety at 3 o'clock after midnight.

Violent anxiety at 3 o'clock in the night ; he now felt hot, now as if he would vomit.

Dread of death coming on suddenly when alone.

The greatest fear and anguish (sees ghosts day and night).

(Great heaviness in the head ; it goes off in the open air ; but returns as soon as he enters the room.)

Burning in eyes.

Eyelids oedematous, often completely closing the eyes.

Corrosive tears, making cheeks and eyelids sore.

Excoriating discharge from nostrils.

Watery discharge from nose—went off in the open air ; watery nasal discharge causes smarting and burning, as if nostrils were made sore by it.

Face expressive of genuine mental agony.

Deathly colour of face. Pale, yellow cachectic look.

Swelling of face, or sunken face.

(Tongue furred, with a red streak down middle) and redness of tip.

Dryness of tongue.

Dry and brown-coated tongue.

Feeling of great dryness in mouth, with violent thirst ; he drinks little at a time.

Burning in mouth along the pharynx and in the pit of the stomach.

Loathing of food.

Excessive thirst : drinking did not refresh him.

Excessive thirst : he drinks much, but little at a time.

(Long-lasting hiccough) at the hour when the fever ought to have come.

Nausea.

(Vomiting violent and incessant) and excited by any substance taken into the stomach.

(Even water is) immediately thrown off the stomach.

Vomiting every time after drinking.

The vomiting brings no relief.

(Frequent vomiting) with apprehensions of death.

Anxiety in the pit of the stomach.

Burning in the stomach.

Violent burning pains in the stomach.

In the stomach fearful burning pains.

Swollen abdomen.

Distention and pain in abdomen.

Pains in abdomen with unbearable anxiety: with intolerable anguish.

Burning pains in abdomen.

The evacuations excoriated the skin about anus.

Burning like fire at anus.

Purging and extreme coldness of extremities. Constipation.

Burning in urethra during micturition.

Involuntary micturition.

Scanty emission, and burning during emission.

Frequent oppressive shortness of breath in every position of the body, causing anxiety. (Chest.)

Oppression : want of breath : a nocturnal asthma makes him spring up at midnight.

Difficult breathing, with great anguish.

Oppression of breath when walking fast.

The heart-beats are irritable.

Palpitation. Irregular palpitation of the heart, but so violent at night that he imagines he hears it.

Palpitation of heart and tremulous weakness after stool : he has to lie down.

Quick, weak, and irregular pulse.

Loss of strength in the small of the back.

Excessive weakness and exhaustion of the limbs, obliging him to lie down.

Uneasiness in lower limbs, he cannot lie still at night, and had to change the position of his feet all the time or to walk about, to get relief.

Very great restlessness, so that she could not lie quiet a minute.

Restlessness and anxiety. Throwing himself from side to side.

The slightest paroxysm of pain is accompanied with an excessive sinking of strength, obliging him to lie down.

He is so weak that he is scarcely able to walk : feels he will fall over . . . scarcely able to walk across the room without sinking down.

Continued weakness and prostration.

Great weariness after a meal.

Faintness and insensibility.

Faint, anxious, weak, early in the morning.

Burning pains, especially in the inner organs, skin and ulcers.

Eruptions round mouth, burning and painful.

Itching, increased by scratching.

Burning pain in the ulcers—as from glowing coals.

Burning like fire around the ulcer.

Burning itching of body.

Startings when falling asleep in the evening.

After midnight (from 3 o'clock on) she tosses about and sleeps only at times.

Shuddering when walking in the open air.

Shuddering without thirst.

Fever at 2 o'clock in the night.

Typhus-like fever with extreme restlessness.

Burning heat internally.

Feels as if burning up internally.

Feeling of heat with anxiety, after midnight.

Cold, clammy sweat.

QUEER *Arsenicum* SYMPTOMS

Sees ghosts day and night.

Fear of killing with a knife.

Runs through house at night in search of thieves.

Imagines house full of thieves : so much fear that he jumps out of bed, and hides in wardrobe—or under bed.

Sees thieves in room.

Sees vermin and bugs crawl about his bed from which he wants to escape.

Excessive vertigo : " the bed is tipping over, I shall fall on the floor."

Brain seems to flap (walking) : as if brain moved and beat against the skull.

ASAFŒTIDA

" A gum resin obtained by piercing the living root of different species of *Ferula*." N.O. umbelliferæ. Ours is *Narthrex asafœtida*.

The fresh oil is said to " smell not unpleasantly : but when decomposed it gives off sulphuretted hydrogen ",—the charming and penetrating odour of electioneering eggs. Political meetings have been before now broken up by the introduction of asafœtida into the hall by rowdy partisans of the rival candidate. Hale White gives another drastic use for the drug:—" cases of malingering may sometimes be cured by making the patient take, three times a day, an effervescing draught containing a few minims each of the tinctures of valerian and asafœtida. The effervescence makes the nasty taste of these medicines ' repeat ' in the mouth for some time after taking them." Old School has a pill of asafœtida, aloes, hard soap and confection of roses : in the margin of our copy of Hale White stands scribbled in pencil,

" Stinks and aloes, one supposes ;
But why hard soap, and why the roses ? "

These silly little things used to make examinations so easy !

And Kent gives yet another popular use—as a supposed protection against disease, hence used in the stables. He says lumps of " fœty " as they called it were put in the corn for the horse, to keep off distemper. And he says " it has been used by the laity as a medicine for fainting, for hysteria, for all sorts of nervous symptoms and complaints :—this use is justified by the proving."

In the *Cyclopædia of Drug Pathogenesy* we find provings and poisonings by *Asafœtida*. In one case it evoked " pressing pain in the cardiac region, as if from over-filling and distension of the heart ". In another there was a sensation of " compression of the brain, as if surrounded and pressed together by a cloth ". " The thorax was seized with spasmodic contractions, till it seemed as if the lungs could not expand completely, respirations being normal." Again, a " sensation as of a cord tied tightly round brain." . . . " Chest so constricted as if squeezed by a heavy body lying on sternum " : and, always, distension of abdomen : " rumbling, gurgling, distension ".

Black Letter Symptoms

Pressive pain in forehead, from within outwards.
Nervous headache of hysterical or scrofulous people.
Nocturnal throbbing pain in and around eye and HEAD.

Extensive superficial ulceration of cornea, with burning, sticking or pressing, from within out. Better rest, pressure, open air. Numbness round EYE.

Discharge of very offensive matter from the NOSE ; *with caries of the bones.*
Swelling of lower lip.

Sensation of a ball rising in throat from STOMACH *to œsophagus.*
Flatus passing upwards : none down.

Heat in spleen and ABDOMEN.

Watery liquid STOOLS *of the most disgusting smell : pains in abdomen and discharge of fetid flatus.*
Watery stools of disgusting odour, profuse and greenish.

URINE *warm and of a pungent, ammoniacal smell.*

Spasmodic tightness of CHEST, *as if lungs could not be fully expanded.*
Asthmatic feeling in trachea, dry cough ; spasmodic dyspnœa as if lungs could not be fully expanded.

Pain and tenderness TIBIA, *almost unbearable at night.*

Nervous PALPITATION *with small pulse, from over-exertion or suppression of discharges.*

HYSTERIA, *with much trouble about throat or œsophagus ; well marked globus ; spasm of lungs, etc.*

Nervous affections after suppressed discharges.
Nervous people.

Some Italic or Curious Symptoms

Swashing and gurgling sensation in brain, especially frontal.
As if a nail or plug were driven into brain : like a pointed plug in left temple, and right parietal.

As if nose would burst.

Heat of face, ear and hands, with chills down back.

Fatty, rancid taste in mouth.

Spasm of œsophagus like that of hysteria.

Winding and twisting in bowels, as of reversed peristalsis.

As if heart would burst.

Has a loathing of beer.

Constriction of chest ; of throat ; about heart.

Cramp in forehead.

Throbbing : head ; in and about eye ; pit of stomach ; big toe.

Numbness : nasal bones ; bones of face ; chin.

* * *

DR. CLARKE gives an excellent little picture of *Asafœtida*. " The symptoms of *Asafœtida* present an almost perfect picture of hysteria of the flatulent order. Reversed peristalsis of stomach and bowels. Excessive abdominal distension, and sensation as if everything in the abdomen would burst through the mouth. After belching of wind, strong rancid taste in the mouth. . . Many of the discharges are fetid ; watery stools of most disgusting odour ; profuse and greenish : fetid flatus . . . *the fetid smell of the drug may be regarded as one of its " signatures "*. . . . Periosteal affections ending in ulcers which are so sensitive that no dressing is tolerated. . . ." (*Hep.*)

* * *

GUERNSEY says : A very great sensitiveness, hypersensitiveness, especially in those in whom the venous system predominates over the arterial. It affects left hypochondriac region ; left abdomen ; left neck, and nape of neck, left upper and lower extremities, left ear. General symptoms left side.

Dissatisfied about oneself. Complains of her troubles.

Fetid or purulent discharges from ears : green and fetid from nose. Ozæna.

Fatty taste : risings in throat. Loathing ; inclination to vomit. . . . Pulsations pit of stomach, perceptible to hand and even eye.

* * *

Asafœtida, then is a drug of very definite localities and modalities. It vents itself on the *mind*, the *nerves*, the *organs of special sense*, the *digestive tract*, the *periosteum*, and especially on the *left side*. Curious how some drugs pick out the right side, some the left. WHY ? But it is the same with patients : one comes whose every ailment is on the left side ; another, on the right. A study of these remedies is often useful in prescribing.

The black type drugs that are very especially left sided are ARG. N., ASAF., ASAR., CAPS., CINA, CLEM., CROC., EUPHORB., GRAPH., KRE., LACH., OLEAND., PHOS., SELEN., SEP., STANN.

The very especially right-sided remedies in black type, are given as ARS., AUR., BAPT., BELL., BOR., CANTH., LYC., PULS., RAN. B., SARS., SEC., SUL. AC.

Then there are others especially *right or left sided*, as APIS, ARG., BRY., CALC., CHEL., COLOC., RAN. S., SULPH.

Some, again (but everyone knows these) start right side, and cross to left, like LYC. : or start left side and cross to right, as LACH. : or go from side to side and then back, as LAC CAN. One has seen this in throats, in diphtheria, and, in the latter case, in ovarian pain. There are so many interesting and intriguing things in homœopathy that help in prescribing.

The *Asafœtida patient* (i.e. the patient most affected by, and therefore most amenable to, the curative action of *Asafœtida*) is described as being of a plethoric appearance, face puffed, bloated, even dropsical—" puffed, venous, purple ". Kent calls it " a very troublesome face, suggesting cardiac disturbance and venous stasis ". (These patients have the extreme sensitiveness that make you think of such remedies as *Hepar*.) " Fat, flabby, purple : and therewith extremely sensitive to pain, full of hysteria." Such persons may have *ulcers*, extremely sensitive, and extremely offensive. *Periostitis*, especially of tibia (*Asaf.* is one of the drugs that affect the tibia, vying with AGAR., LACH., RHUS, etc.—*and* DRŏS.). One remembers a bad case of Paget's disease of the tibia, with atrocious pain, where none of these drugs helped, but DROS., with its *pain in long bones*, acted marvellously, restoring painlessness and sleep. No one seems to have realized the power in bone disease of *Drosera*, except Hahnemann ! It is worth while getting a copy of *Materia Medica Pura*, now that it has been republished in facsimile form at a moderate price. It is a book one would not be without—*anywhere !*

Asafœtida is one of the remedies of " old scars, when they turn purple and threaten to suppurate ", or " take on a venous aspect and become painful and turn black ".

* * *

We keep on quoting KENT : let us run through his masterly picture of the drug, condensing :—

Full of *discharges* ; catarrhal, watery, from different places, even watery stools : and *all these discharges are horribly offensive and ichorous*. Bloody discharges, horribly offensive, from nose, eyes, ears, chest, bowels, fistula openings, ulcers; . . . The phlegmatic person who is purple, who gets no sympathy when sick, and is almost distracted about the horrible fetid discharges. Even the discharge from the eyes may be bloody and offensive.

Most of the pains seem to *bore*, as if they extended from the bone to the surface,—from within out.

Then *numbness :* a general feature of this remedy. Numbness of scalp, or deep in head : numb, dead feeling associated with the pain (*Cham., Plat.*). Often, numbness after sleep. Numbness of nose.

Hysteria : ball rises, as in *globus hystericus*. Hysterical and choreic affections of œsophagus and trachea. This " lump in the throat, or suffocation ", is a sort of hysterical spasm of the œsophagus.

Stomach.—If you have ever seen a typical case of *Asaf.* you will wonder where all the air comes from. It comes up in volumes : choreic jerking of the diaphragm, with expulsion of wind like the sound of a small pop-gun going off almost every second. Loud belching : loud eructations of wind from the stomach. . . . flatus not downward, but all upwards . . . always horribly offensive. Meteorism. And liquid stools of most disgusting smell.

Asaf. is one of the remedies having nightly aggravations.

* * *

The direction of *Asaf.*, then, is *from within, out.* The heart feels over full to bursting. The nose as if it would burst. Abdominal distension, as if everything in the body would burst out through the mouth.

Asaf. has a symptom one has not observed elsewhere, but which one finds recorded in the poisonings, in the *Cyclopædia of Drug Pathogenesy : " undulating twitchings in muscles."* One saw this recently while actually reading up the drug, in a patient ; undulating twitchings in upper arm especially ; ripples, wavelike, in the arm muscles front and back. The patient seems to have seen them first, rather than felt them. She has received *Asaf.* and it will be interesting to hear the outcome. But nerve specialists in London and in Belgium confessed that they had never seen this before : and proceeded to give a rather terrible diagnosis :—which other symptoms did not, so far, seem to bear out.

Asaf. is one of the drugs that affect the secretion of milk ; causing its disappearance* ; its increased flow ; even its appearance in the breasts of non-pregnant, or elderly, women ; as in a woman of 50, where " the breasts swelled and secreted a milky fluid ".

* *Alum. ph.*

AURUM

In his *Materia Medica Pura*, if we turn up Hahnemann's Preface to METALLIC GOLD, we find an account of its checkered medical history—How it was esteemed by the Arabian physicians and the ancients. How it was scorned, condemned and rejected, because of its insolubility and its indestructability, by the Schools* which put a higher store on reasoning than on experiment—sole arbiter in such matters. How it was revealed in its mighty power for good and evil by Hahnemann's methods of trituration, potentization and provings. How he began, following precedents, with low triturations, and later got his best results from the higher potencies.

Some of us could tell tale after tale of patients, in these days of world-wide commercial depression, who, reduced to despair by straightened means and anxiety, threatened suicide, and yet were rapidly restored to life, to hope, to renewed effort by a few doses of homœopathic gold. We say " homœopathic gold " because gold when tested on normal healthy persons has produced just such states of suicidal despair and hopelessness; and again, because by its reduction to infinitesimals the noble metal, thrice noble in these its higher uses, emerges from bulk, weight, visibility and inertness, as a mighty energy to strengthen the will and revive the natural affections—even to the deepest and most fundamental of all—the LOVE OF LIFE.

These are some of the mental symptoms elicited by Hahnemann when he tested the powers of GOLD—to *hurt,* and therefore *to heal.*

Dejected and full of grief : seeks solitude. Imagines he has lost the affection of friends.

Dissatisfied with everything : imagines he sees obstacles everywhere ; partly his own fault, partly occasioned by a contrary fate.

Melancholy : imagines he is not fit for this world : longs for death : the thought of death gives him intense joy.

Great anguish, increasing to self-destruction.

Quarrelsome—peevish—vehement : can't stand the least contradiction. Rash anger and vehemence. And so on . . . .

* In our day Old School medicine, having discovered colloidal gold, uses it —for a blood-test in syphilis : also in the form of *Sanocrysin,* a thiosulphate of gold and sodium, which " may be used in the case of patients " (with pulmonary phthisis) " who have not responded well to other forms of treatment ". It is given intravenously, the dose " according to the weight of the patient and the character of the lesions ". (*Taylor's Practice of Medicine,* 1930. ED.) In the older text-books no mention is made of Gold !

But even so it is not given with Hahnemann's precision and fore-knowledge, in answer to the cry of symptoms, to raise the resistance of the patient and to evoke curative reaction, but merely with the idea of destroying the tubercle bacilli—the dose according to the weight of the patient, and the character of the lesions ! Medicine has a long way to go yet, to catch up with Hahnemann !

Great anguish about the heart. . . .

When BURNETT, after his manner, made a short proving of Gold upon himself " because, to get a concrete conception of what a given drug can do, there is nothing like *trying it on your own body,*" its first effects were "excitant and exhilarating" (Hahnemann has this in black type. " All day long good humour, talkative and contented with himself—alternating action ? ") But in a few days Burnett found himself "not up to the mark ; very depressed and low-spirited ; nothing seems worth while ! " He was having bad nights too, dreaming of death—of the dead—of corpses. . . . " Look and feel ill, weary, yet no inclination to rest or sleep. . . ." His memory was at first so sharp, that, since it was already becoming very bad, he abandoned his provings—" fearing the effects in this direction might be serious". Three or four weeks later, " memory was already getting good again ". But, having taken one grain and six-tenths of triturated gold in twelve days, he says, " I am thoroughly satisfied that it can make *me* ill. My allopathic brethren maintain that GOLD is *inert* ! Sure proof that they have never tried it, properly triturated, on their *own* bodies"

These are some of the things that Burnett has to tell us about GOLD, in his brilliant little monograph GOLD AS A REMEDY IN DISEASE.

" In the treatment of some heart diseases, some bone diseases, and of sarcocele, to know the medicinal value of GOLD or to ignore it, is just the important difference between curing and failing. But of course, the metal must be first triturated, so that it may become remedial."

" The glands, bones, skin, and nose are alike stricken with scrofula, syphilis, and Gold."

" Gold has an important place in the treatment of heart affections of the gravest kinds."

" Gold in *angina pectoris*. With me it is, next to *Arnica* (a grand cardiac !) the most frequently prescribed, and it has rendered me important services. . . "

" No wonder Hahnemann should exclaim : ' Gold possesses great healing properties, the place of which no other remedy can supply.'"

" Gold is no mere function disturber, but a producer of organic change, and hence its brilliant effects in organic mischief. The vascular turgescence of *Belladonna* and that of *Aurum* are very different affairs."

He quotes Hahnemann, " I have cured several cases of Melancholy, similar to those of Gold, promptly and permanently, and they were those of such who went about with the serious intention of committing suicide "

Burnett used Gold *inter alia* for the " non-thriving, pining condition of boys—low-spirited, lifeless, memories bad ; lacking in boyish go ".

NASH says, " I once cured a young lady who tried to commit suicide by drowning " (with *Aurum*). " After she was cured she laughed at the occurrence, and said she could not help it. It seemed to her she was no use in the world. She *felt* so."

(One remembers a man, deeply depressed and hopeless, in the out-patient department, years ago. *Aurum* was prescribed. And as he went out, " You will come and see me in a month's time ? " " I shall not be alive ! " But he *did* come, and he said, " I have forgotten all that nonsense ! ")

Gold is a great remedy for over dosing with mercury in the treatment of venereal disease. Nash says, " There would be a great falling off of business for physicians if the old school could learn to cure their patients without poisoning them with drugs ".

He says, " *Aurum* is one of our best remedies for *bone pains*. Never forget it ".

And now let KENT, that great prescriber and vivid writer, take up the tale. . . .

" In *Aurum* all the affections, natural to healthy man, are per-verted. So great in extent is this that one of the fundamental loves, which is the love of living, of self-protection, is perverted, and he loathes life, is weary of life, longs to die and seeks methods to commit suicide. . . . Absolute loss of enjoyment in every-thing. Self-condemnation, continual self-reproach, self-criticism, a constant looking into self ; she does nothing right, everything is wrong, nothing will succeed, hopelessness. . . . Has neglected something—neglected his friends. . . . He is wrong, is wholly evil, has sinned away his day of grace, is not worthy of salvation—this is the train of thought that runs constantly through his mind. . . . Broods. . . . is wholly unfit for this world, and then he longs to die. . . .

" Now what are the causes of this state of insanity, grief and hopelessness ? Prolonged anxiety and unusual responsibility. Syphilis is a common one : loss of property is another. Persons who in their young days have been repeatedly drugged with *Mercury* and were always taking ' Blue Mass ' in the Spring, as good for the liver, have established upon themselves a mercurial disease, with the enlargement of the liver, and this is almost always attended more or less by melancholy and sadness, and such hopelessness as we find in *Aurum*. *Aurum* produces such affec-tions of the liver as are associated with cardiac affections, endo-carditis, dropsy of the heart, and rheumatic affections that have gone to the heart."

" Notice the peculiar relation between the lungs and the under-standing, and between the heart and the will. With every little trouble located in the heart there comes hopelessness, but when the manifestation of disease is in the lungs there is hopefulness. . . . Heart and liver affections are associated with hopelessness and despair. . . .

" In this remedy the pains wander from joint to joint and finally locate in the heart. *Angina pectoris* is often the ending of an old rheumatism that has wandered from joint to joint."

" The remedy is full of rheumatic affections—with swelling of joints : affections of cartilages and bones, inflammations of perios-teum, thickening and induration of periosteum. . . . Like syphilis and mercury, the complaints are aggravated at night. . . ."

Aurum affects and cures diseases of bones ; especially those of the nose and skull. It is curative of disease-conditions of eyes and nose. One remembers the astonishing curative effect of gold in a small child, with ulceration in nostrils and horrible nasal discharge, where *Sulphur* had failed. As Kent says, " *Aurum* is full of nasal troubles with fœtid discharges. The bones of the nose necrose (like syphilis and mercury). But with all these complaints the patient is bowed down with sorrow ; full of grief ; wants to die ; everything is black."

Kent sums up *Aurum* thus : " *We see this entire perversion of all the loves of mankind, and finally their entire destruction.*"

It is at least curious that Gold supplied in potency should be homœopathic to the loss of Gold in bulk. It alone can restore sanity with the realization, that " *the life is more than meat, and the body than raiment* ".

Dr. H. A. Roberts, in his *Rheumatic Remedies*, sums up the heart symptoms and the sphere of *Aurum* in acute rheumatism, thus :

" Severe pain in heart. Must sit up. Sensation as if the heart stopped, then gave one sudden hard thump. Heart flounders. Loud endocardial bruits. Pulse irregular. In inflammatory rheumatism *Aurum met.* is of value when there is high fever, extreme tenderness to touch, profuse sweat and envolvement of the endocardium with the peculiar heart symptoms."

BLACK LETTER SYMPTOMS

(*Hahnemann, Allen* and some from *Hering*)

Disgust of life, suicidal tendency.
Despondent melancholy. Hopelessness.
Great anguish increasing into self-destruction.

Anxious palpitation and desire to commit suicide.

Peevish and vehement : least contradiction excites wrath.

Moroseness ; indisposed to talk.

All day long good humour ; talkative and contented with himself (alternating action).

Heat and anger, quite forgets himself with quarrelling. Sulky.

Rush of blood to HEAD.

Tearing pressure—left forehead, left crown, right side of crown.

Pressure from within outwards in EYES *: worse when touched.*

Tension in eyes interferes with vision.

Can distinguish nothing distinctly, because he sees everything double and one object seems to run into another : tensive pain worse when he fixes his eyes on something, less severe when he closes them.

Half-sight ; as if the upper half of the vision were covered with a dark body : upper objects remain invisible.

He cannot get air through the NOSE, *for ulcerated, agglutinated, painful nostrils. Soreness both nostrils.*

Right nasal bone and adjoining part of upper jaw painful to touch.

Tickling internally in alae nasi.

Syphilitic ulcers palate and throat.

Tensive pain in hypogastrium just below navel and on both sides lumbar regions, with feeling of fullness, and with call to stool.

Pinching pain in hypogastrium, now here, now there.

Grumbling and rumbling in ABDOMEN.

Discharge of much fœtid flatus.

Discomfort in hypogastrium, as if wanted to go to stool, esp. after a meal.

(Affections of genitalia) : Uterus prolapsed and indurated.

Extreme tightness (chest) : difficulty of breathing at night.

Tightness of CHEST, *also when sitting and not moving : always takes a deep breath and cannot get enough air.*

Great weight on chest : esp. heavy weight on sternum.

Violent beating of the heart.

Awakened by BONE *pains : suffering so great he despairs : does not want to live.*

(Many pains in bones and limbs are detailed.)

Pain in knees as if they were tightly bound.

Remarkable ebullition in the BLOOD *(as if it boiled in the blood vessels).*

Frightful dreams at night.

BAPTISIA TINCTORIA

THIS invaluable remedy is one of the comparatively newer ones. One looks in vain for its most characteristic symptoms in Allen's *Encyclopedia* : but one finds them in Hering's *Guiding Symptoms*, in Hale's *New Remedies*, and its uses are developed and especially described by Kent, Nash, etc.

It seems natural to follow *Gelsemium* with *Baptisia*. They are so alike, and yet so utterly dissimilar that no one could mistake the one for the other, and both are so very useful in *influenza*— that trying complaint that we have " always with us ! "

Of course one associates *Baptisia* especially with TYPHOID— typhoid fever—typhoid conditions in any fever—the cases of influenza that exhibit typhoid conditions.

Remedies have their paces. Kent tells us that *Gelsemium* is slow-paced as regards its onset, but that *Baptisia* is of rapid onset ; the patient sinks rapidly into a stupid typhoid state— dull—drugged—besotted. He considers *Baptisia* more useful in typhoids of unusually rapid onset.

But Dr. C. E. Wheeler, in his *Case for Homœopathy*, tells us something immensely interesting and suggestive in regard to the more recent provings of *Baptisia*. He says, " There is no scepticism in regard to the next experiment. In typhoid fever the blood develops a substance which is not normally present in it, called an agglutinin ; which causes the typhoid bacilli to clump together, and forms a stage in the defence mechanisms against the disease. If healthy people take the drug *Baptisia* persistently, they develop (more or less according to individual susceptibility) this agglutinin in their blood." And *Baptisia* has certainly earned its laurels in the treatment of typhoid ; and it will always act rapidly and surely where its characteristic symptoms are present : *drowsiness, dull red face and besotted condition*, not only in typhoid but in any fever.

One has seen startling examples of the prompt curative action of *Baptisia* in influenzas ; in slight cases, and in serious. In that year of very fatal " typhoid 'flus " following the 1914-18 War, one remembers being sent for urgently by a local doctor to see a case— his worst—of influenza, in a Jewess. He thought she would die. She was dark, almost purple in the face, with the *Baptisia* drowsiness. . . . " *Baptisia !* " " But I only have it in the mother tincture." " Why not ?—give it ! " And in a few hours she was out of the wood, and made a rapid recovery—so one was told.

Another case, less severe. He was red-faced, dull and drowsy (suddenly, one morning) unable to rouse himself or take any interest, his words died away in drowsiness ; high temperature ; just a sudden attack of 'flu, of the *Baptisia* type. Happily getting his remedy, he was found practically well by the afternoon.

Again, in " gastric 'flus " it has seemed to me to be practically specific. As here. . . . Sudden attack of violent diarrhœa and vomiting—frightfully and suddenly ill—and a journey to go ! *Baptisia :*—and in the afternoon, the journey successfully accomplished, and an abrupt end to the trouble. . . .

This is the clinical picture :—Sudden onset, sudden great prostration and distress, apparently almost desperate conditions— with the *Baptisia* symptoms—*Baptisia*, and sudden recovery.

Every medicine has its own job, and can do that job, and no other. As a friend in need, *Baptisia* is worth knowing !

KENT stresses the suddenness of *Baptisia*.

He says : " *Baptisia* is suitable for acute diseases. It is a short-acting remedy. . . . It produces a violent change in the economy like a zymotic state. All its acute diseases and complaints have the appearance of zymosis, like scarlet fever, and diphtheria, and typhoid, and gangrenous complaints. There is one thing that is unusual about it, it brings on this septic state more rapidly than most other remedies—that is, its pace is more rapid than that found in most other remedies. . . . *Baptisia* is suitable for those blood poisons that are highly septic, such as the puerperal state. . . .

" Every medicine has a pace, a velocity. It is an important feature of it. Every medicine must be observed as to its velocity, as to its pace, as to its periodicity, as to its motion, as to its wave. We get that by looking at the symptoms.

" You take an individual who has been down in a mine, in a swamp, down in the mud, in the sewers, who has inhaled foul gases, who goes into bed with a sort of stupor, from the beginning he feels stupid. It is not gradual, but he goes down very suddenly, and he is stupid. He is prostrated.

" His face is mottled. Sordes begin to appear on the teeth much earlier than you would expect them in the regular typhoid. . . . Abdomen distended much earlier than we expect in a regular typhoid. . . . mouth bleeding, and is putrid. His odours are horrible, and he is in a marked state of delirium. . . . Velocity. He is going down towards death rapidly.

" Now it does not matter much whether it is a scarlet fever, or typhoid fever, or a septic surgical fever, or a puerperal fever or what. If you . . . try to rouse him up, he gives you the impression that he has been on a big drunk. . . . His countenance is besotted. It is bloated and purple and mottled . . . it is like an old drunkard.

" His mind seems to be gone . . . he is in confusion. When aroused, he attempts to say something, and utters a word or two, and it all flits away, and he is back in his state of stupor again. . . . No matter what disease that comes in, no matter what inflammation is present, no matter what organ is inflamed, if that state of the blood that can give rise to such symptoms and such sepsis is present, if that state of the mind is present, it is *Baptisia*.

" Discharges putrid. Odour cadaverous—pungent—penetrating. Odour of stool putrid, penetrating . . ."

And then Kent graphically describes the wanderings and delirium of *Baptisia*.

" A strange thing that runs through the remedy is a peculiar kind of mental confusion, in which he is in a constant argument with his parts. He seems to feel that there are two of him. He will begin talking about the other one in bed with him. It is said clinically that ' his great toe is in controversy with his thumb '. Or, ' one leg is talking to the other leg ' . . . or he is scattered around over the bed ; fumbles and you ask him what he is trying to do. ' Why, he is trying to get those pieces together.' . . . It is that dual* idea, that attempt to reconcile something. You see his lips go, and you rouse him to see what he is about, and he is trying to get the pieces together. . . .

" As soon as we come to the face, we begin to realize the *Baptisia* symptoms, that besotted expression. The countenance shows that. The eyes show it, the face shows it. And these are the symptoms, ' Dark red with besotted appearance. Hot . . . flushed, dusky.' "

Even her head " feels as though scattered about, and she tosses about the bed to get the pieces together." (Hale.)

In bad cases, the mouth and tongue—swollen, raw, denuded, stiff and dry, ulcerated, foul—such as we saw in some of those post-war cases of 'flu-pneumonias.

" The darker it is, the more likely would I be to think of *Baptisia*—but never a bright red. I have never seen the *Baptisia* mental state associated with a bright-red appearance. That low form of mental state is associated with blood decomposition, with duskiness, with a dark appearance of the skin, and of the mucous membranes." (Kent.)

---

* A like dual consciousness (Physical) occurs with *Pyrogen* and *Petrol* : a mental one in *Anacard*.

" One peculiar symptom indicates *Baptisia* in some sore throats. The throat may look dark-purple, livid, and *as if* very painful, but it is *not*. Dr. Miner cured an inveterate sore throat which was *not painful* (with the 30th)." (Hale.)

HALE gives indications for *Baptisia* :
" *Soreness all over the body ; mouth and tongue very dry.*

Feverishness, with feeling all over as if bruised ; the parts on which he is lying soon ache, and feel sore and bruised. (*Arn.*)

Typhoid fever, in the *premonitory* stage of bilious, gastric, or catarrhal origin—or from impure exhalations. It will often prevent the *access* of fever.

Typhoid fever in the first stages ; it will often arrest the disease, and bring about a rapid convalescence.

Typhus fever, with heavy sleep, unconsciousness, delirious muttering, etc.

Fevers, with drowsiness ; pulse 120 and thready ; lips parched and cracked ; pasty tongue heavily coated ; great thirst ; mind wandering ; could not give a direct answer to any question ; falls asleep in the middle of a sentence ; delirious at night, and low muttering.

Gastric fevers, with nausea, vomiting, dry, baked tongue, rapid pulse, tenderness of abdomen, diarrhœa.

Scarlet fever, with dark-red eruption ; dry, brown tongue, inclined to be red in the centre ; fetid breath ; stupor ; fever ; dysenteric stools.

Catarrhal fever or influenza, when the prostration is excessive, and the sore, bruised pains and sensations predominate.

Bilious fevers ; gastric fevers ; enteric fevers ; septic fevers.

Puerperul fevers, from absorption of purulent matters, or from infection.

Cerebro-spinal, or spotted fever.

Fevers setting in during dysentery, or any intestinal affection, and assuming a low type. (*Arn.*)

In typhoid fevers, and typhoid conditions, *Baptisia* vies with *Pyrogen* and *Arnica*."

One remembers a very bad case of typhoid, during the 1914-18 War, contracted in France, at a place where a very severe type of typhoid was raging. This patient gave great anxiety, till ".Ça va si bien, Mademoiselle ! si bien." And the symptom, " says she feels well, when desperately ill," led to the administration of *Arnica* which cleared up the case.

Arnica has not the drowsiness, or the redness, or the besotted condition of *Baptisia*, though they both have the hard-bed sensation, markedly. (*Pyrogen.*)

Baptisia has the *Arnica* " sensation, all over body, as if bruised or beaten ". And in one prover, " Lying in one position for a few minutes, or upon the back, caused the sacral region to become exceedingly painful, as though I had lain on a hard floor all night, and induced the conviction that a short continuance of the same position would cause bedsore ; when turning on the other side, the same sensation was produced on the hips." (*Baptisia* should be useful in bedsores.)

Summary of Black Letter and Characteristic Symptoms

Stupor ; falls asleep while being spoken to, or answering ; heavy sleep until aroused : wakes only to fall asleep again in the midst of his answer, which he vainly endeavours to finish.

Confusion of ideas. Confusion as if drunk.

She cannot go to sleep, because she cannot get herself together.

Feels scattered about, and tosses about to get the pieces together.

Aversion to mental exertion. Indisposed to think : mind seems weak.

Dull bruised feeling in occiput.

Face sallow : dark-red ; with a besotted expression : flushed : dusky.

Sordes on teeth and lips : tongue ulcerated.

Fetid odour of mouth (Merc.).

Fauces dark-red : dark, putrid ulcers . . . unusual absence of pain.

Tonsils and soft palate swollen : not accompanied by pain.

Can swallow liquids only. The least food gags.

Œsophagus feels constricted from above down to stomach.

Paralysis of organs of deglutition (Gels.).

Right iliac region sensitive.

Abdominal muscles sore on pressure, with acute intermitting pain.

Fetid, exhausting diarrhœa, causing excoriation.

Drowsy : stupid : delirious stupor.

Cerebral forms of fever.

Typhoid and cerebral forms of fever, with delirium, drowsiness.

Feeling head, or limbs, scattered, etc. Involuntary scanty stool, difficult breathing.

Prostration with disposition of fluids to decompose.

Discharges and exhalations fetid ; breath, stools, urine, sweat, ulcers.

Ulceration, especially of mouth ; also with tendency to putrescence.

BELLADONNA

THIS is another of Hahnemann's Polycrests—drugs of many uses—which has its place (for paramount utility in acute and violent conditions) in every homœopathic medicine chest, however diminutive:—One of those medicines, " without which, we might indeed shut up shop "

Violence runs through *Belladonna*, violence and *suddenness*. We associate *Belladonna* in our minds with sudden violence—violent pain, violent headache, violent throbbings, violent delirium, violent mania, violent starts and twitchings, violent convulsions.

Bell. is a remedy of sudden, acute conditions, like *Acon.*, yet very unlike *Acon.* in its symptoms. Roughly speaking, *Aconite* is *turmoil in circulation ; Belladonna turmoil in brain ;* in the same way that *Chamomilla* provokes and cures ailments associated with *turmoil in temper*.

The cardinal symptoms of inflammation, as we are taught, are heat, redness, swelling, and pain. And all these *Belladonna* has in a violent degree ; therefore *Belladonna* is *palliative* to inflammations in general, and will modify them, if it does no more ; but it is *curative* only where the rest of the symptoms agree. For instance, in inflammations of lung and pleura, its disease picture, as we have shown, is easily distinguishable from that of *Bryonia, Phosphorus*, and other remedies. It is the " totality of the characteristic symptoms " that have to be taken into account if sudden and striking *cures* are to result. Sudden cures in pneumonia ?—in herpes ? How can you suddenly cure a pneumonia with consolidation ?—a herpes with wide vesicular eruption ? With the right medicine, early, the pneumonia should have been aborted, should not have gone on to consolidation. But even so, the sudden drop in temperature and pulse, the sudden possibility of rest and sleep, the sudden well-being of the patient, when he asks for food, the newspaper, and talks and smiles, announce the cure, even though the lungs may take days to resolve. In the same way with herpes, the pain and the redness, the inflammation, suddenly go, the vesicles are seen to be dried up, mere scabs ; the thing is dead, and will give no more trouble. In acute sickness the needed homœopathic remedy declares itself unmistakably and often almost suddenly. When you have hit it, there is no mistaking the fact.

Belladonna has been found to abort whitlows in the early stages, to abort an appendicitis, has doubtless aborted countless pneumonias. The typical *Belladonna* picture is unmistakable when you meet it :—the bright-red face, the dilated pupils, the burning skin, the throbbing pains, the intolerance of pressure and JAR. Those call for *Belladonna*, whatever the disease. *Belladonna* can abort and can cure (as we have seen elsewhere) where drug-picture and disease-picture match. Of course there are drugs, aspirin, genasprin, etc., which abolish the *sensation of pain only*, and cure nothing. Such drugs may be dangerous in acute appendicitis, acute middle-ear disease, because they merely mask symptoms while the disease runs on, perhaps into a gangrenous appendix and general peritonitis, or an " acute mastoid " necessitating speedy operation to avoid cerebral abscess. Beware of analgesics. They are not safe. Homœopathic remedies that fit the symptoms only kill the pain by curing the condition that caused it.

An early experience, never forgotten, of *Belladonna's* rapid curative action was away in the country years ago, where a boy having been exposed to a very hot sun, came down suddenly with violent headache, flushed face, and a very high temperature—as high a one as I had met with in those days, and which filled me with awe—105, or 106. He got some *Belladonna*—and was well by next day. These early striking experiences are not lightly forgotten.

In sunstroke, and in violent congestive headaches, *Belladonna* and *Glonoine* would seem to run almost neck and neck. *Glonoine* (potentized nitro-glycerine) also has throbbing, bursting head-ache—waves of throbbing, bursting headache, waves of intense pain. It has also the flushed, hot face and, like *Belladonna*, cannot bear the least JAR. The great difference between them seems to be, that *Glonoine* is markedly aggravated by heat—can't bear any heat about the head, may even be ameliorated by cold applications, whereas *Belladonna* is very sensitive to cold ; the *Belladonna* head is especially sensitive to cold, and *Belladonna* has complaints from getting the head chilled, or wet—even from getting the hair cut.

One has seen the extraordinary effect of *Glonoine* in the terrible pains of a badly fractured skull. The boy had been for days under morphia; how was he to possibly exist without it ? *Glonoine* soon settled that question satisfactorily.

Belladonna is hypersensitive to LIGHT—with its hugely dilated pupils !—to noise, to motion, to PRESSURE, to JAR, to cold and, as we said, to washing the head and to getting the hair cut.

GUERNSEY says about *Belladonna*, "Manifested under this drug is a remarkable quickness of sensation, or of motion ; the eyes snap and move quickly ; pains come and go with *great* celerity ; a pain may have lasted for some time, then, in a second, it is gone ; may commence suddenly, slowly increase in celerity till the height is reached, then in a second be gone. Much twitching and jerking of the muscles. Dull and sleepy, half awake and half asleep."

In regard to the sudden come and sudden go of *Belladonna* pain, one remembers a capable and much appreciated little housemaid, who began to get sudden, very violent headaches, and, presently, occasional sudden convulsive attacks, for which no cause could be found. As to the headaches, she would go to bed all right, then, some nights, would come down to my room, where I was sleepily preparing for bed, swaying—waving tremulous hands before her head, " Oh, my head ! my head ! oh ! my head ! Oh ! give me something for my head ! " A dose of *Belladonna* ; a few minutes' wait—then, suddenly, " It's gone now ! " and off she would go, happily, to bed. The matter ended, tragically, in a fit, when cleaning the drawing-room grate in the early morning. An under-housemaid discovered her lying forward with her head in the large fireplace, while a black mark across her throat, from the top bar, betrayed the cause of her death—suffocation. The girl who found her made no attempt to pull her out, but ran off in a fright to tell someone else, and time was wasted before any attempt was made to resuscitate her. A *post mortem* revealed a " glioma " of the brain, a small tumour which accounted for the whole condition. But it was curious to see how *Belladonna* would always quickly, suddenly, relieve the severe head pains, even when dependent on such a condition.

Never think that Homœopathy can cure everything : it cannot. But it *can* relieve even the incurable to such an extent that it is difficult to realize, at times, its incurability.

KENT has a wonderful lecture on *Belladonna*, from which we will proceed to borrow . . .

Belladonna stands for *heat—redness—intense burning*.

The *Belladonna* throat burns like coals of fire : the inflamed tonsils burn like fire. The skin burns like fire to the patient, and is intensely hot to the doctor.

Put your hand on a *Belladonna* patient and you want to suddenly withdraw it : the heat is so intense. Kent says the sensation of heat may remain in your fingers for hours afterwards.

The heat is *violent*. " Heat intense. Violent heat."

With the *Belladonna* heat there is *Redness* : bright redness ; going on perhaps later to dusky appearance, or to mottling. But bright-red, shiny skin.

Belladonna has rapid *swellings :* " as if it would burst."

Then *throbbings*—violent pulsations : " a veritable turmoil : an earthquake. Everything is shaken when the patient needs *Belladonna*."

" One of the most painful of remedies " : *pains come suddenly, and go suddenly.*

Motion, with *Belladonna*, means violent suffering : feeling that the head will burst, that the eyes will be pressed out : *hammering* pains.

Worse for touch, which excites violent throbbing.

Worse for JAR. A patient worse if you jar or touch the bed, " will reveal to you the remedy—*Belladonna* ".

Intense pains, then, worse for *light*—for *jar*—for *motion*—for *cold*. Better hot : better wrapped up : worse draught.

Inflammations : especially of *brain, lungs* and *liver.*

Belladonna's pains, its inflammations and sufferings, its nightly attacks of delirium, are violent inflammatory attacks, and are attended by that violent heat.

Spasms : from the twitchings in sleep of teething babies, to the most violent convulsions.

Convulsion of infants, with hot skin and cerebral congestion : attacks which are brought on by light, by a draught, or if the infant gets cold.

Spasms, again, of circular muscles also, of the circular muscles of the bile duct, clutching a little stone. Kent says after a dose of *Belladonna* the spasm lets up and the stone passes, and the agony of gall-stone colic is relieved.

Violence, again, runs through all the mental symptoms which *Belladonna* can cause and therefore cure : " a wild state," says Kent, " perhaps relieved by eating a little food."

With the violent delirium of *Belladonna* there will be its *heat*, its *redness*, its *burning*. Brain burns : head burns : skin burns.

Bryonia, as we saw the other day, has the busy delirium of everyday, common things : the anxiety about business : the desire to get on with it.

Belladonna has the furious delirium that leaps at the bare wall : that tries to escape : that bites—spits—tears. Fears also, of an imaginary black dog—of the gallows, etc.

Kent says that *Belladonna* is not indicated in continuous fevers, such as typhoid. Here it will do actual harm. But here

Hyoscyamus will come in. And Nash says that *Hyoscyamus* is the best remedy he knows for typhoid fever, or typhoid pneumonia, with delirium that lapses into stupor, carphology, silence or muttering.

Belladonna, *Stramonium* and *Hyoscyamus* are botanically related : and they are all " high-grade delirium drugs " in the order given, *Belladonna* being the most violent. They have much in common, yet much that distinguishes.

Belladonna and *Stramonium* have both redness of the face, but *Stramonium* lacks the intense, burning heat. The face of *Hyoscyamus* is pale and sunken. *Belladonna* cannot bear light : *Stramonium* cannot bear the dark, is terrified of the dark : must have light. *Stramonium* wants to pray : *Hyoscyamus* in its delirium or mania has lost all sense of decency and wants to uncover . . . and so on. These are Nash's " trio of delirium remedies ". But of course it does not need delirium, or mania, or convulsions to call for one of these remedies in sickness. These are their extremes of action.

Hahnemann says that a study of the symptoms of *Belladonna* shows that it corresponds in similarity to a number of commonly met with morbid states, and is therefore frequently applicable for curative purposes. That the small-souled persons who cry out against its poisonous character, and let their patients die for want of *Belladonna*, because they " have mild remedies for these diseases " only betray their ignorance, " *for no medicine can be a substitute for another* ".

And he teaches that the most violent poisons will become the mildest of remedies, " provided that they are given in appropriate smallest doses ". He says, by a hundred-fold experience at the sick bed during the last eight or ten years, he could not help descending to the decillion-fold dilution (the 30th potency). Besides its prophylactic powers in scarlet fever, he finds it the best preventive of hydrophobia, given at first every third or fourth day, and then at longer intervals. And indeed *Belladonna* has many of the symptoms of hydrophobia : the fear of water, the attempts to bite : the spasm of the throat that prevents swallowing, the mania, the delirium, in which he is "in terror of dogs"— " surrounded by dogs ", and so on.

ALLEN in his *Encyclopedia*, gives 2,545 symptoms, as caused by *Belladonna*. Of these the black-type symptoms, the much-caused and much-cured by *Belladonna*, are so numerous that we will only attempt to give some of them : they go to show the genius of the drug and its spheres of most-marked action.

Inclination to bite those around them.

She attempted to bite and strike her attendants, broke into fits of laughter, gnashed her teeth. The head was hot, the face red, the look wild and fierce.

Inclination to bite those around him, and to tear everything about him to pieces.

Raging, violent fury. Furious delirium. She pulled at the hair of the bystanders.

Such fury (with burning heat of the body, and open, staring, immovable eyes) that she had to be held constantly, lest she should attack someone : and when thus held, so that she could not move, she spat continually at those about her.

The face was red, the head hot, the look wild and staring : pupils dilated : the arteries of the neck and head visibly pulsating.

In the evening he was seized with such violent delirium that it required three men to confine him. His face was livid ; his eyes injected and protruding ; the pupils strongly dilated ; the carotid arteries pulsating most violently ; a full hard frequent pulse, with loss of power to swallow.

Great intolerance of light and noise.

He sought continually to spring out of bed. When put to bed he sprang out again in delirium, talked constantly, laughed out, and exhibited complete loss of consciousness, did not know his own parents.

Rush of blood to the head : pulsation of cerebral arteries, and a throbbing in the interior of the head. Very intense headache.

The pains in the head are aggravated by noise, motion, when moving the eyes, by shocks, by contact.

Afraid to cough on account of the increase of pain it causes.

Pressive headache, especially in forehead.

Painful pressure in head, especially lower part of forehead directly above the nose, intolerable on stepping or treading.

Three violent stabs, forehead to occiput, whereupon all previous headache suddenly disappears.

Violent throbbing in brain from behind forwards and towards both sides : throbbing ends on the surface in painful shootings.

Jerking headache, violent on walking quickly or going rapidly upstairs . . . at every step it seemed as if the brain rose and fell in the forehead ; the pain ameliorated by pressing strongly on the forehead. (The only " better for pressure " of Belladonna ?)

Stabbing as if with a knife from temple to temple.

The head is so sensitive that the least contact gives her pain.

Eyes projecting and sparkling : pupils dilated.

A staring look. Distorted, with redness and swelling of face.

Eyes dry ; motion attended with sense of dryness and stiffness.
Burning heat in eyes.
Dilated pupils : dilated and immovable.
Everything he sees looks red.
Great sensitiveness of smell.

Great redness of the face : glowing red face, with inexpressible pains in the head. Face, neck and chest much swollen.
Tumefaction and redness of face and lips.
Spasmodic action of the muscles of the face.
Convulsive movements of face, with distortion of mouth.
The tongue and palate dark-red. Dryness of throat and difficult swallowing.
Dryness of tongue and throat, so great as to interfere with speech. Dryness of fauces most distressing.
During deglutition, feeling in throat as if it were too narrow, as if nothing would pass properly.
Scraping raw sensation of epiglottis : raw and sore.

Nausea.
Long-lasting painfulness of the whole abdomen, as if it were all raw and sore.
Excessive tenderness of abdomen, which cannot bear the slightest touch.
Violent cutting pressure in hypogastrium, now here, now there.

Retention of urine, which only passes drop by drop.
Badly smelling hæmorrhage from the uterus.
Violent pressing and urging towards the sexual organs as if everything would fall out there.
Menses too soon and very profuse, of thick, decomposed, dark-red blood.

Catarrh or cough with coryza.
Painful dryness in larynx.
Larynx as if inflamed and swollen.
Hoarseness.
Hollow, hoarse cough.
Pulse full and quick.

(Then numbers of black-type symptoms of extremities.)
Thighs and legs, as if bruised all over, as if rotten.
Shootings and gnawings along the shafts of bones . . . tearing in joints . . .

Epileptic convulsions.
Every moment wished to get out of bed.
The boy wished to escape.

Great irritability and impressiveness of the senses.
Tastes and smells everything more acutely.
Taste, sight and hearing keener; mind more easily moved and thoughts more active.
Excessive nervous excitability with exalted sensibility of all the organs. The least noise—light—annoying.

Redness of the whole body with quick pulse.
Redness like scarlatina of the entire surface of the body.
Pustules break out on cheeks and nose . . .

He starts as if in fright and awakes, when just falling asleep.
Starts as if in a fright, feeling as if she were falling down deep (Thuja), which caused her to shudder violently.
Very restless sleep.
At night the boys became restless, spoke irrationally, and could with difficulty be kept in bed.
The child tosses about, kicks and quarrels in its sleep.

Temperature of the head very much increased.
The skin hot, dry, scarlet, especially intense on face and ears.
Burning heat within and without.

* * *

Whatever the ailment, headache, fever, inflammation, where there is burning heat, redness, pain that will not bear pressure, jar, or motion, think of Belladonna.

* * *

But, after all this, who would dream that *Belladonna* was one of the most commonly useful of nursery remedies?—yet it is.

As FARRINGTON puts it, "The character of the (*Belladonna*) disease is acute, sudden and violent. The very rapidity of the onset should at once suggest *Belladonna*." [Or *Aconite*, he might have added: but their symptoms are very different, as we have seen.] "For example," he says, "a child is perfectly well on going to bed. A few hours afterwards it is aroused with violent symptoms, jerking of the limbs, irritation of the brain, and screaming out during sleep. All these symptoms suggest *Belladonna*." [But to complete the picture, he might have added, that in these cases the face is red, the head hot, the pupils big.]

One consults and quotes from several of our prescribing geniuses, because one man has more completely grasped the inwardness, and has had more experience with one remedy, another with another remedy.   For the same reason it is well to read and study the same drug in several books, to get enlightenment always from the man best qualified to enlighten.   Pick plenty of brains if you want to nourish and stimulate your own.

We will quote a little from Farrington (*Clinical Materia Medica*) . . .

In *Belladonna* poisoning cases, the mouth and throat are distressingly dry, compelling frequent efforts to swallow, with suffocative spasms of fauces and glottis.   Thirst is violent, yet water aggravates : vertigo, confusion, hallucinations and finally stupor. The pupils are so much dilated as to nearly obscure the iris.   Strong coffee is the best antidote,—of course after efforts to get rid of the poison, or the berries that have been eaten.

. . . Our symptomatology from provings and poisonings enables us to employ the drug with mathematical certainty, so far as its selection is concerned . .

It is best suited to persons of a plethoric habit, subject to congestions, especially to the head more than to any other part of the body.   Also suited to precocious children, with big head and small body . . . they learn rapidly ; sleep is unnatural ; hot head ; red cheeks ; screaming during sleep . . .

Belladonna is very often called for in the treatment of convulsions.   Epilepsy is readily modified by it, and at times cured. And spasms of children during dentition, from repelled eruptions, etc., keep the remedy in almost daily demand.   In all these cases the cerebral symptoms must be present, hot head, flushed face, throbbing carotids, starting from sleep in terror, etc., foam at the mouth having the odour of rotten eggs . . .

Convulsions, particularly in children, are very violent, distorting the body in every conceivable manner, opisthotonos predominating . . .

On closing the eyes the patient is apt to see abnormal visions ; these usually disappear on opening the eyes . . . or a sensation of falling . . . as when a child, suddenly rouses from sleep, clutches at the air, and trembles as if from fear . . .

A peculiarity of *Belladonna* is the faculty it has of exciting constriction of the circular fibres of blood vessels, contraction of sphincters, etc. . .   exemplified in the constriction of the throat, worse from liquids ; constriction of the anus, . . . the agony of gall-stone colic, where a small stone is spasmodically

gripped in a narrow duct on its way out into the intestines . . .
the spasmodic constriction of the os uteri, retarding labour ;
ineffectual or frequent urging to pass water, with scanty discharge . . .

In inflammations, if they are violent and come suddenly, and
are almost overwhelming in their intensity, *Belladonna* is again
suggested . . . In abscess, whether this be an abscess of the
tonsil, a boil, or any other kind of abscess, when pus develops with
lightning-like rapidity . . . Indicated by phlegmonous
erysipelas, which goes quickly on to suppuration . . . the
very suddenness of the attack suggests *Belladonna* . . .

Again in inflammation of the breasts. It is here indicated
by the violence of the symptoms, by the radiating redness, by the
throbbing and tendency towards suppuration . . .

In the female, *Belladonna* causes and cures constant violent
" bearing down " with this curious modality, *worse on lying down*,
relieved by standing . . . [The knowledge of such peculiarities
of drug action are all-important, since they make prescribing sure
and easy—comparatively ! *Pulsatilla* has something like this,
" bearing down " *worse lying*. Guided by this symptom one saw
a nasty case of distress and fever, after an abortion, cure up
rapidly with *Pulsatilla*. The more commonly useful drugs for
"bearing down", *Sepia*, *Lilium tigrinum*, etc., are worse from standing, have to sit down—to cross the legs—to support the parts.

One of our best remedies in acute and chronic rheumatism,
pains are cutting, tearing, running along the limbs like lightning
. . . one of the best remedies in rheumatic stiff neck, caused by
cutting hair, getting the head wet, or sitting with head and neck
exposed to a draught . . .

Belladonna is HOT. It may have hot sweat : in uterine
hæmorrhages the blood pours out and feels *hot* . . . In
rheumatic fever, when the whole system seems involved, with pain
in joints flying from place to place, and almost always profuse sour
sweat which gives no relief whatever. The patient seems to soak
everything about him with the sweat, and the more he sweats
the more he does not seem to get any better . . . [*Thuja* has
the strange symptom, *sweat only on uncovered parts*, and this has
led to brilliant cures, suggesting a drug that might not have been
otherwise considered. *Belladonna* has the opposite, sweat *only on
covered parts*.] " On raising the bedclothes there appears to issue
forth hot steam."

Kent's picture of *Belladonna* in rheumatic fever is this . . .
Inflammatory rheumatism when all the joints are swollen, or a
great number of them, and they are hot, red, and burn. We have

in the rheumatism the heat, redness and burning running through,
with the same sensitiveness of the whole patient, and a sensitiveness
of the joints to the jar of the bed.   He wants to lie perfectly still,
is much worse from motion, and has considerable fever . . .
It is especially suitable to those that are very sensitive to cold,
who cannot bear the least uncovering, cannot bear a draught,
very sensitive to the motion of the covers, and ameliorated by
heat. "The very stamp and character of *Belladonna* is in its
rheumatic state, like it is in all its other complaints. · It is the
patient that has given *Belladonna* that character in the provings ;
it is the *patient* that gives disease that character when he has it, and
it is only the fulfilment of the Law of Similars when these come
together, and the remedy annihilates the sickness."

BELLADONNA "ALMOST SPECIFIC FOR SCARLET FEVER."

In March, 1933, we published, together with this *Belladonna
Drug Picture*, the experiences during an epidemic of scarlet fever
in his district, of a doctor who had attended our Post Graduate
Course, and was minded to put what he had heard about *Belladonna* to the test, as a cure and as a prophylactic.

His results were what one would expect, but amazing to the
Sanitary Inspector who, meeting him in the street, asked how he
was treating his scarlet fever cases ? saying that, when he called
in to see them, they all looked very well, with only the merest
trace of rash remaining, and subsequent visits showed how quickly
they recovered.   The doctor asked, and how were the other cases
doing in comparison ?   "Well, they just drag on as usual." The
Inspector said also, that there were no complications and never
more than one case in any household. It was all a mystery to
him.

The doctor details some of his cases in patients whose ages
ranged from eighteen months to twelve years. . . . No
deaths. No complications even, e.g. kidneys, ears, throat, etc. ;
while the disease was cut remarkably short, and there was
practically no convalescent stage. In 80 per cent. *Belladonna* was
the only remedy required. He ends with, "I have never had such
pleasant and happy scarlet fever patients to treat before." He
also tells how he used *Belladonna* with success as a prophylactic
(as was noticed by the Sanitary Inspector). Only in one instance
did a second case occur in the same house—*four weeks later !* (the
incubation period of scarlet fever being from one to eight days).

BELLIS PERENNIS
(The Daisy)

OUR own lovely indigenous bruise-wort—wound-wort : our own *Arnica*, even to the production and cure of boils ! Here we have one of Burnett's own particular remedies, of which, scattered through his telling little monographs, he has so much to say. Clarke, his friend, admirer, and recorder, says, " The daisy is a flower which is repeatedly trodden upon, and always comes up smiling ; and being the day's eye, may be the sign of its too easy waking propensities." He quotes Burnett as saying, " It acts very much like *Arnica*, even to the production of erysipelas."

Clarke gives its relations to other remedies, which are highly suggestive in regard to its uses. He says, " Compare *Arn.*, *Calend.*, *Hyperic.*, *Con.*, *Ars.*, *Hamam.*, *Vanad.*" Which means, when at a loss for one or other of these vulneraries, we can go out into the fields and, in its season—a very long one !—get help from the floweret from which our childish fingers used to weave daisy-chains. You may have to scramble up Leith Hill for *Chelidonium* ; or drag your feet out of squishy marshes to obtain *Equisetum* for urinary difficulties ; but while many precious herbs are difficult to find or recognize, no one can mistake or overlook the unpleasant stinging nettle, or the ubiquitous daisy, which makes the meadows, everywhere, to smile.

Poets have loved this flower. For Shakespeare, it is " Daisies pied " (variegated like a magpie), while Tennyson makes the unfortunate lover of " Maud " sing :

> " I know the way she went,
>   Home with her maiden posy ;
> For her feet have touched the meadows,
>   And have left the daisies rosy."

CULPEPER (1616-54) writes of the " Little Common Daisy " : " The leaves and sometimes the roots, are used, and are reckoned among the traumatic and vulnerary plants, being used in wound-drinks, and are accounted good to dissolve congealed and coagulated blood, to help the pleurisy and peri-pneumonia. In the King's evil the decoction given inwardly, and a cataplasm of the leaves applied outwardly, are esteemed by some extraordinary remedies. This is another herb which nature has made common, because it may be useful." He also speaks of it " just boiled in asses milk, as very effectual in consumption of the lungs ".

But it is Burnett, who has, in our day, revived and rendered scientific its applications. In his *Diseases of the Skin*, he has a good deal to tell us about *Bellis*, and we will quote rather extensively. He says : " In this little volume I am, before all things, seeking to show that Diseases of the skin have, for the most part, their origin, not in the skin itself, but are essentially cutaneous manifestations of some more or less remote organic or organismic wrongs.

" Thus Fletcher mentions *Acne from Cold Drinks* ; and anent this I wish here to quote an interesting and instructive experience of my own of the curative effects of the *common Daisy* in complaints that are due to *wet cold*, e.g. acne of the face.

" As I consider the observation of wider practical importance, I will give the source of my own knowledge.

" Bellis Perennis AGAINST THE ILL-EFFECTS OF WET COLD IN THE OVER-HEATED.

" I refer to *D. Johann Schroeder's Pharmacopœa Universalis*, with Hoffman's remarks, 1748. The Daisy is here commended in Hæmorrhage, Dysentery, as a ' *herrliches Wund kraut* ', internally and externally, i.e., as a vulnerary, for the effects of falls, blows, bruises and the like, pains in the joints, rheumatism (and hence called ' Gicht kraut ') ; in nocturnal cramps, *angina pectoris*, fevers and inflammations ; for lameness ; and he says that German mothers were in the habit of using it for their children as an aperient.

" An ordinary commendation of *Arnica* reads almost in the same terms, but I would specially call attention to this, ' This herb is useful to such as have partaken of a too cold draught of something, for it possesses a peculiar quality, as shown by experience, of being useful in all those terrible and dangerous accidents that arise from having drunk something very cold when the body is in a heated condition.' This important point I have verified as will be seen later on.

" Further, it would appear that Mindererus, in his *Kriegs-Artzeney*, cannot sufficiently praise the Daisy in such cases, for he declares that an account of this action of the herb *should be written up over all gates and doors for the benefit of the poor harvesters who in the hot harvest season get ill from partaking of Cold drink* ; its effect in such cases he affirms is remarkable, and so prompt that amelioration sets in at once.

" Christoph Schorer in his *Medicina peregrinantium*, gives similar testimony, and says that he cured two men of dangerous coughs, with emaciation, that were due to their having drunk something cold when they were heated. And Schroeder affirms that it will cure dropsy due to drinking too much in ' dog days ', i.e. hot weather.

" We know from experience the immense value of certain generalizations in the treatment of disease, as, for instance, *Arnica* for falls and bruises ; *Hypericum* for wounded nerve tissue ; *Dulcamara* for the ill effects of damp, and so on.

" Now we may add this other, that *Bellis perennis* is curative of complaints due to drinking cold drinks when the body is heated, i.e. *effects of sudden chill from wet cold when one is hot.*"

He then gives a case : Woman of 30, acne since 12 years old. Great bumps in the face about every three weeks, at times hardly seen, at times looking like Phlegmonous Erysipelas. Eruption coincided with the commencement of the menstruation. He elicited the following curious fact.

Just before her twelfth year she was out in sultry weather haymaking, and, when greatly heated she fell head foremost into a brook, and some days later broke out all over head and face with an eruption " just like small-pox ". Face and ears were covered, and a handkerchief had to be tied round her neck to prevent the discharge from dropping on her clothes. She was indoors eight weeks with it, and " since had had any amount of medicines and greases and all sorts of things, but they never did me one bit of good. . . .".

Burnett then argues out his reasons for his prescription— *Bellis* 3x, ♏3, *t.d.s.*, and continues,

" In four weeks the face was quite well ; not a speck on it for the past fortnight. Actually menstruating, and her face is quite free for the first time at the beginning of the flow, in her whole menstrual life, which began 18 years ago ! " She had developed symptoms, constipation, and a queer shaking beginning in stomach, as if she had been running fast.

" Another month, and still well of the eruption. Last poorly time not a spot !

" She reported occasionally for two or three months, but so far it has remained permanently cured."

Burnett adds, " My reasoning may be faulty, but I think this case shows that the Daisy is a notable remedy, and this virtue of a common weed lying everywhere at our feet deserves to be made very widely known. People of any experience do not need to be told that the ill effects of drinking cold drinks when the body is heated are very serious at times, and always inconvenient. Of course it is not confined to the drinking, as the idea is *sudden wet chill to heated stomach or body surface.* This property of the Daisy is the more valuable, as we know of no other remedy in our vast Pharmacopœa that possesses it ; and beyond myself, I believe no one is acquainted with it. Most of what I here write has been lying in a drawer of my writing desk for years, and this little clinical tip ought long since to have been published, for it may be a good while before another lover of the fair Daisy stumbles against old Schroeder's generalization in a humble receptive mood. I regard this peculiar property of the Daisy as eminently important, and ask all who may read this to make it known, so that it may be available for such as travellers, tourists, harvesters, soldiers on the march, when they, being heated, have had a cold ducking, or have drunk cold liquids.

"I would recommend it also in the acute and chronic dyspepsia from eating cold ices, as the conditions here are identical, for I have, in such cases, found it an eminent curative agent . . . the facial dermatitis, here, was one that would be classed as a Disease of the Skin, and internal treatment alone cured it."

Five years later, in his *Change of Life in Women*, Burnett again takes up the tale, and tells us more about his beloved Daisy : "This morning I received a letter from a colleague in America, asking me what my indications are for the use of *Bellis per.*" He gives his reply :

"*Bellis per.* is our common daisy ; it acts very much like *Arnica*, even to the contingent production of erysipelas ; it causes pain in the spleen, and generally symptoms of coryza, and of feeling very tired, a person (the writer) wanting to lie down. It acts on exudates, swellings, and stasis, and hence in a fagged womb its action is very satisfactory ; indeed, in the discomforts of pregnancy and of varicose veins patients are commonly loud in its praise. In the *giddiness* of elderly people (cerebral stasis) it acts well and does permanent good ; likewise and particularly in fag from masturbation ; in old workmen, labourers, and the overworked and fagged, it is a princely remedy. In the head-sufferings of elderly working gardeners its action is very pretty. Its action in the ill-effects from taking cold drinks when one is hot is now well-known. It is a grand friend to commercial travellers and in railway spine of moderate severity it has not any equal so far as my knowledge reaches. I think *stasis* lies at the bottom of all these ailings. . . . P.S.—When given at night *Bellis* is apt to cause the patient to wake up very early in the morning, hence I order it by preference to be taken not too late in the day. I have often cured with it the symptom, ' Wakes up too early in the morning and cannot get off again,' and here the higher dilutions act much more decidedly and lastingly, as a rule, and without any side-effects, for here the action is purely homœopathic and not simply deobstruant."

In another of his booklets, *Organic Diseases of Women*, Burnett talks of *Bellis* in the *Inconveniences of Pregnancy*.

" It happens to some ladies when they are *enceintes* that they find it very inconvenient to get about, walking being very irksome and almost impossible. In such cases the Daisy soon sets matters right. I mean of course, when the cause of the trouble lies in the mechanical circumstances, and these are of a remediable kind. One severe case of trouble during child-bearing I treated with many remedies, including *Bellis*, and was greatly disappointed ; however the event showed the cause of my failure, viz., all the trouble arose from the *long legs* of the fœtus, that at birth were very much bent. . . ." He gives a case, far gone in the family way, where it was very difficult to get about, and where, a fortnight later, he got this report ? " The *Bellis* did me so much good. I can walk quite well now, and do not get tired or stiff." Here its action was prompt and satisfactory, with no inconvenient side-effect or after-effect, i.e. truly specific. Why did I give *Bellis* in such a case ? Merely because the inconvenience complained of was due to mechanical pressure ; the tissues were pressed upon, and therefore in a condition precisely like that of a bruise—hence I gave my old friend the daisy—bruise-wort, i.e. it acts on the muscular fibres of the blood vessels, and upon the tissues, and thus clears the line of these mechanical obstructions. *Arnica* 1x and 1, I have used in like manner and with almost identical results. . . . On another page he writes, " In merely organ diseases constitutional treatment is not indicated, and is therefore useless ; but a battered, bruised uterus yields quickly to anti-traumatics such as *Bellis perennis* and *Arnica montana*. And the organ remedies—*Helonias dioica* and *Fraxinus Americanus*—quickly cured the hypertrophy of the organ." " And in the case of organ remedies, small material doses act best—indeed brilliantly ; such remedies also need to be repeated at short intervals. On the contrary, organ hypertrophies from constitutional causes are not curable by organ remedies at all until the constitutional disease has been cured by infrequently repeated high dilutions of remedies closely homœopathic thereto. . . ."

We will not apologize for quoting somewhat lavishly from the unique teachings and experience of a very brilliant prescriber. When our knowledge is perfect, and our methods of pre-scribing give absolutely the results we aim at in all cases, we shall be able to afford to overlook what stands outside our experience.

BORAX

HAHNEMANN, *Chronic Diseases*, discusses *Borax*, which, he says " has for a long time been used as a domestic remedy, against the aphthæ of children, and to facilitate the labour-pains of pregnant women."

Borax is another of those invaluable minor remedies, with very distinctive symptoms and selective tissue-action. It is not easy to forget, when once its peculiarities are mastered. Its great suggestive symptom, which will lead to its use in a variety of conditions, is its *intense dread of downward motion of any kind*. It affects *head*, with vertigo from downward motion. It has a curious action on *hair*, which tangles at the tips and sticks together; and this is re-formed when these bunches are cut off. Its most notable effect on *eyes* is that the lashes turn in (entropion) and of course inflame the eyes : especially are the outer canthi inflamed. The lower lids may be entirely inverted.

One notices the " red nose of young women ". Also the pale earthy, suffering expression of face—especially in young children; and the herpetic eruptions about the mouth, reminding one of *Nat. mur.* and *Sepia*. From the mouth, downwards, all through to the anus, *Borax* can be a torment. It has aphthæ, so tender that they prevent the babe from nursing, or the older victim from eating ; that, in the stomach, prevent peaceful digestion, with vomiting of slime ; that affect the abdomen with pinchings and diarrhœa ; that inflame rectum and anus, even to stricture, with burnings and aphthæ. But *Borax* not only tortures the infant, but the pregnant and nursing mother : with aphthous nipples that will not tolerate suckling ; and milk, too copious, or too thick, or repulsive to the infant by reason of its bad taste.

Borax is one of the remedies of pleurisy when, like that of *Bryonia*, " the patient cannot move or breathe without a stitch".

But we will now let some of the Masters of prescribing take up the tale.

*   *   *

GUERNSEY. Great fear of downward motion of every kind. Afraid to go downstairs ; can't swing, ride horseback, or use a rocking chair. Children spring up suddenly on being laid down in bed : or may be sleeping quietly, when they suddenly wake up, screaming and holding on to the sides of the cradle, without any apparent cause.

Hair rough and frowsy : eyelids turn in upon the eye : distension from flatus after every meal : stool before making water : dingy, unhealthy skin which ulcerates easily on being injured. Smoking may bring on diarrhœa.

FARRINGTON says :

Borax as a medicine won its first laurel in the nursery, where it has long been used in the treatment of sore nipples and children's sore mouth. Like all popular remedies, it has been greatly abused. Homœopathy has rescued it from the nursery and now offers it to the profession as a medicine of great value, telling when it may and may not be used. Underlying this sore mouth, which seems to be the keynote for the use of *Borax*, is a system or constitution which will permit of the sore mouth, that is, an ill-nourished system. Thus the infant becomes pale or of an earthy hue, its flesh grows soft and flabby ; it cries a great deal when it nurses, screams out during sleep and awakens clinging to its mother as if frightened by a dream. It is excessively nervous, so much so that the slightest noise, the mere rustling of paper, as well as a distant heavy noise, will arouse and frighten it. This nervous excitability qualifies the pains (of *Borax*). For instance, in earache, you will find that each paroxysm of pain causes the child to start nervously.

Borax is distinguished from those other remedies, *Belladonna*, *Pulsatilla* and *Chamomilla*, by this starting with the pain or from slight noises, by the paleness of the face and above all by another well-proved symptom, the dread of downward motion. It is not simply the motion that awakens the child, for the child will not awaken if it is moved without any downward motion. It must, then, be the downward motion that arouses it. The reason for this is, that the child is suffering from cerebral anæmia and this downward motion causes a feeling as though it were going to fall. You will also find that ladies, after some exhausting disease, cannot use a rocking chair, because, when they rock backwards, they feel as if they would tumble.

Aphthous inflammation of the mouth appears as a concomitant of the diarrhœa. The mouth is hot, which the mother notices when the child takes hold of the nipple. The child lets go of the nipple and cries with pain and vexation, or else refuses the breast.

BRYONIA has caused and cured infants' sore mouth. But the characteristic symptom in *Bryonia* is this ; the child refuses to nurse or makes a great fuss about it, but so soon as its mouth *is moistened*, it takes hold of the nipple and nurses energetically.

MERCURIUS, with the sore mouth, has profuse salivation.

ARUM TRIPHYLLUM is readily distinguished from *Borax* by the violence of the symptoms, and is accompanied by soreness and scabs around the mouth and nostrils.

I would advise to caution your nurses, not to use powdered borax every time the child has a sore mouth. It may do harm if not indicated. I think that I have noticed after its use that the bowels suffer and the child grows paler and dwindles rapidly, which it did not do before the meddlesomeness of the nurse.

From KENT : abstracts :—

Borax, is one of those domestic remedies, long used for all sorts of local conditions as a soothing substance, and for healing purposes. In " nursing sore mouth " of mother or child borax has been used as borax and honey, as a wash, . . . it is a fact that borax will rapidly heal up a sore mouth, and it is not strange that it does do, for *Borax* in its proving, produces aphthous conditions of the mouth, which extends down the throat and even into the stomach. It cures where the genitalia and anus are covered with these aphthous appearances.

Nervousness, anxiety, fidgetiness and sensitiveness are prominent in *Borax* . . . a state of turmoil and anxiety : aggravated by upward or downward motion. Going up in an elevator nearly drives him to distraction ; but is made worse by going downwards. All complaints are worse from downward motion. sore mouth in children with worse when laid down in bed :—cries out in fright · *Borax* is the remedy. . . . An intensified activity all through the body—hearing intensified ; oversensitive to all surroundings ; over anxious. Aggravation of anxiety till 11 p.m., he has noticed as the peculiar time of *Borax*. " You will notice sometimes in insane people that it seems as if they were possessed of the devil ; and at once a lucid interval will come and they will talk as if nothing had happened. So it is in *Borax* that a great change may occur at 11 p.m. ; this state of anxiety and nervous excitement may stop at that hour. . . .

" Here is another feature, while engaged in thinking at work, strong nausea . . . with the aggravation from mental exertion, from noise, from excitement, from downward motion, we get the mental aspect of *Borax*."

" The *Borax* patient with stomach aphthæ will gag and retch and cough : mothers say, ' It is a stomach cough because the child gags and retches with it.' "

Then the rectum ; thickening of the mucous membrane, with stricture growing smaller and smaller till only a long thin stool is passed . . . this inflammatory stricture has been cured by *Borax*.

The urine burns so that child screams with the desire to urinate. The hot urine burns like fire.

Membranous dysmenorrhœa, with violent labour-like pains before and during the flow, as if the uterus would expel itself from the vagina. I have known *Borax* cure when the membrane was a cast of the uterus : such patients are easily startled from downward motion : let that be your guide in membranous dysmenorrhœa.

When mother could not nurse the child, " The milk is too thick and tastes badly." If *Borax* is given at the beginning of pregnancy to a *Borax* patient it will change the milk, as well as the rest of the constitution, and the mother will be able to nurse the child. This remedy has loathing of the breast in infants, due to the fact that the milk tastes bad . . . the mother needs a dose of *Borax*.

BLACK LETTER SYMPTOMS

The child becomes anxious when dancing ; if one rocks it in arms it has an anxious expression of face during downward motion.

Anxious feeling during downward motion or rocking. Dread of downward motion.

Very anxious when riding rapidly down hill, contrary to his custom he feels as though it would take away his breath.

Anxious feeling during downward motion or rocking. (Diarrhœa.)

VERTIGO *and fullness in head on descending a mountain or stairs.*

APHTHÆ *with salivation.*

Aphthæ in mouth and on tongue, and inner surface of cheek, bleeding easily ; with great heat and dryness of mouth ; with cracked tongue.

Mouth of infant very hot.

Aphthæ are so tender that they prevent child from nursing.

Soft, light yellow, mucous STOOL.

Worse before URINATION.

Frequently cries and screams before the urine passes.

White albuminous, or starchy LEUCORRHŒA.

Leucorrhœa like the white of an egg, with sensation as if warm water were flowing down.

Acrid leucorrhœa, appearing for two weeks, between catamenia, with swelling of labia and inflamed and discharging Duvernis glands.
Sensation of warm water running down thighs.

PLEURITIC PAIN *in right pectoral region ; patient cannot move or breathe without a stitch.*
With every cough and deep inspiration, sticking in the chest.
Children may be sleeping quietly, and awake suddenly, screaming and holding on to sides of cradle without any apparent cause for so doing.
The infant frequently cries out in its sleep, and anxiously grasps its mother, as if it had been frightened by a dream.
She cannot fall asleep again for two hours, on account of heat in the whole body, especially in the head.
Period of dentition and infancy.

SOME CURIOUS, OR ITALIC SYMPTOMS

Fretful, ill-humoured, indolent and discontented before the easy stool in the afternoon ; after it lively, contented, and looking cheerfully into the future.

Easily startled by unusual sounds.

Fright : starts in all his limbs on hearing an anxious cry.

Strong nausea when thinking at his work ; with trembling of body and weakness of knees.

Vertigo and fullness of head descending a mountain or stairs ; driving down hills.

Hot head and chilliness.

Hair tangles at the tips, and sticks together.   If these bunches are cut off, they form again.

Hair rough and frowsy, cannot be combed smooth.

Eyelashes turn inwards towards eye and inflame it, especially at outer canthus, where margins of lids are very sore.

Eyelashes loaded with gummy, dry exudation, stick together in the morning.

Lower eyelids entirely inverted.   Difficult opening of lids.

Tip of nose shiny red : dry crusts in nose reform if removed.

Painful pressing downwards, right nostril, as if all the brain would be forced out.

Cobweb sensation, face.   Sensation of a bug crawling over under lip.

Crawling like insects on the lips.

Redness of gums above roots of teeth, front upper jaw.

Cramp, numbness and stiffness of tongue, impeding respiration.

Mucous membrane of palate in front seems burnt and shrivelled.

Cheerful, contented mood after stool.

Disagreeable sensation of emptiness in mammæ after suckling.

Milk too thick ; tastes badly, often curdles on being drawn. Loathing of the breasts in infants.

Colic of infants : they scream when laid down, or show signs of vertigo when carried downstairs.

Child throws up hands when an attempt is made to put it down.

Arrest of breath when lying in bed ; must jump up.

Sticking in chest when coughing.

Violent cough with slight expectoration of mouldy tastes and smell. Musty expectoration.

Sensation as if heart were on right side and being squeezed.

Phagedenic ulcers on joints of fingers and toes.

Infant cries out in sleep and grasps its mother.

Something pulls from spleen into chest.

BROMIUM

AMONG the drugs one has long desired to study is *Bromium* ; so we will attempt its portrayal for the benefit of all of us.

The one occasion on which its effect was dramatic enough to stamp it on the memory, was the case of a sailor on shore with asthma. In the Repertory one finds it, thus : " Asthma of sailors as soon as they go ashore, BROM.", in black type, and no other remedy given. Anyway it worked promptly. And one has added it as a second remedy in that other rubric, " Seashore ameliorates, *Med.*", which some of our prescribers find an absolutely straight tip to the successful use of *Medorrhinum*. When a case halts, Nosodes (potentized disease products) do help one out in a very marvellous way : or, on the other hand, they may make the subsequent use of the simpler, apparently indicated drug, operative.

With *Brom.*, deep forcible inspirations are necessary from time to time. He cannot *inspire* sufficiently. The glottis may close with a spasm.

Bromium, again, cannot stand dust or draughts. The two " Worse dust " remedies one has been able to discover are *Brom.* and *Lyss.*

Asthma is a very interesting condition, which many doctors find difficult to cure ; and the chemists must appreciate the income it affords them, in its palliation. A second of the halogens, *Chlorum* (Chlorine) has asthma with a very definite indication, DYSPNŒA ; CAN'T EXHALE. Another suggestive symptom is " Great dyspnœa : inspiration through the nose, while expiration was blown from the lips as in apoplexy". Among its modalities are, "Worse lying. Better from motion and in the open air."

In the asthma of *Iodum*, a third of the four halogens, it is the *inspirations* that are difficult (*Brom.*) ; and *Iodum* is markedly better for cold in every form, and worse for heat. It has also " emaciation with a ravenous appetite ".

The respiratory symptoms of *Fluorine*, which we use in the form of *Fluoric acid*, or rather hydrofluoric acid, appears to affect, in a minor degree—in that combination—the organs of respiration, and vents its spleen on scalp, glands, veins, bones and nerves. In regard to its pains, a queer modality was once obtained from a brilliant homœopathic chemist, " *Pain better by shaking the part* ". It was an unconscious memory, as he afterwards traced it, from a burn when etching on glass. The pain in question was a sciatica which had resisted all the prescribing of light and learning : only to yield to that " intuition " or unconscious memory and a few doses of *Fluor. a.* 30.

* * *

Where bromides are long used, to induce sleep in chronic sleeplessness, or for the suppression of epilepsy, the patient is gradually reduced to what one calls a " pimply idiot ". In *Bromism* the skin is first involved, with papules like acne. Then comes a lowering of cutaneous sensibility and of the pharynx ; with loss of powers, general and sexual. The intellect is dulled : the patient is depressed ; easily fatigued and unfit for work. The higher functions of the brain are depressed, before the lower —" in the reverse order of physiological development of the functions—(the Law of Dissolution) ".

Apply all this, in potencies, to just such a patient and you will be able to use *Bromium* curatively.

* * *

We are told that " if *Bromium* is introduced into a cut it becomes unhealthy looking ; a green decay forms about it, with an offensive odour." If you come across such a condition, again use *Brom.* in potency and cure. It will go straight to the spot.

It has pimples on nose, on tongue, on fingers, on anus : boils on arms, etc. It has " continued yawning with dyspnœa " and vivid dreams, of climbing, journeying, quarrels, fighting.

We will now let others, wiser and more experienced, take up the tale.

* * *

GUERNSEY says, *Bromine* affects particularly the internal head, left side. Important in diphtheria and croup, especially in children with thin, white, delicate skins, very light hair and eyebrows.

Mood cheerful, with desire for mental labour. (Primary action.)

Diphtheria begins in larynx and runs up. He talks of croupy sounds, loose rattling in larynx, but no choking with the cough, as with *Hepar*.

Affects chiefly eyes, chest and heart. In females it has a curious symptom, " escape of flatus from vagina ". [We have used this symptom, in prescribing *Brom.* in the " Gynæ. Dept."]

* * *

KENT gives many pages to *Bromium*. We will extract, condensing. He says : " It is so seldom indicated that most homœopaths give it up as a perfectly useless medicine. . . .

They give *Brom.* for diphtheria, and when it does not work, they give *Merc. cy.*, and when that does not work they give something else ' for diphtheria ', always *for diphtheria*.　They do not take the symptoms of the case, and prescribe in accordance with the individualizing method.　They do not prescribe for the *patient*, but for the disease.　You may not see more than half a dozen cases of diphtheria in the next twenty years, but when you see a *Bromium* case, you want to know *Bromium*. . . . An underlying feature, of *Brom.* is especially for individuals that are made sick from being heated.　Also complaints that come on after a very hot day in summer.　Getting overheated. . . . But after the complaint comes on, no matter where it is, he is so dreadfully sensitive to cold that a draught of cool air freezes him to the bones ; but he cannot stand being over-heated.

" Glands become hard, indurated ; but seldom suppurate. Remain hard.　Inflammation with hardness is the idea.　It has cured enlargement and great hardness of the thyroid.　Goitre. *Bromium* with some is a routine goitre remedy, and when that does not work, they try eggshell treatment, and when that does not work they try something else, instead of taking the symptoms of the patient.

" Emaciation—and tendency to infiltration :　it is not strange that it has been a curative medicine in tuberculosis and cancer. Weakness :　legs weak and prostrated ; growing prostration with trembling limbs.　Membranous exudate.　A natural feature of the mucous membrane is infiltration, so that mucous membrane appears to exudate little greyish-white exudations, and beneath them is induration.　That is true in ulcers.　An ulcer upon mucous membrane will eat in deeper and deeper and build beneath it all the time a hardened stratum of tissue. . . . ' Icy coldness of limbs.'　' Heat of head.'　Dyspnœa with great sweating. Croupy manifestations.

" Palpitation :　with nausea, with headache, with nervous excitement.　Aversion to work, to reading.　No interest in household duties.　Indifferent ; tired.　Sad and discouraged.　Ear troubles with parotid enlarged and hard.　Swelling and hardness of left parotid. . . . Flushed face.　Hot-blooded, easily heated. But this is entirely the opposite of the chronic constitutional *Bromium* condition.　Oldish appearance.　Chronic *Bromium* will have the sickly, grey, ash-coloured face.　Or plethoric children have red face, and are easily over-heated.　Of course, where dyspnœa has lasted for hours, or many days, the patient becomes cyanotic and pale :　gasping, and choking, as in diphtheria, in croup, in laryngeal affections.

" *Bromium* fits the most malignant type of diphtheria. The membrane grows like a weed ; shuts off breathing, closes the larynx. Begins in throat and goes into larynx. Great violence : afterwards great prostration. A great many of the cures by *Brom.* have been in left-sided diphtheria : yet it has cured both sides. You will seldom see *Bromium* develop in cold, dry weather : but in hot, damp weather.

" Chronic stomach ulcers. Vomiting with signs of ulceration. Vomiting or diarrhœa are worse after eating. Worse acids ; oysters ; tobacco smoke. Worse warm things, hot tea, hot drinks. ' Pains from taking hot foods.' Membranous stools. Black, fæcal stool ; must go to stool after eating.

" Enlarged veins. Protruding hæmorrhoids : smart day and night. ' Blind, intensely painful hæmorrhoids, with black, diarrhœic stool.'

" Jumps up for want of breath : gasping and suffering for breath. Sneezing, and rattling in larynx. Air passages as if full of smoke, or fumes from sulphur, or tar. . . . Tickling, or sensation of coldness in larynx. As if larynx covered with down, or velvet, but it feels so cold. The air breathed feels cold, as if blown off snow or ice . . . sneezing, hoarseness, irritation in respiratory tract from handling dusty things."

BLACK LETTER SYMPTOMS (*Allen, Hering*)

She does not feel as she generally does, but can't tell why.

PAROTIDS, *mostly left, affected.*
Swelling and hardness of left parotid, warm to touch.
Suppuration of left parotid : discharge watery and excoriating : swelling remains hard and unyielding. (Especially after scarlet fever.)

Long-continued obstinate CORYZA, *with soreness beneath nose and on margin of the nose.*

Grey, earthy colour of FACE.

Stony hard swelling of GLANDS, *especially on lower jaw and throat.*
Diphtheria or croup.

Periodically much pain in left *hypochondrium and iliac regions. Pain violent, as if a sore inside.*

Black, fecal STOOLS.

VARICES, *anus, worse application of cold or warm water.*

Loud emissions of flatus from vagina.

Cold sensation in LARYNX, *with cold feeling on inspiring.*
*Chronic hoarseness.   Hoarseness : loss of voice : he cannot speak
clearly.*
Scraping and rawness provoking dry cough ; in the evening.
A feeling as if the pit of the throat were pressed against the trachea.
Cough with paroxysms of suffocation.
Rattling of mucus in larynx when coughing : cough sounds croupy.
DIPHTHERIA, *when disease commences in larynx and comes up
to fauces ; or in some cases where it runs down to larynx, with croupy
cough and rattling of mucus.*
No choking with cough, as with Hepar.
Much rattling in larynx when breathing : more when coughing.
*Danger of suffocation from phlegm in larynx.   (Ant. tart. has
rattling lower down in chest.)*
*Croupous inflammation formed by exuberant growth of fungi.
(Diphtheria.)*
Constriction of CHEST ; *no cough ; with difficulty of breathing.*
ASTHMA *of sailors as soon as they go ashore.*
Symptoms of croup during whooping cough.

Icy cold forearms.

*Diphtheria : great weakness and lassitude when all symptoms
have passed off.*

Blonde, red-cheeked, scrofulous girls.
*Scrofulous swelling, glands, several already in suppuration :
thyroid ; testes ; submaxillary ; parotid.*

KENT says of *Bromium* :—" Its complaints come on in the
night, after a very hot day ; yet after the complaint comes on, he
is so dreadfully sensitive to cold that a draft of cool air freezes
him to the bone.
" *Bromine* infiltrates glands : which become hard but seldom
suppurate.   Inflammation with hardness is the idea.
" *Bromium* fits the most malignant type of diphtheria.   The
membrane grows like a weed ; shuts off breathing ; closes up the
larynx."

BRYONIA

Bryonia is one of the priceless remedies of Homœopathy, especially useful in acute diseases. *Bryonia* is also a remedy of very definite symptoms that can hardly be missed, therefore it is one of the easiest to prescribe with assurance. It was one of Hahnemann's earliest provings—one of those " without which", as Dudgeon says, " we might indeed shut up shop "

Hence *Bryonia* finds its way into every handbook of Homœo-pathy, and into every domestic medicine chest. But—it behoves us to know when and how to use it, if we want to see the miracle work.

Guernsey says, of Bryonia, " The great characteristic of this drug is *aggravation produced by any motion*. The patient cannot bear a disturbance of any kind, either mental or physical. Can't sit up in bed, as it makes the patient so sick and faint, even when rising to take a drink of water. Moving from one side of the bed to the other is not so bad, but the patient *cannot sit up*."

Let us follow this out into the provings. This *Worse from motion*, with.*Bryonia*, is such a constant symptom with sufferings in all parts of the body, as to have become a *General*.

Motion aggravates the vertigo and headache ;
　　　　　　the fullness in the forehead ;
　　　　　　(worse even from moving the eyes !)
　　　　　　the severe pulsating pains in head ;
　　　　　　the shooting pains in head and eyes ;
　　　　　　the expanding headaches, etc. ;
　　　　　　the pains everywhere.

Worse for movement are :
　　　　　　the vomiting ;
　　　　　　the fullness and pressure in stomach ;
　　　　　　the cutting and constricting pains in
　　　　　　　stomach ;
　　　　　　the burning and stitching in stomach ;
　　　　　　the excessive pain in stomach ;
　　　　　　the griping and cutting in intestines ;
　　　　　　the colic ;
　　　　　　the sticking and shooting pains in abdomen ;
　　　　　　the involuntary passing of urine ;
　　　　　　the after-pains ;
　　　　　　the pains of an inflamed breast.

Worse from motion are :

the pains in lumbar region,
the stiffness, tearing, tenderness there ;
the pains of sprained wrist ,
the pain and swelling of finger joints ;
the sticking pains there ;
the sciatic pains ;
the stiffness and stitches in knees ;
the pains in calf—in ankle—in joints ;
the sweats—the aching—the faintness—the
chills ;
the soreness in periosteum, ligaments, etc.,
etc.

So we can add to the *worse for movement* of the everywhere-present *Bryonia* pains, their character—STITCHING AND STICKING.
Stitchings, deep in brain : in head : in eyes : deep in ear :
in teeth : in throat : in stomach : in abdomen :
in liver : in spleen : in chest :
in intercostal spaces and sternum : in glands :
in heart-region : between shoulder-blades, and
under the left, extending to heart :
in arms, elbow, wrist, fingers, knees, soles, big toe :
in ALL SEROUS MEMBRANES, pericardium, pleura,
meninges, linings of joints.
And all these are also worse from motion.

And now, to complete the *Bryonia* picture, we must add to the WORSE FROM MOTION, and the characteristic STICKING PAINS, the RELIEF FROM PRESSURE. This is, of course, in part at least, a corollary of the *worse from motion :* because pressure tends to keep the suffering parts still.

And here *Bryonia* differs fundamentally from *Belladonna* (both inflammatory drugs) in regard to causation and to cure. *Belladonna* is intolerant of the slightest pressure, or increase of pressure. The throbbing pains of *Belladonna*—in a " felon ", for instance, are intensified with even the extra pressure of blood in the part from every heart-beat. . . . And yet, when a student, I watched a fellow-student, a senior, with horror, as she applied a fomentation to a whitlow in the form of a hot hard pad of wool, bandaged tightly on to *one side* of the finger ! Students and doctors do the best work where they have themselves experienced the agonies they are treating. " Fancy bandaging " is supreme cruelty to a *Belladonna* patient ; for it is difficult to do a really pretty piece of bandaging otherwise than firmly. During the war I used to be told that, at La Panne, the wounded dreaded being bandaged by a certain Queen who helped to nurse them : she bandaged too tightly.

A *Belladonna* pneumonia will never be found lying on the " sore side ". A *Bryonia* pneumonia will lie on the inflamed side, to keep it still, or on the back—never on the good side ; for that would keep the useful side compressed and still, and inflict more active movements on the painful side of the chest.

Another leading characteristic of *Bryonia* is DRYNESS. The dry stage of pleurisy, where the inflamed surfaces rubbing together with every breath, produce the stitching pains. Dryness of inflamed serous membranes—pericardium—pleura—meninges of brain—linings of joints. Dryness also of lips, of tongue ; of intestines, causing constipation with dry, hard, dark stools. Painful, dry, spasmodic cough, with pains as if the head would fly to pieces ; with bursting pains in head and chest, needing support and pressure to limit their intensity.

Kali carb. has also these severe sticking pains in chest with pneumonia and pleurisy ; but the pains of *Bryonia* are only with movement—with respiration ; whereas those of *Kali carb.* come independently of respiration.

One remembers a striking *Kali carb.* case—a severe case of right-sided pleuro-pneumonia in *December* 1917, when pneumonias were common and severe.

Man, 65. Had been taken suddenly ill at his work. Brought into our Hospital on the fourth day of illness : had been unable to rest or to sleep for these three nights because of the pain.

On admission, temp. 104, respiration 39, "prune-juice" expectoration. Great pain, extorting cries. But these stabbing pains were found to be independent of respiration, and the pneumonia was, as said, right-sided. He was given *Kali carb.* 30 two-hourly, and in two hours the pain had stopped, and he had a good night. Next day the temperature was down two degrees, and on the third day its highest was 99·4, and that ended it. He made a good and rapid recovery.

And here is a little *Bryonia* case about the same time. A naval patient, aged 41, was sent in by the Admiralty, with pleuro-pneumonia ; again right base, with a temp. of 103·4, respiration 44, and stained sputum. *His* symptoms suggested *Bryonia*, which was given in the 200th and then 1m potencies. On the second day temp. had dropped a degree, on the third day (the fourth day of his illness) it was already subnormal, with a small rise in the evening :—and that ended the case. He made a rapid and uninterrupted recovery.

With such, i.e. real, Homœopathy, if the case is treated early, one sees again and again that it is possible to abort pneumonia. I suppose many more cases of pleuro-pneumonia call for *Bryonia* than for any other medicine, even *Phosphorus*. One could produce a number from Hospital records, to the few that have demanded *Kali carb.*, . . . that is to say, *whose symptoms have demanded Kali carb.* But in Homœopathy, one medicine will not do for another. Homœopathy is individualization. It is not enough to diagnose pneumonia, and to give a pneumonia medicine. With Hahnemann we must diagnose " a kind of pneumonia— a kind of pleurisy ". And what kind ?—Why, a *Phosphorus* kind— a *Bryonia* kind—a *Kali carb.* kind—a *Natrum sulph.* kind—a *Mercurius* kind—of pneumonia. It is the symptoms, always, that decide, if *curative* work is to be done. One may palliate, and the patient gets well, with perhaps less suffering ; but that is not CURE.

Turning the pages yet further, one is tempted to give one other interesting case, about the same date, of broncho-pneumonia aborted in a child of three years.

She was seen in the out-patient department March 14th, 1918. Temperature at noon was 100·4, resp. 40. Her mother had been up with her all night, she had been burning hot, crying and coughing. Refused food. She " had been burning hot at night for eight days ". There were " creps " at rt. base, and (?) left. She was given *Bryonia* 1m six-hourly. The result was " beautiful rest at night " ; but as there were (the next day)" creps " at both bases and respiration was 48, she was admitted and given *Bry.* 10m. (three doses). Next day the temperature was subnormal, respiration 29-36. The temperature did not rise again, and she made an uneventful recovery.

Broncho-pneumonia is elsewhere found a dangerous and lengthy disease for little children : the statistics of homœopathy in this disease are excellent.

Different remedies pick out different organs or tissues. *Bryonia* especially selects serous membranes, to irritate, and therefore in fine dosage to stimulate and to heal. It has a tremendous effect on pleura and on lung,—and is one of the drugs that has produced pneumonia.

Bryonia's time aggravations are—3 a.m., when its delirium, its profuse night-sweats, and its toothache are worse. 9 p.m. is also one of *Bryonia's* bad hours : and there is apt to be profuse urination from 6-7 p.m. Many of *Bryonia's* symptoms are worse in the morning, and many worse in the evening.

A queer *Bryonia* symptom is given by Hahnemann, " on slight mental emotion (on laughing) there suddenly occurs a shooting (itching) burning all over the body as if he had been whipped with nettles or had nettlerash, though nothing is to be seen on the skin ; this burning came on afterwards by merely thinking of it, or when he got heated ".

Bryonia is a great *East wind* remedy. The " aetiology " of certain remedies is of great importance. For instance, the complaints of *Dulcamara* come on in cold DAMP weather—from the chill of a wetting—or a wetting when hot—or a chill when heated. *Bryonia* and a few others have acute sufferings that come on after exposure to cold, dry EAST wind. Such are *Acon.*, *Asar.*, *Caust.*, *Hep.*, *Kali c.*, *Nux*, *Sep.*, *Spong.*, etc.

Bryonia is one of the remedies of *nosebleed* (but here, *Vipera* is in our experience the especially effective remedy—even when the condition has been life-long). It, *Bryonia*, is the great remedy of vicarious menstruation—nosebleed or vomiting of blood.

Here is a tip from one of our teachers, who speaks from personal experience. In a *Natrum mur.* patient with a severe headache, do not give *Natrum mur.* for the acute condition or you will fearfully intensify the suffering. Give its " acute " *Bryonia* ; and only the *Natrum mur.* in a quiescent period.

Mentally, and in delirium, *Bryonia* is commonplace. Its chief note is ANXIETY : anxiety about the future : about the everyday concerns of life. Dreams, and in delirium talks, about the business of the day. Irrational talking about his business : prattling about the business that must be attended to. *Wants to get out of bed and go home.* Irritable and morose.

It is a great remedy for the breasts. " Breasts heavy, of a stony hardness ; pale but hard ; hot and painful." While in *Belladonna* inflammations there is bright redness, with burning skin, and much throbbing. In one case of cancer of the breast, where *Bryonia* was given because of a big pleural effusion, it astonishingly improved the breast condition as well as wiping out the effusion which one had been afraid to aspirate.

Here are some of Allen's and Hahnemann's black-type symptoms, especially characteristic of *Bryonia*, and which *Bryonia* has much caused and much cured.

ANXIETY ; he is apprehensive about the future.
Irrational talking about his business.
Very ill-humoured ; troubled with needless anxiety.
Morose : everything puts him out of humour.
Dreams full of quarrelling and vexacious things.

Dreams all night very vividly of anxious and careful attention to his business. In his dreams he is occupied with household affairs.

During sleep was continually busy with what he had read the evening previous.

Delirious prattling about business to be attended to.

Confusion of the head.

Vertigo as soon as he rises from his chair.

On rising from bed in the morning, dizzy and whirling, as if head were turning in a circle.

Headache commences in the morning, when first opening and moving the eyes.

Pressive frontal headache, very much increased by stooping.

In the occiput, obtuse pain.

A pressing pain in the occiput, with drawing down into the neck ; relieved towards noon.

Digging pressure in the front of the brain, with pressing towards the forehead, especially violent when stooping or walking quickly. A walk tires him very much.

Headache on stooping, as if everything would fall out at the forehead ; as if everything would press out at the forehead.

Pressive pain above the right eye, followed by dull pressing pain in the occiput, whence it spread over the whole body, and continued more or less severe the whole day : on quick motion and after eating the pain became so severe that it seemed like a distinct pulsation within the head.

An out-pressing pain in both temples.

Pain in left eyeball, especially violent on moving the ball.

Frequent lachrymation.

In the morning eyes as if gummed up with matter.

Nosebleed for a quarter of an hour in the morning.

Red, hot, soft puffiness of the face.

Drawing, sometimes twitching toothache in the molars of left upper jaw, only during and after eating, at the same time the teeth felt too long and as if they waggled to and fro.

Pain as if a tooth were screwed in and then pulled out, momentarily relieved by cold water.

(Toothache about 3 a.m.) which becomes aggravated on lying on the painless side, and then goes away if one lies on the painful cheek.

Very white, coated tongue. Tongue thickly coated white.

Dryness in the mouth : mouth very dry. Violent thirst.

Collection of much soapy frothy saliva in the mouth.

Insipid, sickly taste in the mouth : he has almost no taste.

Offensive, bitter taste. Intensely bitter taste on the tongue.

Frequent drinking of cold water relieved the bitter taste and the inclination to vomit.

Excessive thirst.

Great thirst : obliged to drink much cold water.

Great thirst : she can and must drink a great deal at once.

Excessive hunger.

No appetite for milk ; but when he takes it the appetite for it comes, and he commences to relish it.

Great longing for coffee.

After a meal bitter eructations : or sourish.

After eating, pressure in the stomach, as if a stone lay there and made him cross.

As if a stone lay in stomach, after eating : epigastric region painful to touch : painful to pressure. (N.B., only here is *Bryonia* not relieved by pressure, i.e. in stomach and abdomen.)

Pasty offensive evacuations in the afternoon, followed by burning in anus.

Diarrhœa preceded by cutting in the abdomen.

Obstinate constipation.

Dry, parched stool, with effort.

Urine dark, almost brown.

Fluent coryza for eight days.

Severe coryza without cough.

Viscid phlegm in the fauces that was detached by hawking.

Dry cough.

Irritation to hacking cough : it seems as if some mucus were in the windpipe ; when he coughs for some time he feels a pain there compounded of soreness and pressure : the pain becomes more violent by speaking and smoking tobacco.

When he comes from the open into a warm room he has a feeling as if a vapour were in the windpipe, which compels him to cough. He feels as if he could not breathe in air enough.

Viscid phlegm in the windpipe, detached by frequent hacking cough.

When coughing it always goes into the head like a pressure.

Stitches in the sternum on coughing he was obliged to hold the chest with the hand.

Internal heat in the chest.

Sharp outward shooting pain under the right nipple, in the cavity of the chest, only on expiring.

*   *   *

(Here are some of ALLEN's italic symptoms, which are very important) :

Short, but violent stitches in the right side of chest, so that he was obliged to hold his breath and could not cry out.

Stitches in the right side of chest between the third and fourth ribs.

Tearing stitches in left side of chest, extend from behind forward, are relieved during rest, aggravated during motion and on deep respiration. (Perhaps we are doing wrong to give only the black-type symptoms: those in italics are tremendously important also !)

Weariness and heaviness in all the limbs.

Swelling elbow joint and somewhat below and above it, to the middle of the upper and forearm, and of the feet.

In the wrist-joint pain as if sprained or dislocated at every movement.

In the fingers shooting pains when writing.

Great weakness in thighs ; he can hardly go upstairs : less when going downstairs.

Tensive, painful stiffness of the knees.

Stitches in knees when walking.

Knees totter and bend under him when walking.

Legs are so weak that they can scarcely support him, on beginning to walk, and even when standing.

Hot swelling of the foot.

Hot swelling of the instep, with bruised pain on stretching out. The foot seems tense on stepping on it, and on touch it pains like an abscess.

Very much inclined to yawn. Frequent yawning all day.

On rising, great exhaustion and weakness—had to drag himself about.

On rising from bed he was attacked by faintness.

After the midday siesta he is chilly and dazed in the head.

Great thirst (he must drink much cold fluid) with internal heat, without being hot to the touch externally.

Sensation of heat in the face with redness of it and thirst.

He perspires all over when walking in the cool air.

Profuse nocturnal sweat from 3 a.m.

Sour sweats.

Until Dr. Haehl, of Stuttgart, in recent years, and after long search, discovered Hahnemann's voluminous case books—

relegated to an attic !—and established them in his Hahnemann Museum at Stuttgart, *Bryonia* had the distinction of figuring in one of the very few cases from his colossal lifework that were, till then, available (at all events in his better known publications). It is worth re-telling. He gives it to illustrate his method of *taking the case*, and *finding the remedy*. As such, it may be interesting to republish it *in extenso* some day.

A washerwoman had come from a neighbouring village to ask for help. She was crippled with pain, and had been unable to work for some weeks. Hahnemann took her symptoms with the care he enjoins on us, and then went through them, jotting down the remedies that had caused, and could therefore cure such symptoms, till *Bryonia* was seen to alone cover the entire picture.

In those early days, he administered a dose of *Bryonia* in the strong tincture, and sent her away.

When, a couple of days later, she failed to return, one of his disciples was anxious to know the effect of the remedy. " Go, then, and find out," suggested Hahnemann. The woman was found at her tub, busy and indignant. She said that *the pain had left her the very next day, and that she had remained well. All these weeks she had been unable to earn her livelihood—did the doctor expect her to leave her work and go all those miles to tell him that she was cured ?*

Bryonia was one of Burnett's *Fifty Reasons for being a Homœopath*. Let him tell the tale.

" When I was a lad I had pleurisy of the left side, and, with the help of a village apothecary, and half-a-hogshead of mixture, nearly died, though not quite ; from that time on I had a dull, uneasy sensation in my side, about which I consulted many eminent physicians in various parts of Europe, but no one could help me. All agreed that it was an old adhesive something between the visceral and costal layers of the pleura, *but no one of my many eminent advisers could cure it*. And yet my faith in them was big enough to remove mountains : so faith as a remedy did no good.

" When orthodox medicine proved unhelpful, I went to the hydropaths (they were called " quacks " then !) and had it hot, and cold, and long ; but they also did me no good. Packs cold, and the reverse ; cold compresses worn for months together ; sleeping in wet sheets ; no end of sweatings—Turkish and Russian —all left my old pleuritic trouble *in statu quo ante*.

" The grape cure, the bread and wine cure, did no better. Nor did diet and change help me.

" However, when I was studying what the peculiar people

called Homœopaths have to say about their *Bryonia alba*, and its affinity for serous membranes, I—What ?—abused them and called them quacks ? No !—I bought some *Bryonia alba*, and took it as they recommended, and in a fortnight my side was well, and has never troubled me since.

" There, friend, that is my second reason for being a homœo-path, and when I cease to be grateful to dear old Hahnemann for his *Bryonia*, may my old pleural trouble return to remind me of the truth of his teaching.

" What you and the world in general may think of it I care not one straw : I speak well of the bridge that carried *me* over.

" For my part, I make but one demand of medicine, and one only, *that it shall cure !* The pathy that will cure is the pathy for me. For of your fairest pathy I can but say—

> ' What care I how fair she be,
> If she be not fair to *me* ? ' "

From the above we see that not only is *Bryonia* a great remedy in acute pleurisy, but that it can also cure the chronic condition sometimes left by pleurisy.

NASH says : " It makes no difference what the name of the disease, if the patient feels greatly better by lying still and suffers greatly on the slightest motion, and the more and the longer he moves the more he suffers, *Bryonia* is the first remedy to be thought of, and there must be very strong counter-indications along other lines that will rule it out."

Nash also says : " The dominant school do not know what they have lost in not being acquainted with the virtues of this remedy, as developed in our provings and clinical use, but we know what we have gained."

*　　　*　　　*

And now, to sum up. . . . If you ever get a patient with severe stitching pains : worse for the slightest movement : worse for sitting up : better for pressure : very thirsty for long drinks of cold water : very irritable : angry, and not only angry, but with sufferings increased by being disturbed mentally or physically : white tongue : in delirium " wants to go home " (even when at home) : busy in his dreams and in delirium with his everyday business, you can administer BRYONIA *and—bet on the result !*

CALCAREA

THIS remedy, impure calcium carbonate, is a trituration of the middle layer of the oyster shell. It was proved by Hahnemann; and Clarke calls it " one of the greatest monuments of Hahnemann's genius. . . . His method of preparing insoluble substances " (by trituration) " brought to light, in this instance, a whole world of therapeutic power formerly unknown."

*   *   *

Some remedies are difficult to spot : the difficulty is to *miss* *Calcarea*, when typical.

Calcarea has at least five definite pictures in the provings; they are distinct, yet they merge into one another.

There is the teething picture.
The picture of rickets.
The picture of anæmia.
The picture of tuberculosis.
The picture of mental deficiency, and decay.

In *Calc.* the child is father to the man—or woman. If you know the *Calcarea* child, you realize *Calc.* later on in life.

First, then, the *teething* picture : the fat, flabby baby, with fair hair, a big head (often sour-smelling), that perspires furiously at night in sleep, and wets the pillow far and wide. Dentition is delayed. The teeth that should begin to appear, don't. The gums are swollen, throbbing, sore. You are told that " her milk disagrees " : she vomits, sour water, sour curds ; sour water runs from the mouth. *Calc.* is very sour ; the stools smell sour— sour and pungent—excoriate. (In *Lyc.* it is the urine that burns and excoriates : in *Calc.*, *Sulph.* and others, the stool.) In *Calc.* the stool (in diarrhœa or in constipation) may be white like chalk. Bracelets of fat begin to surround the wrists and ankles, the rickety rosary may be felt. Fontanelles are slow to close— teeth to erupt—bones are slow to bear weight, of poor quality— bend.

Cough: a " teething cough ". (One used to give something for the bronchitis and with it *Calc.* to help the teeth through, till one found that *Calc.* covered both—in a *Calc.* child.)

All this merges into the *rickety child*. The *Calcarea* child of the Provings and the *Materia Medica*, is the typical rickety child.

The fat, fair, pallid child is brought in, and dumped down onto a chair, and *sits there*. No wriggling down to wander about, and touch everything in the room. She sits there, lethargic and dull. Perhaps plays with her fingers and picks them.

With the chalky complexion, goes—

Fatness without fitness.

Sweating without heat.

Bones without strength.

Tissues of plus quantity and minus quality.

Mere flabby bulk, with weakness and weariness.

The *Calc.* head, when you inquire, still sweats exceedingly. Sweats when cold. Sweats in a cold room. Sweats at night and soaks the pillow. (It is *Calc.* and *Sil.* that soak the pillow at night and during sleep ; but their pictures are so different.)

In *Calc.* everything is slow, and late, and heavy, and weak.

You will be told about the night-terrors ; how the child starts out of sleep screaming with terror ; knows no one ; can hardly be pacified. Is trembling with fear. " *Calc.* children have dreadful times in their dreams," Kent says. And *Calc.* has a wonderful record for curing night terrors.

Calc. desires eggs ; eats lime, slate pencils, earth (*Alum.*), chalk, clay, raw potatoes, sweets, ice cream, etc.

And later on, hates coffee, meat, milk (or likes milk which disagrees) ; hates tobacco.

Stomach swollen " like an inverted saucer ".

A third picture—further on in life—" the leucophlegmatic patient ", as she has been called,—fat, fair, flabby. She comes in puffily, and presents you with a froggy hand, that makes you shiver and look round for soap and water—so boneless it is, so moist and cold. You can spot *Calc.* by that hand.

She will give the symptoms of her ANÆMIA : her weariness, her weakness, her palpitation. Her breathlessness on going up the slightest ascent. Her sensation of chest too full of blood ; head too full of blood.

Her chilliness. Her tendency to sweat, especially about head and feet. How she sweats when cold ; in a cold room ; in sleep. How her coldness comes in patches, even spots—cold head, cold feet, cold abdomen, cold thigh, cold scalp ; icy cold.

(*Sulph.* has heat in patches : *Calc.* has cold in patches, and, Kent says, sweat in patches.)

Here you see a great fat woman, without strength, breath, energy, firmness, colour, health. Such weakness! such weariness! such breathlessness! such palpitation!

She will tell you that her menses are too early, too profuse, too long-lasting : are apt to recur with any exertion or excitement.

And then her cramps! She cannot get into a cold bed without cramp. She stretches out her leg in bed and gets cramp : calves, fingers, and toes all indulge in painful cramps (*Cuprum*).

And she is so easily sprained. Has pain in the small of the back as if sprained ; is unable to lift anything heavy ; and sweat breaks out suddenly ; in the morning ; at odd times.

And she has a curious feeling as if tight-laced about the waist. Has rushes of blood to head. Vertigo on turning head.

I once saw *Calcarea* clear up a very bad case of pernicious anæmia for several years. I had tried things on various indications, then gave *Calc.* because her chalky face looked like it. She lived far away and gave up treatment at last, and relapsed and died. But she bloomed and got strong meanwhile.

Then the T.B. type. All foreshadowed in the provings. They tell of submaxillary glands as big as hens' eggs (*Dros.*). Of hard swellings in submaxillary glands. Ulcers, with indurations about them.

Night sweats.

Abdomen very much distended ; hard, swollen glands in both groins.

But all in a "*Calc.* patient, whether adult or child"

Kent describes it thus : "Children with cold feet, emaciated extremities, enlarged abdomen, stomach distended like an inverted saucer, bloated abdomen. Cold, and sensitive to cold. Pale skin. Pale, waxy face."

Then, the chest is so sore—so sensitive to touch and inspiration. So tight. So full up with blood.

And the cough—the tickling cough, with sweetish expectoration and spitting of blood. Yes : the provings suggest rickets, anæmia, tuberculosis.

Then the Calcarea mental picture.

So frightened—so afraid!

The terrors at night ; after sleep ; on waking from sleep.

Fear ; fear ; fear.

Fear that something is going to happen to herself, or to someone else.

Fear that she will lose her reason, and that people will notice.

Fear that people will notice her confusion of mind.

Fearfulness, with restlessness and vague fear. Fear of Death.

Can't help it ! She sits—sits and fidgets with small things—bends pins by the hour.

Broods over little things that have no importahce.

Dread and aversion to labour.

Fear of consumption.

Peevish ; fretful ; obstinate.

Thoughts vanish. Brain feels paralysed—can't think or remember ; with confusion.

Dread of disease and suffering. Despairs of her life and reason.

Calc. epilepsy has for aura the " mouse sensation " Sensation of a mouse running up arm or leg. (*Bell.* has this also, and *Sil.*)

NASH says, " If *Calcarea* has one symptom that not only leads all the rest, but also all other remedies, it is found in the PROFUSE SWEATS ON THE HEAD OF LARGE-HEADED, OPEN FONTANELLED CHILDREN. The sweat is so profuse that during sleep it rolls down the head and face, wetting the pillow far around. Many a little child has been saved from dying of hydrocephalus, dentition, rachitis, marasmus, eclampsia, cholera infantum, etc., where this sweating symptom was the guiding symptom to the use of *Calcarea.*

He also draws attention to malnutrition as one of the disorders calling for *Calcarea.* He quotes from Hering's *Guiding Symptoms :*

" Tardy development of the bony tissues with lymphatic enlargements."

"Curvature of the bones, especially spine and long bones."

" Extremities deformed, crooked."

" Softening of the bones : fontanelles remain open too long, and skull very large."

And he adds, these symptoms " show the lack of, or imperfect nutrition of bones. They are nourished irregularly, or unevenly. One part of a bone, the vertebræ for instance, is nourished, while the other is starved. While all this irregular bone development is going on the soft parts are suffering from over-nutrition. This we have recorded in the pathogenesis, tendency to obesity, especially in children and young people."

By the way—*Calc.* is the chronic of *Belladonna :* i.e. when *Bell.* has again and again helped the acute condition, *Calc.* will be curative, and so, prevent its recurrence.

Now we will conclude with some points from KENT :

" *Calcarea* sweats in spots. . . . When *Calcarea's* feet become cold, they sweat.* . . .

* Cold sweat, feet and legs, sensation of damp stockings, *Sepia* also.—ED.

" Children going through difficult dentition have dreadful times in their dreams : screech out in the night, and the pillow is wet all round the head. . . .

" *Calcarea* produces that kind of anæmia known as chlorosis. It produces a most pernicious anæmia. . . .

" Sensitiveness to cold and weakness run through the remedy . . . fat, flabby, very anæmic subjects. *Calc.* is a very tired patient . . .

" They go into a state of enlarged glands, emaciation of neck and limbs, while abdominal fat and glands increase. *Calc.* has both fat flabby and pale patients, and it has emaciated states too. . . .

" *Calcarea* children long for eggs : and are better for eating eggs.

" They have sour, pungent stools with undigested milk.

" Tickling cough.*

" Relaxation of tissues everywhere—muscles—veins—especially of lower limbs and anus, i.e. hæmorrhoids or varicose veins of legs. . . .

" *Calcarea* grows and cures polypi—in the *Calcarea* patient. And *Calcarea* babies are almost always more or less wormy.

" Indurations in ulcers—base of ulcers—round about ulcers, i.e. its wonderful use in palliating and restraining malignant ulcers, as these have always an indurated base. Old cancerous ulcers are greatly restricted in growth : patient improved : very much more endurance, and the ulcers will take on healing. In cancerous affections that would kill in sixteen months, the patient will live five years with *Calc.*—if *Calc.* is indicated."

Kent says that infants fed with lime water in the milk soon become lime subjects : unable to take lime from their natural food, they grow fat and flabby. But the natural lime cases are born so, with inability to absorb lime from their natural food, and they grow fat and flabby, and produce deficient bone : deficient teeth, or no teeth. He says, " What a foolish notion to feed that infant lime, because he cannot digest lime. . . . Now it is astonishing that one single dose of the potency will make that infant commence to digest its food, and appropriate therefrom all the lime it needs for its bones and elsewhere. All at once the teeth begin to grow, the bones begin to grow, the little

* Here one recalls an old, fat woman, typically *Calcarea*, as described. She had a tickling cough at night for years, which disturbed her neighbours, and got her people up to get her hot water to drink. A dose of *Calcarea*, high, stopped the cough for a whole year.

fellow s legs get stiff enough for him to walk and they will hold him up.

"It is a peculiar feature of *Calcarea*, that the more marked the congestion of internal parts, the colder the surface becomes. With chest troubles, and stomach troubles, and bowel troubles, the feet and hands become like ice, and covered with sweat ; and he lies in bed sometimes with a fever in the rest of the body, and the scalp covered with cold sweat. That is strange. You cannot account for that by any process of reasoning in pathology, and when a thing is so strange that it cannot be accounted for, it becomes very valuable as descriptive of the remedy, and is one that cannot be left out when prescribing for a patient."

* * *

HAHNEMANN first proved *Calc. acet.* His proving of *Calc. carb.* appears in Vol. II of his *Chronic Diseases.* He says : " Take a clean oyster shell, somewhat thick ; of the soft snow-white calcarean substance which is found between the internal and external hard shell, take one grain, which is then to be triturated and dynamized in the usual manner."

He says, *inter alia*, " *Calcarea* generally is indispensable and curative when the catamenia appear a few days before the period, especially when the flow is considerable. But if the catamenia appear at the regular period or a little later, *Calcarea* is almost never useful, even if the catamenia should be rather profuse."

" In affections of persons advanced in age, *Calcarea*, even after other intermediate remedies, can scarcely be repeated with advantage ; a dose which is given after another without any previous intermediate remedy, is almost always prejudicial ; in cases of children, however, several doses may be given in succession, provided the remedy continues to be indicated : the younger the children the more frequently may the remedy be repeated."

BLACK LETTER SYMPTOMS

Thinking is difficult.

Visions of faces and persons, when eyes are closed.

Fears that she will lose her reason, or that people will observe her confusion of mind.

Anxiety, shuddering and dread as soon as evening comes on, with fear of death.

Great anxiety, restlessness and palpitation.

Despairing, hopeless of ever getting well, with fear of death ; tormenting all around, day and night.

Children self-willed, inclined to grow fat.

After exerting mind ; hyperæmia of head ; chorea ; trembling spells.

Excitement brings on dysmenorrhœa ; least excitement endangers return of catamenia, or causes.

Vertigo ; when climbing into high places ; on going upstairs, or up a hill ; on suddenly raising or turning head, even when at rest ; on walking in open air, as if he would tumble, especially on suddenly turning HEAD *; with stupefaction and a sensation of falling (neurosis cordis) with inclination to fall backward or sideways ; with headache ; nausea and vomiting, incarcerated flatulence ; accompanied by nausea and a feeling as though one would fall unconscious ; with unsteadiness in thighs when walking rapidly ; in Addison's disease ; during intervals of epileptic spasms.*

Stupefying pressive pain in forehead, with confusion of senses and dullness of whole head, while reading ; he was obliged to stop and did not know where he was.

Tearing headache above eyes down to nose, with nausea.

Headache begins in occiput and spreads to top of head, so severe that she thinks head will burst, and that she will go crazy.

Concussive, stitching, pulsating pains in head, as if it would split, with cough.

Internal and external sensation of coldness of various parts of head, as if a piece of ice was lying against it, with pale puffed face.

Congestion to head ; with heat and stupefying headache ; with red puffed face ; with toothache ; during night ; < in morning when awakening, and from spirituous drinks.

Chronic hydrocephalus.

Burning in vertex ; also after grief.

Internal and external sensation of coldness of one (r.) side of head, as if a piece of ice was lying there : < weather changing ; in early morning ; from motion in open air ; < on lying down.

Sweating of head very profuse, rolling down face in large, beadlike drops ; the pillow is wet for some distance around child's head. Tinea. Chalk-like stools.

Nocturnal sweats of head.

Head too large, fontanelles not closing.

Rachitis.

Open fontanelles, with large head and with sweating of same ; Children leuco-phlegmatic, very fat and of leaden weight ; abdomen hard and distended, with sour-smelling diarrhœa.

Scratches head impatiently on getting awake or when disturbed in sleep.

Tinea favosa ; thick scabs covered with thick pus.
Crusta serpiginosa ; herpes circinatus.

Great photophobia ; < in evening ; agglutination of lids in morning.
Cataract.
Horrid visions when EYES *are closed.*
Dilated pupils ; often indicated after Sulphur.
Fungus hæmatodes with opacity of cornea.
Dimness of cornea ; opacity ; maculæ.
Pustules on cornea, much lachrymation and excessive photophobia ; < by gaslight, or in morning, and in changes of weather.
Ophthalmia ; from taking cold ; entrance of foreign body ; in the newborn ; scrofulous ; arthritic.

Inflammation and swelling of outer and inner EAR.
Otorrhœa muco-purulent, affecting principally right ear ; enlarged glands.
Ulceration, then granulation, then polypus ; great stench.

Nasal polypi, with loss of smell.
Swelling of NOSE *and upper lip, in children.*

Face looks old and wrinkled.
Face puffed up, in children.
Lips chapped and cracked ; corners of mouth ulcerated.
Chewing motion of jaws during sleep.
Painful swelling of submaxillary GLANDS.
Hard, painful swelling of submaxillary glands ; painful tension when chewing ; sticking pain when touched.

TEETH *cannot endure air or any coldness.*

Difficult dentition. With Rachitis. Eclampsia. Cholera infantum. Hydrocephalus. Crusta lactea. Infantile catarrh. Laryngo-tracheitis. Bronchitis. Bronchial catarrh. Marasmus. Urticaria. Chorea.

TONGUE *dry, does not like to talk.* (Compare Phos. ac. and Bellad.)

Sore THROAT *marked ; cellular tissue around cervical glands swollen ; nose sore ; obstructed.*

Ravenous hunger, with weak STOMACH.

Appetite poor, with an aversion to meat and a craving for boiled eggs.

Complete loss of appetite.

Longing for boiled eggs.

Aversion to meat.

Sour vomiting, especially during dentition.

Vomiting and diarrhœa of teething children.

Pit of stomach swollen like a saucer turned bottom up ; painful to pressure.

Bloating in region of stomach, compelling him to undo his clothing.

Tight clothes about hypochondria are unbearable.

Pains more on left side, especially under left hypochondrium ; tearing stitching pains in left chest to hypochondrium.

Flatulency with gurgling in right side of ABDOMEN.

Abdomen much distended ; hard.

Mesenteric glands hard and swollen in children ; abdomen feels as if filled with stones or ovoid bodies.

Mesenteric atrophy.

Emaciated everywhere, except abdomen.

Soreness of navel ; a moist excrescence like proud flesh from navel of infants. (*Kali carb., Nat. mur.*)

Diarrhœa of sour smell.

Watery stools.

Tapeworm and ascarides with stool.

Tapeworm ; after Graph.

Polypi and varices of BLADDER.

Increases SEXUAL *desire and provokes emissions, but unusual weakness follows indulgence and ejaculation is tardy.*

Impotence.

Consequences of onanism or of too frequent coitus ; pressing pain in head and back ; lassitude and weakness in lower limbs ; knees seem to give way ; sweats easily ; debility ; hands tremble.

Frequent nocturnal involuntary emissions.

Itching and burning of genitals of both sexes.

Menses will not appear ; in plethora.

Menses ; too early ; last too long ; too profuse.

The least excitement brings on a return of profuse catamenia.

Metrorrhagia.

LEUCORRHŒA ; *like milk, with itching and burning. Before or after menses ; during micturition ; profuse at times ; in fits and starts ; worse after exercise ; with great debility ; with stinging in os and aching in vagina ; with burning in cervical canal ; with accumulation of mucus between labia and thighs ; with chlorosis ; in scrofulous women.*

Leucorrhœa with pruritus ; white, milky, but not thick ; heat of parts.

Leucorrhœa thick, yellow ; < by day, when urinating.

Frequent leucorrhœa between menses, which are too early and profuse.

Vaginal polypi and fistula.

Clumsy, awkward, easily falls ; tired from short walk, from a general feeling of lameness in pelvis. Cramp in toes, or soles of feet, during pregnancy.

False labour pains, running upward.

Secretion of MILK *too abundant ; galactorrhœa.*

Excessive lactation ; also hectic and sweat ; debility as a consequence.

Breasts distended, milk scanty ; she is cold ; feels cold air very readily ; there is a want of vitality to secrete milk.

Deficient milk ; mammæ not swollen.

Breasts hard, but not red.

Milk disagrees with infant.

Crusts on head in nursing children.

Inflammation of eyes with newborn children.

Difficult teething of children.

Painless hoarseness ; could scarcely speak ; < in morning.

HOARSE, *hardly audible voice.*

Loud breathing through nose.

Shortness of breath after walking and on going up slightest ascent.

Mucus rattles in CHEST *on expiration ; < when lying and in evening.*

Night cough.

Cough ; < in morning on rising and in early evening.

Acts upon upper and middle portion of right lung.

Sore pains in chest, as if beaten ; < during inspiration.

Tuberculous consumption.

Chest painfully sensitive to touch, and on inspiration.

Cervical glands swollen.

GLANDS *of neck swollen, with eruption on head.*

Easily overstrains himself from lifting, from which NECK *becomes stiff and rigid, with headache.*

Pressure between and under shoulder blades.
Weakness and trembling in legs, especially above and below knees.
Swelling of knees.
Cold, damp feet.
Sensation in feet and legs as if she had on cold damp stockings.

Child is very BACKWARD *in learning to walk, or children seem to forget how to walk.*

EPILEPSY ; *before the attack sense of something running in arms, or from pit of stomach down through abdomen into feet ; sudden attacks of vertigo ; loss of consciousness without convulsions ; pharyngeal spasms, followed by desire to swallow. Causes : vexation, fright ; onanism ; protracted, intermittent ; suppression of chronic eruption. Worse at night, during solstice and full moon, with hallooing and shouting.*

Great weakness.
Easy relapses, one does not continue to convalesce.
Great loss of power on walking, especially in limbs, with exhausting sweat.
She was unable to go upstairs, and became very much exhausted from it.

The same disagreeable idea always rouses the sick as often as they fall into a light slumber.
When closing eyes, horrid visions.
Child chews and swallows in SLEEP.

Hectic FEVER ; *with alternate chills and heat ; frequent attacks of flushes of heat, with anguish and palpitation of heart, or constant shuddering in evening, with red cheeks ; skin dry, withered ; sweats easily ; great debility ; after prolonged or profuse lactation, loss of fluids, tuberculosis, etc.*
Partial sweats ; nape of neck ; chest ; hands.
Intermittent fever after abuse of quinine ; chronic forms with scrofula ; chill commences in stomach, agonizing weight, increasing with chill and disappearing with it ; with people who work much in cold water ; cachectic constitutions ; suppressed eruptions ; desire for eggs.
Typhoid fever, during aggravation which precedes rash (14th day), palpitation, tremulous pulse, anxiety, red face, delirium, jerks ; short, hacking cough ; excessive diarrhœa.
Morning sweat.
Cold feet at night in bed.
Aversion to open air ; the least cold goes right through.

Worse during full moon.

Chlorosis.

Varicose veins ; burning in veins.

Inflammation, painful swelling and induration of glands.

Cystic swellings

Tardy development of BONY TISSUES, *with lymphatic enlargements.*
Softening of bones ; fontanelles remaining open too long, and skull very large ; swelling of joints.
Curvature of bones, especially of spine and long bones.
Extremities deformed, crooked. (Rachitis.)
Hip disease ; second stage ; scratches head on awakening ; craves boiled eggs ; swollen glands ; diarrhœa, etc.

MUSCLES *soft and flabby.*

Nutrition impaired, with tendency to glandular engorgements.

CHAPS, *or rhagades, especially in those who work in water.*

Eczema, thin, moist scabs upon head, with swollen cervical glands ; eczema behind ears. (Graph.)

Diseases of children, especially during DENTITION.
Leuco-phlegmatic temperament in childhood.
Constitution. CHILDREN ; *self-willed ; fair, plump ;* FAT, *flabby, with red face, sweat easily, and readily take cold ; large head and abdomens, open fontanelles and sutures, and crooked legs.*
The young who grow too fat and heavy.
During dentition. Eclampsia.
Nervous, hæmorrhoidal, plethoric and lymphatic constitutions ; disposed to grow fat.
Leuco-phlegmatic ; light complexion, blue eyes, blonde hair, fair skin.
Compatible : before *Lyc., Nux, Phos., Plat., Sil. ;* after *Cham., Nit. ac., Nux, Puls., Sulph.* (especially if pupils dilate).
Incompatible : before *Nit. ac.* and *Sulph.,* according to Hahnemann.

CALCAREA PHOSPHORICA

ONE looks upon this powerful medicinal agent as one of Schuessler's Tissue Remedies, having been " adopted by him ", as Clarke puts it : though previously potentized and proved by various homœopathic doctors, among them Constantine Hering.

Though we reproduced a short paper on *Calc. Phos.*, by Dr. E. P. Cuthbert, U.S.A., at the end of our Drug Picture, *Calcarea carbonica*, in 1934, yet we seem never to have ourselves attempted its portrayal, which we will now endeavour to do.

When we are treating babies and little people in evident need of their vital stimulus to enable them to assimilate the lime they need for teeth, bones, etc., we have to ask ourselves, shall it be the *Calcarea* made famous by Hahnemann, or the *Calcarea phosphorica* ascribed to Schuessler, which, with many symptoms in common, yet, owing to its phosphorus element, presents in the provings and in its range of action many striking differences. Because we must remember that, when it comes to *curative* work, one remedy will not do for another, and we are always thrown back on the actual symptoms of the provings as our only sure guide.

Let us contrast the two drugs in the effort to help ourselves as well as others ; extracting from Nash, that accurate observer and distinguished and brilliant physician, and also from H. C. Allen's *Guiding Symptoms*.

Calc. carb. Deficient or irregular bone development. (Fontanelles open, crooked spine, deformed extremities. Fair, fat, flabby, obese.)

Calc. phos. Tardy closing or re-opening fontanelles, in slim, emaciated children, with sweaty heads (though he says later, that in *Calc. phos.* the sweaty head is not a prominent symptom, as in *Calc. carb.* and *Silica*).

Instead of " fat, fair, flabby, obese ", the *Calc. phos.* is typically anæmic and dark-complexioned ; dark hair and eyes ; thin and spare, instead of fat. Children : emaciated, unable to stand, slow in learning to walk ; sunken, flabby abdomen.

Both are invaluable in rickets : and in delayed or complicated teething.

In *Calc. carb.* the head sweats profusely during sleep, wetting the pillow far around (*Silica*).

It is only Hahnemann who has taught us how to make a correct choice, and hit the mark every time.

Both drugs affect the same organs and tissues, bones, glands, lungs, etc., but the individuals differ markedly.

Black Letter Symptoms from different authors

She wishes to be at home, and when at home to go out ; goes from place to place. (Compare *Ars.*)

Headache of school girls with diarrhœa.

Sensation in eye, as if something were in it ; renewed if others talk about it.

Slowness in teething ; also in closing of fontanelles ; complaints during teething.

Chronic enlargement of tonsils.

Relaxed sore throat.

Craves bacon, ham, salted or smoked meats. Much flatulence. Cholera infantum.

At every attempt to eat, bellyache.
Flabby, sunken abdomen.

Fistula in ano, alternating with chest symptoms, or in persons who have pain in all the joints from any change of weather.

Uterine displacements with rheumatic pains.

After prolonged nursing.

Chest difficulties associated with fistula in ano.

Stiffness of neck after draught of air.
Rheumatism of joints with cold or numb feeling.

Weariness on going up stairs.

Pains with sensations of crawling, numbness, coldness.

Copious nightsweats in phthisis.

Chronic gonorrhœa in anæmic subjects.

Rheumatism pertaining particularly to cold weather, getting well in Spring and returning next Autumn.

Cannot get awake in early morning.

Anæmia and chlorosis.
Non-union of fractured bones.

Acute affections of the lungs.

Large pedunculated nasal polypi ; polypi of rectum and uterus.
Rachitis ; fontanelles wide open ; diarrhœa, emaciation.
Flabby, shrunken, emaciated children.
Phosphatic diathesis.
Child refuses the breast ; milk has a saltish taste.
Involuntary sighing.

*   *   *

GUERNSEY.   *A subject for this remedy does not present so clear and white a complexion as is called for by Calc. carb.   Patient more of dirty white or brownish colour.*
Worse cold ; change of weather.

SOME ITALIC AND NOTEWORTHY SYMPTOMS

Likes to be alone.

Children scream and grasp with hands ; cold sweat, face ; body cold ; with open fontanelles.

Anxiety of children, in pit of stomach ; with bellyache, with chest complaints ; with palpitation.

Feels as if she had been frightened.

Feels complaints more when thinking about them.

Old people stagger when getting up from sitting.

Heat in head, burning on top, running down to toes.

Acute and chronic hydrocephalus.

Sensation as if brain were pressed against skull.

Sore pain, drawing, rending, tearing in bones of skull, mostly along sutures.

Crawls over top of head ; as ice lying on upper occiput.

Head is hot, and with smarting of roots of hair.

Skull soft and thin, crackling like paper when pressed upon.

Fontanelles remain open too long, or close and re-open.

Non-union of bones in fracture of skull, especially in the aged.

Cannot hold head up ; moves it from place to place ; head totters.

Eyes misty : shimmering, glittering ; fiery circles ; veil over eyes.

Eyeballs hurt, ache as if beaten. Cool feeling back of eyes.

Squinting distortion of eyeballs, as if from pressure : they seem distended, and protrude somewhat.

Sweat of brows and lids. Spasm of lids.

Large pedunculated nasal polypi. Swollen nose with sore nostrils.

Point of nose icy cold : itching.

Face ; pale, sallow, earthy ; full of pimples.

Coppery face, full of pimples.

Flabby, sweetish taste.

Disgusting taste : bitter taste in morning.

Tongue swollen, numb, stiff, with pimples : little blisters, sore and burn, tip of tongue.

Diarrhœa from juicy fruit or cider.

Colic from eating ices.

Nausea from smoking or coffee.

Motion in belly as of something alive. (Compare *Croc.*, *Thuja*.)

Abdominal wall : tingling ; numb ; quivering or aching.

Diarrhœa after vexation with headache; of schoolgirls ; offensive pus with stools.

Watery, very hot stools.

Stools green, loose, sometimes slimy ; soft, passed with difficulty ; hot and watery ; white and mushy.

Morning, copious soft stool ; renewed urgency directly on wiping. Very offensive diarrhœa.

Two provers experienced, a small furuncle to right of anus-with much pain ; cannot sit ; has to stand, or lie on left side.

Discharge of bloody pus, leaving a small painless fistula.

Fistula alternating with chest symptoms. Fistula ani with pains in joints every spell of cold, stormy weather.

Fistula ani alternating with chest symptoms.

Fissures of anus, in tall slim children, who form bone and teeth slowly.

Violent pain kidney region when lifting or blowing nose.

Large quantities of urine with sensation of weakness.

Has been found useful in diabetes mellitus where lungs are implicated ; of very great service not only to lungs, but in diminishing quantity of urine, and lowering its specific gravity.

Difficulty in preventing escape of urine.

Wetting bed, with general debility.

Uterine polypus.

Milk changeable, from alkaline to neutral or to acid ; watery and thin.

Mammae sore ; feel large.

Child refuses breast, milk has a saltish taste.

Constantine HERING tells us that buttermilk and koumiss are invaluable foods for the aged, because the lactic acid in them dissolves the phosphate of lime and prevents the ossification in tendons, arteries and elsewhere.

* * *

SCHUESSLER tells us how this drug was prepared by Dr. Hering. He says " It is absolutely essential to the proper growth and nutrition of the body. It is found in blood-plasma and corpuscles, in saliva, gastric juice, bones, connective tissue, teeth, etc. ; has a special chemical affinity for albumen, which forms the organic basis for this salt in the tissue cells, and is required wherever albumin or albuminous substances are found in the secretions. It also supplies new blood cells, becoming the first remedy in anæmia and chlorosis. It is of the greatest importance to the soft and growing tissues, supplying the first basis for the new tissues, hence necessary to initiate growth. Is curative in diseases depending upon a disturbed action of the lime-molecules in the body : such as occurs in the tardy formation of callus around the ends of fractured bones, the unnatural growth and defective nutrition of bone and other textures found in rickets, etc., . . . it is an essential food to soft and growing tissues, in cases of malnutrition and defective cell growth : hence its use during dentition, in convulsions and spasms occurring in weak, scrofulous subjects, stimulating nutrition."

If not the most modern teachings, the above may be useful in suggesting the practical applications of the drug.

" Schuessler has no use for Hahnemann's greatest of polycrests, *Calc. carb.* He limits his " calcareas " to *Calc. phos.* and *Calc. fluor.* because it is only in these combinations that lime is found ultimately in the body. But life does not need, much less prefer, requirements ready-made. She has her own adequate bio-chemical laboratory, whose function is two-fold, to break down and to build up. She chooses her materials, however provided, tearing to pieces and extracting her requirements, and pushing out useless or harmful refuse. And when she falls on evil days, she has her own way of demanding the stimulus needed for regeneration, in the symptoms she puts up, and which the Law of Similars permits us to appropriately counter.

As said, one remedy can never take the place of another. In the treatment of infancy and youth—and age ! one or other will be more specially indicated in different cases of unflourishing growth and development or nutrition, according to the actual, individual symptoms. No two drugs are alike : it is a case here of the one or the other, if we are to do brilliant work.

Later on, Schuessler threw out one of his original tissue remedies, *Calc. sulph.*, " because ", as Clarke says, " it was not an actual constituent of the tissues, and he distributed its functions between *Silica* and *Natrum sulph.* But homœopaths having no Biochemic theory to support, may continue its use without scruple, especially as it has been proved by Hering and others."

*   *   *

NASH gives *Calc. phos.* in a nutshell :

Tardy closing or re-opening fontanelles in slim, emaciated children, with sweaty heads. But he says, further on, that in *Calc. phos.* the sweaty head is not a prominent symptom, . . .

Rheumatic troubles, which are worse in Fall or Spring, when the air is full of melting snow.

Calcarea phos. has also a very peculiar desire; the little patient, instead of wanting eggs (*Calc. carb.*) wants " ham rind ", a very queer symptom, but a genuine one. (*Mag. carb.* craves meat, in such children.)

Diarrhœa is very prominent, and the stools are green and spluttering. . . . I have made some very fine cures in such cases where there seemed little hope for the child and hydrocephaloid seemed impending.

An excellent remedy for broken bones, where the bones refuse to knit. . . . Feels complaints more when thinking of them.

*   *   *

A doctor friend, points out in regard to RICKETS : " The orthodox treatment is based on the fact that vitamin D is necessary for the absorption of calcium. Therefore cod liver oil and sunlight treatment are given to supply vitamin D.

But why is it that of two children in the same environment, and having the same food, one will develop rickets and the other will not ?

" Of course the answer is, *constitutional defect* ; which can be readily cured by the appropriate remedy, such as *Calcarea carb.*, in high potency."

One remembers well the cure of perhaps one's worst case of rickets, years ago, with a single dose of *Calc. carb. cm.* It was luckily not repeated, because the child, living far away, did not re-appear at out-patients for many months. Sometimes our best prescriptions have been saved by the non-reappearance of the patient. The safe rule is, where there is definite improvement and continuous, nature has got the matter in hand, so just put yours behind you till the reappearance of symptoms demands further attention.

CALCAREA SULPHURICA

Gypsum. Plaster of Paris.

A VERY useful remedy of, often, severe conditions, but not too well proved, or known. One of the indications on which one has prescribed it with success is, when the case works out almost equally to *Sulphur* and *Calcarea* ; some of the important symptoms making appeal for the one remedy, some for the other, and one suddenly realizes that there is a drug *Calc. sulph.*, which fills the picture.

Calc. sulph. was one of Schuessler's Twelve Tissue Remedies. But Clarke tells us that, in his last edition, Schuessler discarded it because it was not an actual constituent of the tissues, and that he distributed its functions between *Silica* and *Natrum phos.* Our indispensable *Calcarea carb.* shares the same banishment, probably for the same reason, that it is not met with, as such, in the tissues of the body. . . . Just as if the body could not take what it needs from other combinations, breaking down and reconstructing, in a manner which not even a bio-chemist can emulate.

Schuessler's calcium salts are, or were, three : *Calc. sulph.*, *Calc. phos.* and *Calc. fluor.* It is interesting to observe that they all affect the tongue, but in different ways. In *Calc. fluor.* the tongue is, typically, cracked and indurated. In *Calc. phos.* it is swollen, stiff, pimply, and white-furred ; while in our *Calc. sulph.* it is flabby, looks like a layer of dried clay, with the *Calc. sulph.* essential yellow coating at the base. It may even be inflamed and suppurating—the taste sour, soapy, acrid.

THE PRESENCE OF PUS WITH A VENT is, we are told, the general indication for *Calc. sulph.*

This drug greatly resembles *Hepar*, which it follows, " taking up the case when the latter ceases to act ". But, surely, one should be able to diagnose between them, so as to be actually on the spot from the first, and save time.

The two drugs are alike in being combinations of *Calcium* and *Sulphur*, but the one, *Hepar*, is to some extent an animal product, being, according to Hahnemann's precise directions, " A mixture of equal parts of finely powdered oyster shells and quite pure flowers of sulphur, kept for ten minutes at a white heat, and stored up in well corked bottles."

Farrington calls *Hepar* " an impure calcium sulphide ". He says it is a valuable addition to the powers of lime and sulphur, used separately. It possesses many similarities and marked differences from its components.

Now let us try to compare and to differentiate between *Calcarea sulph.* and *Hepar sulphuris calcareum.*

Both are intensely sensitive to draughts and to touch : but one great distinction between them is, that *Hepar* is very sensitive to DRY cold, and better in damp weather; whereas *Calc. sulph.* is worse in WET cold weather.   *Hepar* is also intensely sensitive mentally— angry at the least trifle, and almost murderous in its rage.

Both have unhealthy skins that " will not heal " ; while, with *Hepar*, every little hurt festers.

Cold, foul footsweats are a feature of *Hepar*, while *Calc. sulph.* has, characteristically, the burning soles of *Sulphur.*   And *Calc. sulph.* has also the *Sulphur* intolerance of clothing.   Like *Camph.* it throws the covers off when cold ; while *Hepar*, though it can scarcely bear a wound to be covered, because of its extreme intolerance of touch and pressure, yet must be wrapped up warmly all the time, and cannot endure the least uncovering.

The pains of *Hepar*, again, are very distinctive ; of a sticking, splinter-like character (*Nit. ac.*).

No drug will do equally well for another—*curatively*, while several may be more or less *palliative*, which is quite another matter.

DR. OSCAR HANSON (Copenhagen) has a good deal to say in regard to *Calc. sulph.*   Valuable in suppurations, when the abscess is perforated, or after incision, and *the pus is yellow and thick.* Suppurations of the tonsils.   Abscesses of the cornea.   Suppurating wounds.   Suppurating processes in the lungs.   Deeper-acting than *Hepar sulph.* ; acts after that remedy ceases to have effect. . . . Much recommended by Dr. H. Siemson, of Copenhagen, in fibroma and myoma uteri, inoperable and with very offensive hæmorrhage.   Also impetiginous eczema (crusta lactea) and torpid glandular swellings. . . . " I have found it very valuable " (Hanson says) " in dry eczema in children."

NASH says this remedy (*Calc. sulphurica*) is not well understood as yet, but acts much along the lines of *Hepar sulph.*, so far as we do know.   He tells of a case where there was great pain in the kidneys for a day and a night.   Then there was a great discharge of pus in the urine, for several days, which weakened the patient very fast.   A specialist had examined the urine a short time before and pronounced the case Bright's disease.   Nash finally gave *Calc. sulph.* 12, and under its action she immediately improved and made a very rapid and permanent recovery.   He says that he had since found it a good remedy in profuse suppurations in different kinds of cases.

CAMPHORA

Camphor is another medicine that should be in every house for emergency use :—but—keep it in the bathroom! Don't let camphor come near any of your medicines, for it antidotes most of them.

Especially is it useless to attempt to cure whooping-cough with *Drosera* in a child smothered with camphorated oil. One has tried it! *Camphor* antidotes *Drosera*, and the child will return " no better "

In our young days there was always a small flask of whisky with a lump of camphor at the bottom, ready for sudden severe chills and for diarrhœa. The whisky dissolves all the camphor it is capable of dissolving, and the lump at the bottom ensures a " saturated solution " Of this, a drop on a piece of sugar, quickly repeated if necessary, restores warmth to people chilled beyond easy recovery, and may avert illness. One has seen this rapid transformation many times.

A child of ten, after long, happy hours of blackberrying— and gormandizing—was vomiting unhappily for days, till at last a drop of camphor on sugar cured.

Give camphor always on sugar. In water it nauseates. On sugar it is delightful to take. And the sugar, also, stimulates and warms.

Poisonings by camphor produce sudden intense coldness—as we have seen in our article on Cholera. Hence it is homœopathic to chills.

And, as Hahnemann tells us, its impression on the human body, " though powerful, is more transient than that of any other drug : therefore it needs very frequent repetition till reaction. In cholera every five minutes, till warmth is restored." In influenza, repeated doses, or constant inhalations, he says.

We have also spoken elsewhere of the extreme rapidity of action of camphor : of its dreadful depressant powers, mental and physical ; its icy coldness and blueness ; its dreadful sufferings.

Its restorative action is *equally rapid*, given in small doses, repeated till warmth is restored.

Camphor, of course, is stimulating and warming, in small doses, BECAUSE it is so chilling and depressing in poisonous doses.

One cannot reel out memories of the curative effects of camphor because they are so prompt as to be promptly forgotten.

The triumphs of camphor in cholera are given in the article on CHOLERA, a good part of which should properly be included in this drug picture.

The mental symptoms of *Camphor* are extraordinary. They run into several pages of Allen's *Encyclopedia*: though other Materia Medicas give very little idea of the extreme mental sufferings that can be evoked by *Camphor*. It was a puzzle case, many years ago, that drew one's attention to these symptoms, and, once realized, they are not easily forgotten.

Woman of forty-nine : ill for five months. Floodings : then " cardiac set in ", as she expressed it. Then influenza—three times in five months. *Nerves terrible !* Heart as if it would burst. Feels as if she were going to die every minute. Very chilly. No energy. Nothing to live for. Every effort exhausts. Worse from a bath ; has to " wash piece-meal ". Was found in a faint in her last bath. *Anguish at night : feeling that she is dying. Her relief at realizing, " Why, I am still alive !"*

Heart's action was poor, but there was no disease, in spite of several attacks of rheumatic fever, the first at eighteen.

Luckily she was asked, " What do you take for these attacks ? "

She took Camphor—eight drops of the spirit of camphor in water as often as from seven to eight times a day. Had done so for five or six years. She took it every time she had a heart attack. Her doctor knew of this, and he said it would not hurt her.

The totality of her symptoms worked out to *Lycopodium* or *Phosphorus*. And in spite of the fact that *Phosphorus* antidotes *Camphor*, she was given *Lyc.* 30, *three doses.* (This was in one's very early days of prescribing.) And of course she was to take no more camphor.

In a fortnight her husband came in great distress. She had seemed more cheerful for a few days after the *Lyc.* but her nights were still very bad. " Going to die ! " Sobs very much. What was he to do ? Supposing she did die ?—they had left their local doctor ! He did not think that she would die ; but they had fearful scenes every night. She was pretty well by day, but the nights were terrible.

Among the camphor symptoms in Allen's *Encyclopedia* are these: "*Precordial anxiety. Great anxiety and restlessness.* Suffocative dyspnœa." " I am dead !—No, I am not dead !—Yes, I must be dead ! " " By day, quiet : night and solitude are my terrors." " Attacks of terror by night. Afraid to go to sleep at night." " I suffered such fearful anguish as no fancy can comprehend." Some of the *Camphor* ravings were read out to the husband, who said they might have been written of his wife. This time she got *Phos.* 12, *three doses.*

A week later she came, so much better as not to be at first recognized. For the last four days, better nights. Nervous feelings all going away. (Says that after her first husband's death she had "nerves": saw mice all over the bed. It was then that she was first given *Camphor* and, finding that it helped her, she had used it ever since.) Most decidedly better. Appears normal!

Another week, and she came again. "So well! Sleeps well. Feels quite well." Looks a vigorous and healthy woman—absolutely changed. Brings another patient.

She continued well.

There are certain symptoms, peculiar to one drug only, which should lead to the consideration of that drug when they crop up in a patient.

Camphor produces this curious condition :—

Great coldness of surface, with a desire to uncover. Great heat or sweat, with aversion to uncover

*   *   *

Or, as KENT puts it, "In camphor, during the heat and when the pains are on, he wants to be covered up. The coldness is relieved by cold, he wants more cold."

"The camphor patient," he says, "is a most troublesome patient to nurse. Coldness, frenzy and heat very often intermingle. . . . From the shock of the suffering, the mind is almost gone, or is in a state of frenzy. Coldness then comes on and the patient wants to be uncovered, wants cold air, wants the windows open; but before all this can be done a flash of heat comes on and then he wants the covers on, and the register turned on, and wants hot bottles; but this stage now passes off, and while the nurse is bringing the hot bottles he wants her to throw them away, open the windows and have everything cool. . .

"The more violently the patient suffers, the sooner he is cold, and when he is cold he must uncover, even in a cold room."

In cases of any disease, with such strange alternating and contradictory symptoms, camphor in small doses, or in potency, will be curative.

No other drug has quite these symptoms. The nearest is *Secale.* Here the patient, though cold to touch, cannot bear to be covered, because of his sensations of intense burning, as if sparks were falling upon him. This may be seen in Gangrene. The burnings of Arsenic, on the contrary, are relieved by *heat.*

Another of these strange and unaccountable symptoms that has led to wonderful curative results, is the *profuse sweating only on uncovered parts*, of *Thuja*.

Camphor may be used to antidote many poisons. Hahnemann says, " The rapid exhaustion of its action and the quick change of its symptoms render it incapable of curing most chronic diseases."

But, with later and fuller knowledge, Kent says, " Camphor *in potentised form* will cure a great many complaints." And others also speak of the virtues of potentized *Camphor*.

Black Letter Symptoms

Better when thinking of the existing complaint.

Throbbing, like beats with a hammer, in cerebellum, isochronous with pulse, head hot, face red, limbs cool, > in standing ; mostly with such as were deprived of sexual intercourse.

Contraction as if laced together in cerebellum and glabella, with coldness all over. Very sensitive to cold air.

Nose cold and pointed (in diarrhœa and cholera).

Cold sweat, with vomiting.

Tongue, cold, flabby, trembling.

Anxiety and restlessness, absence of evacuations, frequently chilly or feeling as if cold air was blowing on covered parts ; great sinking and collapse. (Cholera.)

Burning during urination.

Newborn children ; asphyxia ; hard places in skin on abdomen and thighs, quickly increasing and getting harder, sometimes with a deep redness spreading nearly over whole abdomen and thighs ; violent fever, with startings and tetanic spasms, with bending backward ; they make no water.

Influenza.

Cool breath, as from the grave, playing upon hand held before mouth. (Carbo veg.) Coldness of limbs.

Congestion to CHEST. *All sequela of measles.*

Cold, clammy, weakening sweat.

PULSE : *weak ; not perceptible ; frequent and scarcely perceptible ; accelerated without fever ; very much accelerated, but undulating, and without strength ; very rapid ; full and rapid ; full and irritable ; irritable in evening ; hard or soft ; extremely*

. . . *small and slow ; small and hard, becoming slower and slower ; small, weak and quite frequent ; could not be counted. Icy coldness all over, with death-like paleness of face ; diminished circulation to parts most distant from heart. Effects of shock from injury; surface of body cold ; face pale and bluish, lips livid ; diarrhœa ; pulse feeble, nervous anxiety and stupefaction ; sighing respiration ; great exhaustion.*

*   *   *

In the cholera epidemic of 1831 Hahnemann faced the problem, How it was to be met ; and wrote papers, widely distributed, on its treatment. He had followers, even in those days, all the world over. When an idiotic censor banned his teachings he wrote, *They seem to prefer delivering all mankind to the grave digger to listening to the good counsel of the new purified medical art."*

Camphor poisoning displays all the symptoms of early cholera, and Hahnemann says, It is only when given alone at the first invasion of the disease, that it is so marvellously useful. The patient's friends must employ it, as this stage soon ends in death or in the second stage, more difficult to cure, and not with *Camphor."* He gave " one drop of the strong spirit of *Camphor* on sugar (or in water) every five minutes. Where jaws are locked and nothing can be swallowed, it can be rubbed into the skin, given as a clyster, or its fumes inhaled, when evaporated on hot iron. The quicker this is done, the more rapid and certain the patient's recovery. In a couple of hours warmth, strength, consciousness, rest and sleep return, and he is saved. Even in the case of persons laid out for burial, where only a finger was seen to move, *Camphor* spirit mixed with oil, introduced into the mouth, had recalled the apparently dead to life."

Results—briefly. The Russian Consul-General reported that of 70 cases in two places, all were cured ; elsewhere of 1,270 cases only 108 died. In Vienna hospitals, two-thirds treated homœopathically recovered, while two-thirds in the other hospitals died. In the South of France, where allopathic mortality was 90 per cent. the homœopathic mortality was 5 to 7 per cent. A missionary (South America) was imprisoned for gratuitously curing a number of cholera patients, when the hospital treatment did not cure one. Even in this country, our results were suppressed till demanded in Parliament, " *as they would give an unjustifiable sanction to an empirical practice, alike opposed to the maintenance of truth, and to the progress of science."*

7

CANNABIS INDICA

(*Hashish*)

THIS drug is said to be botanically identical with *Cannabis sativa*, " the difference in soil and climate being responsible for the difference in their properties ". Indeed, many writers " lump " them together, as if there were no differences !—but it is *Cannabis indica* which provides such an extraordinary wealth of mental symptoms, and which is so astonishingly curative wherever these provide the indications.

Our writers seem to have given up *Cannabis ind.* in despair, probably because of the redundancy of its mental aberrations : but Allen (*Encyclopedia*) devotes twenty-seven long pages to its 275 mental symptoms ; while of the rest, Hughes (*Pharmacodynamics*) is the most illuminating. We will quote, before going on to others, and to " Allen " :

HUGHES says: "Some provings of the Indian hemp, made upon seven persons with the tincture and lower attenuations, were published by the American Provers' Union in 1839. Since then scores of persons have tested its curious effects upon themselves ; and the experiences of haschish-eating have been put on record— by one writer with a descriptive power and gorgeousness of diction hardly inferior to that of the English opium-eater. Of the results thus obtained Dr. Allen has made an exhaustive collection ; and 918 symptoms of the drug, including the mental phenomena described at full length, stand in his *Encyclopedia*.

" To possess yourselves of the characters of the haschish intoxication, it is necessary that you should study it thus in detail. No outline can adequately present it. It is a condition of intense *exaltation*, in which all perceptions and conceptions, all sensations and emotions, are exaggerated to the utmost degree. Distances seem infinite and time endless : pleasure is paradise itself, and any painful thought or feeling plunges at once into the depths of misery. Hallucinations of the senses are common ; and the least suggestion will set going a train of vivid mental illusions. All the time a dual consciousness is present ; the experimenter feels ever and anon that he is distinct from the subject of the hashish dream, and can think rationally. The bodily sensations accompanying these phenomena are not many. Headache, sense of dryness of the mouth and throat, and anæsthesia of the surface, are not uncommon. The headache is very commonly a sensation as of the brain boiling over, and lifting the cranial arch like the lid of a tea-kettle. The anæsthesia may be preceded by sensations over the body like those produced by slight electric sparks. In the motor sphere there is experienced at times the peculiar condition known as cataleptic. Dr. O'Shaughnessy thus describes the effect of the resin on a native of India : ' At 8 p.m. we found him insensible, but breathing with perfect regularity, his pulse and skin natural, and the pupils freely contractile at the approach of light. Happening by chance to lift up the patient's right arm, the professional reader will judge of my astonishment, when I found that it remained in the posture in which I had placed it. It required but a very brief examination of the limbs to find that the patient had by the influence of this narcotic been thrown into that most strange and most extraordinary of all nervous conditions—into that state which so few have seen, and the existence of which so many still discredit—the genuine catalepsy of the nosologist. . . .'

" Dr. Ringer and others recommend it in headache, the former esteeming it the most useful medicine we possess for diminishing the frequency of the paroxysms of migraine. . . .

" It should be remembered if we ever come across a case of catalepsy. I myself had a patient in whom attacks, probably hysterical at bottom, assumed a cataleptiform character, and here *Cannabis indica* proved rapidly curative. . . .

" The effects of *Cannabis indica* on the brain may be advantage-ously compared with those of *Agaricus, Belladonna, Camphor, Crocus, Hyoscyamus, Opium* and *Stramonium*. In its power of causing catalepsy its only rival is the *chloride of tin*.

*   *   *

KENT has a vivid little description of the action of *Cannabis indica*, in the 2nd edition of his *Lectures on Materia Medica* (omitted with some other good things from his third edition, where he evidently wanted room for new drugs). We will quote from it :

" A strange ecstatic sensation pervades the body and senses. The limbs and parts seem enlarged. A thrill of beatitude passes over the limbs. The limbs tremble. Great weakness spreads over the body. The symptoms resemble catalepsy. Anæsthesia and loss of muscular sense. Complaints ameliorated by rest. Exalta-tion of spirits with mirthfulness. Wonderful imaginations and hallucinations. Wonderful exaggerations of time and space. He seems to be transported through space. He seems to have two existences, or to be conscious of two states, or to exist in two spheres. Delusions. Incoherent speech. Laughs at serious remarks. Laughs and weeps. Fear of death ; of insanity ; of the dark. Anguish and sadness. Mental symptoms ameliorated by walking in the open air. An opposite phase prevails with his weakness. He loses his senses and falls. Passes from the rational to the irrational in rapid succession, back and forth. Forgets words and ideas. Unable to finish his sentences. Thoughts crowding upon each other in such confusion prevent rational speech. His mind is full of unfinished ideas and phantoms. Wonderful theories constantly form in the mind. Loquacity. He cannot control the mind to reason rationally upon any subject. Any effort to reason is interrupted by flights of wild imagination and theory. Vision upon vision passes before the perception. Hears voices, bells, music in ecstatic confusion."

* * *

" Epilepsy, with exaltation of all powers of mind and body before the fit."

* * *

FARRINGTON, when one gathers up the fragments scattered through his *Comparative Materia Medica*, has some valuable clinical hints. He says it is one of the best remedies in delirium tremens, *with errors of perception as to space and as to time*. . . . In *delusions as to distance and time*, as when a patient tells you he is hungry, and has eaten nothing for six months, when the dishes from which he has just partaken are yet by his bedside. . . . Or, on looking out of the window, he says that objects a few feet off are many yards distant. . . . Then the *urinary symptoms* : " Burning, stitching, aching in kidneys ; pains when laughing. Also uraemia with sensation as if vertex were opening and shutting." And again, " Paralysis with tingling of affected part."

* * *

NASH has little to say about *Cann. ind*. But he gives a case which illustrates one of its phases, i.e., " *Forgetfulness : begins a sentence then cannot finish it, because he forgets what he intends to speak or write*."

This is the case : A lady with dropsy, consequent on valvular heart disease, after being relieved of the bloating, was suddenly unable to talk. In answer to a question she would begin a sentence, but could not finish it, because she could not remember what she intended to say. She was very impatient about it and would cry, but could not finish the sentence ; but could signify her assent if it was finished by some one else for her. This continued for several days, or until she received *Cannabis indica*, when she rapidly recovered her power to express herself."

One recalls two vivid experiences in regard to *Cannabis indica*, one curative, the other, apparently, causative.

A nice little fat, healthy-looking girl, fair haired and with rosy cheeks (before these mad days of " make-up "), arrived at " *Out-patients* " in great distress. We have already told the tale previously, but it will bear repeating.

She was a typist, working for a big railway company. She said, " I do not know quite how to tell you, but I have been living in a dream and I have lost my employment because of it. I used to go home every night and tell them ' I am dead tired, because I have been all day long in the trains, working my typewriter.' It needed the hardest proofs to convince me that this was not true. I believed it. Sometimes a rhinoceros followed me about, and into shops, and I told people so. I believed it. What am I to do ? If, in the street, I pass a motor car, it is all I can do to prevent myself from saying to someone with me, ' Come, and I will take you for a drive in my car ' : and of course I have no car, and I cannot drive. *What am I to do ?* " I was puzzled. I went across to the man I was working with. He suggested *Cannabis ind.* and she got a dose, and only came up once or twice more. She had " forgotten all that nonsense," and was quite well.

The other concerns a luckless country parson, with an astute, unscrupulous, determined enemy, vowed, for reasons connected with religious practices, to drive him out of his parish. The monkey tricks that were played on this unhappy man were past imagination, and savoured of romance and melodrama. But we are concerned with only one of them.

One day his parish clerk (in the employ of the enemy) tempted him with some wonderful tobacco, given him by his master. The parson said he had no pipe, but the man produced a new one. The parson put the chunk into his pocket, and having business some miles away from home, set off across country on foot. At the top of a steep hill, he rested, and remembering the gift, fished it up from the bottom of his coat to which it had migrated through a hole in his pocket, and proceeded to cut it up on the top of a gate. But with difficulty, for it was hard, and unlike any tobacco he had ever come across. Then he filled and lighted his pipe, and started to smoke it.

He began to " feel queer ". Then, almost immediately there was violent vertigo : terrifying when he attempted to move. . . . . And—

He must have been helpless there for several hours· before passers-by in a car befriended him, and took him home, where the local doctor was called in. But he was delirious all night—in a most alarming state : " counting elephants all night ", as he afterwards expressed it.

Two minor attacks occurred, after smoking certain cigarettes : while the rumour went round that the rector was very ill, and would have to resign and go away. But the attacks ceased when he eschewed the cigarettes of the village store, and bought his smokes elsewhere, beyond the reach of mischief.

Curious !—these delusions of elephants and rhinoceri. How on earth does a drug manage to evoke these things ? They remind one of the fears and delusions and dreams of snakes (*Hyoscyamus* and *Lac caninum* and a few others).

BLACK LETTER SYMPTOMS

Imagines he hears music ; shuts his eyes and is lost for some time in the most delicious thoughts and dreams.

Incoherent talking.

Fixed ideas.

Exaltation of spirits, with excessive loquacity.

Laughs immoderately.

Uncontrollable laughter, till the face becomes purple and the back and loins ache.

Anguish accompanied by great oppression, ameliorated in the open air. He was in constant fear he would become insane.

Very absent-minded.

Every few moments he would lose himself, and then wake up, as it were, to those around him.

Vertigo.

Frequent involuntary shaking of the head.

On regaining consciousness, violent shocks pass through his brain.

Fixed gaze.

Injection of the vessels of the conjunctiva of both eyes.

While reading, the letters run together.

Throbbing and fullness in both ears.

Ringing and buzzing in the ears.

He looks drowsy and stupid.

His lips are glued together.

Dryness of the mouth and lips.

White, thick, frothy, and sticky saliva.

The throat is parched, accompanied by intense thirst for cold water.
Increased appetite.
Ravenous hunger.
Pain in the cardiac orifice.

Burning and scalding before, during and after urination.
Stinging pain before, during and after urination.
Profuse colourless urine.
The urine dribbles out after the stream ceases.
On squeezing the glans penis, a white glairy mucus oozes out.
Satyriasis.

Rough cough, which scratches the breast under the sternum.

Pulse below the natural standard, as low as 46.

Pain across the shoulders and spine, forcing him to stoop, and preventing him from walking erect.
Paralysis of the lower extremities and right arm.
Agreeable thrilling through the arms and hands.
Entire paralysis of the lower extremities.
Agreeable thrilling in both limbs from the knees down, with a sensation as if a bird's claws were clasping the knees.
Thoroughly exhausted from a short walk.

Excessive sleepiness.
Sound sleep.
Profuse sticky sweat, standing out in drops on his forehead.

*   *   *

And now, since an adequate conception of the action of *Cannabis indica* can only be obtained from Allen's *Encyclopedia*, we will condense from his twenty-seven long pages of its mental symptoms, merely pointing out that these provings or poisonous effects are from some forty different sources, which he gives : while the same experiences and even series of sensations were detailed almost in the same words by different persons.

Very excited : dancing about the room : laughing : talking nonsense, knew it, but could not stop without effort which he did not care to make. Shouts : leaps into the air : claps hands for joy. Sings : extemporizes words and music. On becoming conscious, finds himself dancing, laughing and singing before a looking-glass.

Incoherent talking. Tendency to blaspheme.

While visiting patients, great difficulty to refrain from saying, or doing unusual things. . . . Must keep himself sober, or might do something foolish.

Accents the last syllable in all words and laughs immoderately.

Quickness of ideas and pleasant sensations : constant succession of new ideas, each of which was instantly forgotten.

Mind filled with ridiculous speculative ideas : *fixed ideas.*

Vivid thoughts in rapid succession, forgotten at their very beginning.

Constantly theorizing. Reveries : delightful reveries.

Had the one idea that he should soon die and be dissected.

Did not know whether he himself existed : whether men generally existed; or for what purpose they existed.

Possessed with the idea that he was about to die.

Fancies thieves in the house : that he hears strange noises. Hunts under beds and tables : unlocks and relocks doors.

Imagines men are bribed to kill him : that he can fly like birds. Said he had been transported to heaven, and his language, usually commonplace, became quite enthusiastic.

All around and within, a great mystery, and terrifying.

Despair : fear of being eternally lost. On hearing the name of God, cried, " Stop ! that name is terrible : I cannot bear it. I am dying."

Demoniac shapes, cloaked in inky palls, clutched at him ; glaring at him with fiery eyes from beneath their cowls. Seemed to be walking in a vast arena encircled by tremendous wall. Stars regarded him with pitying human aspect : the sun was reeling and the clouds danced round him like a chorus.

" I could trace the circulation of the blood along each inch of its progress : I knew when every valve opened and shut. The beating of my heart was so clearly audible, I wondered it was not heard by others."

Seems possessed of a *dual existence*; one of which from a height watches the other as it passes through the phases of the Hashish delirium. Had a feeling of duality, one of his minds would be thinking of something, while the other laughed at it. Felt as if he were a third person, looking at himself and his friend.

The soul seemed to be separated from the body, to look down on it, and view all the motions of the vital processes, and to be able to pass and repass through solid walls.

Extreme protraction of time, and *extent of space :*—a few seconds seem ages ;—the utterance of a word as long as a whole drama, and a few rods, a distance which can never be passed, it is so great. The room expands : the ceiling is raised : he is in a vast hall.

The sitting room seemed to be of an immense depth below him (it was really on the same floor). Time was indefinitely prolonged. Minutes seemed to be days. A friend in the same room seemed a long way off. A strange feeling of isolation, with a great sense of *loneliness*, though surrounded by friends.

Imagines that he is *possessed of infinite knowledge and power of vision :* then that he is the Christ come to restore the world to perfect peace. Believes there is creative power in his own word ; that he has only to speak, and it will be done. That he possesses the wealth of the world, and showers riches on all the needy around him.

Feels that he is *transparent :* feels the blood in his veins : " the fire in the grate was shining through me, to warm the marrow of my bones ". Imagines he is gradually swelling, his body becoming larger and larger. That he is on horseback ; hunting ; seeing blue water ; swimming ; is captain of a vessel ; travelling ; that he has no weight.

Illusion that he was a pump-log, through which a stream of hot water was playing, and threatening his friend with a wetting. That he was an inkstand, and that, as he lay in bed, the ink might spill over the white counterpane : he opened and shut his brass cover, it had a hinge ; shook himself, and saw and felt the ink splash against his glass sides. Now he is a huge saw, and darts up and down while the complete planks fly off him on either side : then a bottle of soda water : then a huge hippopotamus ; then a giraffe : then a fern, surrounded by clouds and perfume. Laughs because his leg is a tin case filled with stair-rods, which rattle as he walks : then the other leg elongates till he is raised hundreds of feet in the air, and has to hop along beside his friend.

All impressions extremely exaggerated.

Walls of room are suddenly covered with dancing satyres and nodding mandarins. Sees numberless diabolical imps with bloody faces and immense black eyes, which terrify him ; till a cold sweat breaks out, and he is suffocating.

All the *events of his past life*, even those long forgotten, and most trivial, were thrown in symbols from a rapidly-revolving wheel, each recognized as an act of his life, and each in its correct order of sequence.

Ludicrous visions of old, wrinkled females who are found to be composed of knit yarn.

Illusions of the senses : hears voices and the *most sublime music* ; sees *visions of beauty and glory*, only to be equalled in Paradise : landscapes of sublimest beauty ; profusion of flowers of brilliant colours : architecture of magnificent beauty and grandeur, giving a consciousness of happiness.

A silent army passed him in the street : the plain suddenly expanded and was covered with a band of Tartars, who rushed by in mad haste, their caps streaming with plumes and horsehair. Houses suddenly take to nodding, bowing and dancing.

When walking in street the muffled figure of a man starts from the wall : excites utmost horror,—every lineament of his face stamped with the records of a life black with damning crime. " It glared on me with a ferocious wickedness and a stony despair. I seemed to grow blasphemous, looking at him." Wakes to see on a bier a fearful corpse, whose livid face was distorted with the pangs of assassination. Every muscle was tense, and the nails pierced the dead man's palm by the force of his dying clench. Two tapers at the head and two at the feet made the ghastliness of the bier more luminously unearthly. A smothered laugh of derision mocked the corpse from some invisible watcher, " then the walls began slowly to glide together, the ceiling coming down, the floor ascending : nearer and nearer I was borne towards the corpse. Tried to cry out, but speech was paralysed, the walls came closer, till my hand lay on the dead man's forehead. I was stifled in the breathless niche, touched on all sides by the walls of the terrible press : then a crash, and I felt all sense blotted out in darkness. I awakened : the corpse was gone, but I had taken its place on the bier, and the room had grown into a gigantic hall, with roof of iron arches . . . then demoniac forms and faces . . . suddenly the nearest fiend thrust a pitchfork of white-hot iron into my side and hurled me into the fiery cradle,—' let us sing him ', said one of the fiends, ' the lullaby of hell ' ; as I lay unconsumed, tossed from side to side by the rocking of the fiery engine. . . . Presently was in a colossal square surrounded by houses a hundred storeys high. Ran in bitter thirst to a fountain carved in iron, every jet of which was sculptured in mockery of water, yet as dry as the ashes of a furnace. I called for water, when every sash in all the hundred storeys of that square flew up, and a maniac stood at every window. They gnashed at me, glared, gibbered, howled, laughed, horribly hissed and cursed. I became insane at the sight, and leaping up and down, mimicked them all."

The scene became theatrical, and he, an actor, improvised his tragedy and held his immense audience entranced. Suddenly a look of suspicion came over every face . . . " they knew my secret, and one maddening chorus broke from the whole theatre, ' Hashish ! Hashish ! he has eaten Hashish ! ' I crept from the stage in unutterable shame. I crouched in concealment : looked at my garments and beheld them, foul and ragged as a beggar's : from head to foot I was the incarnation of squalidity. Children pointed at me ; loungers stood and searched me with inquisitive scorn : the multitude of man and beast all eyed me : the very stones in the street mocked me with a human railery, as I cowered in my besmeared rags."

Imagines someone calls him. Hears music of the sweetest and sublimest melody and harmony, sees venerable bards with their harps, who play as it were the music of heaven. A single tone seemed like the most divine harmony. *Imagines he hears music : shuts his eyes, and is lost in the most delicious thoughts and dreams.* Hears numberless bells ringing most sweetly. For fully two weeks after, when sitting in his office, he would hear most magnificent harmony, as if some master-hand were playing an organ, and using only the softer stops. There was this peculiarity about the hearing of the music, one must be in a state of half-reverie, then the divine strains, soft and marvellously sweet, followed one another in a smoother legato than any human fingering ever accomplished. If one roused the attention and strained the ear, to be sure of catching every chord, *silence came at once.*

Heard the noise of colours, green, red, blue and yellow sounds coming to him in perfectly distinct waves.

After such experience of ecstasy, when emerging from a dense wood, heard a hissing whisper, " Kill thyself ! Kill thyself ! " and unseen tongues repeated it on all sides, and in the air above me, " The Most High commands thee to kill thyself." But an invisible hand struck at the knife which he was aiming at his throat, and sent it spinning into the bushes.

Physical sensations of exquisite lightness and airiness, and *mentally* of a wonderfully *keen perception of the ludicrous in* simple and familiar objects. Objects by which he was surrounded assumed such strange and whimsical expression, and became so inexpressibly absurd and comical, that he was provoked into a long fit of laughter.

It seemed to him as if he existed without form throughout a vast extent of space. *His body seemed to expand*, and the arch of his skull to be broader than the vault of heaven.

His enjoyment of the visions was complete and absolute, undisturbed by the faintest doubt of their reality ; while in some other chamber of his brain, reason sat coolly watching them and heaping the liveliest ridicule on their fantastic features. One set of nerves was thrilled with the bliss of the gods, while another was convulsed with unquenchable laughter at that very bliss. His highest ecstasies could not bear down and silence the weight of his ridicule, which in turn was powerless to prevent him from running into other and more grotesque absurdities.

He *laughed* till his eyes overflowed profusely, every drop that fell became immediately a large loaf of bread and tumbled upon the shop-board of a baker : the more he laughed, the faster the loaves fell, till such a pile was raised about the baker that he could hardly see the top of his head. His throat was as hard as brass : his tongue a bar of rusty iron: Though he seized a pitcher of water and drank long and deeply, his palate and throat gave no intelligence as to his having drunk at all. . . . He tore open his vest and tried to count the pulsations of his heart, but there were two hearts, one beating at the rate of a thousand beats a minute, the other with slow dull motion. His throat was filled with blood and blood was pouring from his ears. (On recovering, after several days, there was no taste in what he ate, no refreshment in what he drank, and it required a painful effort to comprehend what was said to him or to return a coherent answer.)

" The *unsteadiness of gait of one who tries to keep down :* for I felt as if there were springs in my knees, and was reminded of the man with the mechanical leg that walked away with him."

" There were present real objects, as well as imaginary ones ; but at times I doubted which was which, and floated in uncertainty."

A weakness of the whole body came on, his legs would not support him : his arms became heavy : he was obliged to throw himself on the sofa, his limbs became rigid, he entirely lost his sensations, *becoming cataleptic :* anæsthesia again extended over his body and now was added an automaton-like and rapid movement of the hands, one hand placed on the breast was rubbed on the back with the palm of the other. By turns the right arm or leg, or the right half of the face, and then all these parts together would seem petrified, so that he could not move them, and would then relax. Suddenly the mass of his brain, all except a small portion, seemed changed to marble ; (his right eye, for a long time, retained the sensation of marbly hardness).

Was a prey to *extreme loquacity and mobility of ideas :* and feared for the fate of his companions, for whom he feared the dose had been excessive and might prove poisonous.

Seized with gesticulary convulsions in arms and legs, and his symptoms assumed the appearance of those which characterize *hydrophobia* :—outbreaks of fear at the sight of bright objects, at any little breath of air, or at the approach of any one. He asked for water, but only to thrust it away without drinking, unable with the greatest effort to swallow a single draught. A sensation that tongue and throat were covered with a dry, soft body.

An urgent desire to be held, guided, taken care of, lest he should get out of bed to commit some foolish act.

Hands carried automatically to his head and held there, as though there were a difficulty in detaching them.

Cramp in calves which made movements impossible ; or caused them to be distended, or take a sudden jump.

Curious, alarming thrills. Went upstairs, seemed not to touch the steps : " I trod the air as a swimmer treads water : my feet came near the steps but did not strike them."

" Thought of *catalepsy*—I must keep my soul in my body by force of will, or perhaps it would never return, I felt it was trying to wing itself away. A feeling of *loneliness* overcame me. I hurled my body through a seemingly impenetrable invisible barrier. Pushing my way through a resistent atmosphere— an ethereal fluid it seemed to be, not as dense as water nor rare as air, yet it resisted. *The two parts of my being were acting separately*, my will or spiritual existence was separate from my bodily existence and spurring it onward, pushing it forward, using it as an artificer uses a tool : onward it forced my body, seeming to exult in its supremacy.

All was unreal ; I myself was unreal ; even my voice did not seem my own.

Being persuaded, I ate a piece of meat : to do so I had to recall the various processes and *modus operandi* of " feeding ". " First," I reasoned, " they put the substance in the mouth, and by moving the under jaw down and up and mixing the saliva with it by motion of the tongue, they masticate it." This was easily accomplished. The spittle seemed to have legs and arms, I could feel it scrambling through the meat, but when it was thoroughly masticated, I could not remember, or rather date back to the time I put the meat in my mouth. Chewing seemed to have been my regular business for ages. It was time to swallow, but to get command of the muscles of my throat wholly baffled all my endeavours."

" If the disembodied ever return to hover over the hearthstone which once had a seat for them, they look upon their friends as I then looked on mine. A nearness of place with an infinite distance of state—an isolation none the less perfect for seeming companionship."

" A fitful wind had been sighing down the chimney, it grew into the steady hum of a vast wheel in accelerating motion . . .

its monotonous din was cnanged for the reverberating peal of a grand cathedral organ. The ebb and flow of its inconceivable solemn tone filled me with grief that was more than human."

"At last I was in the street. Beyond me the view stretched endlessly away—an unconverging vista whose nearest lamps seemed separated from me by leagues. A soul setting out for his flight beyond the farthest visible star, could not be more overwhelmed with his newly-acquired conception of the sublimity of distance than I was. I began my infinite journey. I dwelt in a marvellous inner world : existed by turns in different places and various stages of being. Now I swept my gondola through the moonlit lagoons of Venice : now Alp on Alp towered above my view, and the glory of the coming sun flashed purple light upon the topmost icy pinnacle. Now in primeval silence of some unexplored tropical forest I spread my feathery leaves, a giant fern, and swayed and nodded in the spice-gales over a river whose waves sent up clouds of music and perfume. My soul changed to a vegetable essence, thrilled with a strange and unimagined ecstasy."

"My voice seemed to reverberate like thunder from every recess of the building. I was terrified at the noise I had made. (I learned in after days that this impression is only one of the many due to *the intense sensibility of the sensorium as produced by Hashish.*)"

"I stood in a remote chamber at the top of a collossal building and the whole fabric beneath me was steadily growing into the air. Higher—higher—on, on forever into the lonely dome of God's infinite universe we towered ceaselessly. The years flew on ; I heard the musical rush of their wings in the abyss outside me, and from cycle to cycle, from life to life I careered, a mote in eternity and space."

"Now through the street, with measured tread, an armed host passed by. The heavy beat of their footfalls, and the grinding of their brazen corslet-rings alone broke the silence, for among them there was no more speech nor music than in a battalion of the dead. It was the army of the ages going by into eternity. A godlike sublimity swallowed up my soul. I was overwhelmed in a fathomless barathrum of time, but I leaned on God, and was immortal through all the changes. . . . Looking at his watch he realized he had travelled through all that immeasurable chain of dreams in thirty seconds. ' My God,' I cried, ' I am in eternity.' In the presence of that first sublime revelation of the soul's own time, and her capacity for an infinite life, I stood trembling with breathless awe. Till I die, that moment of unveiling will stand in clear relief from all the rest of my existence. I hold it still in unimpaired remembrance as one of the unutterable sanctities of my being."

Then follow more and more ecstasies, with celestial music " such as I shall never hear again out of the Great Presence ".

Under the same circumstances, the same dose of Hashish will produce diametrically opposite effects. Or from a large dose may result a scarcely perceptible phenomenon, yet a dose of but half that quantity may cause the agonies of suffering of a martyr, or rejoicing in a perfect frenzy. But if, during the Hashish delirium another dose, however small, is taken to prolong the condition, such agony will inevitably ensue as will make the soul shudder at its own possibility of endurance without annihilation. The use of it after any other stimulus will produce consequences as appalling.

" I began to be lifted into that tremendous pride, so often characteristic of the fantasia. My powers became superhuman ; my knowledge covered the universe ; my scope of sight was infinite.

Repeatedly I have wandered past doors and houses which in my ordinary condition were as well known as my own, and have at last given up the search for them in utter hopelessness, recognizing not the faintest familiar trace in their aspect. Certainly a Hashish eater should never be alone.

Then an extraordinary case of *clairvoyance* is detailed. . . . Threw himself on a sofa and asked a pianist to play him some piece of music, without naming any in particular. The prelude began : and the dreamer was at once lifted into the choir of a grand cathedral. The windows of nave and transept were emblazoned, in the most gorgeous colouring, with incidents culled from saintly lives. Far off in the chancel monks were loading the air with essences that streamed from their golden censers : on the pavement of inimitable mosaic knelt a host of worshippers in silent prayer. Suddenly behind the great organ began a plaintive minor, like the murmur of some bard relieving his heart in threnody. This was joined by a gentle treble voice among the choir. The low wail rose and fell with the expression of wholly human emotion. One by one the remaining singers joined in ; and now he heard, thrilling to the very roof of the cathedral, a wondrous miserere. At the far end of the nave a great door swung open, and a bier entered supported by solemn bearers. On it lay a coffin covered by a pall, which being removed, as the bier was set down in the chancel, discovered the face of the sleeper. It was the dead Mendelssohn ! The last cadenza of the death-chant died away, the bearers with heavy tread, carried the coffin through an iron door to its place in the vault ; one by one the crowd passed out of the cathedral till the dreamer stood alone. He turned to depart and, awakened to complete consciousness, saw the pianist just resting from the keys. " What piece have you been playing ? " he asked. The reply was, " Mendelssohn's Funeral March." This piece he had never heard before. . . . " Certainly it is as remarkable an instance of sympathetic clairvoyance as I ever knew."

" A colossal music filled the whole hemisphere above me, and I thrilled upwards through its environment on visionless wings. It was not song, it was not instruments, but the inexpressible spirit of sublime sound—like nothing I ever heard—intense ; the ideal of harmony, yet distinguishable into a multiplicity of exquisite parts. . . . Like a map the arcade of the universe lay bare before me. I saw how every created thing not only typifies but springs forth from some mighty spiritual law as its offspring, its necessary external development, not the mere clothing of the essence, but the essence incarnate."

" From the ethereal heights I had been dropped into the midst of Acherontian fog. . . . I awaited extinction. The shapes that moved about me in the outer world seemed like galvanized corpses : the living soul of nature had gone out like the flame of a candle. The very existence of the outer world seemed a base mockery, a cruel sham of some remembered possibility which had been glorious with speechless beauty. I hated flowers, for I had seen the enamelled meads of Paradise : I cursed the rocks, because they were mute stone ; the sky, because it rang with no music ; and earth and sky seemed to throw back my curse."

*   *   *

Truly *Cannabis indica* is a great medicine—for those who know how to use it for the cure of that which it can induce.

Among its sensations one notices the unreality, the loneliness, the dual consciousness, the levitation, and senses its value in delirium, in delirium tremens, in the grandiose delusion of G.P.I., in hydrophobia, in catalepsy, where being" of the stuff that dreams are made of", it should be useful for such persons as suffer terribly with frightful dreams—and that from year's end to year's end. One such came to Out-patients only yesterday !

CANTHARIS

ANOTHER vehement drug of storm and stress, tamed by Hahnemann, till it acts as veritable oil on the waters, is *Cantharis*.

Cantharis is very like *Lilium Tigrinum* in some of its symptoms, mental and physical, and very unlike in others. It is far more inflammatory, and is rapid and destructive in its action. *It is therefore curative in intense inflammatory, rapid, and destructive conditions.* It should be compared with *Merc. cor.* and *Arsenicum*.

Let us first give the black-type symptoms from Allen's *Encyclopedia*, that is to say, the symptoms repeatedly *caused* and *cured* by *Cantharis*.

It will be observed that, while *Cantharis* produces intense inflammations and burnings on mucous membranes generally, and on the skin, its great action is on the genito-urinary system, and especially on kidneys and bladder.

Diarrhœa, consisting of blood and mucus.
Violent diarrhœa, with intolerable burning ; and intolerable burning in the anus.

Violent pain in the bladder, with frequent urging to urinate.
Fearful pain in the bladder.
Intolerable tenesmus (straining).
Tenesmus and strangury (spasm of bladder) ; the urine squeezed out drop by drop.
Violent, burning, cutting pains in neck of bladder.
Before, during and after urinating, fearful cutting pains in the urethra.
Urine scalds him. It is passed drop by drop.
Urging to urinate, with burning in urethra.
Constant urging to urinate : urine was passed drop by drop, with extreme pain.
Priapism.

The above are only the black-type symptoms, out of Allen's 1,650 symptoms of *Cantharis*—many of them in italics. We may summarise here by quotations from Kent and Nash. These writers give graphic and not easily forgotten pictures of the action, and curative reactions of this magnificent medicine.

* * *

NASH says, " If I were to select the one remedy with which to prove the truth of the formula, *Similia Similibus Curentur*, I think this would be the one.

" There is no remedy that so surely and so violently irritates and inflames the urinary organs, and no remedy that so promptly cures such irritation when it puts on the *Cantharis* type or form, as it so often does."

It is amusing (or pathetic !) to remember that we used to be taught in our student days, " *Cantharides is hardly ever used internally, as it is such a powerful irritant.*

" It produces severe gastro-intestinal irritation, the patient suffering from abdominal pain, diarrhœa and vomiting. . . . The active principle is absorbed into the blood, and in a few hours the patient complains of great *pain in the loins and strangury—* that is to say, there is urgent desire to micturate, the effort is very painful from vesical tenesmus, and the quantity of urine passed is very small : it may contain *albumen and blood.* In severe cases of poisoning there may be . . . .

" *Post mortem. Intense gastro-intestinal inflammation,* consequently swelling, ecchymoses and hyperaemia of the mucous membrane of the alimentary canal. *The kidneys are found to be very congested and in the early stages of acute nephritis.* Also much inflammation of the genito-urinary mucous membrane."

Old School still uses *Cantharis* chiefly *externally* to raise a blister and as a counter irritant. Even so, it has, in these days, to be cautiously used, lest it should be absorbed from the skin. " It is the basis of many preparations whose object is to stimulate the growth of hair." (*Hale White.*)

Alas for the poverty of Old School in actual curative remedies !

KENT gives one of his most vivid pictures of the action of *Cantharis*. " The most important feature of this medicine is its inflammatory condition, and the most important characteristic in the inflammation is the rapidity with which it develops a gangrenous state . . . the inflammatory state terminates in death of the part with such rapidity that it is surprising.

" Taken internally it proceeds almost immediately to attack the urinary tract and establish a uraemic state which brings about the mental symptoms. . . . It brings the patient down violently sick in a great hurry. Sudden loss of consciousness with red face. Thoughts run riot, and go whatever way they will, as if possessed by outside influence. Frenzy, delirium, great excitement and rage, paroxysms renewed by dazzling or bright objects. . . . The mind often runs towards subjects that the inflamed parts would suggest. The bladder and genitals are inflamed and the excitement and congestion of the parts often arouse the sexual instinct, so that there are sexual thoughts and sexual frenzy."

" Running through all the remedy there is BURNING. *Burning* in head, throbbing, stabbing. Eruptions *burn* when touched. Erysipelas of the face with large blisters : of the eyes, with gangrenous tendency. In erysipelas *Rhus* has the blisters and the burning, but in *Canth.* between your two visits it has grown black ; it is dusky, a rapid change has taken place, and it looks as if gangrene would set in. . . . *Canth.* corresponds to the lowest forms of disease, even gangrene and violent inflammation of bowels, bladder, brain, spine, lungs, with sinking and hippo-cratic countenance. Inflammation of lungs, gangrenous type, and the affected lung *burns* as if full of boiling water, or *burns* like fire. (Kent says) ' I left a patient—he had just come out of a prolonged drunk, in such a state as I have described. Urine was suppressed. He was drooling a bloody saliva from his mouth, and he was dying. This condition had come on in one night, from being nearly frozen in a drunk. It would be *Cantharis* or death before morning, but by morning he was expectorating a rusty sputum and went on to a good recovery. . . . These violent remedies are needed in those cases that will die.'

" *Intensity and rapidity are the features of this remedy.* It brings on a state of pain and excitement found in no other remedy.

" Whenever there is rapid inflammation of the bowels there is diarrhœa of bloody mucus or serum : the same watery bloody fluid from the eyes. Wherever this watery fluid comes in contact with the skin, it *burns* and takes the skin off. The whole urinary organs and genitalia are in a state of inflammation and irritation and threatened gangrene. . . ."

These, then, are things that *Cantharis* can cause, and that *Cantharis* only can cure.

Nash quotes H. N. GUERNSEY, " *It is a singular fact, though known to most practitioners, that if there be frequent micturition attended with burning cutting pain, or if not so frequent and the cutting burning pain attends the flow,* Cantharis *is almost always the remedy for whatever other suffering there may be, even in inflammation of the brain or lungs.*" And Nash says, " he might have added in the throat, and mucous membranes all through the intestinal tract, even to the rectum and anus, and in the pleura or on the skin."

Guernsey also wrote, " *Cantharis* should always be remembered and studied in treating affections of the air passages, when the mucus is tenacious."

This, Nash says, he verified in the case of a lady who had long suffered with bronchitis. The mucus was so profuse, tenacious and ropy that he thought of *Kali bich.* which did not even ameliorate. She got worse all the time till one day she mentioned that she had *great cutting and burning on urinating, which she must do very frequently.* " On the strength of which (for I knew nothing of its curative powers on the respiratory organs at that time) I gave her *Cantharis.* The effect was magical."

The mental symptoms of *Cantharis* are as violent as its physical symptoms.

" Furious delirium, with crying, barking and biting. . . .

" Paroxysms of rage, renewed by sight of dazzling, bright objects (*Bell., Hyos.*), or touching the larynx when trying to drink water." (These are indication for the use of the drug in hydrophobia.) " Frightful satyriasis."

* * *

Cantharis is one of the remedies to be considered in pruritis. It has all the burning and itching, and inflames the vulva and vagina. It is one of the remedies that proves curative here.

Cantharis burns and vesicates, and causes painful blisters. Hence, with us, it vies with *Urtica urens* in the treatment of BURNS. And, like *Urtica*, it almost instantly relieves the pain of burns. Nash says that " Hering used to challenge sceptics to burn their fingers, and then cure them by dipping their fingers into water medicated with *Cantharis*, so great was his faith in it."

And a doctor, once a student in Chicago, was greatly struck by a case of painful burns, whose pain quickly vanished after a few globules of *Cantharis*, high, given on the tongue by Dr. Kent. *Cantharis*, internally, in Homœopathic potency, is a very old tip for charming away the pain of burns.

In our Out-patient Department persons who come up with inflammation of the bladder (cystitis) in great distress from the frequent passage of drops of scalding urine, get a few doses of *Cantharis* 200, and that soon ends the trouble.

" Homœopathy knows no specifics " except the specific remedy for the individual. Yet, as Hahnemann tells us, some remedies so exactly reproduce a disease condition, as to become specific. Such are *Canth.* in cystitis, *Bell.* in scarlet fever, *Merc. cor.* in dysentery, and *Latrodectus* in angina pectoris.

But it is well to remember that *other drugs have produced a like condition, with, always, distinguishing symptoms to give the casting vote between them.*

Again, in such minor troubles as GNAT BITES. . . . I am permitted to reproduce somebody's personal experience, recorded at the time, since these things stick in the memory and give confidence when one is prescribing for others.

This is the record. . . . " Last Tuesday, 10 p.m., a fine

sharp stab just above right wrist, and a flimsy little demon flew gaily off. Almost immediately thereafter a hard wheal appeared, pricking and extending. At night, awakened by a stab in finger of left hand, and then a second finger wounded. All Wednesday —*those bites !* By Thursday, absolutely obsessed, to the exclusion of thought or interest in anything else, by the incessant urgent necessity of handling and nursing the torment, and struggling against the impulse to scratch and tear. Wrist ; round wrist ; up arm ; farther and farther round wrist ; higher and higher up arm ; round fingers ; over back of hand : everywhere, burning, itching, swelling ; spreading more and more widely. On Thursday afternoon, things were at their worst, when, starting for Wembley, a friend-in-need produced a few globules medicated with *Canth.* 30, which were obediently sucked ; and a second dose, to be taken later on, was provided. The rapidity of the relief was unbelievable : the suffering was soon negligible, then forgotten. Able to concentrate again !—able to experience the thrill of the Wembley Tattoo. And on this (Friday) morning, arm and fingers are again normal—except for a few scratch-marks. But why record all this ? Because such airy demons are not the last of their kind, and because someone else, some day, may be glad to prove the merits of *Cantharis*, in potency, for GNAT BITES.''

A private detective had been standing and watching for hours in an unpleasant spot, legs soaked with wet salt-petre. Came in distress to exhibit them—red, swollen, very painful,—severe cellulitis nearly up to the knees. One wanted to get the patient into hospital ; but that was " not possible ! " So *Cantharis* 200 was given—just a few doses—and it all vanished astonishingly, and there was no further trouble—to the great relief of the doctor !

Cantharis being so frightfully rapid in its evil action—i.e. in the production of destructive inflammations, is equally rapid in its benign action, when used curatively.

It is well to remember that even *in pace of action, disease and remedy must match.*

BLACK LETTER SYMPTOMS

Great amativeness ; amorous frenzy.

Inflammation of EYES, *particularly when caused by a burn.*

Burning sensation in THROAT, *which feels as if on fire.*

Passage of white or pale red tough mucus with STOOL, *like scrapings from intestines, with streaks of blood.*

Paroxysmal cutting and burning pains in both KIDNEYS, *the region very sensitive to slightest touch, alternating with pain in tip of penis ; urging to urinate ; painful evacuation, by drops of bloody* URINE, *and at times, of pure blood.*

Violent tenesmus vesicæ and strangury.

Painful discharge of a few drops of bloody urine, causing very severe sharp pain, as if a red-hot iron was passing along urethra : this pain was most acutely felt at membranous portion of canal, and in meatus urinariius.

Violent burning, cutting pains in neck of bladder, extending to fossa navicularis, < before and after urinating.

Violent pains in bladder with frequent urging ; intolerable tenesmus.

Urging to urinate from smallest quantity of urine in bladder.

Dribbling discharge, reddish, sometimes mixed with blood.

Ardor urinæ.

Before, during, and after urinating fearful cutting pains in urethra ; she must double herself and scream from pains.

Burning, when urinating, and when not.

Retention of urine, causing pain. Suppressed gonorrhœa.

SEXUAL *desire ; increased ; disturbing sleep at night.*

Frightful satyriasis ; violent, painful priapism, with excessive pains.

Retained placenta or membranes, usually with painful urination.

Burning in chest.

Pain in loins, with incessant desire to urinate.

Pain in loins, kidneys and abdomen, with such pain on urinating that he could not pass a single drop without moaning and screaming.

In third stage, when there is complete insensibility ; cramps in abdomen, muscles and legs ; suppression of urine ; hæmorrhages from stomach and intestines ; cold sweat on hands and feet. (Yellow fever.)

Scalds and BURNS.

Burns, before blisters form, and when they have formed.

CAPSICUM

Cayenne or Red Pepper (Hering)

" HAHNEMANN says, this 'spanish pepper' as it is called, was introduced as a spice to season the sauces at the dainty tables of high
livers (the pulverized seeds of the still more pungent 'cayenne
pepper' being often used as a substitute) in order to stimulate
the palate to an unnatural appetite, and thus—ruin the health.

" In the meantime but little was heard of the medicinal use of
this powerful substance. Bergius alone mentions having cured
several agues of long standing with two grain doses of capsicum.
But he did not give it alone, for the old original sin of traditional
medicine induced him to combine it with bay berries. . . . He
does not describe the agues cured by it according to the totality of
their symptoms, but only employs the expression 'old agues'
after the manner of his other old school colleagues, so that the
virtus ab usum of the mixture prescribed is shrouded in darkness.

" On the other hand the homœopathic physician proceeds much
less doubtfully and with much greater certainty in his cures with
Capsicum; for, guided by the peculiar, pure morbid states produced
by this powerful medicinal substance in the healthy body, he only
attempts the removal of those natural diseases the sum of whose
symptoms is contained in the greatest possible similarity among
those of *Capsicum*.

" The diseases curable by *Capsicum* are rarely met with in
persons of tense fibre."

*　　*　　*

One notices that .the burning pains of *Capsicum*, which so
greatly affect mucous membranes, are the " burnings, as of cayenne
pepper, sprinkled on the part ". They affect especially mouth,
tongue, stomach, abdomen, bowels, rectum and bladder. But
chest, lungs, and skin may also be thus affected.

Then one notices pressing pain in eyes : to protrusion : with
burning, redness and lachrymation.

And, not only deafness and pains in ears, with otitis : but the
mastoid process is specifically affected : with swelling, periostitis and
even caries. This seems to us especially worthy of notice. Kent's
Repertory gives only *Capsicum* here. There are also bursting
pains, head, abdomen, etc. We are told, by an ex-R.M.O. of our
Hospital, of a patient with early mastoid trouble (and with marked
home-sickness) who got *Capsicum*. It worked.

It is one of the sea-sickness remedies : and a unique remedy for *home-sickness*.   One of our young " residents " when he found a recently admitted child inconsolable ; screaming, or sobbing its heart out ; would give a dose of *Capsicum*, and come back shortly afterwards to find it playing happily with toys.

Then, a curious symptom, coughing causes pain in some distant part.   This also we have verified.

These remedies of limited, but curious and unique action are most useful, where they fit ; one may need them seldom : but yet nothing on earth will take their place, where symptoms demand them.   Happily they are easy to remember.

Black Letter Symptoms

Home-sickness.

Of a contented disposition :. is jocular and sings, and yet on slightest cause, gets angry.

Disposition to start.   After emotions, fever with red cheeks.

Intoxication.

Confusion of HEAD *: or, all the senses are more acute.*

When moving head and when walking, headache as if the skull would burst.

Throbbing, beating headache : in one of the temples : in the forehead.   Pressive pain in forehead.

Drawing, tearing pain, left side of head.

A shooting headache, worse at rest, better by movement.

An outstretching headache, as if the brain were too full.

Drawing, tearing pains frontal bone, more on right side.

Aching pain in eyes as from a foreign body.

Swellings ' of MASTOID *process : painful to touch :*
Periostitis and caries of mastoid.

Tearing pain in concha of ear.

An itching or aching pain quite deep in ear.

Epistaxis.

Burning blisters in MOUTH.

Tough mucus in mouth : or dryness.

Taste foul : like putrid water.

Chaps on the lips : fissured lips.

Tough mucus in posterior nares on rising : difficult to dislodge.

Tonsillitis, with burning, smarting pain.

Great soreness in THROAT, *with smarting.*

Pain when swallowing, burning and other pains in throat, worse between acts of swallowing.

Throat inflamed, dark-red, burning, pressing.

Heartburn.
Dyspepsia from torpidity ; especially in old people.
STOMACH *ice cold : or burning in stomach.*
Inclined to vomit.
Thirst : drinking causes shuddering ; drawing pains in back.
Burning, cutting pains in ABDOMEN.
After every stool, thirst, and after every drink shivering.
Aching tension, ABDOMEN, *especially in stomach, worse movement :*
with aching tension lower part of back.
Tensive pain, abdomen to chest, as from distension.
Abdomen feels distended almost to bursting, impeding breathing,
to suffocation.
A drawing and turning over in abdomen.

After flatulent colic in hypogastrium, small frequent STOOLS *of*
mucus mixed with blood, which cause tenesmus.
Tenesmus : violent tenesmus.
Burning pain in anus.
Dysentery : tenesmus and stranguary : pain worse from a
current of air, even if warm.
Smarting and burning pain in the anus and rectum.
Tenesmus of rectum and bladder at the same time.
Hæmorrhoids, burning as if pepper were sprinkled on them,
swollen, itching, throbbing : with sore feeling in anus : bleeding or
blind with mucus discharge ; with bloody mucous stools ; with drawing
pain in back and cutting pain in abdomen.
Small frequent stools of mucus, at times with blood : cause
tenesmus.

Burning in bladder.
Burning, smarting after urination.
Strangury : tenesmus neck of BLADDER *: urging to frequent,*
almost ineffectual urination.
Scalding of urine.
Gonorrhœa : second stage : white discharge : excessive sensi-
bility of parts to contact : cordee only suppressed by cold water.

Creeping and tickling in NOSE, *as in stuffed coryza.*
Hoarseness, from straining voice, in singers, preachers, etc.
When coughing, headache as if skull would burst.
COUGH *expels an offensive breath from lungs.*
Nervous, spasmodic cough.
Tightness of CHEST *: appears to come out of stomach.*

Chest constricted, with oppressed breathing : worse very slight movement.

Throbbing pain in chest.

Drawing tearing pain in and near spine.
Tensive pain in knees.

Coldness beginning in back.
Shivering.
Lack of reactive force, especially in fat people.
Is wide awake at night : cannot sleep.
Sleep full of dreams.
Yawning.
Great desire to lie down and sleep.

So awkward that she runs into everything.
Sea-sickness.
Lazy, fat, unclean persons who dread open air.
Children who are always chilly,
Shivering with chilliness after every drink.
As if cayenne pepper were sprinkled on parts !
Relaxed fibre : obesity.
Shuns all movement.
Burning in skin.
Hæmorrhoidal constitutions

SOME ITALIC, AND STRANGE, RARE AND PECULIAR SYMPTOMS

Children become clumsy and awkward.
Home-sickness, with red cheeks and sleeplessness.
Wakes in a fright, screams : remains full of fear.
Senses obtuse.
Brain too full. Bursting pains in head. Head feels bruised.
Pressing headache in forehead, as though pressure in occiput would force brain out through forehead.
Violent, deep-penetrating stitches, vertex.
Head seems too large.
Affects especially mastoid process.
Flickering before eyes : or objects look black.
Eyes very prominent, with pale face. Eyes protrude from sockets.
Pressing pain in ear with every cough : as if abscess would open.
Aching in ears when coughing.
Tip of nose very red and hot : worse towards evening.
On coughing or sneezing, cutting in one or other limb.
Pain internal or exterior of face, with biting as if from salt.

Dry throat without thirst.

A remedy of cancrum oris.

White spots in throat, with red halo.

Malignant or gangrenous pharyngitis.

After every stool, thirst, and after every drink shivering.

After a drink, must go to stool.

Hæmorrhoids burn, as if pepper were sprinkled on them.

Needle-stitches, in forepart of urethra, when not urinating.

During pregnancy, affections of ears, etc.

Tickling in trachea causes violent sneezing.

Cannot get air deep enough into lungs.

Cough in sudden paroxysms : convulses whole body.

Cough, as if head would fly to pieces.

With every explosive cough, pungent, fetid air escapes.

Coughing or sneezing causes sudden pain in a limb.

Stitches in suffering parts, with cough.

Splitting pain in head, with cough : or pain chest, back, bladder, neck or ear. Inclined to vomit : or pain in knees, legs, ears, throat.

Cough : worse anger, warm drinks, evening, night, when lying, dry cold weather, draught, warm or cold.

Pain in chest, as if it were too full : not room enough in it.

Fatty degeneration of heart in obese persons.

Violent pulsations of arteries of abdomen.

Clucking, rapid pulsation in some of the larger arteries.

Chilliness between scapulæ : " cold water dropping down back."

*   *   *

NASH summarizes its peculiarities thus :

Burning pains, especially on mucous membranes, or *smarting*, as from red pepper, on the parts.

Cough with pains in distant parts, as head, bladder, knees, legs, etc.

Chill or shuddering *after every drink*. Begins between the shoulders and spreads all over.

With above symptoms, it is a good remedy for dysentery, or the later stages of gonorrhœa, or in throat complaints. A remedy to be remembered in all affections, with the red pepper *burnings*.

He says, I cured a very bad case of years' standing. The patient would cry out and grasp head with both hands at every cough. It finally became so bad that he had to lie in bed, because the hurt was so much worse when sitting. *Capsicum* cured very quickly

*   *   *

Guernsey. It affects mucous tissues in a *very* prominent degree.

Head, aches as if it would burst : beats : throbs ; darts. Better in motion. Biting, burning, stinging itch, scalp, as if it had been rubbed with cayenne pepper. . . .

Abdomen as if it would burst. . . . Yawning by day, and sleeplessness by night. Sensation as if falling from a height during sleep (this occurs especially with *Thuja.*). . . . Eructations of red pepper feel and taste :· sensation of cold water in stomach. Symptoms generally left sided ; for light-haired people : tendency to get fat : lax muscles : bloated skin.

*   *   *

Farrington speaks of the marked irritating properties of *Capsicum* : it takes but little of the drug to produce irritation. He says it is eliminated through the kidneys, producing strangury with burning when passing water. He says it acts best on stoutish persons of lax fibre. Weak stomach, weak digestion, whole man weak. Adults and children alike are irritable and get angry : are worse from the least draught, even of warm air : clumsy.

He is thirsty, yet drinking causes shivering.

An unusual symptom : very offensive breath during cough. In diphtheria, carrion odour from the mouth.

Throat feels spasmodically closed : worse when not swallowing.

*   *   *

Now for some extracts from Kent. He says :

Most of the substances that are used on the table as seasonings in foods will in the course of a generation or two be very useful medicines, because parents poison themselves with these substances, tea, coffee, pepper, and tobacco (though tobacco cannot be said to be on the table, yet it might as well be if it is used at all), and these poisonous effects in the parents cause in the children a predisposition to diseases, which are similar to the disease produced by these substances.

In the fat, flabby, red-faced children of beer drinkers and pepper eaters, with poor reaction, a relaxed and flabby constitution, red face and varicose condition, those that have been over-stimulated, children of overstimulated men, we find the sphere for *Capsicum* very often. The face looks rosy, but is cold and not warm, and is seen to be studded with a fine system of capillaries. . . . Plump, round, with no endurance, a false plethora, like *Calc.* End of nose red, cheeks red, redness over cheekbones, red eyes. These constitutions react slowly after diseases, do not respond to remedies, are sluggish, tired, lazy. Schoolgirls who cannot study, and get home-sick. Gouty joints, stiff, clumsy, weak. . . . Chilly in the open air : worse for bathing.

Mental state : home-sickness . . . oversensitive : suspicious : always looking out for an insult. Obstinate in the extreme : it is devilishness. If she wants a thing will oppose it, if suggested by someone else.

Tormented by persistent thoughts of suicide.

Headache : as if skull would split when moving head. Feeling as if skull would fly to pieces : holds head with hand. Head feels too large. As if brain would be pressed out and eyes pressed out on stooping.

Capsicum has a peculiar action on the bones of the external ear and the mastoid process.* Abscesses round about and below the ear, and caries: petrous portion of the temporal bone necrosed. It has been a frequently indicated remedy in mastoid abscess which worries the old school doctors so much that they bore down and remove the cells for fear of basilar inflammation : a devilish practice, for, after they do all this and nearly kill the patient and spasms come on in spite of it all, the indicated remedy comes in and cures the patient, and the spasms, and the ear disease.

Old catarrhs . . . when no reaction seems to come after the most carefully chosen remedies, and all at once the doctor wakens up to the realization that the patient has a red face, and it is cold, and the end of the nose is red and cold, and the patient is fat and flabby and has not much endurance ; never could learn at school : and if she exerts breaks out into a sweat and freezes in the cold air. . . . When he gives *Capsicum* to that patient it rouses her . . . it may not cure, but after it *Silica* or *Kali bich.* or other remedy which was perhaps given before and did not act, takes hold and cures. . . .

The parts you touch are loose and flabby, red, fat, and cold.

Dysentery. After stool tenesmus and thirst, and drinking causes shuddering. . . . Hæmorrhoids sting and pinch, as if pepper had been sprinkled on them . . . with plethora : plump, flabby ; sensitive to cold, red face. . . . Chronic hoarseness : and he is rotund, chilly, red-faced and the hoarseness disappears under *Capsicum*.

Cough in sudden paroxysms, convulsing the whole body ; every cough jars the affected part. Stitches in the suffering part with the cough.

---

* *A girl has been seen at Hospital with a constant temperature of about 100° since a mastoid operation some years ago. A dose of* Capsicum *given after working on this Drug Picture has resulted in a normal temperature ever since, i.e. three months.*

CARBO VEGETABILIS

(*Wood Charcoal*)

FROM the earliest times, Hahnemann tells us, physicians considered charcoal to be non-medicinal, and powerless.

Then came the curious discovery of the chemical properties of wood charcoal in especial, its power of removing from putrid and mouldy substances their bad smell, and preserving fluids from fetid odours. Then physicians began to employ it externally. In fetor of the breath they caused the mouth to be rinsed with powdered charcoal, and applied powdered charcoal to putrid ulcers, and in both cases the fetor was immediately removed. Again, administered internally in autumn dysentery it removed the evil odour of the stools.

But, he tells us, this is merely a chemical use of wood charcoal, which takes away the foul odour of putrid water when mixed with it in coarse lumps, and does so most effectually in coarse fragments.

But this was merely a chemical, not dynamical employment, penetrating the inner vital sphere. The mouth rinsed only remained free from fetor for a few hours. The old ulcer was not improved, and the fetor, chemically removed for the moment, always recurred. The powder taken in autumn dysentery removed the fetor of the stools only for a short time ; the disease remained, and the disgusting smell of the stools soon returned.

Pulverized wood charcoal, he says, can exercise almost none other than a chemical action. And a considerable quantity of wood charcoal may be swallowed without producing the slightest alteration in health.

And yet *Carbo vegetabilis* is one of our most powerful and precious remedies : at times " a veritable corpse-reviver ", as one has seen : and it is one of the striking proofs of the value of Hahnemann's great discovery in regard to the liberation of power, in inert substances, by dynamization or sub-division of particles.

He puts it thus . . . " It is only by prolonged trituration of the charcoal (as of many other dead and apparently powerless substances) with a non-medicinal substance, such as sugar of milk, that its inner, concealed, and, so to speak, slumbering medicinal power can be awakened and brought to life," and he found that a minute quantity of the " millionth-fold power-attenuation, injested, produced great medicinal effects and derangement of the human health ". He did not advise the use of a stronger potentization than the millionth-fold (the third cent. potency). And his provings were made with this " Million-fold power-attenuation."

KENT says of *Carbo veg.* " It is a comparatively inert substance made medicinal and powerful, and converted into a great healing agent, by grinding it fine enough. By dividing it sufficiently, it becomes similar to the nature of sickness and cures sick folks . . . It is a great monument to Hahnemann. It is quite inert in the crude form and the true healing powers are not brought out until it is sufficiently potentized . . . A broad-acting, deep-acting, long-acting medicine . . . It affects the vascular system especially ; more particularly the venous side of the economy—the heart and the whole venous system. Sluggishness is a good word to think of when examining the pathogenesis of *Carbo veg.* : sluggishness, laziness, turgessence . . . Everything about the economy is sluggish, lazy, full, distended, swollen, puffed. The hands are puffed ; the veins are puffed ; the body feels full and turgid ; the head feels full . . . the limbs feel full, so that the patient wants to put the feet up to let the blood run out. The veins are lazy, relaxed and paralysed. Vaso-motor paralysis . . . varicose veins.

" The mental state, like the physical, is slow . . . Slow to think ; sluggish ; stupid ; lazy . . . The limbs are clumsy . . . the skin is dusky. The capillary circulation engorged. The face is purple and dark."

Carbo veg. has BURNINGS—and COLDNESS. Burnings in-veins, in capillaries, in head, itching and burning of skin. " Burning in inflamed parts. Internal burning, and external coldness. Coldness with feeble circulation, with feeble heart. Icy coldness. Hands and feet cold : knees cold : nose cold : ears cold : tongue cold. Coldness in stomach with burning. Covered with cold sweat : collapse with cold breath, cold tongue, cold face. (*Camph.*) Looks like a cadaver, yet in all these conditions the patient wants to be fanned."—Kent.

Or, as NASH has it . . . " Vital force nearly exhausted ; complete collapse. Blood stagnates in the capillaries ; venous turgessence ; surface cold and blue.

" In the last stages of disease, with copious cold sweat, cold breath, cold tongue, voice lost, this remedy will save a life."

One has seen that—in one extreme case, in especial : the sort of case one does not forget, and which one quotes to show what *Carbo veg.* can do in the most desperate conditions, *where the symptoms agree.* It was a small girl with heart disease, and an acute exacerbation supervening that was abruptly ending her young life. She had a pneumonia with pleural effusion, an endocarditis with pericardial effusion, and one morning, when the Physician was going his round accompanied by several other doctors, she was found lying forward on the supports that had had to be provided, because she could not rest otherwise, cold, white, unconscious ; just alive, because she was still giving the infrequent sharp gasps of the dying. *Carbo veg.* (I think 200) was quickly administered, while one of the doctors of wide experience exclaimed, " I'll eat my hat if that child lives ! " But before the ward round was finished she had regained warmth and consciousness—death had passed on ! And, under *Kali carb.* (the complementary remedy, by the way !) she got well, so far as the damaged heart would permit. It is such experiences that have gained for *Carbo veg.* the name " *corpse reviver* ".

It· is curious and important to note that these *Carbo veg.* patients, even *in extremis*, with the coldness of death already present, have air-hunger, and want to be fanned.

But apart from such desperate conditions, *Carbo veg.* is one of the useful remedies of everyday life—where symptoms demand its use.

For instance it is one of the most FLATULENT* of remedies (*Lyc., China*). Stomach feels full and tense, with great accumulation of flatus : this is worse at night : worse when lying down. In one's experience there may be belching and belching by the hour, with great distress, and then a dose of *Carbo veg.* and it all subsides, without any more coming up. We know that vegetable charcoal in the crude state has an extraordinary capacity for absorbing gases—the amounts it can absorb are phenomenal : but one does not expect this strange power to be carried into the realm of the potencies ! Explanations may be difficult : but it is facts that count every time. In the same way *Carbo veg.* in the potencies will banish fetor far more effectually than in the crude form. But here a word of warning. *Carbo veg.* will work its miracle on flatulence night after night, and will need to do it again and again, night after night—*if it is not a Carbo veg. case.* Whereas some other drug—perhaps *Argentum nit.*, whose symptoms *do* correspond to those of the patient, will act curatively, and the condition will not return ; certainly not for some thirty days and then not with the same intensity. To the correct remedy the reaction will be curative, not merely palliative.

GUERNSEY tells us that *Carbo veg.* has also " complaints from *obstructed* flatulency (may be pains in the head, around the heart or

---

* *For excessive flatulence* Carbo animalis *seems equally, if not more effective, than* Carbo veg. *Nothing could be more striking than its prompt relief of flatulent distension after operations on the abdomen. One has seen this more than once.*

anywhere, which are relieved by the discharge of flatus). Flatus has a putrid and very stinking smell ".

In regard to its stomach conditions, Kent has a telling little paragraph—Kent's Lecture on *Carbo veg.* gives a wonderful picture of the drug and its uses ! He says : " The *Carbo veg.* patient has a longing for coffee, acids, sweet and salt things. Aversion to the most digestible and the best kinds of food. Now if I were going to manufacture a *Carbo veg.* constitution, I would commence with his stomach. If I wanted to produce those varicose veins and the weak venous side of the heart, this fullness and congestion, and flatulence, this disordered stomach and bowels, and head troubles and mind troubles—sluggishness of the whole economy—I would begin and stuff him. I would feed him with fats, I would feed him with sweets, with puddings and pies, and sauce, and all such indigestible trash, and give him plenty of wine—then I would have the *Carbo veg.* patient. Do we ever have such people to treat ? Just as soon as they tell their story you know enough about their lives to know that they are mincepie fiends : they have lived on it for twenty years, and now they come saying, ' Oh, doctor, my stomach ; just my stomach : if you will simply fix up my stomach.' . . . He has burning in the stomach, distension of the stomach, constant eructations, flatulence, passing of horribly offensive flatus . . ."

Nash, and others, quote H. N. Guernsey " one of the best prescribers that ever lived " to the following effect . . . " No truer remark was ever written than that *Carbo vegetabilis* is especially adapted to weak and cachectic individuals whose vital powers have become weakened. This remark is made particularly clear in the light of those cases in which disease seems to be engrafted upon the system by reason of the depressing influence of some prior derangement. Thus for instance the patient tells us that asthma has troubled him ever since he had the whooping cough in childhood ; he has had dyspepsia ever since a drunken debauch which occurred some years ago ; he has never been well since he strained himself so badly (*Rhus tox., Calc.*), the strain does not now seem to be the matter, but his present ailments have all appeared since it happened ; he sustained an injury some years ago, no traces of which are now apparent, and yet he dates his present complaints from the time of the occurrence of that accident . . . It will be well for the physician to think of *Carbo veg.* in similar cases which are numerous, and may present very dissimilar phenomena, as these circumstances being suggestive of *Carbo veg.* it in all probability will be found to be the appropriate remedy, *which the agreement*

8

of other symptoms of the case with those of the drug will serve to corroborate."

The italics of the last phrase are ours, and for this reason: one used to " try " *Carbo veg.* where the illness dated from, or was ascribed to, a previous sickness or accident. But the results were poor, and the idea dropped out. But where such a history makes you think of *Carbo veg.* and you find on reference to Materia Medica that *the symptoms agree*, you will inevitably get your results. That is quite a different story. And that is what Guernsey emphasizes in his last sentence. Often a strange symptom, or a tip, such as the above, suggests a drug which would not have otherwise occurred to you, *and when*, by reference to Materia Medica, *the symptoms are found to agree*, you will succeed. There are more ways than one of finding the remedy : and the ultimate court of appeal is MATERIA MEDICA. No Repertory can possibly supersede the actual provings. And it is the peculiar symptoms, when they agree in drug and patient, that lead to a consideration of that drug, and a successful prescription.

One has seen, or knows of, the amazing effect of even a dose of *Carbo veg.* in GANGRENE, in one case with the most appalling fetor. Kent says of *Carbo veg.*, " Ulceration, with relaxation of the blood vessels and feebleness of the tissues, you need not be surprised if there is no repair, no tissue-making. So when a part is injured, it will slough . . . An ulcer, once established, will not heal. The tissues are indolent . . . Poor tissue-making or none at all. ' *The blood* stagnates in the capillaries.' You can see how easy it would be for these feeble parts to develop gangrene. Any little inflammation or congestion becomes black or purple, and sloughs easily—that is all that is necessary to make gangrene."

But short of such end-processes as gangrene, one finds *Carbo veg.* extraordinarily useful in some cases of VARICOSE ULCERS, and VARICOSE VEINS. In the *Carbo veg.* cases there are blackish patches or areas, caused by stagnation in venules and capillaries. It is here that *Carbo veg.* especially helps (*Thuja* has something of the sort). The blackness vanishes and the ulcer heals.

Here are some of the uses of *Carbo veg.* all suggested by, or brought out in, the provings.

Indifference ; heard everything without feeling pleasantly or unpleasantly, and without thinking of it.

Headaches : all the provers had headaches, mostly occipital. Headaches, and can't wear a hat. Hair falls out by the handful.

Face pale : cold : cold sweat on face (*Verat.*). Tongue cold and contracted ; white ; coated ; bluish ; parched ; sticky ; black

(*Ars.*). Looseness of teeth and bleeding gums. Foul taste and odours from mouth.

One of the mumps medicines (*Pilocarpine*).

Much catarrh.

Coldness : " cold limbs : cold knees : cold nose : cold feet : cold sweat. Face pale : cold, covered with sweat."

In chest conditions with much dyspnœa, copious expectoration, exhausting sweat, great coldness—and the patient must be fanned.

Cold breath, coldness of throat, mouth and teeth, but desires to be fanned. Must have more air.

Cold knees at night. Ulcers burn at night ; discharge offensive.

Hæmorrhages : indolent oozings . . . " Even the tongue piles up that black exudate, that oozing of black blood from the veins." " Vomiting of blood with icy cold body and breath."

Kent says that the abdominal fullness aggravates all the complaints of the body. There may be " even flatulence in the tissues under the skin, so that it will crepitate ".

" Extremely putrid flatus : incarcerated flatus : collects here and there as if in a lump." " Diarrhœa horridly putrid, with putrid flatulence."

" One of the greatest medicines we have in the beginning of whooping cough."

" Attacks of violent spasmodic cough in paroxysms, with cold sweat, cold, pinched face."

" Pneumonia, third stage, with fetid expectoration, cold breath, cold sweat, desire to be fanned."

" Feelings of internal heat and burning, with external coldness —a common feature of *Carbo veg.*"

Burning in stomach. Great accumulation of flatus : distension of stomach and abdomen.

ASTHMA. Kent gives the *Carbo veg.* picture of asthma . . . " We see the patient propped up in a chair by an open window, or some member of the family may be fanning him as fast as possible. The face is cold, the nose pinched, the extremities cold, and he is pale as death. Put the hand in front of the mouth and the breath feels cold. The breath is offensive, putrid . . . Internal burning with external cold is a common feature with *Carbo veg.*

BLACK LETTER SYMPTOMS

Indifference ; heard everything without feeling pleasantly or unpleasantly, and without thinking of it.

Anxiety ; as if oppressed with heat in face ; accompanied by shuddering ; on closing eyes ; in evening, after lying down ; on awakening.

FAINTING *after sleep ; after rising, or while yet in bed, mornings ; belching ; caused by debilitating losses, or abuse of mercury.*

Dull headache in occiput ; violent pressive pain in lower portion of occiput ; feeling of weight.
HEAD *feels heavy as lead.*
Hat pressed upon head like a heavy weight, and he continued to feel the sensation even after taking it off, as if head was bound up with a cloth.
Sweat on forehead, often cold.

Burning in EYES.

Parotitis.

Looseness of TEETH, *with bleeding of gums, which are very sensitive.*
TONGUE *turns black.*
Tongue cold.
Stomacace.

Great accumulation of flatus in STOMACH.
Stomach feels tense and full ; flatulence.
Distension of stomach and abdomen.

Burning in RECTUM.
Itching of anus.

Rawness and chafing of children in hot weather.
Cholera Asiatica, stage of collapse.
After sexual excesses and onanism.

Soreness, itching, and burning and swelling of pudenda.
Debility from nursing. Gastralgia.

Great roughness in larynx, with deep, rough voice, which failed if he exerted it, though without pain in throat.

Breathing short, with cold hands and feet.
Desires to be fanned, must have more air.
Weak, fatigued feeling of CHEST, *particularly on waking.*

Pneumonia ; third stage, fetid sputum ; cold breath and sweat ; wants to be fanned ; threatened paralysis of lungs.

Fine itching eruption on HANDS.
Cold knees, particularly in night.
Ulcer on leg burns at night ; discharge offensive ; mottled, purple.

Awakens often from COLD *limbs, especially cold knees.*

Adynamic and gastric fevers, occurring in hot weather from abuse of ice-water and other summer beverages.
Typhoid and yellow fever patients ; cyanotic, and coldness of limbs, almost in agony of death ; impending paralysis of heart and collapse.
Yellow fever ; third stage, hæmorrhages, with great paleness of face, violent headache, great heaviness in limbs and trembling of body.

Swelling of GLANDS, *in scrofulous or syphilitic persons.*

SEPSIS, *sunken features, sallow complexion, hectic, typhoid symptoms.*
Blue colour of body, with terrible cardiac anxiety and icy coldness of whole surface. (Cyanosis.)

ULCERATIONS, *with burning pain.*

Vital powers low, VENUS SYSTEM *predominant.*

CAULOPHYLLUM
Squaw-Root : Papoose-Root : Blue Cohosh.

WHEN the conventional practitioner saturated with the learning of the Schools, finds his lot cast for him among " natives " and " savage tribes " of sorts, he is apt to brush aside impatiently the inherited lore that surrounds him—whether malign or benign ; perhaps often the former—but far from always ! Secure in his comparatively easy methods, sanctioned, as they are, by Authority, he is apt to despise and trample out, in his lordly way, much that it were greatly to his advantage to explore and study.

His beloved *antiseptics*, for example, oust for him the invaluable " wound-herbs " of the district. These (instead of his clumsy and anxious efforts to destroy, or at least deter, the dreaded " organisms " more or less at the expense of the inherent healing powers of the tissues) would work for him, gently and effectively, after the manner of such herbs ; routing the enemy by the simple method of stimulating healthy healing in damaged tissues. Or again, armed with quinine (one thing he did obtain, by observation of native healing), and some few stock drugs chiefly of a palliative nature, he is apt to consider that all knowledge is with him ; that what he does not know about medicine is not worth knowing, or, for him, no subject for orthodox speculation. Forgetting that,

> *Knowledge is proud because she knows so much :*
> *Wisdom is humble that she knows no more.*

Far other, thank God ! is the attitude of the Homœopath,—always on the prowl for that which heals. His insatiate thirst for *power* has taught him to not despise but investigate. Hence he has introduced, from the world over, from North American Indians—from South America, especially from Brazil—from Martinique and the West Indies—from everywhere—not only precious herbs of healing, but those magnificent reptilian venoms —of snakes—spiders—toads—lizards—which give to homœopathy a much wider range of healing than is dreamt of by Old School. Some of his native remedies have been slowly filtering through to the laggards in Materia Medica : for instance *Hamamelis—Witch Hazel*, introduced by Constantine Hering in 1850, and now common property. . . . In glancing down the lists of medicines in *Hale White*, who instructs the cramming student in " Mat. Med.", one can always spot the imported homœopathic remedies, because they are set down as simple tinctures, and not wrought into the compound prescriptions of hoary antiquity. But—it *is* amusing to find oneself occasionally warned off our everyday stand-bys—and for this imperative reason, as Clarke points out, that *curative* remedies work under a double Law : and that of Dynamization must be added to the Law of Similars, if they are to be, not only safe, but effective. It stands to reason that, if you are using that which can *cause* mighty evil to *cure* something similar, it requires delicate handling and prescribing. You cannot pour it in from a bucket.

And now Old School has at last got its teeth into the snake venoms, and is lost in admiration of the vast possibilities envisaged. But here again, the snag !—*for these most potent of potent homœopathic remedies will have to be used according to the methods of Hahnemann, if they are to do the maximum of good and the minimum of damage.* And, again, it is only by their " provings " that it can be discovered what actually they are capable of, as well as which is to be used for this case—this purpose—and which for that !

But, to revert to our subject, the Squaw-roots of America are wonderful aids in the treatment of the pangs and diseases " which " (female) " flesh is heir to." One notices that, coming from such source, they have often, at all events to begin with, been used in low potencies and in substantial doses. But, as a case we quote presently, from Nash, shows, they may do even better service in the potencies.

* * *

DR. BORLAND (*Homœopathy for Mother and Infant*), says :

It is an experience common to homœopathic doctors everywhere, who are conducting a general practice, that their patients do not suffer from difficult labour. That does not prove anything, but it is a fortunate fact for the patients. There are two factors which have a bearing on this happy experience. A pregnant woman who is treated throughout her pregnancy with homœopathic medicines will approach her confinement freed from the physical and mental ailments which so often are factors in the production of an unsatisfactory confinement. Secondly, there is a drug—*Caulophyllum*—which has the power of regulating the processes of labour. This is a fact which was known and used by homœopaths many years ago, and is equally true to-day.

I have a patient, recently confined of her first child. Years ago her mother was given *Caulo.* before this patient was born. Now the patient herself was put on *Caulo.* before the birth of her child. During her confinement she was attended by an obstetrician of very wide experience. She had a large child and it was her first pregnancy, labour had started, and she was examined. The attending lady gynæcologist said that everything was going well, but that many hours must elapse before anything could be done

to help, and went off home. She got into her own door as the
telephone bell rang, asking her to return at once, and got back
to the nursing home just in time to see the child born. The
mother was saved trouble, forceps delivery, hours of suffering, and
prolonged labour with its increased danger for the child. She had
been taking small doses of *Caulo.* daily for a month before.
Coincidence, perhaps, but a coincidence one has come to expect.*
    And again,

IN PREPARATION FOR UNCOMPLICATED LABOUR

Caulophyllum.   (" *Squaw-root* " of the North American Indians.)
                   Fretful—apprehensive.
                   Uterus feels congested.   Tension and fullness.
                   Spasmodic pains, uterus : and during menses.
                   Leucorrhœa : with bearing down pains.
                   Threatened abortion (*Vibrum*).
                   Spasmodic rigidity of os, delaying labour.
                   Labour pains, short, irregular, spasmodic,
                       no progress being made.
    Caulophyllum has not been extensively proved : but taken,
a dose daily, during the last two or three weeks of pregnancy,
it is found to make labour easy.   12th or 30th potency.

                    *   *   *

    IT was HALE, in his *New Remedies,* who first drew attention to
this invaluable remedy. He says :

    This is one of a class of remedies whose virtues seem to have
been well known to the aborigines of this country.   They called it
" squaw-root " by which name it is known to the common people.
Early pioneers, lay as well as professional, all bear witness to the high
estimate placed on it by the Indians for the relief of the sufferings
and weaknesses of the women of that race.   It has another name,
"Blue Cohosh", the origin of which I have not been able to ascertain.

    Its sphere of action, as near as can be stated at present, is not
extensive, but confined to the small muscles and joints, the muscular tissues of the generative organs, and possibly the motor
nerves and mucous membranes.

    The provings made do not throw much light on its general
powers.   Its clinical uses afford us almost all the data upon which
we base our knowledge.

    Its most prominent value seems to be its power of causing
intermittent contractions of the gravid uterus, and possibly of the
unimpregnated.   In this it differs from Ergot, which causes, or tends
to cause, persistent contractions.   The remedies which most resemble
it in this respect are *Viburnum, Cannabis indica,* and *Cimicifuga.* . . .

    * N.B.—*At our farm it helps the cows also in their calving.*—ED.

It is a powerful agent for the prevention of premature labour and of miscarriage, provided the premonitions are pains of a spasmodic character.

The aborigines and earlier settlers claimed for it the power of preventing tedious and painful labours. This testimony has been substantiated by many prominent and trustworthy physicians of the eclectic school, as well as of the homœopathic. . . .

My experience has been so uniform and conclusive on this point, that I do not hesitate to assert that it prevents not only a too painful labour, but it prevents those premature labours which are so common among the weakly women of this age.

It seems to be homœopathic to rheumatism of the short muscles and small joints of the extremities, and a few cases of that character have been reported.

* * *

FARRINGTON (*Clinical Materia Medica*) says : " Another remedy to be compared with *Pulsatilla* is *Caulophyllum*. This is a remedy that we have had not many years, and yet it is so useful that we would not now be able to get along without it."

Its main characteristic is *intermittency of pains*. If they are neuralgic and reflex from uterine disorder, they are intermittent in character. They are usually sharp and crampy and appear in bladder, groins and lower extremities.

During labour *Caulophyllum* is indicated when there is extreme uterine atony. The pains may be as severe as ever, yet there is apparently no expulsive effort. It is often indicated in nervous women in whom pain seems to be intolerable. The pains are spasmodic and fly about from place to place, now in the groins, then in the abdomen and next in the chest ; but not going in the direction of the normal pains. The patient seems to be exhausted, There is great exhaustion of the whole system. She can scarcely speak at times, so weak is the voice. These are the symptoms which call for *Caulophyllum*. It has been used here by most physicians in the low potencies, although all potencies may be used. It may also be indicated during the last weeks of pregnancy when the patient suffers from false labour pains, these consisting of painful bearing-down sensations in the hypogastrium. I have known a single dose stop them after they had lasted for hours. . .

Another remedy that I have found very valuable in the *leucorrhœa of little girls* is *Caulophyllum*, when the discharge is profuse and weakens the child very much. . . .

We find that in uterine spasms, *Caulophyllum* and *Actea racemosa* act like *Magnesia mur*. I must say that I believe *Caulophyllum* heads the list. I know of no other drug that produces

such continued spasmodic condition of the uterus unless it be
Secale. . . .

Caulophyllum is especially suited to rheumatism of the
phalangeal and metacarpal joints, particularly in females.

* * *

GUERNSEY (*Keynotes*) has also a few words of appreciation for
Caulophyllum.

Rheumatism of small joints. In labour we find deficient pains
on account of the exhaustion of the patient ; *Cauloph.* will at once
brace up her strength and produce efficient pains.

His summary of the uses of *Cauloph.* in diseases of women is
worth reproducing.

Extraordinary rigidity of the os uteri.

Spasmodic and severe pains, with no progress made.

Pains become very weak from exhaustion of the patient, on
account of long labour.

Thirst and feverishness.

False pains : spasmodic, in various parts of abdomen.

Patient much exhausted, and pains very inefficient.

Menorrhagia, or hæmorrhage after labour, especially hasty
labour. Flow very profuse, due to want of tonicity of uterus,
which is relaxed and contracts feebly.

Convulsions with very weak and irregular pains. Feels very weak.

Retained placenta, with characteristic sense of weakness or
exhaustion, and pains too weak.

After-pains after protracted and exhausting labour : spasmodic
pains across lower abdomen, may extend to groins.

Lochia bloody lasts too long : passive oozing from relaxed
uterus with great exhaustion.

Abortion threatened, with want of tonicity ; uterine contraction feeble.

Neuralgia of vagina, when vagina is excessively irritable, and
pain and spasm are intense and continued.

Hysteria and uterine displacements with above characteristics.

Leucorrhœa burning, producing characteristic weakness.

Extremities : Very severe rheumatic pains, aching, drawing,
erratic, now in one place, now in another.

Especially in *small* joints, fingers, wrists, toes, ankles. Great
painful stiffness of affected joints.

Worse in open air : from coffee.

* * *

Weakness : *exhaustion* : *want of tone*, as one sees, are the Keynotes of the remedy.—KENT (*New Remedies*) brings this out.

Weakness in the reproductive system of the woman.

From weakness she is sterile, or she aborts in the early months of gestation.

During parturition the contractions of the uterus are too feeble to expel the contents, and they are only tormenting.

Labour-like pains during menstruation with drawing pains in the thighs and legs, and even the feet and toes.

Uterine hæmorrhage from inertia of the uterus.

Relaxation of muscles and ligaments.

Heaviness, and even prolapsus.

Subinvolution.

Excoriating leucorrhœa.

Menses too soon, or too late.

She is sensitive to cold, and wants warm clothing, quite unlike *Pulsatilla*.

She is hysterical, like *Ignatia*.

She is fretful and apprehensive.

She is rheumatic, like *Cimicifuga*, only the small joints are likely to be affected.

Later she suffers from after pains, and they are felt in the inguinal region.

Rheumatic stiffness of the back, and very sensitive spine.

She is sleepless, restless, and withal very excitable.

This remedy has cured chorea at puberty when menstruation was late.

*   *   *

There is always a good deal of repetition in quotations from several prescribers, yet each one is able to stress some important point, " Learn from many, if you would know more than a little."

Lastly NASH speaks of *Caulophyllum* as another very valuable " women's remedy " because of its specific action upon the uterus. He says it deserves a thorough proving.   And in regard to its curious action on *uterus and small finger joints* he gives an instructive and suggestive case.   We will abbreviate.

Married lady of 40, with wry neck of long standing, was seven months pregnant.   She was attacked with *severe pains and swellings of all the finger joints*.   Intense pain, and only relief, in order to get sleep, by enveloping her fingers in mustard.

Nash gave *Cauloph.* 3*d*, which relieved the finger pains, but brought on severe labour pains, and was discontinued for fear of premature labour.   Then the bearing-down pains ceased, and the finger pains returned and continued in full force until she was delivered of her child, when they ceased for two or three days.

Then the lochia, instead of decreasing, increased till it amounted to a metrorrhagia. *The flow was passive, dark and liquid.*   There was a great sense of weakness and *internal trembling*, and now the terrible finger pains returned again.

Nash was afraid of *Cauloph.* which seemed indicated, because it had brought on the bearing-down pains. He gave *Arnica*, *Sabina*, *Secale* and *Sulphur*, without the least improvement : then concluded to give *Caulophyllum high.* He did so in the 200th potency, and cured the whole case promptly and permanently. He says, " Now this was a perfect *Cauloph.* case, and had I given it properly in the first place I have no doubt I would have saved that woman all unnecessary suffering."

He adds : " I have given this remedy in long-continued passive hæmorrhage from the uterus after miscarriage when I had the characteristic weakness and sense of *internal trembling* present. It has often regulated irregular spasmodic labour pains, and relieved pains of the same character in dysmenorrhœa."

Many cases of rheumatoid arthritis in women begin at the menopause. Whenever that is the case, and the small joints of hands and feet are involved, *Caulophyllum* should be one of the drugs that comes up for consideration. Also in any non-menopausic cases where *uterus and small joints* are affected.

* * *

Here is a LITTLE CASE that came up again the other day at Out-patients and, reminding one of the drug, suggested that, as it was little known, and could be frightfully useful, it should be Drug-pictured. Hence this attempt !

Mrs. X, 52, came to Out-patients in April 1936 complaining of rheumatoid arthritis. Hands and feet deformed. Symptoms suggested *Causticum* or *Medorrhinum.* She had one after the other, without improvement. Later, because of the very marked " *Worse thunderstorms* ", she got *Rhododendron*, for some months, in different potencies, and improved very much.

In February 1937, hands were " less good " and there was more pain. And now *Rhododendron* failed, and, again, *Causticum.*

March 1937. Finding that hands were " worse during her periods and for three days before ", and " nice afterwards " she got *Caulophyllum*, a dose of the 30*th* potency.

April. " MUCH better and knuckles less swollen."

May. Much better.

July 20th. " Ever so much better " ; and in herself also. " Not so down-hearted now she can use her hands."

August 17th. Says, " When she first came her hands got much better, then bad again. They are fine now." She feels and looks very well ; and the movements of her hands are normal, with very little to show their original condition.

CAUSTICUM

ONE of Hahnemann's flashes of genius : an outcome of Hahnemann the Chemist, and Hahnemann the Physician.

FARRINGTON says, " *Causticum* is evidently a potash preparation, but its exact composition I do not know. Hahnemann was not able to define it and chemists since his time have not been able to tell of what it is composed. Nevertheless it is a unique remedy and is one that we cannot do without in practice."

HAHNEMANN calls it a *hydrated caustic*, but what is more important, he gives full directions as to the preparation of " *this powerful drug* ". He says :—

" Take a piece of recently burnt lime weighing about 2 lbs., immerse it for a minute into a vessel full of distilled water, and then lay it in a dry cup, where it soon becomes pulverized, giving out much heat and a peculiar odour. . . . Of this fine powder you take 2 ounces, place it in the mortar which had been previously warmed, and then mix it with a solution of 2 ounces of bisulphate of potash in 2 ounces of boiling hot water, the potash, before having been dissolved, having been exposed to a red heat, melted and cooled again, and then pulverized. This thickish preparation is inserted into a retort, to the open end of which the receiver which ought to be dipped in water to half its height, is hermetically fastened. The liquid is distilled over by gradually approaching a coal-fire to the retort, and until the preparation is perfectly dry. The liquid in the receiver is about one ounce and a half, as clear as water, and containing the *Causticum* in a concentrated form, which smells like the lye obtained from potash, and has an astringent and burning taste on the back of the tongue. Its freezing point is below that of water. It promotes the putrefaction of animal substances which are placed in it. With the salts of baryta it gives out no trace of sulphuric acid, nor any trace of lime-earth with the oxalate of ammonium.

" One or two globules of the 30th potency are given at a dose, which often acts for upwards of fifty days."

HERING'S *Guiding Symptoms* says : " Whatever diversity of opinion may exist theoretically in regard to the chemical nature of this substance . . . the unquestionable good results obtained by its use, in potentized form, by a majority of our best practitioners stamp it a polychrest of the highest order."

And NASH calls it " A very unique remedy, proven by Hahnemann. . . . Its exact chemical composition is not known but it is supposed to be a kind of potash preparation. It has quite a long list of peculiar symptoms, which are very reliable."

Causticum, mentally, is unhappy : weeps, cries : is melancholy —hopeless : looks on the dark side : has forebodings and apprehensions. Is peevish, irritable, censorious : very suspicious and distrustful. It is a remedy of mental alienation after suppression of eruptions.

Affects especially persons dark-haired, dark-eyed, and of darkest mood and temper. No suspicion of brightness or gaiety here. Kent says *Causticum* " has cured insanity : not acute mania with violent delirium, but mental aberration of the passive kind, where the brain has become tired. The constitution has become broken down with long suffering and much trouble and finally the mind can be no longer co-ordinated : it is in confusion."

*   *   *

FARRINGTON says : " Especially suited to patients who are timid, nervous and anxious, full of fearful fancies especially in the evening at twilight, when shadows grow longer and fancies more rife. The child is afraid to go to bed in the dark."

We will quote further from Farrington : " The patient has rather an odd sensation, one not frequently met with, a feeling of an empty space between the brain and the cranial bones—relieved by warmth. Odd as this symptom may seem, it is not too uncommon for you to make a note of. . . .

" Very characteristic of the drug is paralysis of single parts or of single nerves . . . facial paralysis, especially when the result of exposure to *dry, cold winds.* . . ."

" These paralyses may be caused by deep-seated nervous disease or, very characteristically, by exposure to cold, particularly to the intense cold of winter when patient is of the rheumatic diathesis." (*Acon.* from the same cause—*bitterly cold, dry winds*). " In facial paralysis, from this cause *Acon.* will often cure, but if it threatens to become chronic, *Causticum.*"

" Children, emaciated, especially about the feet, with abdomen large and tumefied. With eruption on scalp, and inflamed eyes ; often otorrhœa, purulent ; and the child stumbles when it attempts to walk. . . .

" Aphonia or failure of voice. N.B., the hoarseness of *Phos.* is worse in the evening ; that of *Caust.* worse in the morning. . . .

" The paralytic condition extends to the cough also ; cannot cough deeply enough to raise the phlegm ; or phlegm, partly raised, slips back into pharynx ; and, again, the urine may spurt during cough." (" This inability to expectorate is found in every species of cough ; whooping cough, etc.")

Farrington also says he has cured Ménière's disease with *Caust.* (*Salicylic acid.*)

Again : " Epilepsy, especially petit mal. Of course, during the unconscious stage the patient passes urine. Convulsions, especially when they recur at the full moon. (*Sil.*). . . .

" Rheumatism, rheumatoid arthritis, especially where joints are stiff and tendons shortened, drawing the limbs out of shape." (Here one remembers an old body, much benefited by *Caust.*, who finally got *Drosera*, and rapidly recovered movement in almost all the joints that had been " set " for years. She had developed pain in the tibia also, which then suggested *Dros.* *Dros.* has particularly " pain in the long bones ".)

Rheumatoid conditions then, with contractions and deformity ; worse cold, dry winds, better warm wet weather.

* * *

KENT says : " *Causticum* is a very searching medicine, suitable, too, in old broken-down constitutions, suffering from chronic disease. Its complaints are progressive, slow, and accompany a declining state of the economy. Gradual decrease of muscular power. A *paralysis.*

"Paralysis of the œsophagus, paralysis of the throat, such as occurs after diphtheria " (*Gels.*) ; "paralysis of the upper eyelids, paralysis of the bladder, paralysis of the limbs, of the lower limbs; great lassitude, muscular relaxation, indescribable fatigue and heaviness of the body " (*Gels.*). " And there is a tremulousness " (*Gels.*), " a quivering, jerking, twitching of the muscles, twitching in sleep. . . ."

Then, " *contractures of tendons and muscles*, when the limb is drawn up. . . .

" Also a rheumatic state of the tendons and ligaments about the joints, with perhaps swelling, but pain and shrivelling of the joint, which becomes tightened up and ankylosed. Stiffness, with weakness and melancholy ; hopelessness ; something going to happen.

" With this rheumatism, he can stand neither heat nor cold ; and he is always worse in dry weather ; worse cold, dry winds. (*Acon.*). Facial paralysis from exposure to cold, dry wind (*Acon.*). Such paralysis will almost always recover under *Causticum.*"

" Then, hysteria ; startled easily ; crampings. Convulsions if frightened. Epilepsy from fright, from being chilled or exposed to some great change in the weather ; or from bathing in a cold river. Passive mental aberrations of a tired mind. Timorous anxiety: ' something going to happen '. Lacks balance. Everything excites him.

"The suppression of eruptions is apt to bring out mental symptoms. . . . He was fairly well while he had the eruption, but when it disappeared his mind gave out . . . the driving in of a facial eruption will frequently result in facial paralysis. Violent headaches . . . associated with rheumatic and gouty ‧conditions which also affect the scalp: which contracts and tightens up in places like the contractures in other parts.

"Torticollis. *Causticum* is a curative remedy in this shortening of the tendons and muscles.

"Paralysis of optic nerve. . . . Deafness from paralysis of auditory nerve. . . .

"Fissures seem to form upon the least provocation. . . . fissures about the lips, the wings of the nose, the corners of the eyes : fissures of the anus, of the skin about joints : old cases of salt rheum with fissures in the bends of the joints. . . .

"Stammering from paralytic condition of tongue. Complete paralysis of pharynx and œsophagus—as after diphtheria : food goes down wrong way, or enters larynx, or posterior nares. Paralysis of organs of speech : awkward at talking, awkward at chewing : bites tongue and cheeks when chewing.

"The *Caust.* patient sits down to the table hungry, but thought, sight or smell of food takes away the appetite (*Ars., Sep., Cocc.*). A common symptom of pregnancy. . . .

"A queer sensation in stomach, as if lime were slaking there.

"Many symptoms are better for a swallow of cold water. The violent, spasmodic cough may be stopped at once by a drink of cold water. Cold water seems to tone up the paralytic condition.

"Paralytic weakness also in rectum : it is inactive and fills up with hard fæces which pass involuntarily and unnoticed (*Aloe.*). Stool passes with less straining when standing : retention of urine except when standing (compare *Sarsaparilla*).

"This remedy has two kinds of paralysis of the bladder, one affects the muscles of expulsion and the urine is retained: the other, centring on the sphincter, when the urine passes involuntarily.

"It is a deep-acting medicine : cures phthisis, especially ' quick consumption '. Cough with the sensation ' cannot cough deep enough to start the mucus ': cough relieved by a swallow of cold water. Cough worse by bending forward. Cough continual, with each cough escape of urine. . . ."

One finds it difficult to stop condensing and quoting from Kent !

*   *   *

Then WARTS. *Causticum* is one of the great remedies for warts (*Thuja, Dulcamara*, etc.). Glance down the black-letter symptoms—warts—warts—warts. Old warts on eyelids, eye-brows, nose. . . . Warts on face. . . . One remembers experiences here. One year on our farm in Surrey a number of calves took to sprouting warts about their faces, noses, ears, necks. My father used to go down on Saturdays, and he took *Caust.* in lowish potency to medicate a tumbler of water with which he soaked bran for their delectation. This soon finished the warts : and the same thing, since, with other animals.

One has proved that *Caust.* and *Thuja* can both produce warts and cure them. A horse, accidentally proving *Thuja* in φ sprouted warts amazingly about anus and genitalia—the favourite localities of *Thuja* for these excrescences : while a girl to whom one gave *Caust.* with more zeal than discretion in those early days, instead of one or two warts on her hand, produced them by the dozen on hands and arms ; but when the drug was discontinued, the whole lot disappeared, including the original ones which were brought for cure.

FARRINGTON records a similar experience. He writes :— " *Causticum* also acts on the skin, one of its most characteristic symptoms being warts, . . . useful when they occur on the hands and face. I remember once giving *Caust.* to a child who had two warts on the under eyelid. At the end of the third week after taking the remedy, there was a string of warts over the inner canthus of the other eye : I believe that these resulted from the *Caust.* Of course I stopped the medicine. At the end of several weeks more, all the warts had disappeared and the child has had none since. This shows you that *Caust.* really produces and cures warts."

NASH says : " *If Hahnemann had never given to the homœopathic school any remedy but* CAUSTICUM, *the world would still be to him under lasting obligation.*"

ODDS AND ENDS, AND CHARACTERISTICS

" Intense sympathy for the sufferings of others."

" Apprehension of impending danger, with urging to stool." (Compare *Arg. nit., Gels.*)

" Cicatrices, especially burns " (*Urtica urens*) " scalds, freshen up, become sore again ; old injuries re-open ; patients say they have never been well since that burn."

" *Caust.* may be called for in colic, after the failure of *Colocynth.* The pains are griping, cutting, relieved by bending double. All the sufferings cease entirely at night."

" Menses too early ; too feeble ; *only during the day* ; cease on lying down."

" Better in damp, wet weather ; warm air."

" Coffee seems to aggravate every symptom."

" Must not be used before or after *Phos.* Always disagrees."

And Hahnemann gives a curious mental symptom—what we have come to call " Spoonerisms". Confounds letters and syllables, for instance, says " cluent foryza, instead of fluent coryza " for several days—after proving *Caust.*

" Hæmorrhoids—burning, raw, sore ; worse walking, thinking of them, from preaching or straining the voice ! " Nash says all these symptoms have been verified over and over again.

BLACK LETTER SYMPTOMS

MENTAL. *Hysterical weeping after spasms.*

The least thing makes the child cry.

Melancholy mood ; sadness, hopelessness, from care, grief or sorrow.

Peevish, irritable, censorious.

Mental and other ailments from long-lasting grief and sorrow.

Excessive anxiety. Full of apprehension in the evening.

Very much vexed.

Indisposed to work.

Weakness of memory. Absence of mind.

Inattentive and absent.

Rheumatic pains in HEAD *so severe as to cause nausea.*

Tinea capitis in occipital region.

Inclination to close EYES *; they close involuntarily.*

Sensation of heaviness in upper lid, as if he could not raise it easily, or as if agglutinated to lower lid and could not be easily loosened.

Paralysis of eye muscles, especially if from exposure to cold.

Burning in eyes : visible jerking of the lids.

Sight obscured, as if a thick fog were before the eyes.

Incipient cataract

Pressure in eyes as if sand in them.

Dryness ; photophobia.

Words and steps re-echo in EARS.

Deafness.

Accumulation of ear-wax, sometimes offensive.

Dry coryza with stoppage of NOSE.

Fluent coryza with pain in chest and limbs.

Itching tip of nose and alæ, as well as inside.
Pimples, ulcers, crusts on tip of nose ; inflamed, swollen, scurfy.
Old warts on nose.
Violent bleeding of the nose.

Acne rosacea on cheeks and forehead, in dispersed groups.
Paralysis of one side of FACE.
Prosopalgia and rheumatism of face.
Warts on face. Yellowness of face.
Tightness and pain in jaws ; difficult to open mouth and to eat.
Arthritic pains in lower jaw.

Pain lower back tooth extending to nose and eye.
Painful looseness and elongation of TEETH.
Stitching and tearing toothache. Throbbing toothache.
Pain in sound teeth on drawing in cold air.
Swelling of gums, readily bleeding and tedious suppuration.
Frequently recurring abscesses of gums.
Sore place in the upper part of the palate.

Stuttering, difficult, indistinct SPEECH.
Speechlessness from paralysis of organs of speech.
Tongue coated white on both sides, red in middle.

Burning pain in THROAT, *not from swallowing ; on both sides,*
seemed to rise from chest.
Rawness and tickling in throat with dry cough and some expectora-
tion after long coughing.
Pain in throat, worse by stooping.
Must swallow continually, throat feels too narrow.
Mucus collects in throat, cannot be raised by hawking ; is obliged
to swallow it.
Hawking of mucus, with pain in pit of throat.
Dryness of throat, constantly obliged to swallow.

Bread causes pressure in STOMACH.
Violent thirst for many days.
A swallow of cold water relieves spasms (whooping-cough).
Sour vomiting followed by sour eructations.
Cramp in stomach.
Pinching, clawing in stomach on deep breathing.

HÆMORRHOIDS *sore, painful ; unendurable on walking.*
Hæmorrhoids : impeding stool : sticking, burning, painful if
touched : when thinking of them : from preaching or straining voice.

The STOOL *passes better standing.*

Frequent ineffectual efforts to stool, with anxiety and redness of face.

Pain and strong pulsations in perineum.

Frequent emission of a large quantity of URINE.

He urinates so easily that he is not sensible of the stream : can scarcely believe in the dark that he is urinating till he makes sure with his hand.

Involuntary passage of urine when coughing, sneezing or blowing the nose ; at night when asleep.

Retention with frequent and urgent desire, occasionally a few drops or a small quantity may dribble away.

Itching, orifice of urethra.

Pressive pain in testicles.

NIPPLES *sore, cracked, surrounded with herpes.*

Sudden loss of VOICE.

Hoarseness, especially evening, with scraping in the throat.

Muscles of larynx refuse to perform their function : unable to speak a word in spite of every exertion.

COUGH *with sore sensation in a streak down along trachea, where it pains on every paroxysm of cough.*

Shortness of breath.

Cough with sensation as if he could not cough deep enough to start mucus, with tickling and rawness.

Hollow, racking cough.

Cough relieved by a swallow of cold water.

Cough better from bending forward.

Continual annoying cough, with each cough escape of urine.

Influenza with tired sensation, limbs as if beaten ; rheumatic pain.

CHEST *tight ; must frequently take a deep breath.*

Soreness in chest.

Stitches in sternum from deep breathing or lifting.

Painful compression of chest from both sides towards sternum.

Sensation (chest) as if clothing were too tight.

PULSE *excited towards evening with orgasm of blood.*

Stiffness and pain in NECK *and throat, pain in occiput : muscles felt as if bound, could scarcely move head.*

Painful stiffness of BACK *and sacrum, especially rising from a chair.*

Pressing cramp-like pain in small of back, region of kidneys.

Bruised or darting pain in coccyx ; or dull drawing pain.

Dull drawing and tearing in ARMS AND HANDS.

Paralysis of right arm with glossoplegia.

Paralysis of upper extremities.

Paralytic feeling in right hand.

Trembling of hands.

Sensation of fullness in hand, when grasping anything.

Drawing pains in finger joints.

Contraction and induration of tendons of fingers.

Warts on tips of fingers ; fleshy warts close to nails.

Soreness between THIGHS *high up.*

Drawing and tearing in thighs, legs, knees and feet : worse open air, better in warmth of bed.

Bruised pains in thighs and legs, mornings in bed.

Marbled skin of thighs and legs.

Cracking in KNEES, *when walking or descending.*

Tendons of knees seem too short.

Gonagra. (Gout of knee joint.)

Gouty tearing in region of LOWER LEG, *especially in small joints of foot, with swelling.*

Cramp in feet, toes and soles.

Emaciation of feet.

Children are slow in learning to walk, with unsteady, tottering gait.

Unsteady walking and easy falling of little children.

Paralytic weakness of LIMBS. *Weakness and trembling of limbs.*

Intolerable uneasiness of limbs in evening.

NERVES. *Chorea, even at night, right side of face and tongue may be paralysed.*

Weakness and trembling. Faintlike sinking of strength.

Paralysis : of vocal cords ; one sided ; of tongue ; of eyelids ; of face ; of extremities ; of bladder.

Gradually appearing paralysis.

Tearing PAINS.

Terrible sensation of tearing, paroxysmal : often moving forward, then remitting, again starting from same spot : neuralgia moving from occiput, upwards and forwards, over vertex.

CONTRACTION *of flexor tendons ; tension and shortening of muscles.*

Disturbing functional activity of brain and spinal nerves, resulting in paralysis.

During first SLEEP *wets the bed.*

Intense sleepiness, can scarcely resist it, must lie down.

Yawning and stretching.

Sleeplessness at night : on account of dry heat. Cannot rest in any position.

Bad effects from night-watching. (Cocc.)

At night he can get no quiet position : cannot lie still a moment.

SKIN. *Subacute and chronic eruptions, similar to blisters from burns.*

Burns and scalds.

Large, jagged, often pedunculated warts, exuding moisture and bleeding easily.

Warts and scrofulous affections.

Varicose and fistulous ulcers.

Dark-haired persons with rigid fibre most affected.

Children with black hair and eyes.

Antidotes poisoning by lead (paralysis). Paralysis of tongue from type held between lips (compositors). Abuse of Merc., *and* Sulph. *in scabies.*

But remember *Causticum* in those difficult " Rheumatoid " cases of arthritis, where there are deformities and contractions, and the patient suffers more in cold, dry winds, and less on warm, wet days.

CEANOTHUS AMERICANUS

HERE we have one of Dr. James Compton Burnett's very special remedies. He was a genius of the first order where the treatment of the sick was concerned, and also in the writing of his telling little monographs. We owe much to his intuition, his enterprise, and his indefatigable industry. He had a very large practice on his London days, as well as in Brighton—his home. We are told that, in Town, he would be literally besieged in the early hours of the morning : and that, when he was discovered lying dead in his hotel room, it was a terrible blow to the many he had helped and cured of difficult and, apparently, hopeless conditions.

In Hale's *New Remedies*, where *Ceanothus* appears as *Ceanothus virginiana*, there is, in the 1880 edition, a lengthy quotation of five long, closely printed pages from a Homœopathic Journal of the previous year from Dr. Burnett's pen. Hale says, " It remained for an English physician, Dr. J. C. Burnett, to discover the affinity of *Ceanothus* for splenic disorders." And in Dr. Burnett's booklet, *Diseases of the Spleen and their Remedies* (1900), *Ceanothus* figures largely, with a number of detailed cases, not only of enlarged spleen, but also of pain deep in the left hypochondrium ; some of which cases had even been diagnosed as heart disease, but which cured rapidly and completely under *Ceanothus*. The whole is a record of the triumphs of a physician who knew just a little more than his fellows, and who joyfully applied his knowledge for the relief of suffering and the removal of grave disabilities.

Burnett always gave honour where honour was due : to the washerwoman who added to his knowledge by curing one of his malaria patients with stinging nettle tea. From time to time " Organotherapy " or " Organopathy " was of great help to him, in regard to which he writes, "The real father of organopathy, in essence and substance, is Hohenheim, an eminent and learned physician called Paracelsus, for proof of which see his works, and hereafter in this little volume on *Diseases of the Spleen*, if space permits." Burnett contends that organotherapy is included in the wider generalization known as Homœopathy ; for whereas organopathy claims only that certain drugs affect certain parts curatively, preferentially, or specifically, as for instance, digitalis the heart, Homœopathy claims that not only does digitalis affect the heart . . . but to be curative the natural disease of the organ must be *like* in expression to the therapeutic organopathy, or drug action. Homœopathy, he adds, " may be said to be based upon organopathy, for a drug to cure the heart of its disease specifically must necessarily affect the heart in the *same* manner. . . ."

Burnett says that previous to reading a short account of *Ceanothus* in an early edition of Hale, he had frequently felt a difficulty in treating a pain in the left side, having its seat, apparently, in the spleen. " *Myrtis communis* has a pain in the left side, but that is high up under the clavicle ; the pain that is a little lower is the property of *Sumbul* ; still lower of *Acidum fluoricum*, a little farther to the left of *Acidum oxalicum* ; more to the right of *Aurum* ; right under the left breast of *Cimicifuga rac.* These remedies promptly do their work when left sided pains are a part of the disease picture, but they will not touch the pain that is deep in behind the ribs of the left side . . . the real splenic stitch requires *China, Chelidonium, Berberis, Chininum sulph.* or *Conium,* or *Ceanothus Americanus.*"

In low potencies, in which Burnett used it, he found, " It frequently relaxes the bowels, and I have known this even amount to diarrhœa."

One patient had been taking it for about a fortnight, when one day she felt a great nervous excitement. This passed when she left the medicine off : then recurred when it was resumed, to again cease when it was discontinued. Her bowels were relaxed, and her menses were two days too early and very profuse ; a thing that had never happened to her before.

We will give a few of Burnett's gleanings and deductions, in regard to *Ceanothus*, quoted from his little Spleen book.

" Death," he says, " is often, at the start, in a particular organ, i.e. *local*, and if the part be saved in time life may be preserved. In the acute processes the value of a particular organ strikes one often very forcibly, there may be no need of any constitutional treatment ; the one suffering part may be the whole case. And in many chronic cases certain organs claim and must have special attention."

" To avoid misapprehension in one or two particulars . . . 1st, what I understand by an organ remedy is *not* a drug that is topically applied to a suffering organ for its physical or chemical effects, but a remedy that has an elective affinity for such organ, by reason of which it will find the organ itself through the blood. Further I do not regard organopathy as something outside Homœopathy, but as being embraced by, and included in it, or co-extensive with it. I would say—*Organopathy is Homœopathy in the first degree.* Finally, I would emphasize the fact, that where the homœopathic simillimal agent covering the totality of the symptoms, *and also the underlying pathologic process causing such symptoms* can be found, there organopathy either has no *raison d'être* at all, or it is of only temporary service to ease an organ in distress."

" I am much struck with the teaching of Rademacher* that a very large percentage of dropsies are curable by spleen remedies."

" Since writing the foregoing in 1879 I have found a good many chronic cases of spleen affections, and those for the most part previously unrecognized."

In one of his cases, " the spleen would not leave off swelling at certain times till I had cured the vaccinosis. That prince of splenics, *Ceanothus Americanus*, readily cured the splenic engorgement, but did not touch the blood disease which caused it. This is the inherent defect of organopathy, that it is not sufficiently radical in its inceptive action ; but the like remark applies to every other pathy more or less, because the primordial cause is more or less elusive and generally quite beyond positive science, which only admits of what it knows, and will not seek to encompass the unknown, by the processes of thinking and reasoning. Because in former times philosophy made science impossible, the votaries of science now round upon philosophy and sneer it out of view. To trace back proximate effects to remote causes is now ridiculed because *mere* science is productive of a gross mindedness, incapable of following the *fine* threads of the higher perception."

In another of his cases there was a pain on the left side, which had lasted for quite twenty-five years. It came suddenly, especially if she drank anything cold. She would get an indescribable pain under the left ribs, and she would have to fight for breath, and the dyspnœa would be so severe that it could be heard in the next room, frightening everybody. She had had ague thirty years ago. . . . Before taking the *Ceanothus*, for many years she was compelled to lie down when dressing in the morning on account of the beating of the heart. This was a case of much enlarged spleen, with tenderness that could not bear any pressure—from clothing even. *Ceanothus* cured ; and Burnett records one of the " sweetest things of his whole professional life—the old lady (and what a lady !) put a tiny packet on my desk, tried to say something, burst into tears, and rushed out ! He says, " I never saw her again, and have often wished I had kept that particular

---

* Rademacher, the exponent of organopathy, had disciples who formed a school and published a journal in 1847. Burnett says they wandered off into the field of experimental pharmacology, but found it already occupied by whom ? by the homœopaths ! The wanderers, he says, never came back, but remained in the *field of provings*, side by side with the followers of Hahnemann.

sovereign and had it set in diamonds." (The patient was a char-woman he had been asked to help, since she was said to be suffering from an incurable disease of the heart. He had promised, after examination, to cure her ; and the lady who had asked his help for the poor old creature, accused him of cruelty for " raising her hopes, when he must have known it is impossible ! " His explanation that it was an enlarged spleen, and not the heart at all, was not believed. " She had been under various doctors, and all had declared it incurable heart disease." It was cured, nevertheless !)

In regard to heart troubles, he tells us that, " Where the heart is perturbed consentaneously with a spleen affection, the relief obtained from the use of *Ceanothus* (and other splenics) is very often noteworthy."

And, " With regard to dropsies, in so far as they are not due to organismic affections, I ascribe, according to a rough calcula-tion, about one-third to the spleen."

Other useful suggestions are :

" Some cases of varicosis will not get well till you cure the spleen of its, perhaps slight, enlargement."

Again, " In one case, where the patient has been under good symptomatic homœopathic prescribing, which had failed, because the symptoms treated were secondary to the enlargement of the spleen. . . . It must be manifest that vomiting due to an enlarged spleen can never be cured by remedies that physiologically produce vomiting, but by such as will bring a large spleen back to the normal."

Hale quotes an American doctor as saying, " During the late Civil War I used this plant for splenitis and so well satisfied have I been with the results that for six years I do not remember using anything else for enlarged spleen. I have used it in the worst cases I ever saw, from infancy to old age. I have yet to hear of its failure in a single case, however inveterate."

Hale says " this is pretty strong and positive testimony, and the author fully confirms my idea that a remedy which cures is homœopathic always, for he further says :

" In chronic cases, when the organ is no longer tender, under the use of the tincture, even without friction, it soon becomes painful and tender, then sinks rapidly to its normal size, and so remains, the patient being no longer conscious of its presence.

" We see here a true homœopathic aggravation, showing that the drug has a specific affinity for that organ. I advise you to use it when you meet with cases of ague-cake, so common in malarious districts.

" Dr. Carroll Dunham informs me that a physician of his acquaintance cured an enormous enlargement of the spleen by the use of this remedy."

Dr. Oscar Hanson gives the therapeutics of *Ceanothus.* " Chronic inflammation and hypertrophy of the spleen, pain in the whole left side, with violent dyspnœa. Persistent pains in hypochondrium, profuse menses and yellow leucorrhœa."

Boger's *Synoptic Key*, adds a little thereto : " Periodic neuralgias. Pain in left side, with dyspnœa, diarrhœa or leucorrhœa. Swelled spleen or liver. Worse cold weather ; lying on left side. Complementary to *Nat. mur."*

Clarke's *Dictionary* also includes this valuable remedy in its wide range of medicaments.

You may say, " Ah ! but whoever sees cases that need *Ceanothus* ? " In the last ten days we have had to prescribe it twice : apparently splenic pains are not so rare as one might suppose.

CHAMOMILLA

MODEST little weed which flourishes about this time of the year in rick-yards among the litter of thrashings, with its acrid scent, and its white petals that bend backwards, as if putting their little hands behind them. This distinguishes it from rather like flowers. As my " herb-woman " used to say, " there are two of every kind ", i.e. the " herb " of great utility, and the counterfeit weed that looks so like it, but is useless. But, as a rule, it is scent, or the want of scent, that distinguishes them easily.

An excellent name for *Chamomilla* is " *Cannot bear it* ".

" Can't bear himself."

" Can't bear other people."

" Can't bear pain " (*Coffea, Acon.*).

Can't bear things : wants them, and hurls them away.

Everything is simply intolerable.

You look at the *Chamomilla* baby and often see one brilliant cheek : you touch its head, and find it warm and wet.

Cham. is one of Clarke's " Nursery A.B.C. drugs "—*Acon.*, *Bell., Cham. Aconite* is turmoil in circulation. *Belladonna* is turmoil in brain. *Chamomilla* is turmoil in temper.*

If *Cham.* is a sick baby he is easily spotted. He will whine and howl and insist on being carried. The moment the tired mother or the jaded father tries to sit down, or to set him down, the music starts afresh ; and the trouble is worse at night.

Or, short of this, he stretches out his little hand for thing after thing, and when it is offered pushes it away in disgust. " He does not know what he wants " (says Nash), " but the doctor knows—it is *Chamomilla*."

When a little older *Cham.*, when sick, will order his nurse or mother out of the room. We have seen a mother crouching outside a closed door, inside which her small sick son was raving if she dared to poke her nose inside.

When still older he will refuse to see the doctor. I think it is Nash who says, when you know you have to see an " ugly " patient, who will refuse to see you, or will be rude to you, send on first a dose of *Cham.* and find peace. *Cham.* is definitely uncivil.

The *Chamomilla* pain is intolerable. One has seen a person tramping the floor in agony, after a bad tooth-extraction ; when a small dose of *Cham.* gave almost instant and complete relief.

---

* *Acon.* and *Cham.* have many characteristic symptoms in common : but the mentality decides between them.

One has seen a person with 'flu, not getting well as quickly as desired, and suddenly impatient and irritable to a degree. A dose of *Cham.* and the temperature promptly came down.

Some time ago we published a case of asthma, with such irritability that *Cham.* stared the doctor in the face. It was given, and cured.

Hahnemann said, " Do not give *Acon.* where sickness is borne with calmness and patience " ; and of *Cham.* he wrote, " It is unsuited for persons who bear pain calmly and patiently."

In acute cases where *Cham.* is urgently demanded by the mental state, you can pull out your watch and count the very few minutes to complete relief. The nature of the ailment matters little, it is the mentality that simply shouts for *Chamomilla*.

Cham. has not only bad temper, but *bad effects of bad temper*.

A *Cham.* woman flies into a temper and gets a hæmorrhage from the womb. Or a *Cham.* woman flies into a fury, and is rewarded with an attack of jaundice. One has seen these. Or a nursing mother has a fit of anger, and her milk poisons her baby.

And Hahnemann says in a footnote, *Mat. Med. Pura*, " The sometimes dangerous illness resembling acute bilious fever, that often comes on immediately after a violent vexation causing anger, with heat of face, unquenchable thirst, taste of bile, nausea, anxiety, restlessness, etc., has such great homœopathic analogy with the symptoms of chamomile, that chamomile cannot fail to remove the whole malady rapidly and specifically, which is done as if by a miracle by one drop of the above-mentioned juice."

Cham. is one of the " out-of-proportions " drugs. *Ars.* has *prostration* out of proportion (seemingly) with the malady, and *Cham.* has *pain* out of proportion (such as pains of labour—tooth-ache—rheumatism, etc.).

A tip for *Cham.* is *numbness with pain*. (*Plat., Cocculus.*)

Hahnemann, footnote *Mat. Med. Pura*, says, " The paralytic sensation of chamomile in any part is never without accompanying drawing or tearing pain, and the drawing or tearing of chamomile is almost always accompanied by paralytic or numb sensation in the part."

Another thing *Cham.* can't stand is BED.

Cham. thrusts the feet out of bed (with *Sul., Puls., Med.*).

Is driven out of bed by pain or intense discomfort and misery.

" The chamomile pains have this peculiarity as a rule, that they are most severe in the night, and then often drive the victim almost to despair, not infrequently with incessant thirst, heat, and redness of one cheek ; sometimes also hot sweat in the head, even in the hair."

Twice *Cham.* has brilliantly cured trench fever, to our knowledge. In one case the officer had been ill for a year, and his fever
was at 9 a.m. (the *Cham.* black-type hour), and the turmoil in his
temper was such that he had to live away from his people, in
a hotel. He only wanted to smash tables and chairs.

Recently an out-patient was complaining of rheumatism,
she could not sleep for it, but got up and walked the room, and
was frightfully irritable. She got *Cham.* 200. On her next appearance, " Much better : feeling better than for months " ; and
now she confessed that she had been so frantic that she had
" wanted to break something ". When pain or fever wants to
smash things, remember *Chamomilla*.

BLACK LETTER SYMPTOMS

Dullness of senses, diminished power of comprehension.

*Joyless obtuseness of the senses : understands nothing properly,
just as if he were prevented doing so by a sort of dullness of hearing,
or a waking dream.*

Child cries ; quiet only when carried.

Child does not wish to be touched.

Very irritable and fretful ; child must be carried.

Piteous moaning of child because he cannot have what he wants.

*Whining restlessness ; the child wants this and that, which, when
offered, is refused or pushed away.*

Averse to talking, short and snappish.

*Cannot endure being spoken to, or interrupted while speaking,
especially after rising from sleep.*

Patient cannot bear anyone near him, and answers snappishly.

Peevish disposition, nothing pleases.

*Peevishness ; she seeks a cause for being peevish at everything ;
can't return a civil answer.*

Irritable, impatient mood.

*Howling on account of a slight, even imaginary insult, which
occurred long ago* (*Staph.*).

Easily chagrined or excited to anger.

*Extreme restlessness, anxious, agonized tossing about, with tearing
pains in abdomen.*

The pains sometimes made him very peevish.

*Oversensitiveness to pain, which seems unbearable and drives
to despair.*

Throbbing HEADACHE. *Semi-lateral drawing headache.*

Transient attacks of throbbing in one-half of brain.

Congestion to head : following anger ; with pressure while lying down ; on vertex ; with heat in face and oppression of chest ; with stitches in head and chest.

(Pain head) increased as soon as attention was directed to it.
Warm sweat on head, wetting hair.

EYES *swollen in morning ; agglutinated with purulent mucus.*
Violent pressure in orbital region, sensation in eyeball, as if it was tightly compressed from all sides, with momentary obstruction of vision.

Roaring in EARS, *as from rushing water.*
Single large stitches in ear, especially when stooping, with ill humour and peevishness about trifles.
Pressing earache in spells, with tearing pain, extorting cries.
Particularly sensitive to open air about ears.

Heat in FACE *after eating (and sweat).*
Redness of one CHEEK, *returning in paroxysms, without shivering or external heat.   Hemicrania.*
Red face, or redness and heat of one.(l.) cheek, the other being pale.
One cheek red and hot, the other pale and cold.

Lower lip parts in the middle in a crack (Nat. m., Sep., Graph.).
Face sweats after eating or drinking.
On and under tongue vesicles with shooting pains.

Toothache if anything warm is taken into MOUTH ; *after coffee, < by talking ; in open air, in room ; getting warm in bed ; during menstruation and pregnancy ; most l. side and lower teeth ; < at night.*
Toothache recommences when entering the warm room, or drinking anything warm.
(Toothache) seems intolerable and makes him very peevish.
Teeth feel too long.
Gums red and tender.   Dentition.
Teething children ; with watery, greenish, and also chopped diarrhœa, smelling like rotten eggs ; jerking of limbs, or starting convulsions, child bends double and draws legs upon abdomen : moaning, wanting to be carried : dry cough, restless at night ; wants to drink ; quick rattling breathing.
Bitter taste in mouth, in morning.
Heat in mouth, pharynx and œsophagus, to stomach.
Collection of saliva, of metallic, sweetish taste.
Fetid smell from mouth.

Spasmodic constriction of pharynx.

Sore THROAT, *with swelling of parotid or submaxillary glands, or tonsils.*

Want of APPETITE.

Great thirst for cold water and desire for acid drinks.

Likes to hold cold water in mouth for a long time, when drinking. Dentition.

After eating and drinking, heat and sweat of face.

Thirsty and hot with the pains.

Fruitless efforts to vomit.

The pains present are aggravated by eructation.

Pressure in STOMACH, *as from a stone pressing down.*

Constrictive gastralgia in coffee drinkers.

Colic returns from time to time, flatus accumulates in hypochondria and stitches shoot through chest. Gurgling in side extending into ABDOMEN.

After a meal abdomen becomes distended.

Wind colic, abdomen distended like a drum, wind passes in small quantities without relief : > by applying warm cloths.

Children have spasms in consequence of nursing milk vitiated by a fit of anger.

Abdomen tympanitic and sensitive to touch.

A white slimy DIARRHŒA *with bellyache.*

Green, watery, corroding, with colic, thirst, bitter taste, and bitter eructations; like chopped or stirred eggs, smelling sour; hot, smelling like rotten eggs; changeable, containing undigested food; mucous and bloody.

A forcing towards inguinal ring, as if that part too weak, and a hernia would come or constipation from inactivity of rectum.

Ulcerating fissures at anus.

MENSTRUAL *colic, following anger.*

Membranous dysmenorrhœa.

Profuse discharge of clotted blood, with severe labour-like pains.

Drawing from sacral region forward, griping and pinching in uterus, followed by discharge of large clots of blood.

Yellow, smarting leucorrhœa.

Labour pains press upward; she is hot and thirsty, cross and inclined to scold.

Rigidity of os; scarcely able to endure the pains.

After-pains, very acute and distressing.

Puerperal convulsions, after anger; or has one red cheek, the other being pale.

Rash of lying-in women and nursing infants, caused by heat or errors in diet, with watery, greenish, chopped egg diarrhœa, corroding anus.

Mammæ hard and tender to touch, with drawing pains, is fretful, sleepless and cross.

Suffocative tightness CHEST, larynx constricted with constant irritation to cough.

Almost uninterrupted tickling irritation to cough under upper part sternum : does not always result in coughing.

Tickling in pit of THROAT, causing dry, scraping cough. Voice hoarse.

Sensation of rawness and scraping in larynx.

Hoarseness from viscid mucus in larynx only brought away by violent hawking.

Suffocative attacks from repercussion of measles eruption, by taking cold.

Needle-like pricks in CHEST : or single severe stitches.

Asthma after a fit of anger.

Scraping, dry cough, caused by tickling in pit of throat, < at night, even in sleep, especially with children after taking cold in winter.

Drawing pain in BACK : pain sacrum especially at nights.

ARMS immediately go to sleep, if she grasps anything firmly : she is obliged to let them sink down.

Cracking in joints, especially lower limbs : pains as if bruised.

Cramp in legs and calves.

Burning of soles, at night ; puts feet out of bed.

Violent rheumatic pains drive him out of bed at night, and compel him to walk about.

SLEEPLESS and restless at night.

Child gets relief from being carried.

Oversensitiveness after abuse of coffee or opium.

Child suddenly stiffens body and bends backwards, kicks when carried, screams immoderately and throws everything off. Dentition.

Tremulous starting up ; twitches of limbs and eyelids.

Single twitches of limbs and of head during morning nap.

Moaning in sleep. Weeping and howling in sleep. Starts up, cries out. Tosses and talks in sleep.

Sleepy, but cannot sleep.

Pains are aggravated by heat, which relieves abdominal colic.

9

CHILL *and coldness of whole body, with burning heat of face and hot breath.*

Feeling of external heat, without actual external heat.

Internal heat with shivering.

Heat and shivering intermingled, mostly with one red and one pale cheek.

In evening, burning cheeks with transient rigor.

Burning heat face which comes out of the eyes like fire.

Long-lasting HEAT, *with violent thirst and frequent startings in sleep.*

Hot and thirsty with the pains.

Fever.

Profuse SWEAT *of covered parts.* (THUJA *of uncovered parts.*)

Sweat during sleep, most on head, usually sour smelling.

Sweat, with smarting sensation in skin.

Oversensitiveness of senses, especially if produced by coffee, or narcotics.

Paralytic sensations are always accompanied by drawing or tearing pain, and drawing or tearing pains rarely occur without paralytic or numb sensation in the part.

Especially helps children newborn and during period of dentition.

Adults, even aged persons with arthritic or rheumatic diathesis.

*   *   *

DR. BOERICKE characterizes *Chamomilla* thus :—

Chamomilla is sensitive ; irritable, thirsty, hot and numb. A disposition that is mild, calm and gentle contra-indicates *Chamomilla.*

*   *   *

One would like to add the following, which comes from America, to CHAMOMILLA, our " Drug Picture ".

In the discussion on an interesting paper on *Chamomilla*, the following delightful and illuminating sidelights flashed out :—

DR. FARRINGTON : Many years ago I read a story about Wesselhœft and Lippe, and when those old boys got together, they had some very good talks on materia medica, and it was too bad that they couldn't have been recorded or that we couldn't have listened in. Occasionally they vied with one another and tried to see who used it most.

Old Wesselhœft thought he had Lippe at a disadvantage. He said, " Dr. Lippe, I had a woman patient who got this peculiar symptom : she felt as though she were walking around on the ends of the bones of her legs* and didn't have any feet, as though the feet were gone. What remedy did I give her ? "

* A symptom of *Cham.*

Lippe said, " You gave her de *Chamomilla*, by Gott."

Well, about a year ago I went to see a woman of eighty, who complained about her feet, that they hurt her, and her corns " always twinging in the damp weather", and she said, " The funny thing is that I feel as though I were walking on the ends of the bones of my legs."

I gave her *Chamomilla* and it not only removed that sensation, which possibly someone might say is imagination, but it cured her corns.

DR. GRIMMER : I want to relate a case of strychnine poisoning. Shortly after I graduated, I was called in the early hours of the morning to a young lady in the throes of strychnine convulsions. I had no antidotes and couldn't get any because the drug-stores were locked up. I didn't even have a stomach pump and wouldn't have done any good with it if I had, because she had got this by taking strychnine given to her, I think, in 1/12 grains. She had been given a vial and the doctor told her to take two or three for headache, but she kept taking them until she got a big dose.

Her teeth were clenched and her head was drawn back and she was pale, not flushed. I started to ask a few questions and she said through her teeth, " Why don't you do something ? I can't bear this any longer. Do something ! "

Well, I had *Chamomilla* in the thousandth potency, so I put a powder of *Chamomilla* on her tongue ; and I want to tell you no chemical antidote would bring the results that that did. She soon relaxed, in about five minutes she vomited and a few minutes later she had a call to go the other way, and by morning, except for tremendous soreness from the muscular convulsions, she was all right, but she broke out with a lot of herpetic eruptions around the mouth, which *Rhus tox.* took care of, as well as the muscular sorene

DR. EDWARDS : Dr. Tyrrell said once to me, " When the husband complains of the wife's being cross and irritable, and he can't get along with her, give him a dose of *Chamomilla*," and it has worked. I have done it many times.

Homœopathic Recorder, U.S.A., No. 4, 1934.

CHELIDONIUM MAJUS

(The Greater Celandine)

" A PERENNIAL plant with a sharp, bitter and burning taste, yielding, when pressed, a yellow, corrosive, milky juice. It grows in hedges and waste places, amid stones and rubbish."

One of our good old chemists (many of them prepared their own homœopathic medicines), used to make pilgrimages to Box Hill in Surrey, where the *Greater Celandine* flourishes, in order to get the best tinctures of the plant in its chosen habitat. Tinctures are made from the root, or from the whole plant.

HERING says : " This remedy, famous in antiquity, preserved its repute through the Middle Ages. It was administered in serious complaints, particularly in hepatic derangements, according to the law of *signatura*, the yellow juice of the plant against the yellow bile and the jaundiced look. It was proved by Hahnemann and later more extensively. . . . Its place in the *Materia Medica* is well defined by numerous clinical reports, verifying the provings."

CULPEPPER, 1616-1654 (*Complete Herbal*) tells us " It is called *Chelidonium*, from the Greek word *Chelidon*, which signifies a swallow, because they say that if you put out the eyes of young swallows when they are in the nest, the old ones will recover them again with this herb . . ." (And *Chelidonium* has had a reputation of *eyes*, and for *cataract*.) Culpepper says " it is one of the best cures for the eyes "—" in an ointment to anoint your sore eyes with " . . . " in my experience and the experience of those to whom I have taught it, the most desperate sore eyes have been cured by this medicine " and he suggests that " it is far better than endangering the eyes by the art of the needle ". And *Chelidonium* IS a great eye medicine : for the provings brought out about 130 eye symptoms.

HAHNEMANN, in his prefix to the provings of *Chelidonium*, says :
" The ancients imagined that the yellow colour of the juice of this plant (*Chelidonium majus*) was an indication (signature) of its utility in bilious diseases. The moderns from this extended its employment to hepatic diseases, and though there were cases where the utility of this plant in maladies of that region of the abdomen was obvious, yet the diseases of this organ differ so much among one another, both in their origin and in the attendant derangements of the rest of the organism ; moreover the cases in which it is said to have done good have been so imperfectly

described by physicians, that it is impossible from their data to tell beforehand the cases of disease in which it must certainly be of use ; and yet this is indispensably necessary in the treatment of diseases of mankind which are of such serious importance. Hence a recommendation of this sort (*ab uso in morbis*) is of but a general, undefined and dubious character, especially since this plant was so seldom given simply and singly by physicians, but almost always in combination with heterogeneous, powerful substances (dandelion, fumitory, water cresses) and along with the simultaneous employment of the so-called bitters, which vary so much in their effects.

" The importance of human health does not admit of any such uncertain directions for the employment of medicines. It would be criminal frivolity to rest content with such guess work at the bedside of the sick. Only that which the drugs themselves unequivocally reveal of their peculiar powers in their effects on the healthy human body—that is to say, only their pure symptoms— can teach us loudly and clearly when they can be advantageously used with certainty ; and this is when they are administered in morbid states very similar to those they are able to produce on the healthy body.

" From the following symptoms of *Celandine*, which it is to be hoped will be completed by other upright, accurate observers, a much more extensive prospect of the real curative powers of the plant is opened up than has hitherto been dreamt of. It is, however, only the physician who is conversant with the homœopathic doctrine who will be able to make this advantageous employment of it. The routine practitioner may content himself with the uncertain indications for the employment of *Celandine* to be found in his benighted *Materia Medica*."

It will be interesting to run through CULPEPPER'S recorded dicta and experiences, and to compare them with the provings of *Chelidonium*, whose " Black letter symptoms " will be found at the end of this small résumé.

He says : " The herb or root boiled in white wine, a few aniseeds boiled therewith, Openeth obstructions of the liver and gall, helpeth the yellow jaundice ; and often using it helps the dropsy and the itch, and those that have old sores on their legs or other parts of the body. . . . The juice dropped into the eyes cleanseth them from films and cloudiness that darken the sight, but it is best to allay the sharpness of the juice with a little breast milk (!). It is good in old filthy corroding ulcers wheresoever, to stay their malignity of fretting and running, and to cause them to heal more speedily ; the juice applied to tetters and ring worms and other spreading cankers will quickly heal them ; and rubbed often upon warts will take them away. . . ." He describes its use in toothache, and says " The powder of the dried root laid upon any aching, hollow, or loose tooth, will cause it to fall out "(!).

Eyes—liver—jaundice—ulcers . . . Culpepper was there all right—as the provings show !

BURNETT (*Greater Diseases of the Liver*) makes great play with *Chelidonium*. Hahnemann tells us to avoid having favourites among the medicines, but *Chelidonium* was undoubtedly one of Dr. Burnett's favourites. . He says, that " In this country it is the greatest liver medicine we have, and there is, in all conscience, no lack of hepatics. Some of my early success in practice was due to my use of *Chelidonium*. . . . My conception of its true seat of action is that it affects the liver cells. . . . It must not be regarded as a liver cure-all, which it is not."

And of *Chelidonium* he says, " Its use has trickled down to us through the ages from the primary source of the Doctrine of Signatures." He says that " it is *kindly and gentle in its action, which action is fully set up with only a very small dose.*"

He tells us that it is one of the *Organ Remedies* of Paracelsus and Rademacher, and quotes from the latter.

" Unweighable and unmeasurable doses of remedies can produce wonderfully curative effects when the conditions of the body in regard to its environment have been altered by disease and thus rendered susceptible thereto, and have thus nothing at all to do with the so-called homœopathic theory."

Rademacher seems to have been jealous of, and to have thought to rival Hahnemann. But poor Rademacher ! he survives for us chiefly in the writings of Dr. Compton Burnett.

In regard to *Chelidonium* NASH has little to say, but it is, as usual, concise and to the point.

" The centre of action of this remarkable remedy is in the liver, and its most characteristic symptom is a *fixed pain* (dull or sharp) under the lower inner angle of the right shoulder blade. This very characteristic symptom may be found in connection with general jaundice, cough, diarrhœa, pneumonia, menses, loss of milk, exhaustion, etc., in fact, no matter what the name of the disease, this symptom present should always bring to mind *Chelidonium* and close scouting will generally reveal hepatic trouble or complications, as would naturally be expected with such a remedy.

" Bitter taste in mouth, *tongue thickly ,ated yellow with red margins showing imprints of teeth*, yellowness of whites of eyes, face, hands and skin ; stools gray, clay-coloured, or *yellow as gold ;* urine also yellow as gold, lemon-coloured or dark brown, leaving a yellow colour on vessel when emptied out ; loss of appetite, disgust and nausea, or vomiting of bilious matter, and especially if the patient can retain nothing but hot drinks, we would have a clear case for *Chelidonium* even if the infra-scapular pain were absent."

Jaundice. One remembers hearing of a man, long ill with jaundice, for whom the local doctor had not done anything, but which was promptly cured with a few doses of *Chelidonium* by a youthful unqualified upstart, who was thereby even more encouraged to think that it was easy and pleasing to "wipe the doctor's eye" And, again the Manager of an Ironworks, most inconveniently ill with jaundice and not making any recovery, " What shall I send him ? " asked the Chairman, himself a good and experienced homœopathic prescriber. " *Chelidonium.*" And *Chelidonium* again lived up to its reputation.

In regard to gall-stone colic, one has had cases (one from years ago turned up at outpatients only the other day) where *Chelidonium* 6 for a time, and then occasional doses of *cm.* caused a cessation of the trouble—and in this case, at any rate, it never returned.

HUGHES quotes Dr. Buchmann's provings, experiments and observations, which have added much to our knowledge of the action of this drug . . . " showing that this remedial power obeys the law of similars. The action on the liver is very strongly marked in his provings. Pain, both acute and dull, and tenderness of the organ ; pain in the right shoulder ; stools either soft and bright yellow, or whitish and costive, and deeply tinged urine appeared in nearly every prover. In three, the skin became yellow or dark ; and in one regular jaundice was set up . . . it has become my own stock remedy for jaundice. . . . .

" Next the experiments of Tests led him to credit *Chelidonium* with a specific affinity for the *respiratory organs*. The two disorders to which he thought its symptoms specially pointed were pertussis and pneumonia. Subsequent experience has confirmed his predictions of its value. . . . Dr. Buchmann shows that in animals poisoned by the drug the lungs are found generally engorged, sometimes hepatized. He develops in several of his provers all the symptoms of an incipient pneumonia. And he contributes from his own practice cases of the disease, in which the beneficial action of the drug was most manifest."

An old homœopathic text-book on Diseases of Children—given away and its author .forgotten—laid it down that most cases of pneumonia in children yielded readily to *Chelidonium*, with which the author always started his cases. *Chelidonium* is one of the great pneumonia medicines, especially pneumonia of the right base. It will be observed that *Chelidonium* is almost exclusively a right-side medicine. It will be useful here to give Dr. KENT'S graphic picture of a *Chelidonium pneumonia*.

" It is generally of the right side, or right-sided spreading to the left. The right-sidedness is marked, and but small portions of the left are involved in the inflammation. The pleura is generally involved, and so there are stitching, tearing pains. You may not practice long before you will find a *Chelidonium* patient, sitting up in bed with a high fever, bending forward upon his elbows, holding himself perfectly still, for this medicine has as much aggravation from motion as *Bry*. All of the aches and pains and sufferings are extremely aggravated from motion. This patient is sitting with a pain that transfixes him ; he cannot stir, he cannot move without the pain shooting through him like a knife. The next day you will see that his skin is growing yellow. If you see him at the beginning *Chelidonium* will relieve him and you will prevent that pneumonia. It is not uncommon in children, and it is extremely common in adults. It is one of the pneumonia medicines."

He adds, " *Bryonia* wants to lie on the painful side, wants to have that pressed, wants to lie on the back if the pneumonia is mostly in the posterior part of the right lung ; he wants pressure and wants to lie on it. In *Chel*. he is worse from touch, as well as motion. *Bell*. must lie on the other side, and he cannot move a muscle. One cannot touch that right side with pleurisy. Cannot stand a jar of the bed, because of the extreme sensitiveness to motion."

BURNETT further says, in regard to lungs : " I would, however, just dwell upon the fact that *Chelidonium* will very frequently cure engorgements of the right lung even when it is a concomitant of true phthisis, but it has no influence over the general phthisical state, other than what pertains to, and results from, the lower half of the right lung and liver. As an intercurrent remedy in the hepatic complications of phthisis it is capable of rendering important service."

Chelidonium has also a very violent spasmodic cough, and is found useful, the indications agreeing, for whooping cough.

Rheumatism also . . .—but space forbids !

HUGHES mentions its " hitherto unknown influence on the kidneys: renal irritation, tube-casts, increased uric acid, diminished chloride of sodium—œdematous swellings of extremities."

The headaches that *Chelidonium* can cure may be very severe. One remembers from many years ago a cottage woman in the country with such frantic headaches that she was impelled (heaven knows why !) to chop off her hand. The indication for the use of *Chel.* are forgotten, but *Chelidonium* quickly cured.

A little symptom-complex that spells *Chelidonium*, in the nondescript cases that come to outpatients, and is useful, is this : Pain at right shoulder-angle ; tooth-notched tongue ; great drowsiness by day. To this one may add : better for milk ; better for hot drinks ; especially better for hot milk.

We will close with the dictum of GUERNSEY (*Guiding Symptoms*) : " The strongest characteristic calling for this drug, is a very severe pain in the *inner lower angle of the right shoulder-blade*, running into the chest. This indication furnishes a keynote for the cure of an almost endless variety of complaints ; also a very specific action on the liver and portal system."

BLACK LETTER SYMPTOMS OF PROVINGS

(From *Hahnemann*, *Allen's Cyclopedia* and *Hering's Guiding Symptoms*)

Great laziness and drowsiness, without yawning. Lethargy.

Great discomfort ; feels not at all well, without knowing what is actually the matter with him. Debility and lassitude.

Distaste for mental exertion and conversation.

Weary, indolent disposition.

Vertigo : with bilious vomiting and pain in liver, with stumbling as if to fall forward ; on closing eyes, etc.

Pain over left eye ; seemed to press down upper lid.

Pressive pain right side forehead.

Heaviness in the occiput.

(Headaches, sick headaches, neuralgias.)

Curious symptom : cranium feels too small ; a forcing in the cerebrum, as if it had not room in the skull, and would be forced through the ear, with noises.

Right supraorbital neuralgia.

A long-lasting stitch in right EAR.
Intolerable sensation in both ears, as if wind rushed out of them.
In both ears, thundering of distant cannon.

Whites of EYES *dirty yellow.*
Stitches above left eye.
Increased secretion of meibomian glands.

Remarkably yellow colour of the FACE, *especially forehead, nose and cheeks.*
The usual redness of the cheeks has a mixture of yellow of a dark colour.
Greyish-yellow sunken countenance.

TONGUE *thickly coated yellow ; with red margin ; showing imprint of teeth.*
Mucus in mouth with tough mucous saliva.
Bitter taste in the mouth.

Great tension on and in the THROAT, *above the larynx, as if it were constricted, whereby, however, only the gullet was narrowed.*
Sensation as if the larynx were pressed upon the œsophagus from without, whereby not the breathing but the swallowing was rendered difficult.
A choking in throat, as if too large a morsel had been too hastily swallowed.

Loss of APPETITE *with disgust and nausea.*
Hiccup.
All complaints lessen after dinner.
Nausea in hepatitis, and in the vomiting of pregnancy.
Bilious vomiting.
Constriction, tension and sensitiveness in pit of STOMACH *and right hypochondrium.*
A sharp painful stitch in pit of stomach, which extends through body to the back.
(Queer sensation, as of an animal wriggling in epigastrium.)

Stitches in region of LIVER. *Pressive pain, liver.*
Pains from region of liver shooting towards back and shoulder.
Pains transversely across umbilicus, as if abdomen were constricted by a string.
Abdominal plethora. Hæmorrhoids. Liver affections.
Continued cutting in BOWELS, *immediately after eating : food however was relished.*

Diarrhœa and constipation alternately.
Thin, pasty, bright yellow STOOLS.

URINE *dark yellow, clear.*
Urine turbid on passing it, brownish-red, like brown beer.
Urine stains the diaper dark yellow.

Short, quick BREATHING *with oppression, > deep inspirations.*
Nightly attacks of asthma, with constriction in chest, region of diaphragm.
(Hindrance to breathing as by a tight girdle.)
Stitches beneath the right ribs.
Deep-seated pain in whole of right side of CHEST.
Oppression of chest, clothing seemed too tight.
Soreness in right lower ribs.
(Hepatization of lungs : hæmoptysis ; pneumonia.)

Stiffness of NECK.
Stitches beneath right scapula. Pains in right scapula.
Stitches : pain, beneath right shoulder blade.
Tearing lowest lumbar VERTEBRÆ, *extending to neighbourhood of os ilii ; as if vertebræ were broken away from one another, only when bending forwards, and on again bending backwards.*

Pain in right shoulder.
Tips of fingers cold, yellow " dead " ; nails blue ; esp. right.
Drawing pain hips, thighs, legs, feet ; especially right side.
Loss of power left thigh and knee when treading.
Hard pressure, below both patellæ.
Pain right knee with burning and stiffness ; < moving.
Neuralgia in limbs : rheumatism, least touch exceedingly painful sweat without relief.
Limbs heavy, stiff and lame ; flabby. Tremble and twitch.

Burning HEAT *of hands, spreads over body.*
SWEAT *during sleep, after midnight towards morning > waking.*

TISSUES. *Chronic, gastric and intestinal catarrhs.*
Hepatitis ; jaundice ; fatty liver ; painful enlargement of liver ; gall stones ; bilious conditions.
Distension of veins ; abdominal plethora ; hæmorrhoids.
Yellow-grey colour of skin.
Itching of skin.- Red, painful pimples and pustules.
Old, putrid spreading ulcers.

CHINA

THOUGH Hahnemann wrote in his wonderful preface to the Provings of CHINA—*Cinchona Bark—Cinchona officinalis—* " Excepting opium I know no medicine that has been more and oftener misused in diseases, and employed to the injury of mankind, than cinchona bark," yet, *it was quinine that revealed Homœopathy to Hahnemann.*

This is how he describes that epoch-making discovery :—

" As long ago as the year 1790 (see W. Cullen's *Materia Medica,* Leipzig . . .) I made the first pure trial with cinchona bark upon myself, in reference to its power of exciting intermittent fever. With this first trial broke upon me the dawn that has since brightened into the most brilliant day of the medical art ; that it is only in virtue of their power to make the healthy human being ill that medicines can cure morbid states, and, indeed, only such morbid states as are composed of symptoms which the drug to be selected for them can itself produce in similarity on the healthy.

" This is a truth so incontrovertible, so absolutely without exception, that all the venom poured out on it by the members of the medical guild, blinded by their thousand years old prejudices, is powerless to extinguish it ; as powerless as were the vituperations launched against Harvey's immortal discovery of the greater circulation in the human body by Riolan and his crew to destroy the truth revealed by Harvey. These opponents of an inextinguishable truth fought with the same despicable weapons as do to-day the adversaries of the homœopathic medical doctrine. *Like their modern congeners they also refrained from repeating his experiments in a true, careful manner* (for fear lest they might be confuted by facts) and confined themselves to abuse, appealing to the great antiquity of their error (for Galen's predecessors and Galen himself had arbitrarily decided that the arteries contained only spiritual air ($\pi\gamma\varepsilon\ddot{\upsilon}\mu\alpha$), and that the source of the blood was not in the heart but in the liver), and they cried out, *Malo cum Galen errare, quam cum Harveyo esse circulator* . . . This blindness . . . was in those days not more stupid than the blindness of to-day, and the present aimless rancour against *homœopathy which exposes the pernicious rubbish talked about ancient and modern arbitrary maxims and unjustifiable practices, and teaches that it is only by the responses given by nature .when questioned that we can with sure prescience change diseases into health rapidly, gently, and permanently.*"

He says the ordinary physicians were guided by an utterly false principle : they confirmed the reproach he had so frequently made against them, that they had hitherto sought in traditional opinions, in guesses prompted by false lights, in theoretical maxims and chance ideas what they could and should only find by *impartial observation, clear experience, and pure experiment, in a pure science of experience such as medicine from its very nature must be.*

He tells us that in his day cinchona bark was regarded as " perfectly innocuous—as a wholesome and universally beneficial medicine in almost all morbid states, especially where debility was observed " : whereas, setting aside all guesswork and traditional unproved opinions, and adopting the method of experiment, he found as with other medicines, that as certainly as it is curative in some kinds of disease, so surely it can develop the most morbid symptoms of a special kind in healthy humans : symptoms often of great intensity and long duration, as he shows by the provings. And " thereby, the prevailing delusion of the harmlessness, the childlike mildness and the all-wholesome character of cinchona bark is refuted."

He tells us that this is one of the most powerful of vegetable medicines. Where it is accurately indicated in a patient suffering from a disease that *China* is capable of removing, he finds that " one drop of a diluted tincture of cinchona bark, which contains a quadrillionth (1/000000,000000,000000,000000th) of a grain of *China*-power, is a strong (often too strong) dose which can accomplish and cure all alone all that *China* is capable of doing in the case before us . . . a second dose being rarely, very rarely, required."

He says, " in the case neither of this nor of any other medicine did a preconceived opinion or an eccentric fancy lead me to this minuteness of dose. No, multiplied experience and faithful observation led me to reduce the dose to such an extent. . . . and these smaller, and very smallest doses proved sufficient to effect a complete cure, and they did not display the violence of larger doses, which tend to delay the cure."

Again he tells us that, " A very small dose of *China* acts for hardly a couple of days, but a large dose, such as employed in ordinary practice, acts for several weeks, if not got rid of by vomiting or diarrhœa, and thus ejected. . . ."

" If the homœopathic law be right—as it incontestably is right without any exception, and is derived from pure observation of nature ", viz. " that medicines can only easily, rapidly and permanently cure, where the disease-symptoms match the drug-disease symptoms discovered by the administration of the drug to healthy persons, then we find, on a consideration of the symptoms of *China* that this medicine is adapted for but *few* diseases, but that where it is accurately indicated, owing to the immense power of its action, one single, very small dose will often effect a marvellous cure."

Then Hahnemann defines CURE. " I say *cure,* and by this I mean a ' *recovery undisturbed by after sufferings.*' "

" Have practitioners of the ordinary stamp another, to me unknown idea of what constitutes a *cure* ? . . . will they call cures the suppression by this drug of agues for which bark is unsuited ? I know that almost all periodic diseases, and almost all agues, even such as are not suited for *China* must be suppressed and lose their periodic character by this powerful drug, administered usually in enormous and oft-repeated doses : but are the poor sufferers thereby really cured ? Has not their previous disease undergone a transformation into another and worse disease. . . . Thus, they no longer complain of their paroxysms appearing on certain days and at certain hours ; but note the earthy complexion of their puffy faces, the dullness of their eyes ! See how oppressed is their breathing, how hard and distended is their epigastrium, how tensely swollen their loins, how miserable their appetite, how perverted their taste, how oppressed and painful their stomachs by all food, how undigested and abnormal their fæcal evacuations, how anxious, dreamful, and unrefreshing their sleep ! Look how weary, how joyless, how dejected, how irritably sensitive or stupid they are, as they drag themselves about, tormented by a much greater number of ailments than afflicted them in their ague ! And how long does not such a china-cachexy often last, in comparison with which death itself were often preferable.

" Is this health ? It is not ague, that I readily admit : but confess—and no one can deny it—it certainly is not health. It is another, but a worse disease than ague. It is the china-disease . . ." And he says, " should the organism, as it sometimes will, recover from this china-disease after many weeks, then the ague (suspended by the superior force of the dissimilar china-disease), returns in an aggravated form, because the organism has been so much deteriorated by the improper treatment . . . then, if the attack be renewed still more energetically with cinchona bark, and continued for a longer time in order to ward off fits, there becomes established a chronic cinchona-cachexy. . . ."

One finds it difficult to stop, but wanders on with sentence after sentence extracted from this delightful and illuminating little preface. But the above picture of what *China* can do to pervert health, is the exact picture of what *China* can cure, provided it be administered after the manner of Hahnemann.

But, why stop ? Why not go on extracting and epitomizing ? for, after all, it is Hahnemann's Drug-picture of *China*. Here, as everywhere, it is the exact and absolute precision of the Master that makes the phrasing, at times, somewhat heavy and involved, and, one tries to catch the meaning and simplify, without sacrificing the idea.

And, in regard to DEBILITY, where he found *China* so useful, and where old school also esteems it, Hahnemann says :—

" How can they ever imagine they can strengthen a sick person whilst he is still suffering from his disease, the source of his weakness ? Have they ever seen a patient rapidly cured of his disease by *appropriate* remedies who failed to recover his strength in the very process of the removal of his disease ? . . . These practitioners cannot *cure* diseases, but they attempt to *strengthen* these uncured patients with cinchona bark. How can such a stupid idea ever enter their heads ? If bark is to make all sick persons strong, active and cheerful, it must needs be the universal panacea which shall at once deliver all patients from all their maladies. . . . As long as the plague of disease deranges the whole man, consumes his forces and robs him of every feeling of well-being, it is a childish, foolish self-contradictory undertaking to attempt to give such an uncured person strength and activity."

He defines the real *China-debility* thus, " There are no doubt cases where the disease itself consists of weakness, and in such cases bark is at once the most appropriate curative and strengthening remedy . . . as where the sufferings of the patient are solely or chiefly owing to *weakness from loss of humours*, from great loss of blood (also from repeated venesections) great loss of milk in nursing women, loss of saliva, frequent seminal losses, profuse suppurations, profuse sweats, and weakening by frequent purgatives, where almost all the other ailments of the patient are wont to correspond in similarity with the *China* symptoms (see footnote in *Materia Medica Pura*) . . . in morbid debility of other kinds, when the disease itself is not suitable for this remedy, the administration of *China* is always followed by injurious consequences . . . although even in such unsuitable cases a stimulation of the strength is produced by it in the first few hours . . ." He says, " if there is no disease in the background to produce or keep up the loss of humours, then for this peculiar weakness, which has here become the disease, one or two doses as small as those mentioned, with nourishing diet, open air, and cheerful surroundings are as efficacious to effect recovery as larger and repeated doses are to cause secondary injurious effects . . ."

A quotation from HUGHES (*Pharmocodynamics*) is of interest here. He says, " Hahnemann found *Cinchona* in use for two great purposes—as a tonic, and as a remedy for intermittent fevers. He proved it to discover on what principle it so acted. That it caused a febrile paroxysm was the Newton's apple which led him to formulate *similia similibus* as the law of specific therapeutics. . . . He also found that it produced in the healthy a peculiar kind of debility ; and that its tonic properties in disease, when analysed, were demonstrably applicable to weakness of this very sort. . . . Where the weakness itself is the disease, *Cinchona* is curative, because homœopathic to it. . . . He acutely pointed out that the best results which were obtained from it were seen in the convalescence from acute disease, and were just correlative to the super-added debility caused by the depleting treatment then pursued. For all this you should read the preface to this proving, which is a masterpiece of observation and reasoning.

" This thought of Hahnemann was as original as it was brilliant and fruitful. It was a pure induction from his provings . . . Hahnemann's doctrine was far more definite, and at once fixed its genuine and certain range of action. It will not cure anæmic debility like *Ferrum*, or nervous debility like *Phosphoric acid* : but in that occasioned by loss of blood ; by diarrhœa, diuresis, or excessive sweating ; by over-lactation, etc., it is a most effectual remedy. ' In all these cases ', said Hahnemann, ' the other symptoms of the patient generally correspond to those of *China.*' In one particular especially they do so, viz. in their tendency to pass into a *hectic* condition. We have here the succession of chill, heat and sweat which we shall see to be characteristic of the drug, and which gives it a place in the treatment of ague. It cannot be too strongly impressed on the mind that *China* is the great anti-hectic. . . . But remember that weakness from drain on the system is the sphere of the tonic action of *Cinchona* ; and within it you will find it manifesting some of the most beautiful curative powers known to the art of medicine. They are seen alike in the most acute and the most chronic forms of debility so induced."

In regard to the *debility of China*, one has again and again proved the value of the drug in patients who, after an attack of influenza, remained chilly and weak, and went crawling about feeling that they would never again be able to wear summer clothing, or go back to normal, and where potentized *China* promptly restored normality and the trouble was forgotten. Other, different cases, when, after. 'flu, the patient would feel indefinitely unwell, with a temperature of about 99° (when one took it) and a feeling of heaviness and shakiness : here the rapid remedy is *Gelsemium.* Or where the legacy is nervous—even mental—*Scutellaria* comes in. Or, again, *Influenzinum* ! One has always used it in the 200*th* potency ; and has seen it clear up such little legacies as furious, unbearable tempers, hitherto unknown in the patient, and epileptic fits. *Influenzinum* has done some pretty work after 'flu, though one cannot define its scope with any degree of accuracy : —except that these things have " only come on after an attack of influenza ". But *chacun a son métier*—even with drugs. You cannot expect a plumber to do the delicate work of a cabinet maker, or a typist to be a Paderewski.

But among the out-patients who flock to us for help, there are quite a number of persons not demonstrably ill, but tired and below par, to whom a dose of *China* in potency is a marvellous pick-me-up. " Oh, that last medicine did me the world of good ! Can I have a repeat ? " If the trouble has been from anxiety, and night-nursing, and broken, or loss of sleep, one thinks rather of *Cocculus* : or if it has been a case of " moving house " and over-exertion and muscular fatigue, then *Arnica* will be the restorative : these are not *China* cases.

It is wonderful what *Arnica* will do for strain of all kinds—heart-strain, even—from over-exertion ; or mental strain from overwork and anxiety—the doctor's overwork, when he begins to wonder, has he done this or that ?—and has to go back and look : here *Arnica* every time. It is not in the big and savage ailments only that Homœopathy comes in : it has great uses in restoring the overwrought, the " *weary with dragging the crosses. Too heavy for mortals to bear.*" It pays to get a grip of the inwardness of our remedies ! And, mind ! the thing that *you* cannot cure, another person may, easily, because he has a grip of the remedy that is needed, which you have not : whereas, another case, impossible to him, is child's play to you—for the same reason. Some of our drugs are mere bowing acquaintances : we know their names, and have met them. Others, friends, have become " grappled to our souls with bands of steel ", because they have stood us in stead in desperate situations, and we have learnt their powers, and can trust them with life and death. But all these things come only with use.

In regard to DIARRHŒA where one sees some of the most outstanding curative actions of *China*, Hahnemann says:

" As cinchona bark in its primary action is a powerful laxative (see the symptoms 497 *et seq.*) it will be found to be very efficacious as a remedy in some cases of diarrhœa when the other symptoms of *China* are not inappropriate to the rest of the morbid symptoms." The symptoms of the provings referred to are these :—

" Three times soft stool with smarting, burning pain in the anus, and with bellyache before and after each stool.

" Looseness of the bowels, like diarrhœa.

" Frequent diarrhœic, blackish stools.

" Severe purging.

" Diarrhœa of undigested fæces, like a kind of lientery.

" Diarrhœa : as if the excrement contained undigested food . . . it comes away in separate pieces and when it is passed, there still remains desire to go to stool, but no more passes. . . ."

As to the extreme HYPERÆSTHESIA of *China*, Hahnemann has this to say :

" Those attacks of pain which can be excited by merely touching (or slightly moving) the part and which then gradually increase to the most frightful degree, are, to judge by the patient's expressions, very similar to those caused by *China*. I have sometimes permanently removed them by a single dose of the diluted tincture, even when the attacks had been frequently repeated. The malady was homœopathically (see note to 685) as it were, charmed away, and health substituted for it. No other remedy in the world could have done this, as none other is capable of causing a similar symptom in its primary action." (The footnote referred to reads, " It is peculiarly characteristic of *China* that its pains are aggravated not only by movement, and especially by touching the part " (here a number of the symptoms of the proving are referred to) " but also that they are renewed when not present by merely touching the part, as in the symptoms 749, 772 and then often attain a frightful intensity, hence this medicine is often the only remedy in cases of this description.")

All the writers since Hahnemann lay special stress on this extreme susceptibility to touch, as affecting pain : and often relief from hard pressure. As Guernsey expresses it, " from touching the parts softly ".

Practical tips in regard to the favourable action of *China* in INTERMITTENT FEVER are also given by Hahnemann in this preface. He says, " An intermittent fever must be very similar to that which *China* can cause in the healthy, if that medicine is to be the suitable, true *remedy* for it, and then a single dose of the above indicated minuteness " (i.e. the 12th potency) " relieves—but it does this best when given immediately after the termination of the paroxysm, before the operations of nature are accumulated in the body for the next fit . . ." Hahnemann did not know the

natural history of the malarial parasite : but, as usual, his observation fits the case ! He adds, " Cinchona bark can only permanently cure a patient, affected with intermittent fever in marshy
districts, of his disease resembling the symptoms of *China*, when
the patient is able to be removed from the atmosphere that causes
the fever during his treatment, and until his forces are completely
restored. For if he remain in such an atmosphere he is constantly
liable to the reproduction of his disease from the same
source. . . ."

Another nice little Hahnemannianism :—

" That the ordinary physicians, by mingling iron in the same
prescription with bark, often dish up for the patient a repulsive
looking and unsavoury ink, may be overlooked, but they must be
told that a compound results from this mixture that possesses
neither the virtues of cinchona bark nor those of iron."

The article from which we have quoted is delightful : and
should be read " in its entirety ", as they say when they put
Hamlet, the whole Hamlet, on the stage—occasionally.

GUERNSEY says, " The chief keynote calling for the use of *China*
is found in the sufferings caused by the loss of fluids, such as
hæmorrhage, galactorrhœa, seminal emissions, diarrhœa, etc. :
debility whether much fluid has been lost or only a little . . .
for any disease or troubles occurring periodically, at certain
definite periods . . . extreme sensitiveness and irritability
of nerves, or relaxation of solids.

" A peculiar feature of the diarrhœa of *China*. Diarrhœa very
debilitating : stools acrid, undigested ; watery ; bilious, black ;
involuntary ; painless ; putrid ; profuse."

Here one has found *China* splendidly effective : one remembers
a very hot summer with a great deal of epidemic diarrhœa among
small children. The painless, undigested stools, profuse and
exhausting, very rapidly cured up with a few doses of *China*. One
was able to cure them easily in the out-patient department.

And KENT, . . . " Persons who have suffered much from
neuralgias due to malarial influences, who have become anæmic
and sickly from repeated hæmorrhages, are likely to develop
symptoms calling for *China*. It produces a gradually increasing
anæmia, with great pallor and weakness . . . symptoms are
tending towards the cachectic state, which is avoided by the prompt
action of the remedy. . . . Nerves in a fret : ' doctor what is
the matter with me, I am so nervous ? ' . . . Patient grows
increasingly sensitive to touch, to motion, to cold air : so that he

is chilled from exposure . . . till patient is always catching cold, has liver troubles, bowel troubles, disordered stomach, and is made miserable and sick by nearly everything he does. . . . Weak, relaxed, emaciated, pale, with feeble heart, feeble circulation and tendency to dropsy. . . . A peculiar thing about this dropsy is that it comes after hæmorrhages. In the anæmic condition, directly following loss of blood, dropsy appears. . . ." This is the typical *China* patient.

"*China* has periodicity, but in no greater degree than many other remedies . . . still periodicity is a strong feature in this remedy. Pains come on with regularity at a given time each day. Intermittent fevers appear with regularity and run a regular course. Aggravation at night, sometimes sharply at midnight. (He gives a case of colic and bloating every night at 12. " After suffering many nights, a dose of *China* prevented any further trouble.")

" A chilly patient, sensitive to draughts, cold air, touch, motion." (One remembers a malarial case, where the slightest chill from a draught- brought on an attack, for which quinine was again and again taken, till it ended in a bout of black-water fever.)

In fevers, Kent emphasizes, " Thirst before and after the chill, and thirst during the sweat. During the heat, his thirst subsides, but all through the sweat he can hardly get water enough.

" Flatulent distension almost to bursting—(*Colch., Carbo veg., Lyc.*). Worse from fish, fruit, wine."

Now we will ask NASH to sum up for us :—

" Debility and other complaints after excessive loss of fluids.

" Hæmorrhages profuse, with faintness, loss of sight and ringing in ears.

" Great flatulence, as if abdomen were packed full : not > by eructation or passing flatus.

" Painless diarrhœa (yellow, watery, brownish, undigested).

" Periodical affections, especially *every other day*.

" Excessive sensitiveness, especially to light touch, draught of air. Hard pressure relieves.

" Dropsy following excessive loss of fluids : great debility . . .

" Face pale, hippocratic. Eyes sunken, surrounded by blue margins : pale, sickly . . .

" Hæmorrhages from all outlets (*Crot., Sulph. a., Ferr.*) Blood dark : or dark and clotted, with ringing in ears, loss of sight, coldness—sometimes convulsions.

" Shaking chill over whole body.

" Sweat with great thirst ; during sleep ; on being covered."

CICUTA VIROSA
(*Long-leaved Water Hemlock : Cowbane*)

HAHNEMANN gives " symptoms, which can only be regarded as a commencement of a thorough proving of the peculiar effects of this powerful plant, in altering the human health."

He says, " further and more complete provings will show that it is useful in rare cases where no other remedy is homœopathically suited, and particularly in chronic cases. . ... .

" Traditional medicine has never made any internal use of *Cicuta* ; for when *Cicuta* was prescribed, as it was very often some years ago, it was actually *Conium maculatum* that was meant by that name. . . .

" The juice of the fresh root (for it has little action when dried) is so powerful that ordinary practitioners did not dare to give it internally in their accustomed big doses, and consequently had to do without it and its curative power.

" Homœopathy alone knows how to employ with advantage this powerfully remedial juice in the decillion-fold dilution (30th)."

*   *   *

GUERNSEY says, " Think of this remedy for convulsions which are excessively violent—whether epileptic, cataleptic, clonic or tonic ; eclampsia."

*   *   *

NASH. " Another remedy characterized by its *excessively* VIOLENT convulsions. The patient is thrown into all sorts of odd shapes and violent contortions, but one of the most invariable is the bending of head, neck and 'spine backwards, opisthotonos. It is on this account that it was tried for cerebrospinal meningitis. Dr. Baker, of Moravia, N.Y., cured, during an epidemic of this dreadful disease, sixty cases of all degrees of malignancy without the loss of a single case. . . . He thinks it is as near a specific for this disease as can be. . . ."

Also a good remedy for the effects of concussion of brain or spine, if spasms are in the train of chronic effects, and *Arnica* does not relieve. In the affections for which *Cicuta* is useful the actions of the patient are as violent as the spasms ; moans and howls, makes gesticulations and odd motions, great agitation, etc.

Also wonderful for skin affections, " pustules which run together, forming thick yellow scabs on face, head, and other parts of the body. I once had a case of eczema capitis in a young woman—it was of long standing—which covered the whole scalp, solid, like a cap. I gave her *Cicuta* 200th and cured her completely in a very short time."

Black Letter Symptoms (*Hahnemann, Allen, and Hering*)

Absence of thought, difficulty of recollecting himself, deprivation of the senses.
Anxiety : violently affected by sad stories.
Moaning, whining and howling.
Tranquility of mind ; he was extremely satisfied with his position and with himself, and very cheerful (curative secondary effect).
Likes childish toys : jumps from bed in a happy, childish state.
Very violent in all his actions.
Anxious thoughts of the future : feels sad.
Anxiety : excessively affected by sad stories.
Mistrust and shunning of men : despises others.

Vertigo : staggering.
Pressive, stupefying headache, externally on the forehead, more when at rest.
Concussion of brain and chronic effects therefrom, especially spasms.
Head bent backwards with convulsions.
Violent shocks through head, arms and legs, which cause them to jerk suddenly : head hot.

Pupils first contracted, then very dilated.
Dilated and insensible.
Convergent strabismus in children, if periodic or spasmodic, or caused by convulsions—blow or fall.

Convulsions of facial muscles ; distortions either horrible or ridiculous.

Lockjaw.

After swallowing a sharp piece of bone, or other injuries to œsophagus the throat closes, and there is danger of suffocation.
Inability to swallow.
Hiccough.

Burning pressure in stomach, and abdomen.
Throbbing in pit of the stomach, which is swollen as large as a fist.

Sudden shock in pit of stomach which causes opisthotonos.
Distension and painfulness of abdomen.
Colic with convulsions and vomiting.

Frequent call to urinate.

Trembling palpitation of heart.
Feels as if heart stopped beating ; sometimes faint feeling therewith.

Tension or cramp in muscles of neck : if he turns head, cannot easily turn it back again.
Pain in nape, spasmodic drawing of head backwards, with tremor of hand.
The back bent backwards like an arch.
Painful sensation on inner surface of scapulæ.
Complete powerlessness of limbs, after spasmodic jerks.
Frequent involuntary jerking and stitches in arms and fingers.

A red vesicle on right scapula, very painful when touched.

General convulsions. Epilepsy.
Frightful epilepsy.
Frightful distortion of the limbs and whole body.
Convulsions with wonderful distortion of limbs ; head turned backwards, back bent as in opisthotonos.
Frightful convulsions.
(Epileptic fits, with swelling of stomach, as from violent spasm of the diaphragm.) Hiccough : screaming : redness of face : trismus.
Loss of consciousness, and distortion of limbs.
Tonic spasm renewed from slightest touch : opening door ; loud talking.
An elevated eruption over whole face (and on both hands, as big as peas) which causes a burning pain when touched.*

Vivid dreams about events of day.
Vivid unremembered dreams.
Frequent waking out of sleep, in which he perspired all over, but from which he felt strengthened.

They all wish to come near the warm stove.

---

* Hahnemann says, " I have cured chronic pustular, confluent eruption on the face, with only a burning pain, with one or two doses of a small portion of a drop of the juice, but did not venture to administer a second dose under three or four weeks, if the first was not sufficient."

IMPORTANT ITALIC SYMPTOMS : QUEER SYMPTOMS

Aberration of mind, singing, performing most grotesque dancing steps, shouting.

Represented to himself as dangerous everything that would happen to him.

Feels as if he were in a strange place. (*Opium*—Comp. *Bry.*)

He did not think he was living in ordinary conditions : everything appeared strange and almost frightful. . . .

Depreciation and contempt of mankind : fled from his fellows : was disgusted with their follies.

Want of trust in people and anthropophobia : suspicious.

Or,—he felt like a child of seven or eight years old, objects were very dear and attractive to him, as toys are to a child.

Keeps staring : at the same place ; cannot help doing so. Has not full command of her senses . . . if she compels herself forcibly, by turning away her head, to cease having her eyes directed on the object, she loses consciousness, and all becomes black before eyes.

Staring look. Stares with unaltered look at one and the same place.

Suddenly consciousness returns and she remembers nothing of what has occurred.

Vertigo. Objects seem to move in a circle :—to move hither and thither, though they retain their right shape.

Must seat herself more firmly, because she sees nothing firm or steady about her ; thinks she is herself unsteady. Imagines she is swaying : everything swings backwards and forwards like a pendulum. When she has to stand still, she wishes she could lay hold of something : objects seem to come near, and then recede again from her.

Falls to the ground : falls and rolls about.

Neck feels stiff and muscles too short.

Most violent tonic spasms, so that neither the curved limbs could be straightened, nor the straight limbs curved.

Head retracted or bent forward and stiff.

Heart seems to stop.

Jerking of head.

As if throat had grown together.

Walks with feet turned inward, swings feet with each step, describing the arc of a circle.

Thumbs turned inward during epilepsy.

In epilepsy, spasm renewed from slightest touch or jar. (*Nux, Strych., Bell.*)

On waking, brain feels loose and shaking.

Useful after concussion of brain : after wounding œsophagus, where there is spasm that prevents swallowing.

[Although the epileptic and other convulsions are very violent, yet many of the symptoms suggest *petit mal.*]

" Acts particularly on the nervous system : a cerebro-spinal irritant, producing tetanus, epileptic and epileptiform convulsions, trismus and local tonic and clonic spasms in general."

* * *

KENT says, " This remedy is of most extreme interest because of its convulsive tendency. It puts the whole nervous system into such a state of increased irritability that pressure on a part causes convulsions.

" Convulsions extend from centre to circumference. The convulsions spread from above downwards, and thus it is the opposite of *Cuprum*. The convulsions of *Cup.* spread from the extremities to the centre : the little convulsions, cramps, are first felt in fingers, then hands, later in chest and whole body. In *Cicuta* the little convulsions of head, eyes and throat spread down the back with violent contortions.

" Read the mental symptoms : at times knows no one, but when touched and spoken to answers correctly. Suddenly consciousness returns and he remembers nothing of what has occurred. . . . Imagines himself a young child : everything is confused and strange. Voices—places—strange. After cataleptic state feels like a child and acts like one : plays with toys. Memory a blank for hours or days, with or without convulsions. (*Nat. mur.*) *Nux mosch.* is another remedy that has such a complete blank when going about, doing things.

" Wants to eat coal—raw potatoes.

" Between the convulsions the patient is mild, gentle, placid, yielding, reverse of *Nux* and *Strych*. *Nux* has convulsions all over the body, worse for touch and draught, blueness : BUT, between the convulsions the patient is very irritable. . . .

" Complaints brought on from injuries to skull, blows on the head. . . . Mind and head symptoms after injuries. . . . Cerebro-spinal meningitis. . . . Has cured epithelioma of lips. After swallowing a fishbone, etc., a spasm comes on. After *Cicuta* the spasm will cease and it can be taken out.

" Barber's itch : troubles from shaving."

* * *

One wonders why one has not made more use of *Cicuta*, after one of the amazing experiences of a lifetime. One has recently reproduced it, as " *Effects of the Remedy* ", in the CORRESPONDENCE COURSE FOR DOCTORS.

Cicuta IN EPILEPSY AND MENTAL DEFICIENCY OF TWENTY YEARS' STANDING

It was many years ago : Charlotte E., an epileptic idiot, 23 years old. First seen in 1909.

History.—At 3½ years old had a fall on head. In bed four months, " unconscious and blind ". On recovery, a pustular rash all over head, cured with ointments.

Epileptic fits ever since, with enuresis. Whole body *violently* convulsed   Sleeps after the fits, sometimes all day.

May have 20-30 fits in one night. May go 14 days without fits, then fits every night for a week.

Very intelligent before the fall (at 3½ years old). Just like a baby now, at 23.

Cannot wash or dress herself, but can feed herself now. If asked whether she wants food, says "No,"—then eats it, if set before her.

Can never be left alone.

For the (*a*) *violence of the convulsions*—

(*b*) *the pustular rash*—

and for (*c*) " *after-effects of blows on the head* ", she got *Cicuta* 200, one dose.

The effect was amazing ; it was a revelation !

Three weeks later, the report was—

Much better. Fewer fits, and less violent. No struggling.

Much more intelligent. Remembers things now !

Remembers, as she has not done since babyhood.

Washed and dressed herself to-day for the first time in her life. *No medicine.*

In five weeks—

Better. Goes upstairs to ˙fetch things for her mother.

Fits ? " Nothing near so bad. Only six fits since here " . . . used to have 20-30 in a night !

Actually *talks about things*.

Dressed herself to come up to Hospital. Understands and remembers.

Mother says, " It doesn't seem true that she can talk to them, and say sensible things," as she does now.

Some festery spots have come out on her face.

The girl talks to me. Tells me that " she likes to go and see the girls doing needlework ". Shows me the pennies that they have given her. Mother says, " She couldn't trust her to do anything for herself ; can now ! " *No medicine.*

In two months—

Very much better. Only two slight fits.

Memory improving. Enjoys coming up here. She positively asked her mother not to forget her hospital card !

Helps herself at meals now. Cuts bread.

Again, spots on face. *No medicine.*

In three months—

Still rapid improvement in intelligence.

Remembers that she had forgotten to bring me flowers.

Two slight fits. *No medicine.*

In five months—

No fits at all.

Can make beds, and do cleaning. Sews on buttons. *No medicine.*

In six months—

Has been ill with a bad cold; doctor called it pleurisy ; and one severe fit. *Cicuta* 200, one dose (for the second time in six months).

In seven months—

Am told that this medicine (like the first) produced an aggravation. She was dreadful for two days, and took no notice of anyone.

Much better since. Does housework. Loves needlework. *No medicine.*

In eight months—

No fit, till she burnt her hand. She was taking a kettle off the fire with paper for a kettle-holder. It flared up and burnt her hand. She screamed with the pain. Three fits, not severe, the next day.

She is very useful in the house. Talks to me a lot to-day. *No medicine.*

In eleven months—

" Getting on tremendously." Does needlework.

Goes out and buys vegetables.

One slight attack. *Cicuta* 200, one dose, for the third time.

In twelve months—

One slight attack. *No medicine.*

In fourteen months—

Better than ever before. No fits at all.

Tells me a long yarn about her sister.

Originates conversations.

After wringing the clothes, and hanging them up to dry, said,
" Now I am dead tired. I'm going to bed. Mother doesn't

want me to, but my nerves are going like that, and I'm dead tired !"
No medicine.

In seventeen months—
Understands that her Sunday School teacher is dead. Said,
" She's gone, and we shall not see her any more." Never men-
tioned her again. *No medicine.*

In nineteen months—
Mother wrote up, " Ill, and ten fits." Sent *Cicuta* 200, one dose.

Two years later—
Several rather bad fits. *Cicuta* 200, one dose.

Three years later—
Had been ill with 'flu ; ten bad fits one night. Otherwise
well. Washes up. Cleans the doorstep. Goes shopping. *Cicuta*
200, one dose.
Then for some six months—No fits.

After four years—
Mother says, " She speaks in proverbs now ! She said, ' What
is it, Mother, when your nose itches like this ? ' " *No medicine.*

In five years—
Mends her clothes. Does all the mangling and hangs the
clothes out. Remembers where she has put things.
Has been seen since, at very long intervals. It was a pleasing
and illuminating case. Excitement or sickness may bring on an
attack. But a girl of 23, with less than the mentality of a baby,
unable to say when she wanted food, let alone to wash or dress
herself, was quickly transformed into a useful and fairly intelligent
member of society by a very few single doses of *Cicuta*, in the
200 potency.

*   *   *

One thinks of *Cicuta* for extreme violence of convulsions :
but, as said, it has all the symptoms of *petit mal* : and one might
have made use of *Cicuta* here, and saved oneself a lot of trouble :
for really these *petit mal* cases are often more difficult than the
major attacks.
Looking up that old wonderful case the other day, led to the
prescription of *Cicuta* in another equally difficult and seemingly
hopeless case.
It was this. A thin slip of a " girl ", nearly 40 years old.
Practically an epileptic idiot since a fall at 12 years old, which
rendered her unconscious. Had had a previous fall as a baby,
which left a " dent on the top of her head ". (Has a queer shaped
skull, with a deep dent, wide, running back from vertex.) Makes

extraordinary noises before some of the fits, or falls without noise : enuresis in fits.

She had very frequent major attacks, minor attacks also, " silent fits ". Skin troubles also.

Her symptoms suggested *Sulphur*, which gave a terrible aggravation, then she improved, to a point.

But still a great number of fits : and also shrieking fits. Better and worse, without really much change, *till* January 29th, 1937. *Cicuta* 30, one dose.

In a month the report is, " Ever so much better : two weeks since the last fit—her longest period without. A different creature : now takes interest in everything. Takes interest in her clothes now. Looks better. Has put on weight."

Why did she not get *Cicuta* before ?

*　　*　　*

The *Cyclopædia of Drug Pathogenesy* gives cases of poisoning by *Cicuta*. Here is one. A healthy man of 20 ate of the root, and was soon ill. He went out and was soon afterwards found stretched on the ground, and as if dying. Face congested : eyes protruded ; foamed at mouth ; scarcely breathed. Soon a violent epileptic attack occurred, during which all the limbs in succession were horribly contorted, the breathing interrupted. He never recovered consciousness and soon died. Another :—a child of 6 soon complained of pain in precordia and fell to the ground and passed urine with great force. He looked fearfully ill ; all his senses left him ; he shut his mouth so strongly that it could not be opened, ground his teeth. Eyes much distorted, blood gushed from his ears and a large swelling formed about the precordial region. Hiccough : attempts to vomit. He threw his limbs about and contorted them, the head was often thrown back and the whole back bent in the form of a bow. The convulsions ceased and he cried to his mother for help, but they returned with renewed intensity, he could not be roused by calling to him : and in half an hour he died . . . And so on with other cases.

In one case of proving given, among a host of symptoms, the stools had this peculiarity, that without premonitory symptoms they suddenly came on with urging so severe that they could hardly be kept back, with bruised pain in sacrum and general weakness. Then, almost every hour a stool of black carrion-smelling mucus in large quantity, with straining. . . . When walking, suddenly a peculiar feeling as if the heart stopped. . . . etc., etc.

CIMICIFUGA RACEMOSA (ACTEA RACEMOSA)
(Black Cohosh. Black Snake-root)

SOME confusion may arise because of the different names applied
to this remedy, and therefore the different parts of Materia Medica
where it is to be sought. Hughes says he prefers to call it by
its Linnaean name—*Actea*. Hering (*Guiding Symptoms*) has it
as *Actea :* he says, " It has received so many improper names
that the oldest is preferred ". Clarke, H. C. Allen, Kent and
Guernsey call it *Actea :* Nash, Boericke, Boger, *Cimicifuga*, which
name is more familiar. Allen also, in the *Encyclopedia*, has it
under *Cimicifuga*.

It seems strange that we should never before have tried to
Drug-picture CIMICIFUGA : one of the remedies so very useful
to physicians brought up on Hughes, rather than on Hahnemann
pure and simple,—that painstaking experimentalist and recorder,
whose genius, so far as we have seen, is not improved by modifica-
tion, or in need of apology. Hughes' *Pharmacodynamics*, excellent
in its way, got the nickname " *Homœopathic Milk for Allopathic
Babes* ", for his great object was, evidently, to reconcile Homœopathy, or at least to make it acceptable, to Old School practitioners
of his day. But Old School has recently made great strides in
its basal conceptions : so much so that the Doctrines of Hahnemann are found to be rather explanatory than antagonistic to
present-day thought, and are quite easily swallowed by the latest
qualified : indeed we hear that already it is being said among the
science teachers of one of the medical schools, " Homœopathy is
the coming medicine ". But the strong meat as well as the milk
of Homœopathy remain not easy of digestion to most of the
older men, some of whom shrink from all this new study " at their
time of life ", which means so much unlearning and relearning,
not only in regard to prescribing, but the plunge into that vast,
unknown Materia Medica homœopathica. . . . " If I had
only come across this forty years ago ! " But the more earnest
seekers after truth, the rebellious against ineptitude, are finding in
Homœopathy the explanation of many difficulties, doubts and
misgivings : a something that goes deeper than mere palliation ;
and proves that good work can be done apart from the daring
and often dangerous experimentation of the laboratories. Moreover Homœopathy leaves them no longer subject to the

temptations and dictates of the manufacturing chemists, whose samples pour in by every post, to be tried and adopted for further experiment on a hit, or discarded as useless on a miss. Do such things belong to the *Reign of Law*?—to any *Science of Medicine*: that Inspiration to which Hahnemann dedicated his life, and for which he wrestled with God and nature during all those long, weary years? Are they not merely a counsel of despair: a terrible acknowledgment of ignorance and failure?

But, to go back to *Cimicifuga*:

Nerve, or nerve and muscle—myalgias—seem to be the very special sphere of *Cimicifuga*: as a very interesting case quoted by Dr. Hughes exemplifies. The drug attacks eyes, in a marked degree, but, it is pointed out, that it is through the eye muscles. As Boger gives it, in arresting type, " NERVES AND MUSCLES, Cerebro-spinal, Eyeballs, Ovario-uterine, Heart " and, like *Caulophylum*, " in females ", joints. And everywhere it is better for *warmth* in every form ; for *open air* ; for *pressure*, and for *continued motion*.

It is a remedy of crazy feelings, of chorea, and one of the remedies that affect especially, uterus and all the conditions dependant on uterine abnormalities of function. . . . It is a rheumatic, choreaic, spasmodic, hysterical and uterine remedy. It reminds one, as one reads, now of *Ignatia*, now of *Gelsemium*, now, as said, of *Caulophylum*, now of *Lachesis*. A very useful drug for more or less superficial conditions—though it has also a reputation in phthisis.

Among its contradictory symptoms are its " relief from flow " —bowels, uterus, etc., yet its aggravation during menstruation. Its relief from flow reminds one of *Sepia, Lach., Zinc.*

One thinks of *Cimicifuga* especially in stiff neck and sciatica,— (provided that these are not dependent on small displacements, and therefore only amenable to manipulation) ; in chorea ; in hysteria : as well as in obscure conditions, such as the myalgia of diaphragm, to which Hughes draws attention.

Hering, stressing the importance of provings on men *and* women of the various drugs, shows that in provings by six women, *Cimicifuga* produced nausea, vomiting and much gastric irritation; while in forty men, it hardly affected the stomach in the least. He says, being an important remedy in morning sickness of the pregnant, we may conclude that all the gastric symptoms observed by female provers depended on the uterus. He says further, that it has been observed that *Cuprum* acts more on the female, and *Ferrum* on the male organs.

Black Letter Symptoms

Thinks she is going crazy.

Mania following disappearance of neuralgia.

Puerperal mania.

Incessant talking, changing from one subject to another.

Feels grieved and troubled, with sighing : next day a feeling of tremulous joy, with mirthfulness, playfulness and clear intellect.

Fear of death.

Fullness and aching in vertex.

Severe pains right side of HEAD, *back of orbit.*

Brain as if too large ; presses from within outwards.

Dull constant pain, especially occiput, extending to vertex.

A pressing upwards and outwards, as if not room enough in upper portion of cerebrum : this pain was very oppressive and almost intolerable. A sense of soreness in occipital region, worse motion.

NAUSEA. *Retching, dilated pupils, tremor of limbs.*

Aching pain in both eyeballs.

Sharp pain across hypogastrium.

ABDOMINAL *muscles sore.*

Pains in UTERINE *region, dart from side to side.*

Menses irregular, delayed or suppressed, with chorea, hysteria, or mental disease.

Shivers, of first stage of labour.

Infra-mammary pains, worse left side.

Night COUGH, *dry, incessant, short.*

Head and NECK *retracted.*

Rheumatic pains in muscles of neck and BACK ; *feeling of stiffness.*

A severe drawing, tensive pain at the points of the spinous processes of the three upper dorsal vertebræ.

Excessive muscular soreness.

Rheumatic persons.

Curious, Distinguishing or Italic Symptoms

As if a black cloud had settled all over her, and enveloped her head, so that all was darkness and confusion : it weighed like lead on her head.

Waving sensation in the brain.

Startled by the illusion of a mouse running from under her chair.

Imagines strange objects about the bed : rats, sheep, etc.

Fear of death : fears those in the house will kill him.

Would not answer, or very loquacious at times.

Mental depression, suicidal, after checked neuralgia.

Suspicious of everything, would not take medicine.

Mind disturbed by disappointed love, business failures, etc.

Feels faint at epigastrium when meeting a friend.

Rush of blood to head : brain feels too large for cranium.

Waving sensation. Opening and shutting sensation when moves head and eyes. Top of head feels as if it would fly off.

As if vertex opened and let in cold air.

Sensation of enlargement, eyeballs, as if they would be pressed out.

As if needles were run into left eyeball through cornea.

Coppery taste. Cannot speak a word though she tried.

Dry spot in throat causes cough.

Alternate diarrhœa and constipation.

Shivers in the first stage of labour : during menses.

Puerperal mania : does not know what is the matter with her head : clutches it. Screams, clutches at breast as though in pain : tries to injure herself.

Acute pain, apex to base of right lung, worse inspiration.

Angina pectoris : pain heart region, all over chest and down left arm : palpitation ; unconsciousness, cerebral congestion, dyspnœa, face livid, cold sweat hands ; numbness of body : left arm numb and as if bound to side. (Cured case, Hering.)

Heart's action ceases suddenly ; impending suffocation.

A heavy black cloud had settled all over her : weighed like lead on her heart.

Stiff neck from cold air, with pain from moving hands.

Weight and pain, lumbar and sacral, sometimes extending all round the body.

Severe pain in back, down thighs and through hips, with heavy pressing down.

Severe pain down arms, with numbness as if a nerve were pressed.

Left arm feels as if bound to side.

Cold sweat on hands.

Must change position, to quiet jerking, in bed.

Can scarcely walk, from trembling of legs.

Must walk about, when restless and impatient.

Going upstairs aggravates feeling as if top of head would fly off.

Moving head causes opening and shutting sensation of head : and cramps in muscles of neck.

Moving eyes causes opening and shutting sensation in head.

Irregular motion of legs, worse left.   Legs unsteady (Chorea).

Epilepsy : Hysteric spasms.

Comatose state.

Affects the nerves, especially muscular nerves.   Myalgia.

Similar to *Caulophylum* in uterine and rheumatic affections.

*   *   *

HUGHES (*Pharmacodynamics*) has a great deal, of great interest, to say about *Actea* as he prefers to call *Cimicifuga*.   He says, "It causes no febrile symptoms " (this, however, we must question judging by symptoms of provings and by cases of amelioration of fever during its use) " but it is a valuable remedy for some forms of rheumatism, especially where nervous centres and muscles are the seat of the disorder. . . . In the acute and local muscular rheumatisms, such as pleurodynia, lumbago and torticollis *Actea* has gained commendation from all. . . . In rheumatoid arthritis, where the pains are worse at night and in wet weather, especially if of uterine origin. . . . Another form simulates gonorrhœal rheumatism, but without any history of gonorrhœa.   Here, not only may the pains be almost immediately relieved, but the joints may become supple and useful again.

Then in the sufferings which heart and uterus often undergo from the rheumatic poison. . . . Provings make it evident that *Actea* affects the heart very powerfully.   When rheumatism affects this organ, not setting up inflammation, but as it does other muscles, we have a valuable remedy in this drug. . . . In a case cured, the symptoms resembled *angina pectoris*, the attacks recurring several times a day.   He speaks also of its power over chorea.

Then, cases having the uterus for their starting point :— *Actea* has an undoubted action on this organ—abortifacient and ecbolic.   Its therapeutic virtues in this region are numerous and well established, especially where the uterus is presumably rheumatic.   It relieves dysmenorrhœa, checks tendency to abortion and after pains, and facilitates parturition. . . . When morbid uterine conditions show themselves elsewhere than in the organ itself, by the pains and agitations characteristic of the drug, it comes potently to their relief.   It cures uterine epilepsy and hysteria ; puerperal melancholia ; the nervousness of pregnancy, and the restless and unhappy state of mind so often seen in uterine patients, especially the sleeplessness.   Then the inframammary pain in unmarried females, which is to the uterus what pain in the shoulder is to the liver. Also pains in the mammæ so arising. . . . Also suffering at the climacteric age, relieving sinking at the stomach (one of its marked pathogenetic symptoms), pain at the vertex, and the irritability of disposition, better than any other medicine.

He quotes an interesting and suggestive article by Dr. Madden, in the *British Journal of Homœopathy*, Vol. XXV, in regard to *Actea* for diaphragmatic pain. " Here the doctor was not only physician, but patient." The pain had its centre in the chest ; " it was as if a person were pressing with his fist firmly on the sternum and forcing it inwards towards the spine." Walking would precipitate an attack. When severe it would spread up the œsophagus and pharynx, causing a peculiar tingling at the back of the throat which extended to shoulder and upper chest, and down the arms to finger-tips. A few moments of perfect quiet would remove the pain. It would never come on when at rest, except on two occasions, during strong mental emotion. It was always worse after food.

The condition persisted, unexplained and resisting all attempts at treatment till something read suggested the idea that it might be a myalgia of the diaphragm ; and the explanation seemed to fit. *Arnica* was rejected ; and *Aceta* selected, as producing an effect on nervous system and muscle.

Actea φ 3 or 4 minims relieved : unaccompanied by the diuresis that usually followed the cession of the pain : but the drug had to be stopped since it began to produce the *Actea* headache and aching pressure on eyeballs. *Actea* 12 gave no result : whereas the first centesimal could be taken without distress and soon cured.

[Evidently Dr. Madden was one of the low potency prescribers. Probably a higher potency, and *no repetition till needed*, would have done him even better ? But, he was *cured* !]

❀ ＊ ❀

Among the things that GUERNSEY specially notes in regard to " Actea ", we find. . . . The Mental craziness, and fear of going crazy : imagines all sorts of strange appearances, and that some one is going to kill her. Her incessant talk, changing from subject to subject. Her despondency and the feeling of being under a heavy black cloud.

Pain in head as if top would fly off : or as if a bolt had been driven from neck to vertex. Or pain shooting from occiput down neck. Headache down to nose.

Pains in eyeballs, shootings into eyeballs so severe it seems she would go crazy. Needles running into left eyeball. While, with regard to nose, every inhalation seems to bring the cold air in contact with brain.

Face bluish. Wild, fearful expression. Forehead cold : deadly pale. Suddenly faint, face ashy white.

Pains, uterine region, darting from side to side. Bearing down : and in small of back, as if something were pressing out . . . labour pains with fainting fits and cramps ; convulsions, from nervous excitement. . . . Puerperal mania : feels strange, talks incoherently, screams, tries to injure herself. . . Similar to *Cauloph.* in uterine and rheumatic affections.

*   *   *

CLARKE (*Dictionary*) says, "Given before term it renders labour easier, cures sickness of pregnancy, and prevents after pains and over-sensitiveness ". He says, " According to Lippe a characteristic indication is, ' The recently delivered uterus becomes actually jammed in the pelvis with great pain '. It has ensured living births in women who have previously borne only dead children, from no discoverable cause ; given in daily doses of 1*x* two months before term."

*   *   *

We will let KENT, as usual, sum up for us ; it is often well to let him have the last word.

He says, the remedy is but meagrely proved, but we can perceive that it is similar to diseased states, especially in women, namely *hysterical and rheumatic conditions.*

The patient is always chilly, easily affected by cold and damp, which rouses the rheumatic state, not only in muscles and joints, but also along the course of nerves.

There is a lack of will, balance, or great disturbance in the voluntary system (the underlying feature of hysteria) ; the symptoms intermingled with rheumatism. Soreness, trembling, numbness, jerking. Inability to exercise the will over the muscles. Turmoil in the voluntary system, with stiffness. Sensitive to cold, except in the head.

A terrible mental state alternates with the physical states. Overwhelming gloom : bowed down with sorrow. This may pass off instantly, or be brought on or aggravated by motion or emotion. The rheumatism may change in a day to chorea : the physical and mental are all the time changing. Jerking, soreness and numbness often keep on together.

He notes *re* the *chorea* : jerking when in a state of emotion or from becoming chilled. The part pressed on will have jerkings. The whole of the side lain on will commence to jerk, and prevent sleep. She turns over, and soon the muscles that side will in turn begin to jerk : she becomes so restless and nervous that she is driven to distraction. . . . The mind full of imaginations and the body full of uneasiness because she can find no place to rest upon. Sometimes it is soreness, sometimes numbness, sometimes jerking that prevents her from lying in peace.

Fear : anguish : restlessness. Fear of death ; excitement, suspicion. Will not take the medicine, because there is something wrong about it. . . . " This remedy belongs especially to women, because its symptoms are so commonly associated with the affections of woman. Mental states following the disappearance of rheumatism is a strong feature. Rheumatism better, mental state worse. Relief from diarrhœa—from flow from uterus : 'some flow must be established, otherwise the mind takes on trouble.' "

" A routine saying about *Actea* is that it makes confinement easy . . . but only when the remedy is given in accordance with symptoms. Repeat that over and over again, *when the symptoms agree*, WHEN THE SYMPTOMS AGREE. It cures and makes labour easy when the symptoms agree, and that will apply equally to all other remedies."

Then its bearing-down sensations show that it is a very useful remedy in prolapsus of uterus : it has the relaxation of the parts. . . . Remedies will cure prolapsus when the symptoms agree, and at *no other times*. If it fits the patient in general, these bearing down sensations will go away, the patient will be made comfortable, and examination will finally show that the parts are in normal condition. You cannot prescribe for the prolapsus ; you must prescribe for the woman. You cannot prescribe for one symptom, because there are probably fifty remedies that have that symptom.

Here, with menstruation, the more the flow, the greater the pain : many of the conditions of *Actea* are worse *during* the menses, rheumatic, jerking, cramping, sleeplessness ; epileptic spasms ; soreness of muscles or joints. . . . ' Rheumatic dysmenorrhœa, is not a bad name."

During labour ; shivering ; hysteric manifestations. Pains have ceased or are irregular. . . . A pain comes on, seems to be going to finish satisfactorily, when all at once she screams out and grasps her hip : it has left the uterus and gone to hip, causing cramp. So emotional is she, that if she hears an emotional story in the room, the pain will stop : or the lochia may stop, or milk be suppressed, and she will be sore and bruised and have fever.

Kent says the best results have been from the 30th, 200th, 1,000th and still higher potencies, in single doses.

CINA

(" *Wormseed* " so-called : but not seed—unopened buds)

HAHNEMANN, in the preface to his provings of *Cina*, tells us that " for centuries no other use had been made of this very important vegetable substance, except for the expulsion of lumbrici in children, in doses of 10, 20, 30, 60 and more grains. I will pass over the not unfrequently dangerous, or even fatal effects of such doses, nor will I dwell on the fact that a few lumbrici are not to be considered as an important disease in otherwise healthy children, and are common in childhood (where psora is still latent) and are generally unattended by morbid symptoms. On the other hand, this much is true, that when they are present in large numbers, the cause of this is always some morbid condition of the body . . . and unless this be cured, though large numbers of the lumbrici may be expelled by *Cina*, they are soon reproduced. Hence, by such forcible expulsion of the worms, not only is nothing gained, but such improper treatment, if persisted in, often ends in the death of the tortured children.*

" This vegetable substance has much more valuable curative properties, which may be easily inferred from the subjoined characteristic morbid symptoms produced by it in the healthy.

" Experience of what it can do, for instance in *whooping-cough* and in certain *intermittent fevers* accompanied by vomiting and ravenous hunger, will excite astonishment. . . .

" Formerly I used to employ the tincture potentized to the trillion-fold dilution, but I have found that when raised to the decillion-fold dilution" (the 30th potency) " it displays its medicinal powers still more perfectly. . . ."

Cina and *Santonin* seem to have been used chiefly for the expulsion of round worms, but here one recalls a rather dramatic experience from the use, not of *Cina* but of *Natrum phos.* 6, a few doses. This is Schuessler's great medicine for *rheumatism*— and *round worms*. A housemaid with an acutely swollen and inflamed knee got *Nat. phos.*, one evening, and in the

---

* And Clarke says of Santonin " the favourite anthelmintic of the old school—chiefly against lumbrici "—" from 2-5 grains are the ordinary doses, but these have caused severe and, in one or two instances, fatal poisonings— convulsions, left-side paralysis, delirium, vomiting and purging."

In Lectures on Materia Medica as students, we were warned against the doses of 2-5 grains given in Hale White for Santonin (the active principle of *Cina*). " They had caused the death of children, and we should modify them."

Recently a child was seen who, after dosing with Santonin for worms, had become deaf. Provings showed effects on the ears, but not, apparently, deafness.

morning the knee was practically well, and *she had passed a couple of round worms*. The drug was naturally looked up as to *worms* and remembered. For *thread-worms*, however, with the *Cina* symptoms, restless nights, dilated pupils, grinding of teeth, boring in nose, irritation at anus, one has given, again and again, *Cina* 200 ; and so far as one remembers " worms " have not cropped up again in later reports.

But there is another trick to help to get rid of thread-worms : smear the anus, inside and out, getting well into the folds, with olive oil, or (? better) vaseline. It is said, with what truth one cannot say, that the worms come down to breed, and bite—hence the itching : that where the lubricant is, they fail to get a hold, and are gradually passed, when the trouble ends. Numbers of mothers have been instructed in this simple measure : and, so far as one remembers, either the *Cina*, or the vaseline, or the two combined, have been successful. One does not remember trouble- some cases of worms returning for treatment ; just once complained of and then, either no further mention, or the report, " no more worms seen ".

And while on the subject of " worms " everybody does not know the trick to catch a tape-worm !—simplicity itself !—and it works. The tape-worm seems to have a great liking for pumpkin seed ! Get one ounce of fresh pumpkin seed, take off the shell and pound and mix with two ounces of honey. Give fasting in the morning in three doses one hour apart. The worm may come away or it may need a dose of castor oil. And here a caution : if the worm is coming away, it is necessary not to stir till it is passed, *head and all*, otherwise the worm will grow again from the head. One has had such tape-worms brought in a bottle for examination as to the presence of the small head. The explana- tion given is that the tape-worm gormandizes on the pumpkin seed till stupid and comatose, when its hooks relax, and it gets passed on and out. But, " *a Carrive !* " for that one can vouch.

It is always a mistake, to say the least of it, " to do harm that good may come ", and to use harmful measures, when simple and harmless ones succeed. Give *Cina* 200 to children, with the trying *Cina* symptoms, and they are not only rid of their thread- worms, but of all the nervous symptoms, dependent on them, or accompanying them, or permitting their continuance ; because healthy children probably would make short work with " worms ". A healthy mucous membrane would not provide them with a suitable habitat. As Kent says : " The old routine of giving *Cina* for worms need not go into your notes, for if you are guided by the symptoms, the patient will be cured and the worms will go."

HUGHES, *Pharmacodynamics*, says, " Hahnemann refers to this use of it " (to expel worms) ; " and very justly, as it was then given in doses of from ten to sixty grains, warns against its danger. . . . He says nothing about the dynamic use of *Cina* in helminthiasis. But his experiments and citations revealed the curious fact that *Cina* produces on the healthy body nearly, if not quite, all those symptoms whose presence leads us to suspect the existence of worms. There are the dilated pupils, with dimness of the sight and twitching of the eyelids, the ravenous appetite, the pinchings in the abdomen, the itching at the nose and anus, the frequent micturition, the spasmodic cough with vomiting, the restless sleep, the fever and the twitchings in various parts of the body. General convulsions also have frequently resulted from the large doses of *Cina* or *Santonin* given as a vermifuge. Homœopathic practitioners thus came to give this drug in minute doses to children suffering from worm affections. They calculated that, on the principle *similia similibus* it might at least relieve the symptoms caused by the presence of the parasites, though they themselves remained in *situ*. It fully answered their expectations, and a curious result followed. By some inexplicable influence these infinitesimal quantities of *Cina* not only relieved worm symptoms, but promoted the death and expulsion of the worms themselves. This occurred so often, that at length it became a recognized homœopathic practice to dispense with vermifuges, and to rely upon dynamic remedies alone. . . ."

Cina " seems beneficial in all varieties of the malady, as Dr. Bayes says he has repeatedly killed *tapeworm* with it, as well as the *lumbrici* and *ascarides* for which it is generally given ; and it acts *omni dosi*, from the 12th dilution of *Cina* of this writer to the 20th of a grain recommended by Dr. Dyce Brown."

NASH is quaint in what he says about *Cina*. " Here is a truly unique remedy that none but the homœopath knows how to use. The old school, chagrined at our success with it, and not willing to resort to our small doses, have bungled with its alkaloid, doing more harm than good, and at last have come to sneer at the idea of children being troubled with worms at all. I have known of several instances of the kind and it has become so common in the region where I practice that the people often ask me—' Doctor, do you believe in worms ? Old School doctors don't. I have found several worms that my child has passed, and have come to see if you can do anything for them.' It is a great advantage to *cure the little patients*, whether we *believe in worms or not*." And he says, " Another thing I have proven to my entire satisfaction, and that is, that it is more efficacious for these cases in the 200th or highest potencies than in the alkaloid or lower potencies." Here Nash follows Hahnemann. If you only thought of poisoning worms, you would naturally give the biggest dose you dared risk; whereas if you merely provide the vital stimulus for the patient, the most-like remedy to his symptoms, and so, causing him to cure these, leave no vantage ground any longer for the troublesome parasites, you will have to do this *a la Hahnemann*, in regard to preparation and dosage. The unit dose generally suffices, in our experience, in the incredibly fine potency which we label the 200th.

We will let Nash describe the leading symptoms that spell " *Cina* ". He says: " The wormy child will be very restless at night, ' *screams out sharply in sleep* ', making one think of *Apis*, but other symptoms appear which rule *Apis* out. *The child is cross and ugly like Chamomilla. Kicks and strikes at the nurse, wants to be carried (Cham.) or rocked, or don't want to be touched or looked at (Antimonium crud.), desires things and then refuses them when offered (Bry. and Staphisagria)*, or, unlike *Chamomilla*, if anyone tries to take hold of it or carry it, it cries. Isn't that a perfect picture of the mind of a wormy child? " Then he diagnoses further between *Cham.* and *Cina*. The *Cham.* face is frequently red and hot on one side, and pale and cold on the other. *Cina* has glowing redness both sides, or is pale and sickly, with dark circles round eyes, or red with great paleness round mouth and nose. Then *Cina* has, in addition, boring and picking its nose, gritting its teeth in sleep, jerking in sleep, and frequently swallowing, or even coughing and choking. Such a combination is not found under any other remedy. Then *Cina* has alternating canine hunger and no appetite at all. . . .

CLARKE says, " *It is pre-eminently a worm medicine as it causes all the symptoms which characterize helminthiasis, both mental, nervous and bodily.* There is irritation of the nose, causing constant desire to rub, pick, or press into it. In children there is extreme ill-humour and naughtiness. Nothing pleases them for any length of time. Gritting teeth during sleep, wetting the bed (when accompanied by picking nose, great hunger, restless sleep) tossing all about the bed in sleep; crying out as if delirious. Sherbino has found ' getting on hands and knees in sleep a strong indication for it. . . . Child lies on belly or on hands and knees during sleep. . . ."—[*Medorrhinum* has this also.]

Among the symptoms of *Cina* Hughes also stresses " *Canine hunger :* hungry soon after a full meal. Craves sweets: refuses mother's milk.

" Cough, dry with sneezing : spasmodic : periodic, spring and fall. Child is afraid to speak or move for fear of bringing on a paroxysm."

" Hahnemann indicates it in whooping-cough (in which Dr. Jousset esteems it the principle remedy), and in certain intermittents accompanied by vomiting and canine hunger . . . Dr. Bayes commends it in the gastralgia of empty stomachs."

H. C. ALLEN says, " Compare *Ant. c.*, *Ant. t.*, *Bry.*, *Cham.*, *Kreos.*, *Sil.*, *Staph.*, in irritability in children.

" In pertussis when *Dros.* has relieved the severe symptoms.

" Has cured aphonia from exposure, when *Acon.*, *Phos.*, and *Spong.* had failed.

" Frequently to be thought of in children, as an epidemic remedy, when adults require other drugs."

" GUERNSEY adds, *Complaints that come on whenever one yawns. Troubles that cause a constant desire to rub, pick, or bore into the nose.*" (*Arum triph.*)

BLACK LETTER SYMPTOMS

(From *Hahnemann*, *Allen's Encyclopedia* and *Hering's Guiding Symptoms.*)

Child exceedingly CROSS, *cries and strikes at all around.*
Pitiful weeping, when awake.
Cannot be quieted by any persuasions : proof against all caresses.
Children wake in evening or before midnight with fear or fright. jump up, see sights, scream, tremble and talk about it with much anxiety.

When walking in open air stupifying, internal HEADACHE, *especially in sinciput, afterwards also in occiput.*
Dull headache, affecting the eyes, in the morning.
Looks sickly about the eyes, with paleness of face.
Optical illusions in bright colours, blue, violet, yellow, green.
Palpitation in muscles of eyebrows, a kind of spasm.

In external EAR, *cramp-like twitchings.*
Dull stitches—a pinching pressure, under the mastoid.

Child frequently bores into NOSE *till blood comes.*
Itching of nose. Child picks its nose very much, is very restless, cries and is very unamiable.

FACE *pale and cold.*
White and blue about the mouth.
Burning heat over whole face : rising heat and glowing rednes[s] of cheeks, without thirst, after sleep.

Adherent mucus in LARYNX, *in a.m. on rising : must often hawk.*

Great hunger soon after a meal : feeling of emptiness.
Desires many and different things.
Gnawing sensation in STOMACH, *as from hunger.*

Very short breath, with interruptions : some inspirations are omitted.
A kind of oppression of CHEST : *the sternum seems to press on the lungs, and breathing is somewhat impeded.*
Hoarse hacking cough consisting of a few impulses, with long pauses before exciting irritation recurs : in the evening.
Before coughing child raises herself suddenly, looks wildly about ; the body becomes stiff, she loses consciousness, as if she would have an epileptic spasm, then follows the cough.
After coughing the child cries out, and a noise like gurgling is heard going down.

BACK AND LIMBS. *Bruised pain in sacrum, not worse by movement.*
Drawing, tearing pain downwards through whole spine.
Boring, cramping pain in left upper arm.
Single, small, twitching stitches, in right, or left hand.
Paralytic pain left thigh, not far from knee.
Obtuse stitches here and there in the body.
In body, limbs, arms, feet, toes, sometimes in the side, or on the back, or in nasal bones, but especially on the hip, obtuse stitches or squeezing, or aching, or like knocks or jerks : on pressing the part it pains, as if sore or bruised.

CONVULSIONS *of extensor muscles : child becomes suddenly stiff : there is a clucking noise, as though water were poured out of a bottle, from throat down to abdomen.*
Worm spasms, the child stiffens out straight.

When yawning, trembling of the body with shuddering.

SOME PECULIAR OR CHARACTERISTIC SYMPTOMS

Child wants to be carried.
Cannot bear least touch : cannot bear to have head touched : paroxysms of chorea reproduced by touch.
Taking hold of child, it cries piteously.
Must be rocked, carried, dandled on knee constantly day and night : will not sleep unless rocked or kept in constant motion.

Or, desire to remain perfectly still in the dark.

Child discharges worms ; picks nose or anus ; has a hacking cough ; is continually making attempts as if to swallow something ; is very hard to please.

*   *   *

SANTONIN, a derivative of *Cina*, has produced and cured nocturnal enuresis in children—" not necessarily connected with worms ".

Like *Cina* it disorders vision. Sees colours, especially yellow and green : and it has some reputation for cataract. A few days ago a patient with cataract said eagerly, " Yes, I can always see green," when a green Hospital card was shown her. It remains to be seen whether *Santonin* can help. In her case one eye was lost, after an operation for cataract, and the second was nearly blind.

HUGHES (*Pharmacodynamics*) gives some interesting eye cases and experiments with *Santonin* (see p. 392) where the late Dr. Dyce Brown in conjunction with an occulist, treated forty-two cases, of which thirty-one were cured or improved. They included choroiditis, retinitis, atrophy of the optic disc, pure amblyopia, and retinal anæsthesia. And in one case of undoubted double cataract, vision was greatly improved.

CISTUS CANADENSIS
("*Ice Plant*" : "*Frost Weed*")

THE first thing one notices about *Cistus*, " Ice plant ", is that it has not earned its common names for nothing. CLARKE says "it has a peculiar property of favouring the formation of ice about its roots in early winter ". HERING says, " It is said that in the months of November and December these plants send out near the roots, broad, thin, curved ice-crystals, about an inch in length, which wilt in the day and are renewed in the morning."

HERING refers to various published papers about this plant, showing its uses—in sore throat :—in Colic after acid fruit :—in Chronic Dysentery :—in Mastitis :—in Cough with tumours on neck :—in Goitre and Erysipelas :—in White swelling of knee joint :—in Intermittent Fever :—in Scrofula, etc.

A truly amazing remedy for catarrh of nasal and postnasal passages, throat and larynx. A recent acquaintance—or rather friend : but rapid and deep-acting—*where symptoms agree*.

One's first experience has been already told in HOMŒOPATHY, but must be retold because it belongs here. A wee girl was brought to Out-patients in the summer—August 1931—because she was always catching cold—and these colds lasted such a long time : bad now, but worse in winter. She was worse in cold weather, had an aversion to fat, to meat, to salt. She had one great craving—*for cheese*.

This was so marked that one went to the Repertory for drugs that craved cheese, and found

(Arg. n.) (Ast. r.) *Cist*. (Ign.) (Mosch.) (Puls.)
Cist. being the one, evidently, that had the strong craving.

So one turned up *Cistus* in *Materia Medica*, and discovered that it fitted the case all round.

It has " Frequent and violent sneezing—chronic nasal catarrh. Worse for cold : for inhaling cold air, etc.," and she got *Cistus* 6 *t.d.s.* for a few days. She was speedily better and growing fast. In the winter the report was, " Not catching colds ". Seven months later she came for " a cold again ", when the remedy was repeated. One learns, *inter alia*, that even the low potencies hold—when you get the correct remedy ; or rather, the reaction to low potencies may also be lengthy.

These cases of chronic catarrh, and everlasting colds are sometimes difficult to treat.

Since then, there have been other cases ; another little school-girl, everlasting colds, got *Cistus*—she also had a great love of cheese !—and her mother reported her freedom from colds—her enablement to stick at school without constantly being pulled up by colds ; later, that " all the other children had streaming colds, while she remained free ". Here again, many months later, there had to be a repeat.

In our Journal HOMŒOPATHY we have given other striking cases, but a drug like this is worth further consideration, and chronic catarrh of nose and throat is not the measure of its usefulness, as we shall see.

In regard to *Cistus*, one notices its prominent sensations, COLDNESS.

Forehead cold, with sensation of coldness inside forehead.

Cold feeling (or burning) in nose.

Sensation of coldness of tongue, larynx and trachea : saliva is cool : breath feels cold. Inhaled air feels cold (*Phos.*, *Rumex*) in larynx and trachea.

Sore throat from inhaling the least cold air : not from warm air.

Cool feeling in stomach : in abdomen.

Sensibility to cold air in chest.

Tips of fingers sensitive to cold air. Cold feet.

Very sensitive to a draught of air.

But *Cistus* has also burnings. Most drugs have opposite conditions.

Next the *catarrhal* symptoms :—

Pressure above eyes in forehead.

Frequent and violent sneezing, mostly evening and morning.

Chronic nasal catarrh.

Left nostril more affected : burning sensation in left nostril.

A feeling of softness in throat : or as if sand were in throat.

Continuous dryness and heat in throat ; < after sleeping, eating and drinking.

A small dry spot in gullet : < after sleeping : > eating.

Throat looks glassy with stripes of tough mucus.

Itching throat and fauces. Rawness from chest to throat.

Stitches in throat cause cough.

Tearing pain in throat when coughing.

Tickling and soreness of throat : sore throat from cold air.

Or, fauces inflamed and dry, without feeling of dryness.

Hawking of mucus, tough, gum-like, tasteless or bitter.

Relief from expectoration.

In black type, SCROFULOUS SWELLING AND SUPPURATION OF GLANDS OF THROAT.

Feeling as if windpipe had not space enough.

Chronic itching in larynx and trachea.

Respiration asthmatic in evening after lying down and at night.

Loud wheezing. Sensation as if trachea had not space enough.

A curious sensation: As if ants were running through the whole body (after lying down), then anxious, difficult breathing. Obliged to get up and open window: fresh air relieves. Immediately on lying down these sensations return.

Pressure on chest. Chest hurts when touched.

Cough—with symptoms previously detailed.

Besides the craving for cheese, *Cistus* longs for acid food and fruits, which give pain and diarrhœa. Diarrhœa also from coffee, and in wet weather.

Glands are affected: goitre: has even a reputation in cancer.

Mental excitement and agitation increase all the sufferings, including cough.

* * *

KENT in his small lecture on *Cistus*, adds some interesting points: . . . He says it is a deep-acting remedy; runs close to *Calcarea*, but is milder in action. It has *Calcarea's* exhaustion from exertion—dyspnœa—sweating—and coldness.

He tells his first experience with *Cistus*, because " often what will forcibly call your attention to a remedy will be the curing of a bad and typical case. A girl of nineteen, with glands of neck large and hard, the parotids especially. She had fœtid otorrhœa ; inflamed and suppurating eyes, with fissures at the corners ; lips cracked and bleeding, and " salt rheum " at ends of fingers. He could not make *Calc.* fit, and at last this little remedy seemed just what he needed, and it cured—though she had had an immense amount of Homœopathy. Kent says he has studied it since, and once or twice tried to prove it—without success. " It should be proved."

He says, the glands inflame, swell, suppurate. Causes caries and cures old ulcers. . . . Affects all mucous membranes, which throw out thick, yellow, offensive mucus ; suitable to old and troublesome catarrh. Chest fills with great quantities of mucus, better for expectoration, but *after he empties the chest it feels raw.* Cold feeling or burning in nose ; in acute coryza the nose fills up with thick, yellow mucus, and when this is blown out, it leaves the nasal cavity empty and in a state of irritation : raw—cold or burning. There is relief when the nose fills up again.

In this remedy, when the nose is empty there is burning or rawness, caused by inhalation of air.

Shooting, itching, thick crusts; with burning on right zygoma. Has cured lupus on face; caries of lower jaw; open, bleeding cancer on lower lip. Cures old, deep-seated, eating ulcers about ankle and shin, with copious acrid discharge; worse from bathing, sensitive to open air; only comfortable when very warm.

Every cold settles in throat; hot air feels good everywhere. "He goes to register, and turns the heat on, wants to feel the heat in nose, throat and lungs."

Chronic induration and inflammation of mammae. Growths with enlargement of glands all round. The glands of the neck are enlarged in lines like knotted rope, as in Hodgkin's disease. "Only a limited number of remedies have this knotting": and so on.

*   *   *

Cistus needs further proving. We have stressed what is known and most marked, because, in its sphere, it is evidently a heroic remedy.

By the way, *Cistus* is also a *rheumatic* medicine. One patient, a doctor, who "ate cheese with every meal", and had been cured by *Cistus* of chronic catarrh and sudden uncontrollable fits of sneezing which would last for ten to twenty minutes unless stopped by sniffing up cocaine or chloroform, developed pain in his right shoulder, "unaffected by weeks of treatment, electric, etc., but was getting worse and more distressing". *Cistus* was found to have produced just such pain, and after a dose of *Cistus* "it was gone in an hour".

Clarke says, "*Cistus* is a very ancient remedy for scrofulous affections, and also in scorbutic states with gangrenous ulcerations."

COCCULUS

OF *Cocculus indicus* HAHNEMANN says : " This vegetable substance, hitherto only used for destroying some noxious vermin and
for stupifying fish so that they may be taken by the hand, was
(like *Staphisagria*) first employed by myself as a medicine (after
I had first ascertained its dynamic effects on the healthy human
body). It possesses many curative virtues, as the following
symptoms produced by it show ; and the tincture prescribed
according to the similarity of effect in high attenuation and
potency is indispensable for the cure in many cases of common
human diseases ;—more especially in some kinds of lingering
nervous fevers ; in several so-called spasms in the abdomen,
and so-called spasmodic pains of other parts, where the mental
state is one of extreme sadness, particularly in the female sex ;
in not a few attacks of paralysis of the limbs, and in emotional
derangements resembling those that *Cocculus* can itself produce."

HERING (*Guiding Symptoms*) says : " Tincture of the powdered
seeds is used, which contain a crystallizable principle, *Picrotoxin*,
a powerful poison.

" *Cocculus* was used by the ancients as a poison for fish,
stupifying them, and rendering it easy to catch them.

" It has been, and still is" (so he says) "extensively used for
adulterating malt liquors . . ." A pleasant idea ! Perhaps,
if this use persists, it may account for some of the symptoms
of beer drunkenness. The attitudes and mentality of the reeling
and roaring monstrosities one used to meet in the streets—
anyway before the war, when beer happily became more costly
and more difficult to obtain—are very suggestive of *Cocculus*
poisoning : the difficult, uncertain gait ; the difficult speech and
articulation ; the noisy, quarrelsome mood of the reeling, roaring
songsters—no wonder that " one of the remedies for the diseases
peculiar to drunkards " is *Cocculus*.

But, as Tennyson has it, " Bygones may be come-agains ",
and we may yet see the good old days back now that beer is
blatantly preached from all the great hoardings, " *Beer is
good for you !* " with all the other brewers' slogans. As an
American journal pointed out in regard to patent medicines,
these are put on the market and advertised not for tender love
of the dear people, or for their relief and salvation, but solely
for the juggling purpose of extracting money from their pockets.
. . . However, all these things spell " Industry " and " Divi-
dends" ; and the revenue from beer is increasing, which must be

very gratifying to the Chancellor of the Exchequer. Only—there is the other side to the question ; appetites whetted ; habits difficult, once formed, to eradicate, and, as always, temptations for the weak and wavering at every street corner. But it is a free country ; or was supposed to be till " DORA " came along—and stayed ; and so long as the Boisterous Britisher only gets drunk and not too disorderly or obstructive in the streets, and drinks only before a certain " witching hour of night ", the kindly police will not cause him over much inconvenience. And meanwhile we homœopaths can see *Cocculus* in the spasticity and loss of power of the inebriate's limbs and his clumsy attempts at progression : and learn how to remember its peculiarities and apply them for healing.

Among the mental symptoms, highly suggestive, are :—

Speech difficult : difficulty in reading and thinking.

Thinks and answers correctly, but takes a long time in reflecting.

Slowness of comprehension : cannot find the right word : forgets himself : cannot talk plainly : or is irritable, speaks hastily, cannot bear the least noise or contradiction.

Great talkativeness : witty joking : irresistible desire to sing. A kind of mania.

Melancholy and sad : sensitive to insults, slights and disappointment. Easily affronted. A trifle makes him angry.

Cannot accomplish anything at her work : cannot finish anything.

Frightened look. Little concern for his own health ; very anxious about others' sickness. (*Ars., Phos., Sulph.*)

Fear of death and unknown dangers.

*   *   *

In regard to *Picrotoxin*, the alkaloid of *Cocculus*, and to its effect on fish, CLARKE (*Dictionary*) tells us that " When *Picrotoxin* is added to water in which fish are swimming, they make winding and boring movements of the body, alternating with quiet swimming, open their mouths and gill-caverns frequently, fall on their side, and rapidly die of asphyxia."

And he tells of a doctor who proved *Picrotoxin* on himself with such alarming symptoms that he had to resort to *Opium* and *Camphor* to antidote. He experienced " nausea with tendency to vomit ; violent intestinal pain and purging ; dysenteric diarrhœa and excessive secretion of urine ; cramps and paralytic sensations. Pain in bowels and sensation as if bowels would protrude at left inguinal ring." (*Cocculus* or *Picrotoxin* has been found useful in left-sided inguinal hernia.)

Of *Cocculus* he says : " It has cured a case of delirium at onset of menses ; the patient said, ' I always see something alive, on walls, floor, chairs, or anywhere, always *rolling,* and will roll on me.' " (*Cocculus* is one of the remedies of troubles and irregularities of menstruation—the rest of the symptoms agreeing.)

And he tells of a cure of enlargement of the liver by the great Lippe : it was after parturition, the indication being " *The liver was more painful after anger.*" And, with *Cocculus, the least jar is unbearable* (*Bell.*).

* * *

HUGHES (*Pharmacodynamics*) quotes a case of poisoning by *Cocculus* related by Hahnemann (in *Hufeland's Journal*). " Coldness ; paralytic stiffness of the limbs with drawing pains in their bones and in the back, and sullen irritability, with anxiety, were the prominent symptoms. The patient said that his brain felt constricted as by a ligature. He wished to sleep, but a frightful sensation, as of a hideous dream, came over him directly he closed his eyes, and made him start up again. He had great repugnance to food and drink. This is a frequent symptom of *Cocculus,* and very characteristic of it."

Hughes also says, " The experiments lately made on animals with the alkaloid contained in *Cocculus, Picrotoxin,* show that convulsions, both tonic and clonic, are a special characteristic of its action. The latter present many of those singular features which have been observed as results of injury to the crura cerebri, as semicircular and backward movements, and rolling over on the axis of the body. With these there is great slowness of pulse and respiration, indicating disturbance at the origin of the vagus."

Again, " *Cocculus* thus appears to influence the motor nervous tract throughout the cranio-spinal axis. To such action is referable, I think, the whole range of its curative influence. It is of great service in certain kinds of vomiting. These, when analysed appear to be of cerebral rather than gastric origin. They are such as occur in sea-sickness, and in some persons from riding in a carriage or any similar motion ; they have another instance in the vomiting of migraine, or of cerebral tumours . . . in the former *Cocculus* has no rival." And he talks of " vertigo, where *Cocculus* is a principal remedy . . . and of the abdominal spasms, accompanied by flatulence, not the product of fermentation . . ."

* * *

FARRINGTON (*Comparative Materia Medica*) says in regard to " *Cocculus,* . . . whose active principle is *Picrotoxin,* bitter poison.

" We shall find under *Cocculus* symptoms that are under many other drugs, but in no other drug do they hold the same relation as they do here.

" The general effect of *Cocculus* is its well-known action on the cerebrospinal system : here it produces great debility. It causes a paralytic weakness of the spine, and especially of its motor nerves ; thus we find it a certain or frequent remedy in paralysis originating in disease of the spinal cord . . . especially in the beginning of the trouble, whether from functional or severe organic disease . . . irritation, softening of the cord, or locomotor ataxia. It is especially indicated where the lumbar region of the spine is affected, with weakness in the small of the back as if paralysed ; the small of the back gives out when walking. Weakness of legs : knees give out when walking ; thighs ache as if they had been pounded ; soles of feet feel as if asleep ; first one hand and then the other goes to sleep, or the whole arm falls asleep, and hands feel as if swollen.

" There is a concomitant symptom almost always associated with these—a feeling of hollowness in some of the cavities of the body—head, chest, or abdomen. It is more than a weakness ; it is an absolute feeling as though the parts were hollow.

" The debility is of spinal origin : especially is it apt to follow loss of sleep : the patient cannot sit up even one or two hours later than usual in the evening without feeling languid and exhausted throughout the entire day following. . . .

" The abdomen is greatly distended and tympanic : this tympanites under *Cocculus* is not the same as under *Cinchona, Carbo veg., Colchicum, Sulphur,* or even *Lycopodium.*

" There are several origins of tympanites. It may come from the blood-vessels, from the air swallowed with the food, from changes in the food itself, and also from the retention of flatus. The latter condition is the cause of the tympany under *Cocculus indicus.* It is not to be thought of as a remedy when flatus results from decomposition of food. That calls for *Carbo veg.*"

In regard to the occipital headache of *Cocculus,* Farrington has some interesting contributions. " Some years ago there was an epidemic of spotted fever in this city. During that epidemic many children died, especially in its earlier days. After a while there was discovered a symptom characteristic of the epidemic, and that was intense headache in the occipital region, and in the nape of the neck. Children in a stupor would manifest it by turning the head back, so as to relieve the tension on the membranes of the brain ; others who were conscious would put their hands to the back of the head ; while still others complained of pain in the back of the head, as if the part were *alternately opening and closing*. That symptom was under *Cocculus*. There were very few fatal cases after *Cocculus* was used. Occipital headaches are hard to cure. . . ."

* * *

This is Nash's little summary of *Cocculus* :
Weakness of cervical muscles, can hardly hold the head up.
Weakness in small of back, as if paralysed : gives out when walking ; can hardly stand, walk, or talk.
Hands and feet get numb ; asleep.
General sense of weakness ; or weak, hollow, gone feeling in head, stomach, abdomen, etc. Worse by loss of sleep or night watching.
Great distension with flatulent colic; wind or menstrual colic ; crampy pains ; inclined to hernia.
Modalities ; < sitting up, moving, riding in carriage or boat, smoking, talking, eating, drinking, night watching :—> when lying quiet.

* * *

To epitomize Kent, who is, as usual, the most illuminating of all :—" *Cocculus* slows down all the activities of body and mind, producing a sort of paralytic weakness."
Behind time in all its actions.
All the nervous impressions are slow in reaching the centres. As (he says) if you pinch the patient on the great toe, he waits a minute and then says " Oh ", instead of saying it at once.
Answers slowly, after apparent meditation.
Weak : tired.
First this slowness and then a sort of visible paralytic condition, and then complete paralysis—local or general.
But there are causes :—Nursing : night nursing : worn out by anxiety, worry and loss of sleep.
Cocculus, he says, from the time of Hahnemann to the present time has been a remedy for complaints from nursing; not professional nursing, for *Cocculus* needs the combination of *vexation, anxiety, and prolonged loss of sleep*. At the end of it, prostrated in body and mind, cannot sleep, has congestive headaches, nausea, vomiting and vertigo. That is how a *Cocculus* case begins.

The instant *Cocculus* gets into a wagon to ride, sick headache, nausea, vertigo come on.

Cocculus cannot endure motion : worse talking, motion, motion of eyes, riding.

Wants plenty of time to turn the head cautiously to see things. Wants plenty of time to move ; wants plenty of time to think ; wants plenty of time to do everything. Is slowed down : inactive.

Then the *incoordination*, the *numbness*. He says it has been used with good effect in locomotor ataxia.

In regard to the STIFFNESS of *Cocculus*. Kent makes this clear and rememberable. "Such a strong symptom, and quite peculiar to *Cocculus*—as to some nerve diseases. Limbs straightened out and held there for a little while can only be flexed with great pain. Persons prostrated with anxiety will lie down on the back, straighten out the limbs, and can only get up with great difficulty. The doctor comes, discovers what is the matter, bends the limbs and she screams ; but is relieved after the bending, and can get up and move about." Kent says, "You cannot find that anywhere else. It is entirely without inflammation : a sort of paralytic stiffness, a paralysis of the tired body and mind. A man will stretch out his leg on a chair and he cannot flex it till he reaches down with his hands to assist. . . . Now with all this slowing down of the thoughts and activities, the patient remains extremely sensitive to suffering and to pain."

Spasms like electric shocks : convulsions after loss of sleep. Tetanus, chorea, attacks of paralytic weakness with pain. Paralysis, eyes, face, muscles, limbs—everywhere. Kent gives a case of paralysis of both limbs after diphtheria in a little girl, which was considered hopeless ; but one of the big old men, looking through the case, gave *Cocculus cm* and "it was not many days before the child began to move the legs and the condition was perfectly cleared up", "and I have never ceased to wonder at it", says Kent.

(Here, and in other of the aspects of *Cocculus*, one is reminded again and again of *Gelsemium*. Both paralyse the eyelids and the throat, producing ptosis and paresis of deglutition ; the limbs : and both may help and cure paralysis after diphtheria. One may compare also with *Plumbum* which, as Nash has pointed out, has *hyperæsthesia with loss of power* :—a brilliant and fertile hint, as one has experienced ; notably in a case of Landry's disease, "ascending paralysis", where the condition caused great anxiety as it progressed, and the hyperæsthesia was such that the hospital nurses had to give up taking the pulse. Rare doses of *Plumbum* in high potency sent her back to useful war-work. It was the sort of case that one does not forget. But *Cocculus* has *spasticity with loss of power*, and should be useful in spastic paraplegias.)

Kent says further : In the extreme *Cocculus* state, there is the appearance of imbecility, the mind seems almost a blank. He looks into space, and slowly turning the eyes towards the questioner answers with difficulty. Prostration and nervous exhaustion accompany most of the complaints of *Cocculus*.

Then, as to the vertigo and nausea : A *Cocculus* case cannot look out of the car window, cannot look down from the boat and see water moving, without nausea immediately. Headaches and nausea, with giddiness and gastric symptoms. Cannot accommodate the eyes to moving objects. . . . Headache as if the skull would burst, or like a great valve opening and shutting (or, as we have heard, mysterious feelings as if the head were hollow and empty) . . . prostration and nervous exhaustion accompany most of the complaints of *Cocculus*. . . . You go to the bedside and ask the nurse, " What have you been feeding the patient ? " and the patient gags. The thought of food makes the patient gag. The nurse will say, every time she mentions food the patient gags. The thought of food or the smell of food in the other room or the kitchen will nauseate the patient. (*Colchicum* :—but also *Ars.* and *Sep.*)

Kent also draws attention to : Sensation as though a worm were crawling in stomach :—(" Something alive inside " reminds one of *Thuga* and *Crocus*) and Kent ends with " *Slightest loss of sleep tells on him.*"

*   *   *

Working through *Cocculus*, as mirrored in the experience of different prescribers, is extremely interesting and instructive, and one remembers with regret cases where *Cocculus* might have been useful. As a matter of fact one's most frequent experience with *Cocculus* has been helping persons worn out with prolonged night nursing and loss of sleep : where

> " *Glamis hath murdered sleep and therefore Cawdor*
> *Shall sleep no more ; Macbeth shall sleep no more.*"

BLACK LETTER SYMPTOMS

(i.e. those which *Cocculus* most notably causes and cures)

THOUGHTS *are fixed on a single disagreeable subject : absorbed in thought and notices nothing about her.*

Sits in deep reverie.

Ill effects of anger and grief.
Sudden extreme anxiety.
Easily startled.
Time passes too quickly.

Stupid in the HEAD.
Cloudiness of the head, chiefly after eating and drinking.
Vertigo as if intoxicated, with dullness in forehead : as if a board across head : on rising from lying : had to lie down again.
Vertigo : as if intoxicated : with confusion : with nausea : things whirl from right to left.
With flushed, hot face and head : then palpitation.
Headache as if eyes would be torn out.
Headache with nausea and inclination to vomit.
Sick headache from riding in carriage, boat, train, cars, etc.
Seasickness.

Dimness of SIGHT.

Dryness of œsophagus.
Loss of appetite with metallic taste.

Unusual NAUSEA *and inclination to vomit, while riding in a wagon.*
Extreme aversion to food, caused even by the smell of food, although with hunger.
Frequent empty eructations.
When he becomes cold, or catches cold, there is inclination to vomit, causing a copious flow of saliva.
Inclination to vomit in connection with headache, and a pain as if bruised in the bowels.

Violent spasm in the STOMACH, *clutching in the stomach.*
Spasm in the stomach : squeezing in the stomach.
Griping in epigastrium, taking away the breath.
Thirst especially for beer.

Great distension of the ABDOMEN.
Flatulent colic about midnight ; awakened by incessant accumulation of flatulence, which distended the abdomen, causing oppressive pain here and there ; some was passed without remarkable relief, whilst new flatus constantly collected for several hours ; he was obliged to lie on one side for relief.
Painful inclination to a hernia, especially after rising from sitting.
Watery urine.

Itching in scrotum.

MENSTRUATION *seven days too early, with distension of abdomen and cutting, contracting pains in abdomen on every motion and every breath, together with contraction of rectum.*

Tensive constriction of right side CHEST, *which oppresses the breathing.*

Very violent tickling in larynx, wakes him at 11.30 *p.m., causes cough, with expectoration of much tenacious mucus.*

Expectoration of much viscid albuminous mucus.

PARALYTIC SYMPTOMS.

Weakness of cervical muscles, with heaviness of head.

In shoulder joint and muscles of upper arm, single stitches when at rest.

Stitches in right upper arm.

Numbness and paralytic feelings in arms.

Now one hand, now the other is numb, as if asleep.

Sometimes one hand, sometimes the other is alternately hot and cold.

Hand trembles while eating, and the more the higher it is raised.

Knees sink down from weakness; totters while walking and threatens to fall to one side.

Cracking of the knee when moving.

Soles of both feet go to sleep while sitting.

At one time the feet are asleep, at another the hands.

(And, in italics Weakness in limbs as if paralysed).

Trembling from excitement, over-exertion and pain.

Sensation of seasickness.

Hysteric complaints with sadness.

Convulsions after loss of sleep.

Attacks of paralytic weakness with pain in back.

Here and there in the limbs an acute paralytic drawing, continuous and in jerks, as if in the bone.

Cracking and creaking in the joints.

Painful stiffness of the joints.

Falling asleep of feet and hands alternately, in short paroxysms.

Tendency to tremble.

Great exhaustion of the body, so that it was an exertion to him to stand steady.

Slight perspiration over the whole body on slightest exertion.

Cocculus *excites shooting pains and heat in cold glandular swellings, at least when they are touched.*

All the symptoms and sufferings,, especially in the head, are aggravated by drinking, eating, sleeping, and speaking.

Intolerance of cold and warm air.

SLEEP *disturbed by excessive anxiety and restlessness.*
Sleepless from long continued nursing ; from night watching.
Anxious, frightful dreams.
Ill effects from loss of sleep and night watching.

FEVER SYMPTOMS.

Chill frequently alternating with heat.
Flushes of heat, with burning heat of cheeks and cold feet.
Insidious nervous fevers, particularly in cases which have been produced by frequent fits of anger, or are accompanied by great disposition to anger.

PECULIAR CHARACTERISTIC SYMPTOMS

Great excitement after two glasses of beer.
His accustomed beer caused headache.
Thirst, especially for beer.
Great sensitiveness of mouth and fauces, so that rinsing the mouth caused cough and vomiting thick masses of mucus.
Loud speaking or brushing the teeth caused cough and vomiting.
Constant desire to spit, with sweetish metallic taste.
Pain in liver after anger.
Pain in tendo achillis—only when walking. No tenderness : limped when walking in street : obliged to turn foot outwards : to stop and hold foot up to relieve the pain. Ascending steps was especially painful.
Pain, redness and swelling of great toes, like gout.
Left great toe especially affected : with fine prickings as from splinters of glass, beneath nail, and at tip of toe.
Coldness of stomach : as if cold air were blowing in it.
Spasmodic internal heaving in epigastrium.
Nausea, felt in head : seems to be mostly in mouth.
Hollowness in head : in chest : in abdomen.

Shivering over mammæ.

Chilly feeling through teeth.

Rolling of eyeballs, eyes being closed.

Sleep aggravates all symptoms, especially of head.

Colic as if there were sharp stones rubbing against each other in abdomen.

Occipital headache, occiput alternately opens and shuts. (Vertex opens and shuts. *Cann. ind.*)

Time passes too swiftly (too slowly).

* * *

In regard to the places where nausea is felt, one is constantly adding to them :

Nausea felt in head and mouth, *Cocc.*

In rectum, *Ruta.*

In ears, *Dioscor.*

Besides the more usual localities, stomach, chest, abdomen.

COFFEA CRUDA

ONE of our most useful domestic remedies : since in many persons coffee causes sleeplessness, not from tossings, not from discomfort, not from pain ; but the sleeplessness of a brain too alert and wakeful, from pleasure, or excitement, or mental stress and activity. Here *Coffea*, in potency, gives a sleep that is natural, restful, invigorating, and leaves no after-effects. It is the most beautiful sedative known, the most perfectly homœopathic reaction that can be imagined.

A case in point : we may have told it, elsewhere ? but it belongs here. She was very seriously ill, and so worn and weak that the doctor said, give her a cup of strong coffee. She had it. And during half the following night, one was in and out, always finding a cheerful wakefulness, not in the least distressed, but absolute sleeplessness. At last, in desperation, one went for a dose of *Coffea* 200, and the patient was fast asleep in a few minutes. This holds three lessons. The rapid action, in a *Coffea* case, of *Coffea* ; the power of potentized drugs ; the property of a remedy, in potency, to prove its own best antidote in the crude state.

BLACK LETTER SYMPTOMS

Unusual activity of mind and body.

Full of ideas ; quick to act, no sleep on this account.

Mental excitability.

Sleeplessness on account of excessive mental and physical excitement.

Fright from sudden pleasant surprises.

Pains seem insupportable, driving to despair.

Affections after sudden emotions, particularly pleasant surprises.

All the senses more acute, reads fine print easier, particularly an increased perception of slight passive motions.

Threatening of apoplexy ; over-excited, talkative, full of fear, pangs of conscience, aversion to open air, sleepless, convulsive grinding of teeth.

One-sided headache, as from a nail driven into head (Thuja) ; worse in open air.

Neuralgic toothache entirely relieved by holding cold water in the mouth, returning as this becomes warm.

During labour or after-pains, extreme fear of death.

Great agitation and restlessness.

Affections after sudden emotions, especially pleasant surprises.
Would like to rub or scratch the part, but it is too sensitive.
Bad effects from wine or liquor drinking.
Thirst at night wakes him during sweat, infrequent during heat ;
almost constant thirst after heat and during sweat.

*   *   *

As to the curious symptom : toothache relieved while cold water is held in mouth, and returning as this becomes warm. We have seen this more than once. And *Coffea* has promptly cured.

COLCHICUM AUTUMNALE

IN the scheme of things remedies seem to be placed where and when they are wanted. *Dulcamara* climbs the hedges in the time of hot days and cold nights. *Arnica* grows in the Andes, and mountainous regions, where it eases and helps to remedy the effects of great fatigue, and falls, and bruises,—*Fall-kraut*, " Fall-herb ", as the Germans call it. The snake remedies come in especially for snake bites, and for the violent and rapid diseases of tropical climates. And not for nothing does *Colchicum autumnale* flower in the autumn, for it is a grand remedy for the diarrhœa and dysentery of autumn, as well as for the acute rheumatism of that season.

HERING (*Guiding Symptoms*) tells us that it was proved by Hahnemann and many others, but his proving is not to be found either in *Materia Medica Pura*, or in the *Chronic Diseases*. . . . It would doubtless be found in *Stapf Archiv.* : but it has probably never been done into English, since ALLEN (*Encyclopedia*) quotes none of its symptoms from Hahnemann.

* * *

Old School has greatly used—and abused—this drug : and this is what HALE WHITE (*Materia Medica*), teaches students and the medical profession in regard to *Colchicum*. He heads his small chapter : ' *The sole value of this drug is that it is a specific for gout.''*

He speaks of its *action* (which *we* know to be its curative action, given in small doses, and when symptoms in patient and drug agree). . . . Loss of appetite : purging : nausea : colic. Great abdominal pain. Vomiting. Profuse diarrhœa with passage of blood. Great prostration, the skin cold and bedewed with sweat. Respiration slow. Death due to collapse. (These, as we shall see, are exactly its homœopathic uses.)

In regard to its *therapeutics*, he says, " *Colchicum* is hardly ever used except for gout. . . . It is often very useful for dyspepsia, eczema, headache, neuritis, conjunctivitis, bronchitis and other conditions occurring in those suffering from gout, and probably related to it.

" It is a true specific ; how it acts is not known."

* * *

But one seldom sees the real old-fashioned gout of our grand-fathers. One remembers meeting it once, in a woman who begged for help one Sunday, when she could not get her regular doctor. She showed a swollen, red, shiny foot ; intensity greater about the big toe ; with much pain and tenderness. For a moment one thought of some septic condition, but was enlightened and relieved when she said that she " got these attacks of gout ". The remedy that put her right (by the next day, as one learned) was not *Colchicum* at all, but Burnett's beloved *Urtica urens*,—tincture of stinging nettles. It was because of his successful use of this simple herb in gout, that he won the name, so one is told, of "*Dr. Urtica*", in the London clubs of his day. He used to give some five drops of the strong tincture several times a day, in HOT WATER.

One gleans at once, by glancing down the Black letter symptoms of the provings that the great spheres of *Colchicum*, besides *joints* (which it inflames and stiffens; wandering from joint to joint, often), are *stomach* and *intestines*.

It has the most intense nausea, excited by the sight, or smell, or even thought of food (*Ars., Sep., Cocc.*). This characteristic symptom has led to its successful use, as in Dr. Nash's classical case, of the old lady collapsed and dying of diarrhœa, with sixty-five stools in the twenty-four hours, passed into the bed; so weak that she could not lift her head from the pillow (also a *Colch.* symptom); and so nauseated by the smell of food that all doors had to be kept shut between her and the kitchen. A dose of *Colch.* 200 (she never needed a second) stopped the drain, and, incident-ally, taught Nash the value of potentized drugs.

Diarrhœa, then, and dysentery, especially of the Autumn, and colitis, especially *membranous* colitis, in which it is so often useful.

Colch. is a remedy of metastases, as when gout leaves the joints and attacks heart or stomach : of such cases we hear less in these days ; but in rheumatism or heart or kidney troubles of the children of gouty parents, or grandparents, it should be useful —symptoms agreeing.

In common with *Dulc.*, another autumnal remedy, it is useful in ailments from cold damp weather and from suppressed perspiration.

In common with *Bry.* it dare not move : and its temper is irritable in the extreme.

In pleurodynia it compares with *Arnica* : as also in its bruised sensations.

* * *

Let NASH speak :

This remedy has one of the most positive and reliable character-istic symptoms in the whole materia medica, and one which cannot be accounted for from any pathological standpoint that I know of— "*The smell of food cooking nauseates to faintness.*" I mention this here because there is a seeming desire on the part of some to base all their prescriptions on pathological indications. I have no objection to their doing so if they can, and succeed in curing their patients. But I claim full recognition for the value of those subjective, sensational symptoms and the modalities which cannot be accounted for. Indeed, I feel quite sure that the well-verified subjective symptoms are oftener to be relied on in curing our patients than all the pathological conditions we know." And he gives the case, alluded to, of his old lady.

He points out that *Colchicum* has two opposite symptoms, viz. *burning* and icy *coldness in stomach.*

He and Kent both point out the value of *Colch.* for great meteoric distension of abdomen. " In the 200th potency it is a good remedy for the bloating of cows that have eaten too much green clover."

In regard to its use for rheumatism, articular, migrating, and gouty, Nash has often found it less successful than our other rheumatic remedies.* BUT, in any of these troubles, or others, " should I find its prime characteristics present " (nausea from smell of food and cooking) " I should certainly give it and confidently expect good results."

*　　*　　*

FARRINGTON, on the contrary (*Clinical Materia Medica*), says : " I am persuaded that *Colchicum* has not the place in practice it deserves. True it comes to us from the allopathic school as a remedy highly recommended for gout. We ought not, however, from the exorbitant use of the drug by that school, go to the opposite extreme, and neglect it as a remedy altogether."

He speaks of its use in *debility*, particularly debility following loss of sleep . . . can hardly drag one leg after the other—appetite gone, bad taste in mouth, nausea :—the debility starts from or involves digestion as a result of loss of sleep. In *typhoid* : pupils wide, almost insensitive : cold sweat forehead : when patient attempts to raise head, it falls back again, the mouth wide open. Face cadaveric : features sharp and pointed, nose looks squeezed, tongue heavy and stiff, protruded with difficulty (*Lach.*), may be bluish especially at base. Almost complete loss of speech and breath cold. Restlessness and cramp in legs. But it has not the fearfulness and dread of death of some other typhoid drugs.

Allied to *Carbo veg.* in coldness of breath, tympany and great prostration.

Tympanites : stools watery and frequent, and involuntary :—contain "shreds";—watery, bloody. In *dysentery*, if there is tympany, *Colch.* is far preferable to *Cantharis* or *Mercurius.*

---

* *Other doctors esteem it greatly in acute rheumatism; with a red blush over affected joint ; with tendency to wander from joint to joint : with hyperæsthesia, and pains worse from cold and damp.*

Then *Colch.* in *joints* and *gout*—extremely sensitive to slightest motion. The patient exceedingly irritable and oversensitive to every little external impression—light—noise—strong odours :—and pain seems unbearable (*Cham.*).

Then *metastasis* of gout or rheumatism to chest. In valvular *heart disease* or pericarditis following rheumatism, it is indicated by violent cutting and stinging pains in chest, especially about heart, with great oppression and dyspnœa. Chest feels tightly bandaged. . . .

* * *

GUERNSEY (" *Keynotes* ") says this remedy is to be thought of when we see a patient suffering from the effects of night-watching (*Cocc.* is classical here.—ED.) from the effects of hard study : . . . Arthritic pains in joints, especially when knocking the joints makes the patient scream with pain, or when stubbing the toes hurts *exceedingly*. Affects largely the periosteum and synovial membranes of joints : small joints. Redness, heat and swelling of parts affected. . . .

After evacuation, relief ; but sometimes a terrific spasmodic pain of the sphincter ani comes on after stool. . . .

* * *

KENT—we will briefly epitomize. He says, it is singular that traditional medicine used *Colchicum* so much for gout : in all old books it was recommended for this malady. The provings corroborate the fact that *Colchicum* fits into many conditions of gout . . . but traditional medicine does not tell us what kind of gout to give it in, or what kind of rheumatism. It was merely a medicine of experience. " *If it is gout, try Colchicum.*" What to do with the *patient* when the remedy failed never came up. It was, " Give the prescription and keep at it," and drugs were administered till the patient, growing steadily worse, passed from one doctor's hands into another.

Colch. is aggravated by cold, damp weather, by the cold rains in the Fall . . . it has also a summer rheumatism. Heat will slack up the flow of urine or the quantity of solids in the urine.

A striking feature running through the remedy is its tendency to move about from one joint to another, from one side to another, from below upwards, or from above downwards :—with swelling, or without swelling : first here, then there.

Another striking feature is, the general dropsical conditions. Dropsy when hands and feet swell and pit : dropsy of abdominal cavity : of pericardium, pleurae, of serous sacs . . . *with pale urine.* Whether copious or scanty, still it is pale.

Rheumatic conditions that have gone on some time and end in cardiac troubles . . . the cardiac condition is but a continuation of the rheumatic state.

Colchicum has cured dropsy after scarlet fever.

All complaints—of head—bowel—liver—stomach—are worse from motion : he dreads to move : almost as marked as we find in *Bryonia*. Chilly, sensitive to cold (rev. of *Ledum*). *Colch.* is better for heat, for wrapping up, for being warm. . . .

A curious symptom, touch and motion bring on *a painful sensation in the body as of electric vibrations*.

Is almost constantly sweating, even with fever, and sometimes the sweat is cold.

Then, the nausea, gagging and retching at the bare mention of food . . . he is so sensitive to odours that he smells things which others do not smell (just as *Coffea* hears sounds that others cannot hear). He smells odours from which he gets sick . . . in typhoid, prostrated beyond the usual, he cannot take milk, cannot take raw eggs, cannot take soup, because he gags at the mere thought of them. He has gone on for days, and his family are afraid that he is going to starve. . . . This enters into his very life, because it involves hatred to odour, and becomes a general . . . Do not say " food " in the presence of a *Colchicum* patient, but give him *Colch.* first, and pretty soon he will want something to eat. It removes that hatred of food. What a vital thing it must be when a man hates that very thing that will keep him alive.

He may have much thirst, or no thirst, or these may alternate. . . . Nausea and inclination to vomit by swallowing saliva.

He describes the bloating of the farmer's cows that have got into a fresh clover patch, and become so distended you are afraid they are going to explode. Farmers have been known to put a knife into the pouch of the cow between the last short ribs to let the wind out : but put a few pellets of *Colch.* on the tongue of each cow, and it will be but a few minutes before that wind will get out of there—to your surprise and the farmer's. When the abdomen is violently distended and tympanitic, *Colch.* is often a suitable remedy.

Then the diarrhœic stools that are like jelly—they form in the pan a solid mass of jelly . . . putrid, dark, bloody mucus, watery, jelly-like mucus, passes as a thin watery flow, but soon as it cools, forms a jelly.

*   *   *

Young doctors, poring over the provings of Materia Medica, often think that everything comes under every drug :—they are so much alike—how to distinguish ? But, get their characteristics and peculiarities of action, and each one stands out distinctly as an entity—almost a personality : and when you have once grasped that personality, and as it were made friends with the drug, you will recognize, as with your friends, not only what he looks like, but his little tricks of manner and speech, how he will behave on all occasions—in regard to noises—foods—friendly overtures—rudeness—sympathy—his restlessness or placidity—his extreme neatness and order, or the opposite—his easy emotion—chilliness—meteoric reactions—his attitude, in short, to environment physical and mental. You will see him in friends and patients, when prescribing becomes comparatively easy, and successful.

BLACK LETTER SYMPTOMS

Memory weakened, ideas not so clear as usual : forgetfulness, absence of mind.

External impressions, bright light, STRONG ODOURS, contact, misdeeds of others, make him quite beside himself.

Strong odours make him quite beside himself.

Aversion to FOOD ; loathing the sight, and still more the smell of it. No thirst.

Smell of cooking nauseates to faintness.

Nausea, eructations and copious vomiting of mucus and bile.

Violent retching, followed by copious and forcible vomiting of food and then of bile.

Violent burning in epigastrium.

Very painful urging to STOOL. Only a little fæces passed, then followed transparent, gelatinous, and very membranous mucus, with some relief of the pain in the abdomen.

Extremely painful stools.

Discharge from bowels like gelatine.

Watery, jelly-like mucus passes from anus with violent spasm in sphincter.

Bloody stools with scrapings from intestines and protrusion of anus.

Autumn dysentery, with discharges of white mucus and violent tenesmus ; bloody stools, mingled with a slimy substance.

Bloody discharge from bowels with deathly nausea from smelling cooking. Tenesmus in rectum.

Discharge from bowels containing a large quantity of small white shreddy particles.

Pain in region of KIDNEYS.

Urine like ink.

Stinging and tearing in muscles of CHEST : pleurodynia.

Oppression of chest, dyspnœa, a tensive feeling in chest, sometimes high, sometimes low down.

Oppression of chest with violent palpitation.

Hydrothorax with œdema of hands and feet.

Pulse thread-like, imperceptible.

Effusion into pericardium after inflammatory affections of heart.

A paralytic pain in the ARMS, *so violent he cannot hold the lightest thing firmly.*

Lameness after suddenly checked sweat, particularly on FEET, *by getting wet all over.*

At the beginning of ACUTE RHEUMATISM, *before fully developed.*

Pains in shoulder and hip-joints, and in all bones, with difficulty in moving head and tongue.

Great weakness and exhaustion, as after exertion, cannot move head from pillow without help.

Fall dysentery.

Constant chilly feeling, even when sitting near the stove ; with flushes of heat.

Pain goes from left to right, in gout.

Rheumatic pains excited by or worse for cold, damp weather.

Acute dropsy with renal affections.

Uric acid diathesis.

Gout in persons of vigorous constitution.

NOTABLE SYMPTOMS, IN ITALICS, OR PECULIAR

Can read, but cannot understand even a short sentence : cannot understand the words : vision is heightened, but intellectual faculties dulled.

His sufferings seem intolerable : external impressions, light noise, strong smells, contact, etc., disturb his temper.

Smell morbidly acute ; odour of meat broth causes nausea and that of fresh eggs nearly fainting : excessive sensitiveness of smell to cooking.

Tongue : bright red : heavy, stiff and numb : cold : moved and projected with difficulty.

Enormous appetite—for different things : but as soon as he sees them, or still more smells them, he shudders from nausea, and is unable to eat anything.

Obliged to bend himself up and lie quite still the whole day without the slightest movement, else he was seized with the most violent vomiting.

Epigastrium pierced by a knife.

Stomach deranged after eating too many eggs.

Colic, worse by eating ; after flatulent food, great distension ; better when bending double.

Distension of gas under short ribs.

In inflammatory irritation of abdominal viscera, by metastasis from gout.

Profuse watery stools, in hot damp weather, or in the autumn.

Long-lasting, agonizing pain in rectum and anus, after stool, causing screams and crying.

Hæmorrhage from anus *in autumnal* cold damp weather.

Child falls asleep on the vessel as soon as the tenesmus ceases.

Nephritis : bloody, ink-like, albuminous urine.

Urging to urinate ; discharge of hot, highly coloured urine ; burning and tenesmus.

Night cough with involuntary spurting out of urine.

Stinging pain, or knife pains region of heart.

Serous effusion in chest, in rheumatic or gouty persons.

Hydropericardium.

Heart disease, following gout or acute rheumatism.

Violent writhing in region of loins and urinary passages.

Knees strike together ; can hardly walk.

Feet feel heavy : difficult to lift feet or go upstairs.

Cramps feet, especially soles. Heels contracted.

Pain in ball of left big toe.

Violent pains in arms and legs : cannot use limbs.

Drawing, tearing pains in limbs, changing places.

Stiffness joints, and swelling hands and feet.

Attacks of rheumatism break forth suddenly and disappear suddenly : Pains shifting : acute attacks merging into chronic form, or during chronic form acute attacks set in.

Pains in joints, especially if knocked : stubbing the toes hurts exceedingly.

Great irritability with the pains : very sensitive to touch : the least vibration makes pain unbearable.

METASTASES to internal organs.

Dropsy of internal organs and cavities—hydropericardium—hydrothorax—ascites—hydrometra.

Stands in close relation to fibrous tissues : redness, swelling, heat, etc., not tending to suppuration ; quickly changing location.

Inflammation of joints with excessive HYPERÆSTHESIA, slightest concussion of air, floor or bed renders the pains unbearable. . . . Large joints intensely red and hot . . . acts more on the small joints.

It hastens relapses of gout if abused.

COLLINSONIA CANADENSIS

ONE remembers well one's first introduction to *Collinsonia*, performed by a hospital gynæcologist in whose clinic one worked for many years, and to whom one is indebted for much good training. He had an enormous opinion of the value of the drug *in " gynæ " cases with hæmorrhoids*. And this is where it seems to have been found invariably useful : but the drug seems never to have been adequately proved.

A single proving of the crude drug is to be found in the Appendix to Vol. X of *Allen's Encyclopedia* by an American doctor who took two and a half teaspoonfuls of the powdered root. And Clarke (*Dictionary*) records another proving, of the tincture. Also a number of writers have described its value in *Constipation during gestation, Prolapsus ani, Prolapsus uteri, with pruritis and dysmenorrhœa*, in Dysmenorrhœa with menstrual convulsions ; even *Sympathetic aphonia*, and *Pulmonary hæmorrhage*. Hering's *Guiding Symptoms* from which we take Black Letter symptoms, and curious symptoms, seems to ignore the proving of the powdered root : which we will, however, quote extensively, since it gives a curious picture of its drug action, suggestive of the rather trying conditions (at times) grouped under " nettle rash ", and " angio-neurotic œdema ".

We quote rather at length, because the curious symptoms of this proving are not to be found in Clarke, or in Hering.

First was experienced a warmth in lips, and pain at a spot where the left supraorbital nerve emerges. Some ten minutes later, an increasing warmth spread along internal surfaces of both lips, which rapidly enlarged, with a sensation of the pricking of innumerable needles, darting back and forth. Then face, cheeks, forehead and hairy parts under chin, from ear to ear, were involved, the numbness and needle-like darting to and fro spreading down to the breast-bone. There was no burning, ever, in throat pit or gullet. While inner lips and whole cavity of mouth were experiencing an intensity of excitement, the face seemed to grow broader and broader : the mind being pleasurably excited.

Now the right forearm grew numb and heavy : then the left arm and its fingers : the balls of both thumbs being worse than the fingers. Then came a sense of nausea, almost to vomiting, not better in open air ; while the lips seemed growing larger all the while, and mouth seemed to stand open, like a huge catfish's.: lips dry, no saliva. While lying, the pulse under the finger would become a mere thread, then return with more volume. Hot things seemed to intensify the effects of the medicine. It was as if *Aconite* or *Arum triph.* had been taken : *Nux vomica* proved the antidote and the effects of the *Coll.* seemed to pass away like a vapour or aura from above downwards. First relief was felt in forehead : then cheeks lost their grotesque largeness ; then lips lost their pungent glow, and arms, down to finger tips were severally bettered. But the balls of thumbs persisted in their numbness and felt unnatural even the next day. When walking in the cool open air, feet and limbs felt strangely light, as if he could run like a deer. Then the lower limbs were affected, as if asleep. *Nux* 1c, sipped, felt like removing a swaddling cloth that embarrassed nervous action by its tightness and weight.

BLACK LETTER SYMPTOMS

Mucous or black and fæcal stools, with colic and tenesmus (after confinement).

Hæmorrhoidal dysentery with tenesmus.

Obstinate constipation with hæmorrhoids, stools very sluggish and hard, accompanied by pain and flatulence.

Piles with constipation, or even with diarrhœa, bleeding, or blind and protruding : feeling of sticks, gravel, or sand in rectum : evening and night : better in morning.

Flowing piles, hæmorrhoids incessant though not profuse, with alternate constipation and diarrhœa.

Chronic, bleeding, painful hæmorrhoids.

Dropsy from cardiac disease.

SOME OF THE ITALIC, OR CURIOUS SYMPTOMS

Gastric or hæmorrhoidal headaches with giddiness.

Tongue coated yellow, centre or base, with bitter taste.

Nausea ; with cramp-like pains in stomach ; with chronic constipation ; during gestation.

Dyspepsia with waterbrash and hæmorrhoids.

Congestion of portal system and pelvic viscera, with flatulent rumbling : sluggish stool with distended abdomen. Piles.

Chronic diarrhœa of children.

Light-coloured lumpy stool with hard straining, followed by dull pains in anus and hypogastrium, lasting about half-an-hour.

Congestive inertia of lower bowel.

Weight and pressure in rectum, with intense irritation. Great itching and burning in anus : tumefaction, rectum and anus.

Varicocele with extreme constipation.

Terrible dysmenorrhœa with hæmorrhoids.

Violent convulsions preceded by severe pain in region of womb.

Pruritis vulvæ, accompanied by hæmorrhoids.

Obstinate constipation during gestation.

Severe attacks of dyspnœa with great weakness.   Irritation of cardiac nerves.   Heart's action persistently rapid but weak.

After heart is relieved, piles reappear ; suppressed menses return.

Palpitation in patients subject to piles, dyspepsia and flatulence,

Can neither walk, lie down, or sit, except on edge of chair, parts so swollen and inflamed ; during pregnancy.

The slightest excitement aggravates heart symptoms.

Faintness, oppression, syncope and difficulty of breathing, from irritation of cardiac nerves.

Feeling of sticks, or gravel, or sand, in lower part of rectum and anus.   Extreme tenderness in rectum.

Burning in anus.   Heat, stomach and anus.

*　　　*　　　*

One notices in these " indications ", that they are mostly cured conditions : they are not *" Caused and cured "*.   There was once a big controversy in regard to such.   It was contended that a drug should not be accepted from the scientific homœopathic point of view, unless it was known to have produced also the symptoms it had cured.   Dr. Clarke entered the arena fiercely : he called it a birth by breech presentation ; and later showed that the drug in question had, when proved, evoked the exact symptoms for which it had been found curative.   Let us get it ! *what a drug can cure, that it can cause ; and what a drug can cause, that, and that only, it can cure.*   This is the very essence of Homœopathy.

But there is no doubt about it : *Collinsonia has a tremendous effect on the pelvic organs : and a great sphere in diseases of the rectum.*   It also affects circulation of blood, controlling congestions and hæmorrhages.

*　　　*　　　*

Dr. W. J. GUERNSEY, in " Hæmorrhoids ", describes the hæmorrhoids of *Collinsonia* as with aching, dull pain ; increasing after hard stool.

Burning : heat : heaviness : itching.

Sticking sensation in rectum as from sticks, sand or gravel lodged there.

As bleeding, flowing incessantly, though not profusely.

Blind : chronic : obstinate : external : protruding.

With paralysis, and congestive inertia of rectum.

Worse : evening, night ; during pregnancy : after hard stool.

Concomitants : constipation : pain epigastrium ; loss of appetite.

Much flatulence. Congestion of pelvic viscera with hæmorrhoids : especially in later months of pregnancy.

Catarrh of bladder with hæmorrhoids.

Stools mostly only in the evening..

Severe colicky pain, hypogastrium, every few minutes, with fainting : has to sit down to get relief.

*   *   *

FARRINGTON mentions *Collinsonia*. It is indicated in hæmorrhoids when there is a sensation as of sticks in the rectum. Constipation is usual. The bowel symptoms are worse in the evening and night.

Collinsonia is also useful in prolapsus uteri complicated with hæmorrhoids. It is just as frequently indicated in this condition as is *Podophyllum* in prolapsus uteri with diarrhœa and prolapsus recti.

We find *Collinsonia* has one of the *Opium* symptoms : dry balls of fæcal matter are passed from the rectum; but they differ from those of *Opium* in that they are of a light colour.

*   *   *

NASH says, it is not thoroughly proven, but enough has been learned from what we have, and from clinical experience, to indicate its great value. As a remedy for hæmorrhoids or rectal trouble it may be compared with *Aesculus hipp.*, for both have a *sensation as if the rectum was filled full of sticks* . . . he proceeds to note some of the differences.

Aesc. has a prominent sensation of fullness : *Coll.* has not. *Coll.* piles often bleed persistently.

Aesc., great pain, soreness and *aching in back* : *Coll.* does not, as yet, develop that symptom.

Aesc. sometimes has constipation, sometimes not. *C.* is greatly constipated, with colic on account of it.

He tells of two of his cured cases :—Very frequent, very severe colic for years, which had baffled old school doctors. He chose the curative remedy because of the obstinate constipation, the great flatulence and the hæmorrhoids present.

He also cured one of his most obstinate cases of constipation. The patient, for two years only averaged a movement of the bowels once in two weeks, under the action of powerful cathartics, after which he would be sick two or three days in bed. *Coll.* cured him within a month, perfectly : his bowels moved every day, and the trouble "never returned for several years, i.e. so long as I knew him".

*   *   *

Truly, a remedy worth knowing. Let us, in turn, pass on the introduction.

COLOCYNTH

I SUPPOSE we have, all of us, witnessed the wonderfully prompt action of *Colocynth* in spasm and colic relieved by bending over and pressing hard into the abdomen ; till *Colocynth* has come to mean, for us, just this and nothing more.

But *Colocynth* stands for a great deal more than " the intestines as if ground between hard stones, the pain relieved by doubling up, and by hard pressure."

It has frightful nerve pains, in spine, in limbs, in head, in ovaries, *especially if caused by anger and indignation.*

NASH says, " No remedy produces more severe colic than this one, and no remedy cures more promptly. Dr. T. L. Brown once said to me in substance : If I was disposed to be sceptical as to the power of the small dose to cure, *Colocynth* would convince me, for I have so promptly cured severe colic in many cases, from a child to adults, and even in horses. Of course every true Homœopath can respond *Amen* to that.

" The colic of Colocynthis is terrible, and is only bearable by *bending double, and pressing something hard against the abdomen.* He leans over chairs, the table or bedposts to get relief. This colic is neuralgic in character, and is often attended with vomiting and diarrhœa, *which seems to be the result of the great pain more than any particular derangement of the stomach or bowels."* Kent also emphasizes this point as we shall see later.

Nash contrasts *Colocynth* with *Chamomilla.* " Both *Chamomilla* and *Colocynth* have colic from a fit of anger, or other affections from the same cause. *Chamomilla* succeeds in the colic of children if there is much wind which distends the abdomen ; the child tosses about in agony, but *does not double up like Colocynth."*

GUERNSEY (*Keynotes*) puts things in a nutshell, and this is how he puts *Colocynth.*

" The strongest characteristic, calling for the use of this remedy, is an agonizing pain in the abdomen, causing the patient to bend over double. Relief is obtained by motion, such as twisting, turning and wriggling around, and the motion is kept up steadily while the pain lasts ; the pain is made worse after eating or drinking the least amount. This pain may occur alone, or in dysentery, cholera, etc. The doubling over of the patient and pressing on the abdomen is the chief characteristic. . . .

Sensations, as though stones were being ground together in the abdomen, working upon the soft parts : of muscles being shortened : of tightness in outer parts. . . . . Worse, from mental troubles ; anger with indignation ; mortification caused by offence . . ."

But it is KENT who gives us the most brilliant picture of *Colocynth*, bringing out certain features of the drug that one hardly gets elsewhere, and which are difficult to extract (we have recently tried it !) from the *Repertory*.

He says, " The principal feature of *Colocynth* is its severe, tearing neuralgic pains ; so severe that the patient is unable to keep still. Sometimes they are relieved by motion—at least it appears that they are worse during rest :—better by pressure and sometimes relieved by heat. . . . Pains occur in the face, abdomen, along the course of nerves.

" These pains are often due to a very singular cause, namely *anger with indignation*. Hence persons who are haughty and easily offended or chagrined have *Colocynth* complaints. Anger will be followed by violent neuralgia in the head, the eyes, down the spine, in the intestines. . . .

" Screams with the pains. Walks about the room and becomes increasingly anxious as the pain goes on. . . . His friends irritate him : he wants to be alone.

" He has all he can do to stand those terrible pains. They are often the result of anger with indignation.

" Vomiting and diarrhœa frequently come with the pains, especially if they are in the abdomen.

" Colic comes on in paroxysms that grow in intensity.

" The patient becomes increasingly nauseated till finally he begins to vomit ; and he continues to retch after the stomach is empty. . . .

" The physician asks, ' What has happened to give you these pains ? ' Her answer is likely to be, ' My servant spilled some dirty water on a handsome rug, we had words over it, and this is the result.'

" The vomiting of *Colocynth* is different from that of most other remedies. Nausea does not appear at first, but when the pain becomes sufficiently intense nausea and vomiting begin, the contents of the stomach are ejected, and the patient continues to retch until the severity of the suffering decreases."

While writing this article a case came along which gave the perfect *Colocynth* picture, so graphically depicted by Kent.

The patient had been brought from her bed, doubled up with pain, vomiting bitter yellow fluid on the journey, and her face expressive of great suffering. " She has had many such attacks, and they all begin the same way, and follow the same course. First she gets pain in the back, between shoulders, this extends to head, and all over back, then she begins to vomit. This attack started nine days ago. ' *If she gets worked up, it brings on an attack.* When ill she is all over the bed, and in and out of bed : wants to get up and walk about : but if she gets up she usually vomits.' "

Kent also points out, " The° expression of the *Colocynth* face is one of anxiety from the severity of the suffering. No matter where the pain is, the face is distorted. . . .

" All pains are better from pressure, but this is in the beginning. After the pain has been going on for several days with increasing severity, the part becomes very sensitive and pressure cannot be endured. . . .

" The stomach pains are clutching, cramping and digging, as if grasped by the fingers of a powerful hand.

" Similar pains occur lower down in the abdomen, but they are still better from hard pressure, and from doubling up—which amounts to pressure—they come on in paroxysms of increasing severity, until the patient is nauseated and vomits. . . . The victim bends down over the back of a chair, or over the footboard, or, if unable to get out of bed, he doubles up over his fists. . . .

" Colic from anger with indignation ; better from bending double and worse in the upright position, while standing, or bending backward.

" In the violent ovarian neuralgias of *Colocynth*, the woman will flex the limb of the painful side hard against the abdomen and hold it there.

" Colic of infants when they are relieved by lying on the stomach ; as soon as the position is changed, they begin to scream again. . . ."

Colocynth produces a state of the nervous system like that found in individuals who have for years been labouring under annoyances and vexations. A man whose business affairs have been going wrong becomes irritable, and nervous exhaustion follows. A woman who must watch her unfaithful husband night and day to keep him away from other women gradually assumes a sensitive, irritable state of mind and is upset by the least provocation. This is the state of the *Colocynth* prover.

" You will seldom find this medicine indicated in strong, vigorous, healthy people who have suddenly become sick. . . ."

HAHNEMANN writes : " The older physicians brought *Colocynth* into disrepute by giving it in large dangerous doses as a purgative. Their successors, terrified by this dreadful example, either rejected it entirely, whereby the curative power it possessed was lost to mankind, or they only ventured to employ it on rare occasions, and then never without previous alteration and weakening of its properties by silly procedures, which they called *correction*, whereby its pretended poisonous character was said to be tamed and restrained. With the aid of mucilage they mixed up with it other purgative drugs, or they partially destroyed its power by fermentation or by prolonged boiling with water, wine, or even urine, as had been already stupidly done by the ancients.

" But even after all this mutilation (their so-called *correction*) Colocynth always continued to be a dangerous remedy in the large doses in which physicians prescribed it.

" It is really wonderful that in the medical school there has always been such an absence of reflection, and that, in regard to matters like this, the obvious simple thought never occurred to anyone that if the heroic medicines acted too violently in a certain dose, this was owing less to the drug itself than to the excessive magnitude of the dose, which yet may be diminished to any extent required ; and that such a diminution of the dose, while leaving the drug unaltered in its properties, only reduces its strength so as to make it innocuous and capable of being employed with advantage, and hence must be the most natural and appropriate *corigens* of all heroic medicines.

" It is obvious that if a pint of alcohol drunk all at once can kill a man, this is owing not to the absolute poisonousness of the alcohol but to the excessive quantity, and that a couple of drops of alcohol would have been harmless to him.

" It is obvious that whilst a drop of strong sulphuric acid immediately produces a blister and erosion on the part of the tongue to which it is applied, on the other hand, when diluted with 20 or 100,000 drops of water it becomes a mild, merely sourish fluid, and that hence the most natural, the simplest *corigens* of all heroic substances is to be found only in the dilution and the diminution of the dose until it becomes only useful and quite innocuous.

" In this way, and in this way only, can the inestimable curative powers for the most incurable diseases that have hitherto lain concealed in the heroic—much less in the weaker—medicines called *poisons* by those afflicted with intellectual poverty, be elicited in a perfectly sure and mild manner to the advantage of suffering humanity. By means of the knowledge so obtained we may effect results in the treatment of acute and chronic diseases such as the whole medical school has hitherto failed to effect.

This method, so childishly simple, of rendering the strongest medicinal substances mild and useful never occurred to the minds of physicians, and they were consequently forced to dispense with the aid of the grandest and most useful remedies.

" Guided by the following peculiar pathogenic effects produced in the healthy by *Colocynth*, I have been enabled by means of it to perform extraordinary cures on the homœopathic principle by the administration of a small portion of a drop of the octillion—or decillion-fold dilution of the above tincture as a dose.

" Thus, to mention only a single example, many of the most violent colics may, under the guidance of symptoms 69 to 109, be often very rapidly cured, when at the same time the other characteristic symptoms of the disease, or a portion of them, are to be found in similarity among the symptoms of *Colocynth*."

BLACK LETTER SYMPTOMS (*Hahnemann and Allen*)

i.e. the pre-eminent characteristic symptoms of the drug, produced in the healthy and cured in the sick of a "like" sickness.

Pressing, aching pain in the sinciput, most violent on stooping and when lying on the back.

Tearing pain in the whole brain, which became a pressure in the forehead, as if it pressed out the forehead—more violent on moving the eyelids.

Burning pain in the skin of forehead above eyebrows.

Sharp cutting pain in right eyeball.

Throbbing and digging pain from middle of the left side of nose, to the root of nose.

Pain in lower row of teeth, as if the nerve were tugged and stretched.

Empty eructations.

Constrictive pain in umbilicus, immediately after dinner.

Seized with terrible, contractive, twisting pain in the bowels, immediately about umbilicus.

Griping about umbilicus.

Griping around the navel, increased by eating fruit.

Griping and cutting in umbilical region.

Violent griping in the umbilical region.

Violent colic-like pains, emanating from the umbilicus, with frequent discharge of flatus, which afforded relief.

Isolated deep stitches, as if from a needle, sometimes in the left, sometimes in the right flank, apparently connected with the ovaries.

Abdomen greatly distended and painful.

Griping in the abdomen, especially about the navel.

Griping and pinching in abdomen.

Violent griping pains in abdomen, worst about three fingers' breadth below the navel, obliging him to bend over.

Griping in the intestines as if the bowels would be forcibly gripped.

Pinching pain in the abdomen, as if the bowels were pressed inward, with cutting extending towards the pubic region, so severe below the navel that the muscles of the face are distorted and the eyes drawn together (closed) : the pain is only relieved by pressure upon the bowels with the hands and bending himself forward.

Pinching in the bowels as if the intestines were squeezed between stones.

Cutting in the abdomen.

Colic very violent in paroxysms, obliging him to bend forward. Colic of the most violent character.   Griping colic.

Urging to urinate.

(Heavy weight in lumbo-dorsal region with some increase of temperature) and sensibility on the part affected. . . . The origin of the trouble lay in the sacral region, corresponding to the plexus ischiadicus, thence it extended through the incisure ischiadica major towards the hip-joint, down the posterior portion of the thigh into the fossa poplitea.

Tensive shooting pain in the right loin only felt on inspiration and most violent when lying on the back.

Short cough when smoking tobacco.

Sore pain in left scapula, when at rest.

In region of right scapula, an internal drawing sensation, as if the nerves and vessels were stretched.

Severe drawing, sharp pain in the left cervical muscles, still more severe on movement.

Violent drawing pains in the thumb of the right hand.

Only when walking, pain in the right thigh, as if the psoas muscle that raises it were too short ; on standing it ceased, but on walking it returned.

Tearing pain in the sole of the right foot, most violent when at rest.

Dr. George Royal (Iowa) writes about *Colocynth*, " Few remedies have been as thoroughly proven as *Colocynthis*.   Hahnemann proved it and recorded the result upon himself, six fellow provers and twenty-six authors . . . and we may truthfully say that *Colocynth* has a greater per cent of verified symptoms than any other remedy in our Materia Medica."

CONIUM MACULATUM

(Hemlock)

HAHNEMANN published two provings of *Conium* : one, more brief, in *Materia Medica Pura* ; one, later, in *Chronic Diseases*. We will quote from the introductory remarks of the latter. ·

After describing its homœopathic preparation, he says : " The great medicinal powers of this plant may be inferred from what has been written by Stoerk and his followers on the brilliant results obtained by means of *Conium* in the years 1770, 1771, etc. However, although some good results were obtained, at least in the beginning, in the treatment of some horrible diseases, yet, on the other hand, the repeated use of excessive doses of this drug has done irreparable injury and has destroyed a number of human lives.

" The apparently contradictory statements of honest observers based upon their respective experience, some of which had a tendency to gladden, others to sadden the heart, have been recently reconciled by Homœopathy. It has shown that it is impossible to obtain beneficial effects from the use of heroic remedies by employing large and repeated doses of a comparatively unknown and powerful drug in the treatment of equally unknown diseases, ' but that the drug ought first to be proved upon healthy persons, and ought to be exhibited in the highest potencies in diseases, to the symptoms of which its own pathogenetic effects are homœopathic.'

" Such doses are indeed strange contrasts of the doses which have been employed by allopathic physicians, 140 grains of the extract, or a wineglassful of the recent juice, even six times a day. The true homœopathist has the advantage of never using this drug to the prejudice of his patient.

" Those terrifying examples have prevented me from investigating the effects of that drug until lately : then it was that I discovered its anti-psoric qualities.

" This remedy, in order to act beneficially, has frequently to be preceded by some other drugs, and must then be used in the smallest possible doses. . . ."

*   *   *

One remembers years ago, in Athens, visiting the prison of Socrates, where the old philosopher calmly met death. One can see it now—that excavation, some way up in the solid rock of the hillside : long and shallow (as one recalls it, after all these years) but of special interest to the homœopath, because of the manner of his death. He had been condemned to die by drinking the expressed juice of hemlock. It took time to prepare. He asked his executioner, " What must I do ? " " Walk about," he was told, " and when there is a heaviness in your legs, lie down." He drank the draught of death, while his devoted friends looked on, mourning him ; and he walked to and fro till, motion and sensation failing in his legs, he lay down. His executioner investigated, and found his legs cold and senseless—then, soon, his abdomen—then the deadness rose higher, and with a convulsive flicker he passed out. That is the way with hemlock : it kills from the extremities upwards, while the brain remains clear.

Who was it that taunted his persecutors, " You may kill my body ; you may kill my soul, too—*if you can catch it.*" Something of the sort said Socrates when asked, " In what way are we to bury you ? " " As you please—at least if I do not escape you. When I have drunk the poison, I shall not stay with you. . . . None may say at the burial that he inters Socrates—say you are burying my body ; and bury it as you please."

In thinking of *Conium*, one always remembers Socrates, and how the drug paralyses, and paralyses from below upwards.

* * *

The mentality of *Conium* is dull and uninspiring ; the very antithesis of the mentality of *Cannabis ind.* " Weakness of memory : forgetfulness : inability to sustain mental effort. He is averse to society, yet dreads to be alone. Disinclined for business : dullness : indifference. Hypochondriasis and hysteria from suppression of, or too free indulgence in sexual instinct, with depression, anxiety and sadness. Likes to wear his best clothes, makes useless purchases, cares very little for things, wastes or ruins them ; does not want to work, prefers to play." So we see that mind, also, is slowed down, and its energies blunted and paralysed.

* * *

We will run through what KENT tells us, gleaning and condensing : This medicine is deep-acting, long-acting. Complaints from taking cold, when the glands become affected all over the body . . . infiltration in the region of ulcers and inflamed parts ; in the glands along the course of the lymphatics, so we get a chain like a string of beads.

Conium has been used extensively for malignant, cancerous affections of *glands*, and no wonder, because it takes hold of glands from the beginning and infiltrates, and they gradually grow to a stony hardness, like scirrhus.

(*Re* its action upon the *nerves*.) Nerves in a state of great debility : trembling, jerking, twitching. . . . Gradually growing paralytic weakness, somewhat like *Cocculus*. Liver becomes indurated, sluggish, enlarged. Bladder can only expel a part of the urine : or a paralytic condition and no expulsive power.

Action so deep that it gradually brings on a state of imbecility. *Mind* gives out : tired like the muscles of the body. . . . Inability to stand any mental effort or to rivet the attention upon anything, are some of the most important symptoms in this medicine. Passive forms of insanity. Thinks slowly ;—for weeks and months, if he recovers at all. " Mental cases with more or less violence and activity are such as correspond to *Bell.*, *Hyos.*, *Stram.*, *Ars.*—you will see nothing of that in this medicine. The mind is full of strange things that have come on little by little. *Conium is of a slow, passive character.* Complete indifference."

Great unhappiness of mind, recurring every fourteen days, *showing a two-weeks' periodicity.*

KENT emphasizes this :—" Whenever under homœopathic treatment the physical improves and the mental grows worse, the patient will never be cured." . . . That does not mean the aggravation caused by the remedy. If the mental does not improve, it means that the patient is growing worse. *There is no better evidence of the good action of a remedy than mental improvement.*

Conium patients cannot endure even the slightest alcoholic drink . . . any stimulating beverage will bring on trembling, excitement, weakness of mind and prostration.

Numbness : it is a general. Numbness with pains (*Plat.*, *Cham.*) ; very often numbness with the weakness.

Vertigo. Vertigo when turning the head, like turning in a circle : when rising from a seat. Worse lying, *as though the bed were turning in a circle* : when turning in bed, or looking around :— while lying in bed on rolling the eyes, or turning the eyes (compare *Cocculus*). . . . The *Conium* patient is unable to watch moving things without getting sick-headache. . . . Riding on the cars, watching things in rapid motion, and inability to focus rapidly :— slowness of accommodation.

(Then, *Vision*) : Objects look red ; rainbow-coloured ; striped : double vision : weakness of sight. . . . Aversion to light without inflammation of eyes. Lids indurate, thicken and are heavy and fall. Has cured epithelioma of the lid, and of the nose and cheek. Ulcers of lip with induration. Deep down under the ulcer there will be hardness, and along the vessels that send lymph towards that ulcer there will be a chain of knots.

Paresis of *œsophagus* extending to paralysis : food goes down part of the way and stops :—when about to pass the cardiac orifice it stops and enters stomach with a great effort. Pressure in throat as if a round body were ascending from stomach.

Inability to strain at *stool*, to expel contents because of the paralytic weakness of all the muscles that take part in expulsion : —while *urine* stops and starts : intermits. Stops, and without any pressure whatever it starts again—two or three times during urination.

And KENT says, *Conium* has cured fibroid tumours of the uterus : has restrained cancerous growths of the cervix. *Conium* has actually produced induration and infiltration of the cervix.

The *Conium cough*—almost constant : worse lying in bed : worse first lying down ; from taking a deep breath. Has to sit up and cough it out.

Ill effects from bruises and shocks *to spine* : injuries, especially lumbar.

Conium differs from a great many medicines. It is common for pains and aches to be relieved by putting the feet up on a chair or in bed. But the sufferings and conditions of *Conium* are *better by letting the limbs hang down*. The patient with rheumatism or ulceration of legs and the other strange sufferings of the legs, will lie down and permit his legs to hang over the bed as far up as the knee. . . . " Up to date, we have no explanation."

Another grand feature of the remedy : he *sweats copiously during sleep*. He may say that if he merely closes the eyes he will sweat.

Then, stenoses and strictures. . . .

*   *   *

BURNETT tells a quaint little story : He had prescribed *Conium* for the wife of a certain Bishop who was developing malignant disease of the tongue. On his next visit he " found the lady in a fearful tantrum, and on enquiring, she screeched at me—' I have not taken your medicine, not a single drop of it.' ' Why not ? ' ' Why not, indeed ! It is *Conium*, and you prescribed it because I am an old woman ! ' In vain I protested." Burnett adds a footnote, " To the uninitiated I may explain that in the homœopathic ' little books ' it is stated under *Conium* that it is good for the complaints of old women." One may add that it is also stigmatized as being good for old bachelors and old maids !

But the above exemplifies one of the reasons for not telling patients what you are prescribing. The knowing ones among them, i.e. the possessors of " the little " homœopathic books, look up the medicines, and criticize your prescriptions, approving or disapproving from that dangerous thing, a little knowledge : or they come to wrong, even at times disastrous, conclusions, deduced from what they can find in regard to the uses of the remedy :—or, having found benefit from what you have given, they proceed to abuse it, not realizing that, not only " what a drug can cause, it can cure," but also that " *what a drug can cure, it can also cause.*" The remedy is not everything in Homœopathy, but the manner of prescribing it.

*　　*　　*

Here is a resume of NASH'S contribution to our clinical knowledge of *Conium*. His epitome is that of all the writers on homœopathic Materia Medica. Viz. :—

Vertigo : < turning head, or looking around sideways, or turning in bed.

Swelling and induration of *glands*, after contusions or bruises.

Cancerous and scrofulous persons with enlarged glands.

Urine flows, stops and flows again intermittently ; prostatic or uterine affections.

Breasts sore, hard and painful during menses.

He calls it one of the so-called SPINAL remedies (*Cocculus*). All seem agreed that it paralyses from below upwards (Socrates). He says, . . . It should be a remedy for locomotor ataxia. Its strongest characteristic is its peculiar vertigo. I once treated a case of what seemed to be locomotor ataxia with this remedy.

The patient had been slowly losing the use of his limbs ; could not stand in the dark. In the street he would make his wife walk either ahead of him, or behind him, for looking at her sideways or in the least turning his head or eyes would cause him to stagger or fall. *Conium* cured him. It would always aggravate at first, then he would greatly improve when it was discontinued.

In regard to the EYE symptoms of *Conium*, NASH points out that the peculiar, prominent and uncommon symptom is, *photophobia intense, out of all proportion* to the objective signs of inflammation in the eye.

In its SCIRRHUS affections, he points out, the pains of *Conium* are burning, stinging, or darting (*Apis*).

" *Sweats day or night as soon as one sleeps, or even when closing the eyes*, is a characteristic found under no other remedy that I know of (reverse of *Sambucus*)." Lippe, he says, once made a splendid cure of a complete one-sided paralysis in a man eighty years of age with this remedy, guided thereto by this symptom. " I think it would be difficult to give a correct pathological explanation of such a symptom : but there is a reason, and whether we can give it or not we can cure it if we have a corresponding one appearing under a remedy ;—where a cure is at all possible."

* * *

Conium and *Phosphorus* are remedies that come readily to mind for simple *vertigo* (when not due to subluxation of atlas, and so amenable to a wee, persuasive twist). One has so often worked out a case of vertigo in the Repertory, when one of these two has come through. But, of course, there are a great number of other remedies which, in an equally marked degree, cause—and cure— vertigo.

Of these two, *Phosphorus* has vertigo looking upwards ; looking downwards ; in the open air ; after eating ; in the evening.

Conium when turning ; when turning head or eyes ; when looking to the side ; when lying. Is better when quite still with eyes closed. *Conium*, as we have seen, cannot watch moving objects—*from paresis of accommodation*.

But, talking of giddiness, there is a remedy of what one may call " *transparent vertigo* ". This is a personal experience, as is its cure by *Cyclamen*. On waking and looking ahead, or on sitting up or rising in the morning one sees the objects one looks at whirling unsteadily, flickering away to one side—the right side—while all the time, through the moving whirl, one sees them standing stolidly and immovably. Twice, at different periods, one has had bouts of this : when a dose of *Cyclamen* has promptly finished the unpleasant experience.

Another disagreeable personal experience of vertigo was a proving of *Ceanothus* :—after taking a few doses of the ϕ. On lying down on the left side, nothing happened : but on turning over on to the right side, the most alarming vertigo was experienced ; everything rushing and turning over and over to the right, while one grasped the sides of the bed, in the effort to maintain one's position. This recurred, in a less degree, the next night, then was experienced never again. But it was horribly unpleasant—even alarming. It taught one that vertigo can be *horrible*. I do not think that vertigo is especially noticed as a symptom of *Ceanothus* : but it should be ! Personal experiences are what most impress one, and are best remembered :—therefore Hahnemann says, " The physician should make himself the infallible and undeceptive subject of his own observations."

Then, in regard to *sweat*—even that common symptom, when qualified, can be most useful in pointing to a remedy that may turn out to have the other characteristic symptoms of a patient, and be therefore curative.

" *Sweats the moment the eyes are closed : or at once if he sleeps, day or night.*" As we have seen, *Conium* has this. But, for sweats on closing the eyes, KENT gives also, in lesser type, *Bry. and Lach* (and in still lesser type, *Calc.*, *Carb. an.* and *Thuja*).

Sweat on uncovered parts : no sweat on covered parts : a most curious and inexplicable symptom, which has led to the successful use of *Thuja ;*—as we have seen, and as has been reported in cases.

Profuse sweat on *affected parts*, ANT. TART. (compare *Ambra*, *Merc.*, *Rhus*, etc., for " sweat on affected parts ").

Sweat *of painful parts* (*Kali c.*).

Sweat *only while awake*, SAMBUCUS. The only competitor here is *Sepia*, in lowest type. (*Sepia* being one of the sweating remedies, and especially a remedy of offensive sweat, and offensive axillary sweat.)

Lachesis sweats with palpitation.

" *Cold sweat while eating* : anxiety and cold sweat while eating," MERC. only is given.

Profuse sweat from *music*, *Tarent*.

" On making any motion, sweat disappears and heat comes on," *Lyc.*

Sweat that attracts flies, *Calad*. One has observed this with horror in some poor old almshouse people, where it was impossible to keep the flies off the face !

Then there are the one-sided sweats :—the sweats of single parts, front, back, upper, or lower parts of body. And the sweats that stain different colours :—or *bloody sweats* (especially LACH. and NUX MOS.).

But perhaps the most useful of all these " sweat-peculiarities " are the *head-sweating during sleep, soaking the pillow* of CALC. and SILICA : often priceless symptoms in treating babes and small children.

* * *

One of the paralytic effects of *Conium* is, " cannot expectorate : swallows sputum ".

BLACK LETTER SYMPTOMS

Inability to sustain any mental effort.

Hypochondriasis and hysteria from suppression of or too free indulgence in sexual instinct, with low-spiritedness, anxiety and sadness.

Want of MEMORY.

Excessive difficulty to recollect things: to comprehend that which one reads.

HEADACHE *as if head were too full and would burst.*

Sick headache with inability to urinate. Great giddiness, worse lying, when everything seems to go round.

VERTIGO *as if turning in a circle.*

Intoxication when taking the least liquor.

Accumulation of EAR-WAX: *blood red, or like decayed paper, with pus or mucus.*

Weakness of SIGHT: *amaurosis.*

Objects look red, rainbow-coloured, striped: confused spots.

Weakness and dazzling of eyes, with giddiness and debility of whole body, especially muscles of arms and legs, so that when I attempted to walk I was apt to stagger like a person who had drunk too much strong liquor.

Aversion to light without inflammation of eyes.

Burning in eyes.

Ulcers on cornea, right to left.

Could scarcely raise lids, they seemed pressed down with a heavy weight.

Intermittent flow of URINE *with cutting after micturition.*

Some sexual symptoms. Bad effects from suppressed desire, or excessive indulgence.

Shrivelling of mammæ, without sexual desire.

Dry spot in larynx, where there is crawling and almost constant irritation to a dry COUGH.

Cough, almost only when first lying down, during day or evening: obliged to sit up and cough it out, then had rest.

Powerful spasmodic paroxysms of cough, excited by itching and tickling in chest and throat, or by a dry spot in larynx, worse at night or lying down. Greatly fatiguing patient.

Lying down and taking a deep breath causes cough.

Stitches as with needles in left MAMMA.

Hardness of right breast, with painfulness to touch and nightly stitches in it.

Pain in mammæ, which often swell and become hard.

Hard, scirrhus-like tumours (breast).

Indurated and swollen cervical GLANDS *in scrofulous children.*

Tremulous weakness and palpitation after every stool.

Paroxysms of hysteria and hypochondriasis from abstinence from sexual intercourse.

Great heat internal and external, with great nervousness.

SWEAT *day and night, as soon as one sleeps, or even when closing eyes.*

Swelling and induration of GLANDS, *with tingling and stitches, after contusions and bruises.*

With all his efforts he could not keep off SLEEP : *must lie down and sleep ; or he only gets sleep after midnight.*

QUEER SYMPTOMS : SUGGESTIVE SYMPTOMS : CURED SYMPTOMS

Likes to wear his best clothes, makes useless purchases ; cares very little for things, wastes or ruins them : does not want to work, prefers to play.

Dislike to society, yet a dread to be alone.

Superstitious and full of fear, with frequent thoughts of death.

Feeling at times of a foreign body under skull, in vertex.

Sensation in right half brain as of a large foreign body.

Headache with inability to urinate.

Tremulous look as if eyes were trembling.

Eyes feel as if pulled outwards from nose.

Lids only opened with great difficulty, and when done, a flood of hot tears spurts out.

Smell of animals in back part of nose.

Ulcers on face and lips : cancer of cheek : cancerous tumours lips and face. Cancer lip from pressure of pipe.

Spasmodic constriction of throat.

Lump in throat, with involuntary attempts to swallow.

Craves coffee, salt, sour things. Aversion to bread.

Violent vomiting ; of mucus ; black masses like coffee grounds, of chocolate-coloured masses.

Pain in liver with accumulation of ear-wax.

Acute inflammation of pancreas.

Hypogastric pain goes down legs.

Twitchings right side face, with curious noise in larynx.

Loose cough with inability to expectorate : must swallow what is raised.

Clothes lie like a weight on chest and shoulders.

Tickling behind sternum.

Sharp thrusts from sternum to spine.

Violent palpitation, with pain as if a knife were thrust through occiput with each pulsation.

Itching breast and nipple. Inflammation of breasts with stitches above nipple.

Mammary induration following breast abscess, remains without change for two years.

Hard and painful lumps in mammæ.

Stony hard lumps in breast after contusions.

Hypertrophy of breast, followed by atrophy.

Complete atrophy of mammary gland, leaving a flaccid, bag-like skin.

Peculiar tumour in centre of back, as large as a cherry, on half-an-inch pedicle : tumour and pedicle bluish.

After falling from a height on back, pain in lower part and small of back, worse laughing, sneezing, taking a quick breath.

Axillary glands swollen.

Arms when lifted fall like inert masses and remain immovable.

Painless loss of power, lower limbs : faltering, vacillating gait ; staggers as if drunk : drags legs after him.

Red spots on calves, turning yellow or green, as from contusion ; preventing movement.

Heaviness, weariness, bruised sensation in all limbs.

Paralysed feeling : difficulty in using limbs : unable to walk.

Unpainful lameness : trembling of limbs.

Paralysis of lower, then upper extremities : or reverse.

Numbness of fingers and toes : fingers look as if dead.

Letting limbs hang down relieves pain.

Sick-headache worse when lying in bed :—worse after going to bed : must sit up or walk about for relief.

Violent pain in stomach, better knee-elbow position.

Vertigo downward motion.

Paralysis of old people, especially old women.

Paraplegia after concussion of spine.

Five minutes after falling asleep wakes up bathed in sweat : most profuse on head and upper part of body.

Always feels worse after going to bed : must sit up or walk about.

Blueness of whole body.

Blackish ulcers ; bloody, fetid, ichorous discharges, especially after contusions.

In the *Repertory* we find, " Coldness in anus during flatus and stool, *Con.*" And CLARKE gives a case of the cure by *Conium* of diarrhœa where the stools were cold. (*Nit. acid* has *cold urine.*)

* * *

HALE WHITE, in his *Materia Medica, Pharmacy, Pharmacology and Therapeutics*, discusses *Conium* and its constituents for the benefit of medical students. Its therapeutics, external and internal, occupy about half a page. His main point is the uselessness and unreliability of its derivatives. He ends his little paragraph on its uses and uselessnesses with, " *Conium* has been given in spasmodic diseases, as whooping-cough, chorea, tetanus, asthma, and epilepsy, but in all it does little or no good." . . . No wonder Old School doctors are such poor prescribers. What they are not taught about Materia Medica would fill a whole bookshelf of big volumes.

But the action of *Conium* would, of course, appeal to the unenlightened medical mind, for *spasm*—because it paralyses : to us it makes appeal, *for paralysis.* It is evidently a poor paliative : but a magnificent remedy—*where the symptoms, in drug and patient, agree.* . . . Groping in the dark is poor amusement compared with walking in the light !—that is, if you want to get along. But that mental darkness which hates the light, and refuses to come to it, is the most hopeless of all. For the darkness of night is dispelled by the rising sun : and yields to the glad light of day.

* * *

The *Cyclopædia of Drug Pathogenesy*, gives a number of poisonings, some lethal, by *Conium*. They all bear out *inter alia* the experience of Socrates. . . . Here are some condensed illustrations:

After taking ʒiii of " *succus conii* ", set out walking. After a bit, felt a heavy clogging sensation in heels : distinct impairment of motor power—" the go " taken out of me : as if a drag was suddenly put on me, and I could not have walked fast. . . . On putting a foot on the scraper, the other leg shaky and almost too weak to support me : my movements seemed clumsy, and I must make an effort to control them. At the same time a sluggishness of the adaptation of the eye : vision good for fixed objects, but on looking at an uneven object in motion there was haze and dimness of vision causing giddiness. Accommodation was more or less paralysed—retarded.

In another experimenter,—on raising eyes from a near to a more distant object, vision confused and giddiness came on suddenly : but so long as eyes were fixed on a given object, the giddiness disappeared, and the definition and capacity of vision for the minutest objects were unimpaired : but all was haze and confusion on directing the eyes to another object, which continued till the eyes rested securely on one object again. . . . Then, muscular lethargy with heavy lids and dilated pupils : . . . weakness in legs, which became cold, pale, and tottering. Legs felt as if they would soon be too weak to support me : . . . to complete paralysis as far as hamstrings, and it required a great effort to open the lids. The mind clear and calm, the brain active, but the body heavy and well-nigh asleep. (Symptoms declined rapidly, and disappeared.)

A young woman, remained calm, but without the power to move arms or legs.

Such are, again and again, the effects of big doses : the rapidly extending—upwards—of paralytic phenomena : and not only muscles of the extremities, but all eye muscles affected, with those of the lids. The pulse generally rises, then quickly subsides to normal : and the mind remains clear and calm !

In one prover, with the paresis, he found that even with eyes shut any movement involving the balance of the body was attended with a singular uncertainty, and falling short of the desired effect, invariably accompanied by a fresh rush of sea-sick feelings. He settled himself in an arm chair, and kept absolutely still and relaxed, when the sea-sickness completely disappeared and he lost consciousness of the poison, *till he opened his eyes*, " to find out whether the enemy was still with me, or not."

In some of the poisonings quoted, there was delirium, even convulsions in some. One doctor who experimented with *Conium* found that provided that his eyes were shut, he could walk straight and steadily, whereas when he tried to walk with eyes open, he had giddiness, nausea, and staggering gait (reverse of locomotor ataxia).

* * *

In addition, then, to its action on muscle—even to eye muscles and especially to those of accommodation, one must remember *Conium* as one of the drugs of indurations, infiltrations, stenoses and strictures.

By the way, the *Conium* death is from paralysis of diaphragm and muscles of respiration. It should be useful in some forms of asphyxia.

CROTALUS HORRIDUS

(*Rattlesnake poison*)

THERE are drugs whose malign effects on the human body present an almost perfect picture of some disease. The glaring instances that occur to one being

Belladonna and *scarlet fever* : who will diagnose between them, without some corroborative history ?

Arsenicum and *ptomaine poisoning.*

Mercurius cor. and *dysentery.*

Latrodectus mact. and *angina pectoris.*

Crotalus hor. and *black water fever.*

Where such correspondences occur, Hahnemann tells us that we have *specifics*. Otherwise, merely to attach to disease-names drugs that have sometimes been found useful, or have a reputation for being useful for them, will lead to disappointment. It is only where their drug-pictures coincide that we may confidently expect dramatic results.

Of course any and all of these drugs may prove useful quite outside their complete symtomatology which, in ordinary practice, one seldom gets. You do not wait for the complete scarlet fever picture before prescribing *Belladonna*, which can be useful in a very wide number of common complaints. Only, the peculiarities—the " modalities "—of *Bell.* must be there, to call for the drug. For instance, it is one of our greatest headache remedies : but their characteristics must be those of *Bell.* viz, bursting, throbbing headache, usually with its fiery red hot face ; and here *Bell.* will cure, even where there is no sore throat, no high temperature, no red rash. Or again, a very dry, stiff, smooth, swollen throat will suggest *Bell.*, without the bursting head, or the bright eyes with dilated pupils. But throat, or head, or whatever it may be, must be of the *Bell.* type, or nothing doing. Patchy, septic throats with excessive, perhaps offensive salivation will not be affected by *Bell.* They are outside its picture and its range of action.

Drugs become very dear to memory when one has once seen their extraordinary promptitude in rescuing someone near and dear from desperately threatening conditions. Such a drug is *Crotalus horridus*. We have written of this elsewhere, but cannot omit it from our Drug Picture of rattlesnake.

A young R.E. officer, home from delimitation work on the Gambia and from frequent attacks of malaria and much quinine—

which disadvantages pursued him home, sent down a message one morning, " *I have got black water fever* ". . . . And, oh ! the fearful rapidity of that deadly disease ! In a few hours inability to lift head from pillow : yellow all over ; chest going green : stool black with blood : urine nearly-black jelly.   Then the starting of the dreaded black vomit, supposed to be fatal.   One can never forget the peculiar sound of that constant retching the following night, when we sent to beg *Crotalus* from a grandson of Hahnemann, an old man who lived in the neighbourhood.   Then *Crotalus* with a few doses (in alternation) of *Phosphorus*, prescribed by the homœopathic doctor who had been called in, and who had had more experience of *Phos.* in hæmorrhagic conditions; and the rapid, glorious subsidence of *all* the terrible symptoms : so that the few fateful hours—the very few—gave life for imminent death. But of course the *pace* of remedies is a most important factor, and the pace of *Phos.* would have been quite inadequate for such a disease. . . . A few weeks later, when a large palmar abscess supervened, very fierce and painful, with high fever, *Crotalus* came again to the rescue, and, the " basinful of pus " as the surgeon expressed it, having been let out, summarily finished the matter.   Never did abscess get well more quickly and com- pletely.   No wonder one learnt to regard that particular snake venom with peculiar veneration, and to use it enthusiastically again and again in septic conditions:—septic foci, even in the gums; whitlows, abscesses, especially where there was much " spoilt " dark, uncoagulable blood.   Its rival here being, perhaps, *Lachesis* : but one has an idea that *Crotalus* is more rapid, more deadly, and more *yellow*.

Another case of years ago :—a young girl dying in hospital of malignant disease, her pitiable emaciation dark yellow, almost brown.   *Crotalus* strikingly improved her appearance and her condition ; for the time, anyway.

And yet one more well remembered triumph for rattlesnake : a memory from medical school days.   A surgeon lecturing to the students, faltered, sat down, turned yellow, buried head between knees in the effort to retain consciousness. He explained that he had been operating on a bad septic peritonitis the previous afternoon, when he had pricked the finger of one hand, and cut the other hand.   There were already glands in both axillæ.   The magic effects of *Crotalus*, " one of the homœopathic medicines " was explained to him, and there was a rush to get the promised remedy and to deposit it at his house.   Next morning a glad message came through, " Tell the students that I am much better."   A fort- night later he was lecturing again, and lingered to speak his acknowledgements. " I took your medicine. I also took quinine. *But the man who did the same thing at Charing Cross—died.*"

Hence *Crotalus* stays " grappled to one's soul with hoops of steel ", and in writing of the drug one desires that others should realize what a power resides in the poison of the rattlesnake—one of the deadliest and most rapidly fatal of all the snake poisons. *The Cyclopædia of Drug Pathogenesy* amply attests to that. But —*the greater the poison the greater the remedy,* provided you know how to prepare and use it. And here it is helpful to remember that, as Hahnemann proved and laid down, *no poison is dangerous after the third potency,*—that is " one in a hundred three times ; or one part in a million. But, not just *mixed,* however painstakingly ! The mixture would probably be irregular, imperfect—not safe. It must be " potentized " after the manner of Hahnemann, viz. one drop in a hundred of alcohol or water (according to its solubility) vigorously succussed ; and one drop of that (the first centesimal potency) in another hundred of the medium, again succussed, to make the second centesimal potency ; of which again, one drop in 100, once more well succussed, to give the third centesimal potency : one in a million. And here you may be perfectly happy in prescribing the most virulent remedies. Their power to harm is gone from them, leaving only their power to heal.

Our remedies for sepsis are so many and so convincing that people find it difficult to diagnose between them. The most frequently considered being *Lachesis, Crotalus hor., Tarantula cub., Anthracinum, Pyrogen, Sepsin* : while the less deadly, or at all events the less rapid cases, are brilliantly controlled by *Hepar, Silicea, Mercurius,* etc. But, as said, the pace of the disease must be taken into account : and the most rapidly fatal diseases are those of the tropics, and the most rapidly-acting remedies we have are the tropical snake and spider venoms.

Let us try to give suggestive differentiating symptoms. In *Pyrogen,* ceaseless movement, as a rule ; marked inco-ordination between pulse and temperature, such as a high temperature with low pulse-rate, or, less frequently, the reverse. In axillary abscesses one thinks, after happy experiences, of *Tarantula cub.* ; also for the virulent insect-stings of some hot summers ; and, since *Tarant. cub.* is said to be made from a *rotten* Cuban tarantula, it will probably come into line with *Pyrogen* and *Sepsin.* The latter won its spurs in the South African War, where it proved remarkably curative of the dysentery that there prevailed (See Clarke's *Dictionary*). But one must not forget *Anthracinum,* with its great record not only for anthrax, but for septic states, and for boils and carbuncles with *burning pains.* (*Ars.*)

But our two most usual snake poisons being *Lachesis* and *Crotalus hor.*, let us try to extract their diverse, and their common characteristics, as pointed out by various observers.

ALLEN (*Keynotes*), says, " In *Lachesis*, the skin is cold and clammy : in *Crotalus*, cold and dry. *Crotalus* has the greatest tendency to hæmorrhages: Blood dark, fluid, offensive." " Hæmorrhagic diathesis : blood flows from eyes, ears, nose and every orifice of the body : *bloody sweat.*" " Purpura hæmorrhagica ; comes on suddenly from all orifices ; skin, nails, gums."

But they are both hæmorrhagic remedies : only *Crotalus* is even more so. And they have many other symptoms in common. Both have loquacity : both are worse for sleep, and sleep into an aggravation ; and both are intolerant of pressure and clothing about the abdomen :—*Lachesis* from its intense sensitivity to touch, pressure and constriction : *Crotalus* more probably from its specific effect on the liver. Both have blueness of parts ; *Lachesis* especially so : both have yellowness and jaundice, but *Crotalus* most especially so. *Crotalus more affects the right side ; Lachesis the left.*

* * *

NASH (*Crotalus*) seems to have shown its greatest usefulness in diseases which result in a decomposition of the blood of such a character as to cause hæmorrhages from *every outlet of the body ;* even the sweat is bloody. . . . Useful in diphtheria when the profuse epistaxis occurs which marks many cases of a malignant type.

In hæmorrhages of the nose in an old man of broken down constitution, where none of the remedies usually applied did the least good, *Crotalus* acted promptly and no doubt saved the man's life. This was a patient of my own, and though he had frequent attacks before, he never had another after the *Crotalus*. As would be expected with such a remedy, there is *great prostration* at such bleedings.

BLACK LETTER SYMPTOMS

Yellow colour of eyes.
Blood oozes from ears.
Bleeding from nose and all orifices of body.
Tongue protruded.
Black vomit.
Jaundice : malignant jaundice ; dark hæmorrhages from nose, mouth, etc., dark scanty urine.
Easily tired by slightest exertion.

Sudden and great prostation of vital force.

Yellow fever : hæmorrhagic tendency, oozing of blood from every orifice, and even pores of skin. Skin yellow. Vomiting of bile or blood.

Fetid, bilious or bloody stools ; liver tender ; heart weak ; fainting.

Fevers resulting from septic absorption and in purpuric cases of zymotic diseases ; puerpural fever.

Yellow colour of whole body.

Broken down constitutions.

Some Italic, or Peculiar Symptoms

Delusions : as mistakes in keeping accounts : forgetfulness of figures, names, places. Surrounded by imaginary foes or hideous animals.

Loquacious delirium : desire to escape from bed.

Suspicious and snappish.

Frightful headache. Cerebral congestion.

Epistaxis, in broken down constitutions or depraved state of blood ; blood thin, uncoagulable, dark : (?) with flushes of face, vertigo, or fainting.

Yellow colour of face : or livid, bloated ; purple ; face tumid ; blueness round sunken eyes : chalky : death-like : leaden coloured.

Distended red face.

Tongue and all round throat feels tied up : cannot speak a word.

Tongue swollen to nearly twice the normal size.

Swelling of tongue till there is no more room in mouth.

Tongue protruded.

Cancer of tongue with hæmorrhages.

Tightness, constriction of throat.

Deglutition impossible, from spasm of œsophagus.

Malignant diphtheria : blood poisoning : œdema or gangrene of fauces.

Swelling, angles of lower jaw.

Unquenchable, burning thirst.

Nausea on movement. Bilious vomiting.

Cannot lie on right side or back without dark green vomiting.

Everything looks yellow : at first everything looked blue.

Pylorus constricted. Agonizing pain, or violent cramp, in stomach.

Cannot bear clothes around stomach and hypochondria.

Sinking sensation : craving for stimulants.

Hæmatemesis : little or no tendency to coagulate.

Pain in liver and top of shoulder.

Skin very dark brown.

Jaundice : malignant jaundice.

Red tipped tongue.

Urine jelly-like and red like blood.

Dysentery : of septic origin : excessive flow of dark, fluid blood, or involuntary evacuations. Great debility and faintness.

Urine : extremely scanty, dark red with blood ; jelly-like ; green-yellow from much bile.

Dull, continuous aching pain, region of heart, down left arm and through to left shoulder blade.

Feels a drawing from sole of right foot through bone of leg.

HERING (*Guiding Symptoms*) gives the relationships of *Crotalus*.

Antidoted by *Lachesis*. Compare : *Lachesis, Naja* and *Elaps*. *Crotalus* is preferable in fluid hæmorrhages, yellow skin (hence in yellow fever with black vomit, etc.), epistaxis of diphtheria. *Naja* has more nervous phenomena. *Lachesis* has skin cold and clammy, rather than cold and dry : hæmorrhages with charred straw sediment ; and more markedly ailments of the left side. *Elaps*. is preferable in otorrhœa, and in affections of the right lung. The *Cobra* poison coagulates blood into long strings. The *Crotalus* poison is acid : the *Viper* neutral. The *Rotten snake* causes more sloughing than any other.

* * *

KENT has much to say about *Crotalus hor.*, and he fully realizes its unique importance. . . .

The diseases that call for the use of such a substance as *Crotalus* are very grave. . . . Its symptoms are peculiar. There can be no substitute for it, as there is no other remedy, taken as a whole, that looks very much like it. The other snake poisons are nearest, but this is the most dreadful of all.

Alcohol has been used in great quantities in snake bites, and it has frequently prolonged or even saved life. . . . But, if he lives through the violent attack he goes on forever manifesting the chronic effects. . . . A peculiar periodicity has been manifested, every spring, as cold subsides and warm days begin. . . . The periodicity of the snake poisons is related to the Spring. *The patient sleeps into an aggravation.*

In its earliest manifestation *Crotalus* is like unto the zymotic changes we find in scarlet fever, in diptheria, in typhoid and in low forms of blood poisoning : cases which come on with great rapidity, breaking down of the blood, relaxation of the blood vessels, bleeding from all orifices of the body, rapidly increasing unconscious-ness like one intoxicated and besotted in appearance. . . . Scarlet fever when it becomes putrid : typhoid when it becomes putrid, diphtheria with much bleeding and putridity. The body appears mottled, blue intermingled with yellow. . . . Jaun-dice comes on with astonishing quickness . . . black and blue spots intermingled with yellow. Hæmorrhages (as already noticed). *Crotalus* is indicated in disease of the very lowest, the most putrid type, coming on with unusual rapidity, reaching that putrid state in an unusually short time. . . . As the blood oozes out it becomes black.

Awful nervousness : trembling : tremulous weakness. Sudden and great prostration of the vital powers. The forms of yellow fever with great prostration. Loquacity. But, with *Lachesis* the loquacity is so rapid that if any one in the room commences to tell something, the patient will take it up and finish the story, though he has never heard about it. No one is permitted to finish a story in the presence of a *Lachesis* patient. *Crotalus* does that too, but he will take it up and mumble, and jumble and stumble over his words . . . a low passive state like intoxi-cation ; in *Lachesis* it is wild excitement.

He sleeps into his symptoms. All the snake poisons more or less sleep into troubles. . . . Headaches ; dull, heavy, throbbing occipital headaches : or whole head in a state of congestion. Head feels too full : as if it would burst. Headaches that come on in waves from the back : a surging of blood upwards. Worse change of position.

This is a wonderful bilious remedy : sick headaches, vomiting of bile in great quantities. Cannot lie on right side or back without instantly producing black, bilious vomiting.

Coldness like a piece of ice in stomach or abdomen. Has cured ulceration of the stomach : greatly restrained the growth of cancer of the stomach when there was much vomiting of bile and blood. . . . Cancer of uterus, etc. . . .

Boils, carbuncles and eruptions are surrounded by a mottled blue, splotched or marbled state. But the peculiar feature is the doughy centre. Around the boil or carbuncle for many inches there is œdema, pitting on pressure : and it will bleed a thick, black blood that will not coagulate. In puerperal fever there is a continuous oozing of black, offensive blood that will not coagulate. In abortion, with like bleeding. Or in menstruation during typhoid, with dark, liquid offensive continuous oozing.

Sleep terrible. Rises from sleep in a fright : has horrible dreams of murder, death, dead bodies ; even the smell of the cadaver is dreamed of. Suspicious. Craves intoxicating drinks : delirium tremens. KENT thinks that, properly used, it may remove the appetite for strong drink.

CROTALUS CASCAVELLA

YET another rattlesnake, that of Brazil, is as deadly, which means is as potent for healing the conditions it can cause, as *Crotalus hor.* : but there are striking differences in their pathogeneses.

Mure's *Materia Medica of the Brazilian Empire*, with *Provings and the principal Animal and Vegetable Poisons*, is the original authority for the uses of this snake-venom : Clarke's *Dictionary* reproduces many of the symptoms; and inasmuch as the majority of them are unique, and peculiar to this snake-bite and its provings, we will proceed to detail the most important.

Crotalus casc. differs from the commoner rattlesnake, by affecting the tissues in a lesser degree, but *mentality* and *sensation* to a far greater extent. It is evidently less hæmorrhagic : but has the same sensitiveness and intolerance of clothing about the body as *Crot. hor.* and *Lach.* It also has liver symptoms and yellowness but not so markedly : and bloody serum drips from nose, whose tip feels drawn up and fastened to the centre of forehead.

It induces clairvoyance and " magnetic " states :—

Sees the spectre of death, as a gigantic black skeleton.

Hears strange voices to left and behind her.

Hurls herself against closed doors : attempts to throw herself out of the window.

Sensation as if one were falling out of bed, even while awake.

Hears nothing : or hears groans.

Sensation of a red-hot iron at vertex.

Brain pressed on by an iron helmet.

Sensation as if something alive were walking about in head in a circle.

Fancies her eyes are falling out.

Blue, dazzling light before eyes.

Eyeball pulled to temple by a thread.

Right eyeball as if drawn out.°

Face red ; or yellow.

Paralysis of tongue. Burning, pricking, itching of tongue.

(In *Crot. hor.* the tongue is enormously enlarged.)

Spitting of black blood.

Taste : salt ; of onions ; putrid.

Craves snow.

Sensation of an opening in stomach, through which air passes.

Food falls suddenly into stomach like a stone.

Sensation of a peg sticking in middle of liver.

Feeling of coldness in stomach after eating.

Thorax encased in iron.

Lancinations like needles in dorsal spine.

Constrictive pain round thyroid.

Pains in jugular veins and carotid arteries ; as if blood rises, and a valve were opening.

Sensation of water in chest : as if heart were dipped in liquid.

Sensation of shortening right limb : causes him to limp. . . .
And so on.

CUPRUM

HAHNEMANN, who solved the problem how to give us insoluble substances *pure* and *in solution*, by means of potentization, thus describes the preparation, for healing purposes, of metallic copper.

He says, " A piece of pure metallic copper is rubbed upon a hard and fine whetstone under distilled water in a china vessel. The fine powder which falls to the bottom is then dried, and then triturated for three hours with sugar of milk, in order to obtain the millionth potency,* from which the dilutions are derived by means of alcohol. One or two pellets of the 30th potency are sufficient at a dose."

" The poisonous effects of this metal and its preparations, and the cruel and frequently fatal symptoms resulting from its application, have prevented physicians from using it internally."

He quotes some of the poisonous effects of copper, which are important for us, because *what a poison can cause, that it can cure.* " Loathing, nausea, fits of anguish and vomiting even in a few minutes, troublesome burning in the mouth, unsuccessful retching, violent pains in the stomach a few hours after the metal, obstruction of the intestines, or too violent evacuations, even bloody diarrhœa, constant uneasiness, sleeplessness, exhaustion, weak and small pulse, cold sweat, paleness of face, pains in the whole body, or in a few parts, pain in the thyroid cartilage, pain in the hypochondria, tingling sensation on the top of the head, palpitation of the heart, vertigo, painful constriction of the chest, cough with interrupted, almost suppressed respiration, extremely hurried breathing, hæmoptysis, hiccough, loss of consciousness, wandering look—also convulsions, rage, apoplexy, paralysis, death."

(Here are foreshadowed the principal curative uses of copper : and in diseases, often of a very severe nature, and great suffering. One can see that it would be—what it is—one of the great remedies

---

* *Hahnemann having so frequently explained the preparation of insoluble substances, in order to render them soluble, does not go into details here. But when he says, " the fine powder . . . is triturated for three hours with sugar of milk, in order to obtain the millionth potency," he refers to his usual method of arriving at that millionth potency.*

The procedure is this—One grain of the powder is strongly triturated for an hour with 99 grains of sugar of milk : the result is the 1st centesimal potency— one in 100. One grain of this 1st centesimal potency is again triturated for an hour with 99 grains of sugar of milk, to give the 2nd centesimal potency—one in 10,000. And a third trituration, one grain of the 2nd centesimal in 99 grains of sugar of milk, gives the 3rd centesimal potency—one in a million : " after which, all substances can be dissolved in alcohol or water."

in *cholera*, in *whooping-cough*, in *cramps* and *spasms*, in *convulsions* and *epilepsy*.)

Hahnemann continues, " Homœopathy alone is capable, by means of the peculiar mode of preparation to which it subjects remedial agents, and by means of its doctrine of the degree of potencies, to employ even the most violent substances for the benefit and restoration of the sick.

" Most of those violent symptoms of poisoning usually appear in groups, lasting half an hour or an hour, and recurring from time to time in the same form and combination, such as,—

" Palpitation of the heart, vertigo, cough, hæmoptysis, painful contraction of the chest, arrested breathing—

" Or—aching in the chest, lassitude, vaccillation of sight, closing of the eyes, loss of consciousness, quick, moaning respiration, tossing about, cold feet, hiccough, a short and hacking cough which arrests the breathing, etc. The use of *Copper* is therefore so much more homœopathic as the symptoms appear *at irregular intervals*, and *in groups*.

" Several kinds of partial or general clonic spasms, St. Vitus' dance, epilepsy, whooping cough, cutaneous eruptions, old ulcers ; and likewise spasmodic affections, accompanied with too fine and sensitive senses, appear to be the principal sphere of action for copper ; it was likewise indispensable either to prevent or to cure Asiatic cholera. . . ."

He adds, " *Copper* acts only a few days " : though later experience, perhaps in *chronic* disease, perhaps in the *higher potencies*, gives its length of action as forty to fifty days.

He quotes from Noack and Trinks, " *Copper* is most suitable to relaxed, irritable and nervous constitutions, with weakness and excessive sensitiveness of the nervous system, inclination to spasmodic affections, convulsions and typical diseases, especially of a chronic nature, with *irregular paroxysms*."

GUERNSEY, *Keynotes*, says :—

" One of the strongest indications for the use of this remedy is a *strong, metallic taste* in the mouth. *Rhus.* is the only other remedy that has this symptom in as marked a form. (The Repertory black types for this symptom are, COCC., MERC., NAT. C., RHUS., SENEG.)

" Spasms. Spasmodic affections generally ; whooping cough, where the attacks run into catalepsy. Epilepsy : spasms, particularly which begin in fingers and toes, then spread all over body. . . . Where eruptions strike in, as in scarlet fever, etc., and where excessive vomiting, great stupor, convulsions, etc., appear, *Cuprum* takes high rank to cause the rash to reappear."

NASH : " SPASM is the one word characterizing this remedy. Cramps or convulsions in meningitis, cholera, cholera morbus, whooping-cough, scarlatina, etc.

"Spasms begin in fingers and toes and, spreading from there, become general.

" In cholera, cholera morbus, or cholera infantum, the cramping pains are sometimes *terrible*.

"Dunham said (in regard to cholera): ' In *Camphor* collapse is most prominent : in *Veratrum alb*. the evacuations and the vomiting : in *Cuprum*, the cramps.' "

KENT: "*Cuprum* is pre-eminently a *convulsive* medicine. The convulsive tendency associates itself with almost every complaint that *Cuprum* creates and cures. . . . It has convulsions in every degree of violence :—from little twitchings to convulsions of all the muscles of the body. When these are coming on, the earliest threatenings are drawings in the fingers, clenching of thumbs, or twitching of the muscles.

" Tonic convulsions, where the thumbs are first affected : they are drawn down into the palms and then the fingers close over them with great violence. . . . *Spasms followed by the appearance as if the patient were dead*."

Kent describes the whooping-cough that calls for *Cuprum*, in the language of the mother. " She says, ' that when the child is seized with a spell of this violent whooping-cough, the face becomes livid or blue, the finger-nails become discoloured, the eyes are turned up, the child coughs until it loses its breath and then lies in a state of insensibility for a long time until she fears the child will never breathe again, but with a violent spasmodic action in its breathing, the child from the shortest breaths comes to itself again just as if brought back to life.' You have here all the violence of whooping-cough and a convulsive case. . . . If the mother can get there quickly enough with a little cold water she will stop the cough. Cold water especially will relieve the spasm."

" Whenever the respiratory organs are affected there is dreadful *spasmodic breathing*—dyspnœa. There is also great rattling in the chest. The more dyspnœa there is, the more likely his thumbs will be clenched and the fingers cramped. . . .

" *Cuprum* is not passive in its business. Violence is manifested everywhere. Violence in its diarrhœa, violence in its vomiting, violence in its spasmodic action : strange and violent things in its mania and delirium. . . .

" In the epilepsy calling for *Cuprum*, we have the contractions and jerkings of fingers and toes. He falls with a shriek, and during the attack passes his urine and fæces . . . epilepsies that begin with a violent constriction in the lower part of the chest . . . or with contractions in the fingers that spread all over the body, to all the muscles. . . .

(In puerperal convulsions) " the urine is scanty and albuminous. During the progress of labour the patient becomes suddenly blind. All light seems to her to disappear from the room, the labour pains cease, and convulsions come on, commencing in the fingers and toes. When you meet these cases do not forget *Cuprum*. You will look around a long time before you can cure a case of this kind without *Cuprum*."

Kent also discusses CHOLERA. He says, " Hahnemann had not seen a case of cholera, but he perceived that the disease produced appearances resembling the symptoms of *Cuprum*,* *Camphor* and *Veratrum*† . . . ; and these three remedies are the typical cholera remedies. . . . You will see that the *Cuprum* case is, above all others, the *spasmodic* case. It has the most intense spasms. . . . These three remedies tend downwards into collapse and death. Now, to repeat : *Cuprum* for the cases of a *convulsive* character ; *Camphor* in cases characterized by *extreme coldness* and more or less dryness ; and *Veratrum* when the *copious sweat*, vomiting and purging are the features. That is little to remember, but with that you can enter an epidemic of cholera with confidence." Kent here compares *Podophyllum* and *Phosphorus* with *Cuprum*. He says the profuse stools of *Pod.* (which has also cramps) are frightfully offensive : and of *Phos.* he says, as with *Cuprum* there is *gurgling*. In *Phos.*, fluids gurgle as they enter the stomach, and gurgle all through the intestines. A drink of water seems to flow through the bowel with a gurgle. " Now this gurgling in *Cuprum* commences at the throat : he swallows with a gurgle : gurgling in œsophagus when swallowing."

---

* *In regard to* Copper *for cholera—workers in copper mines are said to be immune from that disease : and little discs of copper are often worn next the skin for a protection. Again, some of the sporadic " cholera " in India, where a picnic party goes down in a few hours with cholera, is said to be sometimes due to badly cleansed copper utensils in which the native servants brew the tea.*

† *For cholera and its remedies, and the marvellous results of homœopathic treatment all over the world in the great epidemics of* 1853-4-5, *and in the Russian Epidemic of* 1830-31, *see our article in* HOMŒOPATHY, *April* 1932. *Everywhere Homœopathy reversed the mortality from two-thirds to one-third : or in some instances, (as in Rubini's cases in Naples) wiped it out.*

He says, " Discharges cease, or are suppressed, and sudden convulsions come on : here *Cuprum* will re-establish the discharge, and stop the convulsions." " Or, inflammations cease suddenly and you wonder what has happened. All at once comes on insanity, delirium, convulsions, blindness . . . metastasis. A perfect change from one part of the body to another." " The same may occur from a suppressed eruption—discharge— diarrhœa, and it goes to the brain, affects the mind and brings on an insanity : a wild, active, maniacal delirium. . . . Convulsions where a limb will first flex and then extend. In a child you will see the leg all at once shoot out with great violence, then up against the abdomen again with great violence, and then again shoot out. It is hard to find another remedy that has that. (*Tab.*) Convulsions with flexion and extension are common to *Cuprum.* . . .

" Jerking of the eyes : . . . snapping of the lids. Face and lips blue :—purple in convulsions. Paralysis of the tongue.

" Many complaints are ameliorated by cold water. The cough is brought on by inhaling cold air, but stopped by drinking cold water, like *Coccus cacti.* . . . A wonderful remedy in *anæmia.*"

One does not know how to stop quoting from Kent ! The more one reads in Kent, the more one marvels at his realization of the *characteristics* of drug action, and his wonderful power of graphic expression. One of our best prescribers carried Kent's *Materia Medica* about with him all through the war, and his powers of assimilation must have been great !—judging by his rapidity in spotting the homœopathic remedy.

For beginners, Nash's *Leaders* is probably the better book to start with : it is less bulky, and (for a beginner) less overwhelming. It teaches one to think homœopathically, and is full of invaluable comparisons between drugs :—but—KENT ! . . . Kent once declared, " I have originated nothing. All the teaching is Hahnemann's." Certainly the mantle of Hahnemann must have fallen on Kent, with a double portion of his spirit.

Coming down to commonplace recollections and experiences. Patients who come to Hospital complaining of severe cramps— especially in calves—very often have to get either *Cuprum* or *Calcarea*. *Calcarea* cramps are especially worse at night in bed, and on stretching the leg in bed. One remembers a case where in malignant disease—I think of uterus—*Cuprum* was given for the violent cramps of which the patient complained, and it not only stopped the cramps, but, for a time, ameliorated the disease-symptoms.

One remembers a wee boy in hospital, very ill with pneumonia, complicated with diarrhœa and severe cramping pains. Here *Cuprum* very quickly brought down the temperature and cleared the lung, as well as disposing of the diarrhœa and cramps.

PECULIAR AND DISTINGUISHING SYMPTOMS.

Child has a complete cataleptic spasm, with each paroxysm of whooping-cough.

Cough worse by inhaling cold air : better by drinking cold water.

Cough in children, threatening to suffocate.

In asthma, clutches air with hands, unable to speak or swallow.

Muscles of calf contracted in knots. Spasms and cramps in calves.

Spasms with blue face and thumbs clenched across palms of hands.

Spasms after vexation, or fright.

Child lies on belly, and spasmodically thrusts breech up.

Convulsions with biting.

CUPRUM ACETICUM AND SMALL-POX

(Reprinted from *The Homœopathic World*)

SIR,—As I visited Gloucester during the late epidemic of small-pox in the Southern half of the city, and took great interest in the methods of treatment pursued there, your readers may like to learn (in the absence of a resident homœopathic medical man in that city) the impressions left upon the mind of an amateur with some slight knowledge of Hahnemann's law.

The fatalities under different treatments varied greatly, as the following approximate list will show :

In Isolation Hospital during the first *regime* ..	54	per cent.
,, ,, under Dr. Brooke	8	,,
With Hydropathy, under Mr. Pickering	10	,,
With Crimson Cross ointment under Captain Feilden	2	,,

I found during my visits that a great and growing confidence had superseded scepticism in regard to the Crimson Cross ointment, which the above rough gauge of results justifies. Feeling sure that if there were any curative effects in the ointment they must be due to our law, I asked Captain Feilden if he would tell me what the ingredients of his ointment were. He readily complied, and I found that the green paint-like unguent, which was smeared over his patients from head to foot, owed its remedial powers to *Acetate of Copper.* On learning last Monday from Dr. Hadwen the approximate results given above, it was evident that it was desirable to compare the symptoms of small-pox with the provings of *Cuprum acet.* The following are the results :

SYMPTOMS OF SMALL-POX, FROM DR. H. VON ZIEMSSEN's *Cyclopedia.*	PROVINGS OF *Cuprum aceticum*, FROM ALLEN's *Encyclopedia.*
Fever and disturbance of general system.	Skin warm and dry, or covered with sweat.
Pulse accelerated.	Pulse accelerated : from 120 to 140.
Frequency of respiration increased.	Respiration accelerated.
Dyspnœa.	Cramping spasms in chest (?) (Suffocative arrest of breathing. Jahr.)
Initial (prodromal) rashes.	Query.
Languor.	Remarkable weakness. Prostration.
Vertigo and syncope.	Exhaustion. Faintness.
Fetor oris. Hoarseness. Aphonia.	Spotted redness of the fauces (Speech is either arrested, or entirely annulled. Jahr.)
Nausea, gagging, vomiting.	Jaundice, with vomiting and eructation. Nausea and vomiting.
Anorexia.	Loss of appetite. Aversion to food.
Constipation, occasional diarrhœa.	Diarrhœa, occasional constipation.
Severe headache.	Agonizing headache.
Face red and bloated : violent pulsation in carotids.	Face very red and swollen, puffy, red, hot.
Delirium, sleeplessness, disquiet.	Delirium. Sopor. Coma.
Pain in the back (less constant than gastric symptoms and Headache).	Pain in the loins and sacrum—at the navel and on the iliac region.
Drawing, tearing pains in the extremities.	Cramps in the calves, tetanic spasms in large toes, most violent pains in the soles of the feet.
Bronchitis less constant.	Query.
Eruption, almost always worse upon face and hairy scalp.	Eruption, seemingly of leprous kinds, consisting of spots of different sizes, the largest white and scaly with moist base, as if something acrimonious had been secreted under the cuticle ; eruption more or less over the body, and very much among the hair of the head.

The above symptoms and provings correspond too closely for the similitude to be altogether fortuitous ; and the startling success of the Crimson Cross ointment points to its being a fresh illustration of the law, *similia similibus curentur*.   The homœopathic branch of the profession have lost a great chance by not unanimously declaring the irrelevancy of vaccination to small-pox ; it may be that, to make up for this lost chance, in *Cuprum aceticum* they have a remedy for variola which may rank with *Aconite* in fever, or with *Camphor* in the early stages of cholera.

I am, Sir, yours faithfully,

A.PHELPS.

Edgbaston, September 11th, 1896.

CYCLAMEN

An experience of years ago, where *Cyclamen* promptly cured, has served to rivet this rather neglected *remedy of visual aberrations* on the mind. It is a drug of great power and prompt action in its special sphere as poisonings, provings and cures testify. Here is the experience, as remembered after all these years.

On waking in the morning and looking across the room one discovered everything in seeming motion : whirling (to right, as one remembers it), while *through* all the movement, solid furniture —a large wardrobe—was seen, normally immovable. It was queer—distressing : but *Cyclamen* took the matter in hand, and forthwith ended it.

One would lay special stress, therefore, on the functional eye symptoms of *Cyclamen* ; nearly all of a " flickering " character. " Flickering before eyes, as from many-coloured glittering needles." " Could not read, on account of burning and flickering of eyes." " Dim vision ; objects seen through smoke or mist. Diplopia."

In the *Cyclopædia of Drug Pathogenesy* a number of cases are detailed, in which vertigo, visual peculiarities, headache, some-times vomiting (bitter, black, yellow or green, occurred, suggesting action of the drug on the liver). Many of the cases had occurred in a Lock hospital where it had been given in big doses for menstrual troubles. Besides the colour visions, the diplopia and misty sight, the vertigo included, objects turning round in a circle, or having a swinging motion, or, in one case, a feeling as if head turned round in bed.

We are told that *Cyclamen* acts upon the cerebrospinal system, affecting sensorium, eyes, gastro-intestinal canal and, more especially, the female sexual organs.

It produces passive, drawing or tearing pains of parts where bones lie near surface.

The provings also suggest that it might be curative in writer's cramp.

BLACK LETTER (Caused and Cured) SYMPTOMS
(From Allen's *Encyclopædia* and Hering's *Guiding Symptoms*.)

Violent headache, with flickering before eyes, on rising in the morning.

Headache, with flickering before the eyes, on rising in the morning.

Vertigo ; objects turn in a circle, or about her, or make a see-saw motion ; when walking in open air ; better in a room, and when sitting ; with dimness before the eyes.

Dimness of vision and spots before eyes, especially on waking. Dim vision with headache.

Flickering before eyes.

Flickering before eyes, as of various colours, glittering needles ; visions of smoke or fog.

Convergent strabismus.

Salty taste of all food. Saliva has salty taste, communicated to all the food eaten.

No thirst the whole day, but it occurs in the evening, when face and hands become warm.

Pork disagrees.

Menstruation : four days too early, with some relief of melancholy mood, and heaviness of feet.

Scanty or suppressed menstruation, with headache and vertigo.

Hahnemann's Black Letter Symptoms

Fine, sharp, itching pricking on hairy scalp, which, when he scratches always recommences on another spot.

Dimness of vision. Dilatation of pupils.

Swelling of upper eyelids.

Drawing pain in interior of right meatus auditorius.

Little hunger and little appetite. No appetite for breakfast. If he takes but a small quantity of food, the remainder is repugnant to him and excites loathing, and he feels nausea in palate and throat.

Complete anorexia, he has no relish especially for breakfast and supper ; as soon as he commences to eat, at these times, he is immediately satiated.

He has dislike to bread and butter.

Food has a flat, or almost no taste.

Hiccup after a meal.

Immediately after a meal rumbling in the hypogastrium : this recurred every day.

Discomfort in the hypogastrium with some nausea therein.

A kind of paralytic, hard pressure on right upper and forearm, as if in the periosteum and quite in the interior of the muscles ; it extends thence into fingers and hinders him in writing.

Painful drawing in the inner aspect of the shaft of the ulna and in the wrist joint.

A kind of paralytic, hard pressure, which commences only feebly in the forearm, but extends into the fingers, where it becomes so violent that it is only with the greatest effort he can write.

Cramp-like pain in thigh posteriorily above the right hough (hock).
A pain, like dislocation, in the right foot.

*   *   *

Besides its black letter symptoms and its visual abnormalities, *Cyclamen* presents some

CURIOUS, NOTEWORTHY OR UNIQUE SYMPTOMS

Head feels bound.

Sensation of brain in motion ; moving within the cranium.

As if brain wobbled about while walking.

Movements in abdomen, suggesting pregnancy. (Comp. *Crocus, Thuja.*)

Running and crawling in bowels, as of something alive there.

Sensation of something alive, running in heart.

Buzzing in region of heart.

Mentally, *Cyclamen* reminds one of *Drosera*, with its illusions of being persecuted by everyone ; or, again, of *Staphisagria*, with ailments from inward grief, or terrors of conscience. As if he had committed a bad act, or not done his duty.

Sensation as if the room was too small, but reluctant to go into the open air.

Sudden changes of humour, as, joy alternating with irritability.

Ill-humoured, morose, fault-finding.

Dullness, as from cotton wool, in ears. Roaring, humming, ringing in ears. Besides the salty taste of saliva or food, taste flat, putrid, offensive, bitter.

A desire for lemonade : aversion to bread and butter ; to beer ; to fatty things ; to ordinary food ; with desire for inedible things.

Constant disgust for meat ; craving for sardines.

Sore pain in heels (*Petr.*).

DROSERA

*(Largely reproduced from a Paper read by the author to the British
Homœopathic Society in 1927.)*

A FEW years ago, I came to the startling conclusion that the only
two people who really knew anything about *Drosera* were Samuel
Hahnemann and myself ; and I have had it in my mind ever
since that I would like to communicate such knowledge as I
possess to my colleagues the world over. I can only hope that
I may be enabled to add something very real to our powers of
fighting one formidable disease—TUBERCULOSIS.

Of course, everybody knows all about *Drosera* ! Has it not
a place in every " Manual of Domestic Homœopathy "—and
a groove in every box of a dozen homœopathic remedies ? For
Drosera is classical, and that for a hundred years, as *a laryngeal
remedy*, and as *our greatest remedy in whooping-cough*.

But when, through a happy accident, I began to realize what
Drosera can do in tuberculous disease of BONE, of JOINT and of
GLAND, I was amazed, and I started hunting homœopathic
literature for my warrant in so using it. Kent knew it not.
Clarke knew it not. But so far as bone and joints were concerned,
I found my justification in black type in the provings of Hahnemann. I wonder why we are content to take most things at
second or third hand ?—why we so seldom go to the fountain-
head ? How many homœopaths of our day read Hahnemann's
" Materia Medica Pura " ? But I may tell you that Hahnemann
gives big black type not only to the laryngeal symptoms that have
made *Drosera* famous among homœopaths, but he gives the same
black type to *joints*, to *shoulder*, to *hip*, and again and again
to *ankle* ; besides to the *shafts of long bones* ; and *pains in
limbs*, and in diverse *muscles*. Hahnemann also, in a foot-note,
especially designates the use of *Drosera* in *laryngeal phthisis*.

But it was only after I had shown some of my gland and bone
Drosera cases to the Society in 1920, that the whole picture of
Drosera began to dawn upon me. I was rather apologetic
about my use of *Drosera* in gland cases ; in fact, I think my
" indications " were demanded of me. But after the meeting,
I was referred to the " Cyclopædia of Drug Pathogenesy " where
the key to the whole position lay, in the experiments of Dr.
Curie. For Dr. Curie proved the homœopathicity of *Drosera*

to tuberculosis in its widest and most important aspect—that is, he showed that *Drosera breaks down resistance to tubercle every time in animals supposed to be absolutely immune to that disease ;* and he also proved to his own satisfaction that *Drosera* was also able to raise resistance to tubercle, by curing early phthisis. And I saw with joy that, in Curie's experiments, GLANDS, especially abdominal and cervical glands, were tremendously affected.

Ancient, non-homœopathic medical literature, as Hahnemann points out, suggests the same fact—viz. the opposite, or homœopathic, action of *Drosera*. It was what Hahnemann had written, together with his further researches in literature, that suggested to Curie to determine " *the exact physiological action of the plant* " and to see " *how far it was connected with the Law of Similars* ". For, among the ancients, *Drosera* had been alternately extolled as a remedy for consumption, and abandoned—as accelerating the disease. Hahnemann explains this. He says, several of the older physicians found this plant useful in some kinds of malignant cough, and in phthisical persons, thus confirming its (homœopathic) medicinal power ; but the moderns, having no knowledge of any other than large doses, knew not how to employ this uncommonly heroic plant without endangering the life of their patients ; hence they rejected it altogether.

And now a word about *Drosera rotundifolia* (Sundew), which Hahnemann describes as " *one of the most powerful medicinal herbs in our zone* ".

Drosera is, I believe, our only insectivorous plant. It sits on the ground in boggy places, with its circle of round leaves studded with glandular hairs, which exude drops of viscid, acrid juice, and which close down on, and digest, any hapless insects that dare to settle on the plant.

Drosera has an evil reputation in regard to sheep fed on pastures where it abounds. They are said to *acquire a very violent cough,* and *to waste away.*

Hahnemann, in a footnote to his black type laryngeal symptoms of *Drosera,* points out " their likeness to some kinds of laryngeal phthisis, *where Sundew is so peculiarly useful,* provided there be no specific cachexy "

In the sixteenth century, the Sundew had a reputation as an excellent remedy " to restore vital moisture in persons labouring under consumption " ; but Gerarde states that " they have sooner perished who used the distilled water thereof, than those that abstained from it ".

Sundew had also a reputation for the cure of madness ; and in the homœopathic provings we find, *restlessness* (in black type), suspicion, *delusions of persecution* (in black type), and inclination to suicide by drowning. It was used also in coughs and diseases of the lungs, and here again it is purely homœopathic. Also in chronic asthma—purely homœopathic—and palpitation of the heart.

Now a word about CURIE'S EXPERIMENTS.

Curie chose cats for his experiments, the cat being, of all animals, least liable to tuberculosis. He says, " it is not certain that tubercles have ever been found in cats."

His experiments were only *three*, " because of the difficulty of obtaining enough of this small plant *for the long time these experiments require* ". " Because," as he says, " it is not a question of exciting functional symptoms, depending on the nervous system." " Tuberculization," he says, " is a work of time ; and a drug capable of producing in its action on the organism the formation of tubercles, will require time in which to do so."*

The results of his three experiments were so conclusive that he felt bound to publish them. For he found that *the prolonged use of* Drosera *induces tuberculization in animals* ; and he states that its power to cure tuberculization has never failed him.

Drosera IN SPASMODIC COUGH, AND IN WHOOPING-COUGH.

Hughes talks of the SPASMODIC COUGH of *Drosera*, and how " Hahnemann's wonted sagacity led him to perceive this, and to recommend the medicine in *pertussis* ".

But we all try to improve on Hahnemann—with consequent loss of power. Hahnemann states that a single dose of the 30th (the decillionth) potency, is quite sufficient for the cure of epidemic whooping-cough (according to the indications given by certain symptoms which he enumerates). " The cure takes place," he says, " with certainty in from seven to nine days, under a non-medicinal diet. Care should be taken not to give a second dose (or any other medicine) immediately after the first dose, for that would not only prevent the good result, but do serious injury, as I know from experience."

---

* *While provings on animals are useless from Hahnemann's point of view in regard to any mental or delicate subjective symptoms so essential to their scientific employment, yet experiments, or accidental effects of drugs, long-continued, on animals may yield valuable suggestive information as to the organs and tissues especially affected by such drugs. It would not be legitimate to press the proving on a human being to the extent of provoking gross lesions ; but it has been elsewhere also recorded that Drosera excites a very violent cough in sheep (fed on pastures where this plant abounds) and Curie's cats prove that it not only breaks down resistance to tubercle in different parts of the body, but leads to enormous swelling of cervical and other glands.*

Hughes, who loves to go one better than Hahnemann, suggests " repeated doses of the 1st, or 1st decimal " (*instead of Hahnemann's decillionth, or 30th*) " to bring uncomplicated cases of whooping-cough to an end in two, three, or four weeks " (*instead of Hahnemann's seven to nine days*) " with mitigation of the severity of the attack meantime ".

But Hughes got called over the coals for this, and had to print a footnote to the effect that homoeopaths truer to Hahnemann in their practice " had recently confirmed the correctness of Hahnemann's observation " (*British Journal*, Vol. xxxvi, p. 268).

I may say that I have been in the habit of curing whooping-cough with single doses of *Drosera* 30 or 200 ; and I saw a good deal of whooping-cough during the 1914-18 war in our Children's Out-patient Department. On a few occasions, one would repeat, after a fortnight, if any cough remained. I can only remember one failure, where I had to give another medicine. It was in a child of four, brought back a week later, no better—worse—and reeking of camphor, which she was wearing in a bag round her neck. This was not quite Hahnemann's " no other medicine " ; in fact, Hahnemann says of *Drosera*, " Camphor alleviates *and antidotes* its effects." The camphor was discarded and with the then indicated remedy, *Carbo. veg.*, the child was practically well in a week.

Here is a typical case. David S., an infant. (His father and mother were among our missionary students.)

> November 1st.—Ill. Temperature 102° F. Coughing and vomiting. *Bry. 1m.*
> November 2nd.—M.B. Better night. Less vomiting.
> November 3rd.—Less well, fits of coughing, with (?) a whoop. *Dros. 1m*, one dose.

It *was* whooping-cough, and the baby was well within fourteen days.

Hughes quotes Jousset as saying that the power of *Drosera* in spasmodic coughs is one of the best illustrations we have of the efficacy of infinitesimal doses. The definition of its sphere of action being, " Cough from tickling in larynx, with vomiting of food." Jousset quoted 107 cases, of which 101 were cured or relieved.

Hahnemann s whooping-cough symptoms include :—

> Cough, coming from quite deep down in the chest.
> Cough, the impulses of which follow one another so violently that he can hardly get his breath.
> Crawling in the larynx which provokes coughing.
> Cough ending in vomiting, etc.

But Hughes, who questions Hahnemann's single dose of the 30th potency, quarrels also with Curie's crude dosage. When Hughes tried to follow Curie with drop doses of the strong tincture of *Drosera* four times a day, he only succeeded " in setting up a most violent spasmodic cough in a phthisical patient, which subsided into the ordinary cough of phthisis when the medicine was discontinued." " Others have had similar experience ", he says.

No ! Hahnemann's way of using " this uncommonly heroic drug " is undoubtedly the safest and most efficacious.

But remember that Homœopathy knows no specifics, and treats no named diseases *per se*. And if you think that *Drosera* will cure every case of whooping-cough that comes along, you will discover sooner or later that it is not so. In one epidemic it is recorded that *Kali carb.* was the remedy, and, once found, cured every case.

The case that opened my eyes, accidentally, to the value of *Drosera* in SPINAL CARIES was one that was sent in to me by one of the Surgeons, when I was running our Children's Department during the War. It was a small boy of four. He had started a T.B. finger at twelve months, and spinal caries six months later. He had been treated by our Children's Physician and by one of our Surgeons, and was lying on a board with double Thomas splint and headpiece. He had improved, on the whole, under treatment, with fluctuations. He got very thin at one time, and there was threatening of lung trouble, and night sweats ; but *Tub.*, *Phos.*, *Calc.*, etc., had helped. The Surgeon now sent him in for whooping-cough : not a desirable occupation for one who was supposed to maintain a restful recumbent position ! He got a dose of *Dros.* 200.

When next seen, two months later, the mother was so enthusiastic as to the good effects of the last medicine on the child's health that I began to " sit up and take notice ". Another two months and he was found to be " eating well ; putting on flesh. Fat and flourishing ". The change in the child was really amazing. The remedy was repeated at long intervals. When last seen some three years later, the note is, " Boy's spine is very good. He has not worn apparatus for nearly two years. Goes to school for the last six months."

One remembers another case of spinal caries (cervical) in a boy of seven years. He started at four years old with a knee, then a finger, then his neck. He had been treated at other hospitals. He had also had fits, and ear discharge, and was brought in a spinal carriage ; never allowed to sit up. He was a happy little fellow, with an extraordinarily deformed neck, which he would move from side to side with alarming jerks. He got *Drosera* 200, and began to improve at once ; and was soon able to turn his head easily, all ways. In two or three months, with the approval of one of our Surgeons, he was allowed to sit up, and he made steady progress, with very intermittent treatment, till a couple of years later it was reported to me that his parents (in spite of warning) " took him flying about the country in the sidecar of a motor cycle—long journeys, sitting up, his neck being joggled all the time ". He rapidly put on flesh, and one of my notes four years after treatment began reads, " Looking very well. Active. Good colour. Father takes him out all day in his van. Does not mind the jolts." And later, I was told that " nothing new in the way of his disease had occurred since first he came here four and a half years ago ". Till then there had been a succession of T.B. manifestation.

One more spinal case—scoliosis in a young woman, with extreme deformity : and—a T.B. history. She was suffering and sickly. She had had a recent fall, and a very gentle manipulation, done in fear and trembling, ended the pain in her back, and *Drosera*, for her family history, made something hardly recognizable of her. She comes for occasional help, and remains robust and healthy-looking.

I am allowed to quote a case, showing the value of *Drosera* in TUBERCULOUS SINUSES. Boy, $13\frac{1}{2}$. For eight months there had been a swelling, constantly recurring in right forearm, followed by several areas left arm. When opened, pus oozed out, but the discharge would not cease. There was a bad T.B. history on both sides of family. The boy had three considerable areas of typical tuberculous-looking tissue, which alternately scabbed and broke down.

Tub. and *Silica* helped. Then *Dros.* 200 was given, and a month later the scars were found to be freely moveable (this is a typical *Dros.* result,—the three drugs one has seen dealing successfully with scar tissue being *Graph.*, *Sil.* and *Drosera* ; and, where tuberculous scars are concerned, the greatest of these is *Drosera*). Treatment was continued till, six months after the first dose, it was so extraordinarily cured that the note is, " Discoloration faint. In certain lights the skin looks almost normal." And—" the boy was well, fat and flourishing."

Where *Drosera* helps, results are very soon seen, and invariably in renewed health and spirits, and in utterly changed appearance. I have seen this so often. The patient who needs *Drosera* and gets it, simply blooms. There is no other word for it.

It was the relief to atrocious nightly pain in a diseased tibia, where a number of remedies had failed, that made me realize that Hahnemann was right when, in his *Materia Medica Pura,* under *Drosera,* he put " pain in the long bones " in big black type ; and that those who followed him in compiling materia medicas, and transcribed these symptoms of his relating to bones and joints, were wrong. They have robbed us of many brilliant results, by reducing the type of what he stressed as so important.

But unfortunately everyone since Hahnemann's day, who writes about, or attempts to practise homœopathy, is always prepared (without the colossal studies, experiments, experience and knowledge of Hahnemann) to go one better.

I suggest that we all, forthwith, open our materia medicas, whether Clarke's, Allen's or Boericke's at *Drosera,* and underline in red all the black type symptoms Hahnemann gives us, of what he calls, " *one of the most powerful medicinal herbs in our zone* ".

In Curie's first cat, killed after six weeks of *Drosera,* besides T.B. lesions of pleura, he says : " I found a very considerable enlargement of the mesenteric glands."

In his second cat, killed after a year, there were also T.B. abdominal lesions—spleen—Peyer's patches—and of the " shut vesicles of the large intestine ". ALL THREE CATS HAD DIARRHŒA.

And Curie says, of his cats :—

Drosera causes the production of tubercular elements in the lungs, and *acts at the same time on the lymphatic system in general.*

And in his second cat, killed after a year of *Drosera,* there were ENORMOUS SUBMAXILLARY GLANDS.

A girl of 19 : " Gets attacks of diarrhœa, and cannot go to business." Had had " fourteen attacks " in twenty-four hours at Christmas, now (in May) gets about five stools a day—loose ; at times, mucous. At Christmas passed blood : not now. Any pain is in left abdomen.

Abdomen was boggy, and a nodule·was felt on left side—a typical " T.B. abdomen."

Some improvement followed with *Sulph., Lil. tigr.* and *Tub. bov.* And in *August* she got a dose of *Drosera* in high potency.

The *September* note is : " Getting on splendidly. Takes food better." " *Goes to business now !* " Was seen at intervals for another year, when an interesting note is, " She never complained of diarrhœa or of indigestion after *Drosera* was first given."

One has had a number of cases of cervical glands doing well under *Drosera,* some of them after long treatment here or elsewhere, and with a great deal of ugly scarring.

What one invariably notices is that the cases that react to this drug, react rapidly, with astonishing improvement in general health and well-being. Where they do not rapidly react, I know that I have not got my remedy. But over and over again I find recorded in *Drosera* cases, and often on the very next visit " patient looks blooming ". I do not think this expression occurs—it certainly does not occur constantly, in my records in regard to any other remedy.

In *Drosera* GLAND cases one notices, as I said, not only the diminution in the size of the gland, but that the old scars fade away, get free, and come to the surface ; that discoloration goes, and that when a gland does break down under *Drosera*, it behaves in a very restrained manner, with a small opening, little discharge, and that it leaves practically nothing to mark what has taken place.

Cases of GOITRE, also, and even EXOPHTHALMIC GOITRE have greatly benefited, or been cured with *Drosera*—cases with a T.B. family history.

The most extraordinary case where this was so, was a boy of 14, sent on, as inoperable, by one of our surgeons. He had marked exophthalmos,* with a pulse of 150, chains of lymphadenomatous glands in the neck : bluish indurated patches on both calves, studded with small ulcerations (typical " Bazin "). He improved under *Tub. bov.* during five months. Legs were nearly well, neck better, right eye prominent. Then *Drosera* 200.

The effect was dramatic, a month later he had started work—engineering. Glands were well ; sores well ; exophthalmos gone ; pulse 80. After that there were fluctuations in pulse, but when last seen thirteen months after treatment began (he was then going abroad to live), he was feeling very well. " No glands," but still some prominence of right eye, and as pulse was again higher, he got his last dose of *Drosera*.

As to *Drosera* in JOINTS . . . occasional cases of rheumatoid arthritis clear up to an astonishing extent on *Drosera*. One remembers an old body of 76. She had been coming up some years before—unable to close her hands : wrists and knuckles especially affected, and ankles and feet, with swelling and deformity. She had an extremely bad T.B. family history. As she had previously improved under *Tub. bov.* and *Causticum* she came again to see if more could be done for her. *Caust.* helped again ; and then, for " severe pain in right tibia ; foot and leg unbearable ", she got *Drosera*.

* *Drosera is in the Repertory for the protrusion of eyes.*

In a month, " Very much better. Pain gone." Says that now her left hand " goes out flat ", and shows it.

Then a succession of visits to boast and rejoice. " Getting back her left wrist, hasn't had it for years ! " (i.e. it is no longer rigid). . . . Later, " can bend her feet, and bend her toes now ; so she knows she is getting better ". . . . " Feels so well now ; does her room, and her washing ! " Later again, " Only comes to show her hands ! Watches herself improving ! Has movement in both wrists now. No pain at all, except in one finger. . . ." Says " she used only to be able to lift a cup between her two clenched hands." Now " stands on tip-toe ". Hands look all gnarled and twisted, with the typical ulnar deflection : but they are pliable, and she is able to extend them flat. (Some Old School doctors who saw her at a clinical demonstration, were very interested in this case.)

A curious fact one has noted is the number of patients who, after months of steady treatment with other remedies and with varying periods of amelioration and relapse, on getting *Drosera*, come back no more, or only after periods of months to years of good health. *Drosera* goes deep.

Now please do not imagine that I want to suggest that *Drosera* will cure all cases of SINUS, GLAND, or BONE disease of tuberculous nature, or in persons of tubercular family history. It will not. But it will revolutionize quite a number of such cases ; and where it acts, as I said, it acts with extraordinary rapidity, and the change in appearance, in general health, and in spirits of the patient is remarkable.

Again, please do not think that I imagine that we have got to the end of the posibilities of *Drosera*.

For instance, *all Curie's cats had diarrhœa*, and the second cat was found to have *hypertrophy of Peyer's patches*. *What about a difficult enteric, with a T.B. history ?*

Drosera has an ancient reputation for *asthma*, and there again the provings are suggestive. *One should certainly think of Drosera for asthma with T.B. history.*

Remember also the effect of *Drosera* on the *spleen*.

In both the dissected cats the *pleuræ* were especially attacked by tubercle.

And I suggest that we should bear in mind, in regard to *Drosera*, its *mental symptoms*, especially in cases of *paranoia*.

Drosera, as Hahnemann says, needs re-proving. It will never repertorize out on general symptoms. It is one of the drugs for which you have to go to materia medica, to see that it fits.

In many cases I am afraid I had little in the way of indications, save the general one, that *a drug that is capable of breaking down resistance to tubercle SHOULD, according to the Law of Similars, be also capable of raising resistance to tubercle*—which happens.

SOME OF HAHNEMANN'S BLACK LETTER SYMPTOMS

Crawling in larynx, which provokes coughing, with sensation as if a soft body was located there, with fine shooting therein to right side of gullet.

Deep down in fauces (and on soft palate) a rough, scraping sensation with dryness exciting short cough, with yellow slimy expectoration and hoarseness of voice, so that it is only with an effort that he can speak in a deep base tone : at the same time he feels an oppression of the chest, as if something there kept back the air when he coughed and spoke, so that the breath could not be expelled.

Quivering in right shoulder, only when at rest.

Paralytic pain in right hip-joint and thigh, and in ankle joint, but in the latter rather as if dislocated, when walking, when he must limp on account of the pain.

A single cutting stitch in the middle of the anterior aspect of left thigh, recurring from time to time.

A fine cutting stitch in right calf, which comes when sitting and goes off on walking.

Tearing pain in right ankle joint, as if it were dislocated, only when walking.

Inflexibility of ankle-joints—they are very stiff.

A pain compounded of gnawing and shooting in the shafts of the bones of the arms, thighs and legs, particularly severe in the joints, with severe stitches in the joints, less felt when moving than when at rest.

Painful shooting pressure in the muscles of the upper and lower extremities at the same time, in every position.

All the limbs are as if bruised and are also painful externally.

Pain in all the limbs. He feels as if all were paralyzed.

He is weak in the whole body, with sunken eyes and cheeks.

Febrile rigor all over the body, with heat in the face, but icy cold hands, without thirst.

Restlessness ; when reading he could not stick long to one subject— he must always go to something else.

He is dejected about the malice of others on all hands, and at the same time disheartened and concerned about the future.

Cough, the paroxysms follow each other so violently that he is scarcely able to get his breath.

Rough scraping, dry sensation deep on fauces, etc., etc.

(Allen, of course, gives all Hahnemann's symptoms, but reduces them to italics, or ordinary type, except those that concern the respiratory organs.)

QUEER AND DISTINGUISHING SYMPTOMS.

Soreness of all the limbs on which he lies, as if the bed were too hard . . . (*Arn., Pyrogen.*)

When at rest, shivering. When moving, no shivering. (Rev. of *Nux.*)

Full of mistrust, as if he had to do with none but false people.

Extremely uneasy, sad disposition. He imagined he was being deceived by spiteful, envious people.

Silent and reserved, with anxiety. He always feared he was about to learn something disagreeable.

Anxiety, as if his enemies would not leave him quiet, envied and persecuted him.

Anxiety, especially about 7 or 8 p.m., as if he were impelled to jump into the water to take his own life by drowning—he was not impelled to any other mode of death.

Anxiety in solitude—he wished to have someone always near him. . . .

Very peevish ; a trifle puts him out of humour.

An unimportant circumstance excited him so much that he was beside himself with rage.

(And Hahnemann ends with the " reaction of the vital power—secondary action—curative action—happy, steadfast disposition ; he dreaded no evil because he was conscious of having acted honourably ".)

N.B.—It was Dr. Curie, father of the Radiums Curie, who brought Homœopathy to this country.

DULCAMARA

(Solanum dulcamara.   Woody nightshade.   Bitter sweet)

ANOTHER of the invaluable medicines whose indications for exact and scientific use we owe to Samuel Hahnemann.   It was, for him, " a very powerful plant ", and he says that its duration of action is a long one.   He used it in the 30th potency.   He was aided in his proving by a dozen doctors, and he quotes a number of authorities in regard to the various symptoms recorded.

Hale White, the Old School text-book for Materia Medica (in my edition, anyway) knows it not.

Even Culpepper (1578-1662) has not a great deal to say about this plant, whose uses, for him, were rather occult than practical. He says, " It is good to remove witchcraft both in men and beast, as all sudden diseases whatsoever.   Being tied about the neck, it is a remedy for the vertigo or dizziness of the head ; and that is the reason that the Germans hang it about their cattle's neck, when they fear any such evil hath betided them : country people commonly used to take the berries of it, and having bruised them, they applied them to felons, and thereby soon rid their fingers of such troublesome guests."

Dulcamara affects subversively and curatively all mucous membranes, besides glands, and skin, and muscles.

The provers of *Dulcamara* suffered especially in cold wet weather : and WORSE COLD WET WEATHER is the grand keynote for the employment of this remedy.   Catarrh—from cold wet weather : diarrhœa—from cold wet weather : urinary troubles— from cold wet weather ; even skin troubles—from cold wet weather : and so on.

Dulcamara affects the entire length of the respiratory mucous membrane.   NOSE—dry coryza, or profuse discharges.   Nose- bleed of clear hot blood, worse after getting wet.   .   .   .   THROAT —tonsillitis from every cold change: hawking up of tough mucus, with rawness.   .   .   .   CHEST, cough from cold damp atmosphere or from getting wet.   Must cough a long time in order to expel phlegm.   Great oppressive pain in the whole chest, especially on inspiration and expiration.

In the stomach it causes eructations—empty or tasting of food, with distension after a moderate meal as if stomach would burst.

A curious regional effect of *Dulcamara* is at, or about, the umbilicus. Here the pinching and shooting pains occur again and again in the provings : and *Dulcamara* has proved marvellously useful in pain, or in skin affections, of umbilicus. The pain is " in the hole " as a wee child expressed it.

Then, MUCOUS DIARRHŒA, ALTERNATELY YELLOW AND GREEN-ISH. The diarrhœas of cold wet weather, or sudden changes from hot to cold. " *Dulcamara* is markedly an Autumn remedy," says KENT. He says, as soon as the cold nights come on and the cold fall rains come, there is (in *Dulcamara* subjects) an increase of rheumatism and an increase of catarrhal discharges . . . catarrhal cases that always stuff up when there is a cold rain.

Kent says our mothers used to make ointments of *Dulcamara* ; and it is astonishing how soothing it is when applied to smarting wounds. Ulcers with an eating condition that spread and do not heal (*Ars.*).

It is a great SKIN medicine. Nettlerash that comes on in cold, damp weather. Crusty eruptions that come especially over the head—the crusta lactea of babies. Head and face covered with this sore, itching, bleeding, crusty eruption.

Ringworm, also. Kent says, " *Dulcamara* will nearly always cure these ringworms in the hair ",—and in other places.

And WARTS. *Dulcamara* is one of the great remedies for warts (*Caust.*, *Thuja*). The *Dulc.* warts are large, fleshy and smooth ; or flat. One remembers a patient with a large wart on the right lower lid, interfering with sight. After a dose of *Dulc. C.M.* it began to dry up, and was gone in a fortnight. " It came away in bits ; they irritated and she rubbed them away." This was in 1927, and there has been no recurrence.

Urinary organs also : turbid urine. Catarrh of bladder from taking cold in cold damp weather.

Muscles ; of the back, especially. In the loin : above left hip. Drawing pain in both thighs, better walking, returns immediately on sitting. Excessive perspiration : offensive.

In *Dulcamara* catarrhs, Kent says the nose wants to be kept warm. The sufferer will sit, in a warm room, with cloths wrung out of hot water, clapped over face and nose to relieve the distress; worse in the open air. Worse in a cold room.

Kent says, in regard to remedies, " We have to observe the time of year, the time of day, day or night aggravations ; the wet and dry remedies, the hot and cold remedies. We have to study the remedy by circumstances."

All the symptoms are worse in cold damp weather, and from getting chilled, better from becoming warm and keeping still.

" So you see whether it is a catarrh of the kidney or a catarrhal state of the bladder, or an attack of dysentery, or an attack of sudden diarrhœa, every cold spell of weather brings on an increase of the trouble."

And Kent says, " There is another *Dulcamara* symptom which will often be expressed in the midst of a lot of other symptoms. The patient will say, ' Doctor, if I get chilled I must hurry to urinate : if I go into a cold place, I have to go to stool, or to urinate.' "

NASH sums up the *Dulcamara* conditions thus : " This remedy, like many others, finds its chief characteristic in its modality. Complaints caused or aggravated *by change of weather from warm to cold*. All kinds of inflammatory and rheumatic diseases may spring from such a cause, and so *Dulc.* comes to be indicated in a long list of them. For instance, after taking cold, the neck gets stiff, back painful, limbs lame, or the throat gets sore and quinsy results, with stiff neck and jaws ; the tongue may even become paralysed."

So we see that with this remedy, it is less a question of locality, or of altered functions that leads us to successfully prescribe : it is the marked *causation* of each and all of the troubles. The patient is the victim of conditions to which he is hypersensitive— COLD, and especially WET COLD.

BLACK LETTER SYMPTOMS

From Hahnemann, Allen's *Encyclopedia*, and Hering

Scald head, thick brown crusts with reddish borders, on forehead, temples and chin ; bleeding when scratched.

Humid eruptions on cheeks.

Thick, brown-yellow crusts on face . . . *crusta lactea.*

Thick crusts all over body.

Warts and eruptions on face.

Warts on hands and backs of fingers.

Warts, fleshy or large, smooth, on dorsa of hands and on face.

Tongue paralysed from cold, yet talks incessantly.

Inarticulate speech from swollen tongue.

Colic : as from taking cold ; as if diarrhœa would occur.

Colic such as is usually caused by wet cold weather.

Yellow, watery diarrhœa, with tearing and cutting colic before very evacuation.

Mucous diarrhœa, alternately yellow and greenish.
Diarrhœa from cold, or change from warm to cold, especially cold damp weather. . . .

Catarrhal troubles caused by cold damp weather.
Cough from damp cold atmosphere, or from getting wet. Must cough a long time to expel phlegm. . . .
A very acute pain . . . *darts through the left side of the chest in fits.*
Great oppressive pain of the whole chest, especially on inspiration and expiration.

Pain in small of back, as after long stooping.
In the loin, above left hip, a digging, shooting pain.
A drawing, tearing pain in both thighs.
Lameness in small of back, as if from a cold.

Eruptions like nettlerash all over the body, without fever.

Chill, commencing in, or spreading from back, not better for warmth, mostly towards evening.
Ill-smelling perspiration.

We have often successfully employed *Dulcamara* for pain, or eruptions in the region of the umbilicus—" The hole ", as a wee girl graphically described her pain-spot. One first discovered this tip in Bœnninghausen years ago. Localities can be important.

*   *   *

YET ONE MORE BLACK LETTER SYMPTOM. *Earache ; nausea ; buzzing : worse at night. Earache the whole night, preventing sleep.*

FERRUM

(*Iron: the Metal*)

THE very word FERRUM suggests anæmia, and, possibly, to many of us nothing else : while perhaps few of us associate *Iron*, apart from anæmia, with digestive troubles. We are wrong : Iron, the Stomach, and Anæmia may form three sides of a triangle. And the eccentricities of the stomach may be causative of the most deadly form of " bloodlessness " ; since pernicious anæmia is said to be curable, as we recently pointed out, when meat, digested in a normal stomach, is withdrawn and administered to a patient with that disease. . . . In pernicious anæmia there is a deficiency of normal gastric secretions ; and we are learning to regard *Ferrum* as one of the great stomach remedies.

One remembers in one " stomach " case, feeling surprised at having to prescribe *Ferrum* : but it filled the picture and therefore worked. And why not ? Consider its symptoms : " *After eating, heat in stomach and regurgitation of food* " (*Phos.*) ; " *spasmodic pressure in stomach after the least food and drink. After fat food, bitter eructations. After eggs, vomiting. Worse from meat, sour fruits, drinking milk, after tobacco, tea, beer. Bad effects from drinking tea. Vomiting of everything eaten, without being digested.*"

As a matter of fact, one has not had a very wide clinical experience of the " virtues " of metallic Iron. In anæmia one has used *Ferrum protoxalate* (said to be more easily absorbed) ; and in early " colds " and even in pneumonias with few discriminating symptoms, one has seen rapid improvement under *Ferrum phos.* That being so, more will be learned from the quotations we have culled to help to its successful use.

But, in future one will take *Ferrum met.* into consideration in attempting to treat *varicose* conditions. Here that other drug so like *Iron* in some of its symptoms—so unlike in others— *Pulsatilla* (which owes some of its properties to the iron that goes to its make-up) is also a most useful drug in varicose veins, especially when inflamed. But *Pulsatilla* likes cold : *Iron*, heat. *Puls.* craves air, from which *Ferr.* shrinks. Likeness in some particulars is not identity ; and, unfortunately for the easy spread of Homœopathy among the work-shy, *one drug will not do for another.*

* * *

HAHNEMANN says " most of the provings of IRON were observed from the employment of a solution of the acetate of iron, yet the symptoms correspond with those of metallic iron ; just as those obtained from dry calcareous earth with those of acetate of lime.

" This metal is said by ordinary physicians to be a strengthening medicine *per se*, and not only innocuous, but entirely and absolutely wholesome ". But, " if iron possesses medicinal power, it must, for that very reason alter the health of human beings, and make the healthy ill, and the more ill the more power-. fully curative it is found to be in disease.

" *Nil prodest, quod non laedere possit idem.*

" . . . The condition of persons residing near waters impregnated with iron, might have taught them that this metal possesses strong pathogenetic properties. . . . In such localities few can resist the noxious influence of the continued use of such waters and remain quite well, each being affected according to his peculiar nature. . . . There we find chronic affections of great gravity and peculiar character, even when the regimen is otherwise faultless. . . . Weakness, almost amounting to paralysis of the whole body and of single parts ; some kinds of violent limb pains, abdominal affections of various sorts, vomiting of food by day or by night, phthisical pulmonary ailments, often with blood-spitting, deficient vital warmth, suppression of the menses, miscarriages, impotence in both sexes, sterility, jaundice, and many other rare cachexias are common occurrences.

" What becomes of the alleged complete innocuousness, let alone the absolute wholesomeness of this metal. Those who are constantly drinking chalybeate waters, called *health-springs* are mostly in a sickly state.

" What prejudice, what carelessness has hitherto prevented physicians from observing these striking facts, and referring them to their cause, the pathogenetic property of iron ?

" How can they, ignorant as they are of the action of iron and its salts, determine in what cases chalybeate waters are of use ? Which of their patients will they send thither for a course of treatment ? Which will they keep away ? . . . Is it blind fancy ? Haphazard conjecture and guess work ? Fashion ? Do not many of their patients come back from the chalybeate springs in a more miserable and diseased condition, showing that iron was an unsuitable remedy for them ? God preserve patients from a doctor who does not know, and can give no satisfactory reasons, why he prescribes this or the other drug, who cannot tell *beforehand* what medicine would be beneficial, what injurious to the patient !

" Only a thorough knowledge of the characteristic primary effects of medicines, and whether they present a great similarity to the symptoms of the disease to be cured (as homœopathy teaches) could protect patients from such fatal mistakes.

" The attempt of the common run of practitioners to produce a purely *strengthening* effect is a capital mistake. For why is the patient so weak ? Obviously because he is ill ! Weakness is a mere consequence and a single symptom of his disease. What rational man could think of strengthening his patient without first removing his disease ? But if his disease be removed, then he *always*, even in the process of the removal of his disease, regains his strength by the energy of his organism freed from its malady. There is no such thing as a strengthening remedy as long as the disease continues : there can be none such. The homœopathic physician alone knows how to cure, and in the act of being cured the convalescent regains his strength."

* * *

Of course *Iron* enters largely into, and has a most important part to play in the body : but in SCHUESSLER'S scheme of " *Tissue Salts* " it only appears as *Ferrum phos.* *Iron*, Schuessler tells us, " is to be found in the hæmoglobin or red-blood cells, and not in such considerable quantities in any other tissue, except in the hair". But he gives it an important place as a constituent of *muscle cells.* A disturbance of the equilibrium of the iron-molecules in muscle fibre, causes relaxation. In the muscular coats of vessels it causes therefore a dilatation and an accumulation of blood :—congestion, with increased blood-pressure, rupture of walls, hæmorrhages. In the muscular coats of the intestinal villi, relaxation, with diarrhœa. In the muscular walls of the intestines themselves, peristalsis is weakened and less active, causing constipation. Anything that causes relaxation of the muscular walls of a vessel, and consequent hyperæmia, such as injury, finds its remedy in *Ferrum phos.*, because this, in minute doses, restores equilibrium to the iron molecules, thus strengthening the muscular fibres. Also, by its power of attracting oxygen, *Iron* and its salts are useful remedies in anæmia.

The *phosphate*, with *Schuessler*, is " *an invaluable remedy in all febrile disturbances and inflammations at their onset, before exudation commences* ".

The provings bear out all these uses of iron, in varices, hæmorrhages, etc.

13 * * *

Black Letter Symptoms

VERTIGO *on rising suddenly ; things grew black ; had to lean against something, or fall : with nausea, prostration, lethargy ; as if balancing to and fro ; as when on water ; when walking over water, like when crossing a bridge ; when descending, with disposition to fall forward.*

HEADACHE : *for two, three, or four days, every two or three weeks : hammering, beating, pulsating pains, must lie down in bed ; with aversion to eating and drinking.*

" Morbus Basedowii " : *especially after suppression of menses : protruding eyes ; enlarged thyroid ; palpitation ; excessive nervousness.*

EPISTAXIS *in anæmic children, with frequent changing colour of face.*

Extreme paleness of FACE, *which becomes red and flushes on least emotion, pain or exertion.*

Face flushes easily on least excitement or exertion.

Canine HUNGER, *alternating with loss of appetite.*

Anorexia : extreme dislike to all food.

Vomiting only of food, immediately after eating.

After eating eructations and regurgitations of food, without nausea or inclination to vomit.

Vomiting of food immediately after midnight, followed by aversion of food and dread of open air.

Cramp-like pain in stomach.

Frequent DIARRHŒA ; *stools watery, with or without tenesmus, and preceded or not by pain, but always with much flatulence, and more frequent after taking food or drink.*

Undigested stools at night, or while eating or drinking.

The threadworms seem to be increased by it.

Involuntary URINATION *at night ; also when walking about by day.*

Nocturnal seminal emissions.

MENSES *too soon, too profuse, too long-lasting, with fiery red face, ringing in ears : flow pale, watery, debilitating.*

Vomiting of pregnancy : suddenly leaves table and with one effort vomits all the food taken, appetite not impaired thereby ; can sit down and eat again.

Difficult breathing, oppression of CHEST, *as if someone pressed, with hand, upon it.*

Contractive spasm in chest and cough, only when moving and walking.

Spasmodic cough after meals with vomiting of all food taken.

Whooping-cough. Child vomits food with every coughing spell : great pallor and weakness.

Scanty, thin, frothy expectoration, with streaks of blood.

Hæmoptysis : of onanists and consumptives : from severe exertion ; from suppressed menses.

Erethitic chlorosis, worse in winter.

ANÆMIA *masked behind plethora and congestions ; pale colour of mucous membranes, with a nun's murmur.*

" Nun's murmur " in veins.

RESTLESS : *must walk slowly about.*

The pain forces him to get up out of bed at night and walk slowly about.

Emaciation.

Red parts become white.

ANÆMIA, *from whatever cause, chlorosis of defective menstruation, or simple poverty of blood induced by hæmorrhages, deficiency of air, light and suitable food, or of exhausting diseases.*

Chlorosis after great loss of blood.

General hæmorrhagic diathesis. Hæmorrhophilia.

Sleeps uneasily : is long awake before falling asleep again.

SOME ITALIC, CURIOUS, OR NOTEWORTHY SYMPTOMS

Prone to weep or laugh immoderately, with choking sensation.

Anxiety as after committing a crime.

Fear of apoplexy.

Irritable : little noises, crackling of paper, drive to despair.

Many symptoms, better for moderate mental exertion.

Head muddled, with cold feet and stiff fingers.

Giddy as if drunk, as though would fall over obstacles (walking).

On looking at running water, as if everything went round with her. Staggering : reeling sensation on seeing flowing water.

Stitches as with a pen-knife in temples, especially at 3 a.m.

Headache, vertex, as if skull were pushed upwards.

Hammering, pulsating headache : congestion to head.

Head dull and full, eyelids heavy : apt to sleep when reading.
Head hot, feet cold.

Capability to see in the dark at night.

Pressure in eyes as if they would protrude.

Redness of eyes and swelling of lids.

Bleeding from nose, in the morning, on stooping.

Face becomes suddenly fiery red, with vertigo, ringing in ears ;
palpitation of heart and dyspnœa.

Persistent diarrhœa in morbid dentition, stools of mucus and
undigested food : face flushes or has a red spot on each side.

Unbearable taste of food : taste like rotten eggs.

Bread tastes dry and bitter.

Appetite voracious : double amount of ordinary meal in evening
hardly sufficient. Or, extreme dislike to all food.

Appetite for bread. Better for wine, except acid wines.

Vomiting after eggs, fat ; worse for meat—milk ; beer.

Vomiting when food has been taken, never at other times, not
as a symptom of disease, or any organic affection of stomach.

Vomiting : easy ; better from ; of food, with a fiery red face.

Pulsation in stomach and through œsophagus : as if a nerve
quivering : as if a valve rose in throat.

Marked swelling of liver : which is sensitive to touch.

Urging to urinate with tickling in urethra, extending to neck
of bladder. Burning in urethra, as if urine were hot.

Oppression chest : hardly moves when breathing : nostrils
dilated in expiration. Difficult inspiration : want of air in
coughing out, and drawing in. Spasmodic cough : whooping
cough.

Asthma : difficult, slow breathing. Better walking and
talking, or by constant reading or writing. Worse sitting still :
most violent lying, especially in the evening.

Cough, with copious purulent, blood-streaked expectoration.

Hæmoptysis : blood bright red, coagulated.

Inflammation of lungs with roof of mouth white.

Women who blush easily.

         *   *   *

KENT points out that the strange thing, in *Ferrum* is that the
complaints—the palpitation, the breathlessness, the weakness
even, come on during rest. The patient is better moving about :
yet exertion tires and causes faintness. Rapid motion aggravates :
but there is amelioration from gentle, slow, quiet motion.

Often patient is puffed up and dropsical : flesh pits, skin is pale, yet face has the appearance of plethora and flushes. And during chill the face becomes quite red ; flushes with wine also. Patient, though flabby, relaxed and tired gets no sympathy. She has palpitation, dyspnœa and weakness, feels she must lie down, yet face is flushed :—a pseudo-plethora.

Blood vessels distended, veins varicose and their coats relaxed : therefore easy bleeding. Hæmorrhages from all parts of the body —nose, lungs, uterus . . . " green sickness ".

Heat in head and face not at all in proportion to the red appearance. Face may be red and cool.

Like *China*, complaints from loss of animal fluids :—prolonged hæmorrhage, with long-lasting weakness. No repair : no digestion : no assimilation. Bones soft and bend. . . . Sudden emaciation with false plethora.

Pains relieved when moving about gently and quietly, like *Pulsatilla* : but *Ferrum* is a very cold medicine : dreads fresh air or a draught.

Slight noises drive the patient wild. . . . Nothing in stomach digests, yet no special nausea. Food goes in and is simply emptied out. Or, eructations of food, like *Phos.* As soon as stomach is empty vomiting ceases till he eats again. *Ferrum* is an interesting medicine, because of this peculiar stomach ; it is like a leather bag, will not digest anything. (Compare *Sepia*. ED.)

Relaxation everywhere : i.e. prolapsus of rectum, of vagina, of uterus. . . . As if organs would come out, and sometimes they do. Bladder also :—This relaxation runs all through the remedy and gives it character.

* * *

NASH. This is another of the abused remedies. It stands with Old School for anæmia, as does *Quinine* for malaria. Each can and does cure its kind of both conditions, but can cure no other ; and each, when it is the true curative, is capable of doing its work in the potentized form. . . . Let no man prescribe *Iron* or any other remedy for anæmia, without indications according to our therapeutic law of cure. I have seen better cures of bad cases of anæmia by *Natrum mur.* in potentized form than I ever did from *Iron* in any form, although *Iron* has its cases, as have also *Pulsatilla, Cyclamen, Calcarea phos., Carbo veg., China*, etc.

Here is Nash's summary of *Ferrum*.

Anæmia with great paleness of all mucous membranes ; with sudden fiery flushing of the face.

Profuse hæmorrhages from any organ : hæmorrhagic diathesis : blood light with dark clots ; coagulates easily.

Local congestions and inflammations, with hammering, pulsating pains : veins full ; flushed face alternates with paleness.

Canine hunger, alternates with complete loss of appetite.

Regurgitation or eructations, or vomiting of food at night that has stayed in the stomach all day : undigested painless diarrhœa.

Worse after eating and drinking ; while at rest, especially sitting still : better walking slowly about.

Ferrum is one of our best remedies for cough with vomiting of food. It is also one of the very few remedies *having a red face during chill,* and has led to the cure of intermittent fever on that symptom.

NASH also says, Palpitation of the heart, hæmoptysis and asthma are relieved in the same way by walking slowly about. It would seem hardly possible that such complaints should be so relieved ; but there are many such curious and unaccountable symptoms in our Materia Medica which have become reliable leaders to the prescription of certain remedies.

*   *   *

By the way, *Ferrum* is one of the four black-type drugs of *obesity* : they are CALC., CAPS., FERR., GRAPH.

It is also a drug to consider in *exophthalmic goitre.* One has hunted for remedies for *blushing. Ferr.* is one.

A very ancient experience has it, that ill-sleeping persons may find rest, by ordering the position of their beds, so that they shall sleep North and South, i.e. in the magnetic field, with head to the North. Personal experience suggests strongly, TRY IT. The feeling of peace that streams down blissfully on the first occasion when this position is tried is not easily forgotten. And why not ? In the blood, *Iron* is incessantly circulating. It is conceivable that its molecules will cruise placidly in the long axis of the body, instead of finding themselves butting about in agitation when the body lies crosswise to the polar current.

FERRUM PHOSPHORICUM

" ONE of the organic tissue-salts introduced by Schuessler. Needs proving. Prepared by trituration. Good results with the 200th potency have been obtained." (HERING, *Guiding Symptoms*).

About the year 1875, Schuessler, a homœopathic doctor, introduced his twelve *Tissue Salts*, or *Bio-chemical Remedies*. Two of the twelve, *Silica* and *Natrum muriaticum*, were old homœopathic drugs, previously proved and given to the world many years earlier by Hahnemann. Of the rest, some have since been proved (on the healthy) or partially proved ; and, as we know, by experience, many of them are invaluable.

Schuessler, looking upon them as tissue foods, gave them in the lower potencies (6*x* usually) and seems to have fed them in at frequent intervals. But, where they are homœopathic to the condition we desire to cure, i.e., where they provoke and cure identical symptoms, the higher and highest potencies give as good, or even better results. For instance, his magnificent *Magnesia phos.*, acts like a charm in the *c.m.* potency in a dysmenor-rhoea of like symptoms ; sometimes a single dose has ended the trouble. Its sphere, here, is the agonizing, crampy pains that cause the victim to double up (*Coloc.*) and to hug a very hot water-bottle. We are told that it is to their *Mag. phos.*, that such remedies as *Coloc.*, *Viburn.*, *Bell.*, etc., owe their griping, abdominal pains. And yet, practically, *one will not do for the other* !

Schuessler discarded all but the actual salts in their tissue-combination ; he even discarded later, *Calc. sulph.*, believing that *Calc.* does not appear thus in the tissues. But vitality has a way of breaking down and building up for itself, and by no means requires that its wants shall be supplied in the exact form, in which they are to be utilized. He passed by that most precious of remedies, *Calc. carb.* and substituted *Calc. phos.*, but—the wide difference in their symptoms ! The soft, lethargic *Calc. carb.* baby, with sweating head, sourness, " plus tissue of minus quality " everywhere—even in bones, is utterly distinct from *Calc. phos.*, equally valuable in its place, but no substitute for the other : the *Calc. phos.* baby is often emaciated and generally dark ; more wiry ; and the sweating head, so characteristic of rickets, is absent. For precise work—alas ! neither will do for the other. And *chemical* and *life-processes*, as Hahnemann showed, are by no means identical.

Another point :—to feed in your drugs upon a hypothesis is one thing, and may advantage the patient. Whereas, to stimulate the organism to take what it needs from ordinary foods by which the want can, and should be supplied, is surely a far higher aim. The stimulative dose of *Calc. carb.* when symptoms agree, will cause the babe to supply its calcium-need from milk—provided the vitality of the milk has not been destroyed by modern methods; just as the infinitesimal dose of *Natrum mur.* (potentized salt) will stimulate an (e.g. asthma patient—we have seen it)—to take the salt he craves and starves for, from the usual food sources that supply ordinary mortals, and so end, with his asthma, his inordinate appetite for salt.

Science means *knowledge.* But the science of any day is never ultimate knowledge, and is apt to be pushed off the board by the science of to-morrow. And always we admire and extol it ; yet, looking back, the science of many days seems to have been but a see-saw of sense and folly.

For instance, to safeguard milk from being a possible vehicle of contagion, it has to be " sterilized "—" pasteurized ", till the poor babes fed thereon, semi-starved of its more occult yet indispensable ingredients, lack the power of resistance to those very disease-organisms from which we have striven to protect them. Then "science advances," and decrees orange juice, lemon juice, or the " cheap raw juice of swedes "—never intended for the up-building of infants—to be added. Again, babes are brought to us, fed on bone-marrow ; on dried milk ; on peptonized milk ; on predigested foods, considered by the experimental, boastful, advertising chemist as proper substitutes for mother's milk, often to the inhibition of necessary gland-activity. Then science, advancing still further, discovers VITAMINS (mark you ! *always* present in normal foods *and in proper quantities*, since the dawn of creation, and available for all except the children of civilization). These " vitamins " being destroyed in drying and sterilizing preparations, it now becomes necessary to supply them artificially : and (the next problem) not to over-supply them, as science is already discovering in regard to " Vitamin D ".

Natural foods contain, in requisite proportions, the elements from which we may draw health and life. Clever, clever scientists !—when the chemistry of life in its perfection has been in operation since man strode the earth and women nursed their babies ; and is still in operation, unless interfered with by ephemeral " science ". And infants have lived delightfully, and flourished exceedingly, and grown into the robust men and women ; whose descendants we are.

> *Knowledge is proud because she knows so much.*
> *Wisdom is humble, that she knows no more.*

One thinks of the old home life ; the fat, happy, rosy babies ; away in the country, because town-life—and in these days, flat-life—is not good enough for children :—The selected cow, whose unboiled milk reared them ; the rushing and exciting games in garden and woods ; the discipline of contact, of the clash of wills and tempers that bred self-control, and provided such ideal training to meet the trials and troubles of the wider life later.

* * *

The tissue-salts one knows best (besides the aforesaid *Natrum mur.* and *Silica*), are four in number, and curiously enough, the *phosphates*: *Calc. phos.* as said; *Ferrum phos.* for somewhat non-descript acute inflammations in their early stage—colds—pneumonias—which lack the well-defined indication that would call for *Acon.*, *Bry.*, *Phos.*, etc. ; *Mag. phos.* for the terrible nerve pains, where previously we had only *Spigelia*, *Coloc.*, etc. ; but with the very definite *Mag. phos.* cry for pressure and HEAT ; *Natrum phos.*, so useful in acid-muscle conditions, whether from fatigue (*Arn.*) or sickness, as in the " growing pains " of small children, indefinite and disregarded often, but ominous where there is with them a small rise of temperature, and perhaps the suggestion of a blowing heart-murmur.

To these many doctors would add *Kali phos.* But this last, for some or no reason, not having taken much hold on one's imagination, and never having become an intuition, it may be well, later on, to *Drug-Picture* it :—a grand means of grasping the real inwardness of a remedy, and learning its uses.

Well, now—to revert to our subject—FERRUM PHOS.

Here is Schuessler's THEORY in regard to it. He says in his last Edition (quoted by Clarke in his *Dictionary*) : " Iron and its salts possess the property of attracting oxygen. The iron contained in the blood corpuscles takes up the inhaled oxygen, thereby supplying it to all the tissues of the organism. The sulphur contained in the blood corpuscles and in other cells, in the form of sulphate of potassa, assists in transferring oxygen to the cells containing iron and sulphate of potassa. When the molecules of iron contained in the muscle-cells have suffered a disturbance in their motion through some foreign irritation, the cells affected grow flaccid. If this affection takes place in the annular fibres of the blood-vessels, these are dilated ; and as a consequence the blood contained in them is augmented. Such a state is called hyperæmia from irritation ; such a hyperæmia forms the first stage of inflammation. But when the cells affected have been brought back to the normal state by the therapeutic effect of iron (*Phosphate of Iron*), then the cells are enabled to cast off the causative agents of this hyperæmia, which are then received by the lymphatics in order that they may be eliminated from the organism." Again, " When the muscular cells of the intestinal villi have lost molecules of iron, then these villi become unable to perform their functions ; diarrhœa ensues." And, once again, " When the muscular cells of the intestinal walls have lost molecules of iron, then the peristaltic motion of the intestinal canal is retarded, resulting in an inertia, with respect to the evacuation of faeces." . . .

" When the muscular cells which have grown flaccid through loss of iron receive a compensation for their loss, the normal tensional relation is restored ; the annular fibres of the blood vessels are shortened to their proper measure, the capacity of these vessels again becomes normal, and the hyperæmia disappears, and in consequence the inflammatory fever ceases."

Schuessler says " *Iron* will cure :

" The first stage of all inflammations.

" Pains and hæmorrhages caused by hyperæmia.

" Fresh wounds, contusions, sprains, etc., as it removes the hyperæmia.

" The pains which correspond to iron are increased by motion, but relieved by cold." (No ! *Ferrum* is better for gentle motion.)

Schuessler recommended trituration and dilutions from the 6x to the 12x. As said, his idea seems to have been to feed in the drug, probably in a potency in which it could be utilized. But, for the more subtle purposes of stimulation, the higher potencies, in less frequent repetition may do even more brilliant work.

*   *   *

So much for theory : now for the practical experiences of successful prescribers.

NASH has a page of appreciation for *Ferrum phos.* We will glean.

A valuable remedy in some inflammatory diseases.

In keeping with its element of iron, it presents the *local congestive tendencies* of that remedy ; in its *Phosphorus* element its affinity for lungs and stomach ; and in its combination proves a great *hæmorrhagic remedy.*

The hæmorrhages are of bright blood, and may come from any outlet of the body.

He also says, further provings and clinical use will enable us to employ it more scientifically than now.

So far as he has observed, it is less adapted to the full-blooded, sanguine arterial subjects, with an over-plus of red blood that *Aconite* cures, but rather to the pale and anæmic, who are subject to sudden and violent congestions and inflammations, like pneumonia, or sudden congestion to head, bowels, etc., or to inflammatory affections of a rheumatic character. It is only useful in the first stage of such attacks, before the stage of exudation appears. . . . In dysentery, in the first stage with a good deal of blood in the discharges it is valuable and often cures in a very short time.

" A very valuable remedy ; and ought to receive a thoroughly Hahnemannian proving."

* * *

BOGER (*Synopsis*) :
LUNGS. *Ears.* Worse at night (6 a.m.). Motion. Jar. *Checked sweat.*

FULL, SOFT, FLOWING PULSE. (rev. of *Acon.*)

Excited and talkative.

Violent earache.

Frequent stools of bloody water.

Laryngitis of singers.

Chest congested.

Fevers.

Pneumonia.

Hæmorrhagic measles, etc., etc.

MARKED SYMPTOMS

from Hering's *Guiding Symptoms*, and from Boericke and Dewey's *Edition of Schuessler's Work.*

" Sows eat up their young ; a transient mania depending upon hyperæmia of brain."

All febrile disturbances and inflammations at their onset, before exudation commences.

Vertigo from congestion to parts of brain or head.

Frontal headache, followed and relieved by nose-bleed.

Congestion to brain ; early meningitis.

Top of head sensitive to cold air, noise, jar, or stooping.

Perhaps a feeling as if head were pushed forward, with danger of falling.

Severe headache with soreness ; can't bear hair touched ; with hot, red face, and vomiting of food.

Rush of blood to head. (Comp. *Bell., Glonoine.*)

Eyes inflamed, red, burning, sore.
On stooping cannot see ; as if all blood ran into eyes.

First stage of otitis.

Epistaxis. (*Vipera.*)

A florid complexion.

Ulcerated throat, to relieve congestion, heat, fever, pain and throbbing (*Bell.*). " First stage of diphtheria."

Worse after meat, herring, coffee, cake.
Toothache relieved by cold.

Vomiting of blood.

Hæmorrhoids, inflamed or bleeding.
Stools of pure blood.

Hæmorrhage from bladder and urethra.

Initiatory stage of all inflammatory affections of the respiratory tract.
Pneumonia with expectoration of clear blood.
Hæmoptysis after concussion or fall.
Pleuritis and pneumonia, first stage.
Coughs clear blood, with nose-bleed.
" Full pulse, less bounding than *Aconite*, but not so flowing as in *Gels.*"

Articular rheumatism. Acute. Attacking one joint after another. Joints puffy but little red ; worse slightest motion.

Felons, at the commencement (*Bell.*).
High fever. Skin hot and dry. Scarlet fever. (*Bell.*).
Copious night sweats, not relieving the great pains of rheumatism, driving out of bed. Sweat between 4 and 6 a.m.

* * *

All febrile disturbances at their onset, especially before **exudation** commences.

" In many inflammatory and some eruptive fevers, it seems to stand between the intensity of *Acon.* and *Bell.*, and the dullness of *Gels.*"

" In anæmia compare with *China*, with which it has many symptoms in common. . . . The tree from which *China* is obtained is always found in a ferruginous locality."

" Measles with conjunctivitis and photophobia (35 cases)."

* * *

One has seen very rapid curative action with *Ferr. phos.* in many early colds without very definite symptoms ; and also astonishing cures of pneumonia, without the definite symptoms that would call for *Acon.*, *Bry.* or *Phos.*

Not having been extensively proved, *Ferrum phos.* has not yet taken the place it richly deserves in homœopathic literature. Its sphere seems to be, *simple, active hyperæmia.* It should be useless in septic cases.

" *Ferr. phos.* is a constituent of *China, Gels., Verat., Acon., Arn., Ailanth., Anis., Stil., Phyto., Berb., Rhus, Asaf., Viburn., Secale* (.25 per cent.), *Graph.* (2.74 per cent.)." BOERICKE.

GELSEMIUM

Gelsemium—Yellow Jessamine—or " Yellow Jasmine ". A climbing plant native to the Southern States of America.

We owe *Gelsemium* as a remedy to Dr. E. M. Hale (U.S.A.), who was proud of the title his colleagues gave him, " Father of the New Remedies ", because he added valuable medicines to our pharmacopœia, and because of his important text book, Hale's *New Remedies*.

CLARKE'S description of *Gelsemium* and its action is excellent. He calls it a drug of importance in Homœopathy, not for the great number of symptoms it causes, but because of the number of its well-marked and clearly characteristic symptoms, which correspond to symptoms constantly met with in everyday practice. We will extract.

" *Gelsemium* is *a great paralyser*. It produces a general state of paresis, mental and bodily. The mind is sluggish, the whole muscular system is relaxed : the limbs so heavy he can hardly move them. . . . The same paretic condition is shown in the eyelids, causing ptosis ; in the eye muscles, causing diplopia ; in the œsophagus, causing loss of swallowing power ; in the anus, which remains open . . . Post-diphtheritic paralysis. . . . The mental prostration is typified in ' funk ' as before an examination ; stage fright ; effects of anger, grief, bad news ; and is accompanied by drooping eyelids. . . . Hysterical dysphagia or aphonia, after emotions. . . . *Tremor* is a key-note of the remedy."

One remembers after an attack of *diphtheria*, prickling in finger-tips and in soles of feet, as if shoes full of little sharp stones, and one uncomfortable moment, when something swallowed went, not down, but up, into the nose. *Gels.* promptly finished all that. It should. One of its characteristic symptoms is paralysis of œsophagus and of the muscles of deglutition. It has proved a great remedy in post-diphtheritic paralysis.

And then *Influenza*. There is one form of 'flu of which *Gels.* makes quick work—where chills are playing up and down the spine ; where legs are too heavy, almost, to lift, and head and brain too languid, and weighty, and dull ; and here a dose of *Gels.* will straighten things up, often in a couple of hours.

Again, patients come—sometimes after an epidemic, several in an afternoon, complaining, " Never well since 'flu some weeks ago ; tired, languid, heavy—*can't* get well." The temperature is found to be about 99 ; and there are chills. . . . GELS. soon restores all things.

Gels. has also proved prophylactic against 'flu. One remembers hearing how a big school was completely protected in a bad 'flu epidemic, which was working havoc in such institutions. But, to successfully use *Gels.* for 'flu, you must see its symptoms ; the heaviness—the weakness—the tremor, often—the chills—the terrible occipital headache, perhaps. Here no remedy is so entirely reliable as *Gels.*

Gels. is one of the few drugs that has " fear of falling ". (*Borax* has something like it ; but this is rather a fear of downward motion, as when a child, being laid down in its cot, clings in terror to its mother.)

This is how the *Gelsemium* fear is expressed in the *Materia Medica* :

" *Child dizzy, when carried seizes hold of nurse, fearing it will fall.*

" *Sensation of falling in children ; child starts and grasps nurse or crib, and screams out for fear of falling.*"

One remembers a hospital child, so in terror of falling (one was told) that it was not enough to cling to her mother, it had to be some solid piece of furniture. After *Gels.* the next report was, that the child was climbing trees. These cases teach one *Materia Medica*.

Gelsemium is apt to be thirstless.

Gelsemium is a great headache remedy. It has *excruciating headache—nervous headache—sudden headache with dimness of sight, or double vision*—and especially *occipital headaches.*

We see little of *measles* at Hospital, and we desire to see less, because, in these days, measles cases are rushed away, while the wretched measles quarantine renders the children's ward useless for weeks at a time. Why don't we treat it, and cure it ! We used to treat and brilliantly cure all these infectious diseases at the Hospital in its early days ! Anyway, *Gelsemium* has a great reputation for measles among doctors who treat the disease, and who do not hurriedly banish it. One remembers a fish-poisoned family who appeared at Hospital with measly faces, eyes almost closed with swelling and distress, the dull-red rash, and even albuminous urine, when *Gels.* cleared the lot in the course of a few hours. It was the likeness to measles that led to the prescription.

Then, that unpleasant and incommodious symptom, ANTICIPA-TION. There are two drugs in the Repertory that have " *Diarrhœa from anticipation* " (painless " psychic " diarrhœa), viz. ARG. NIT. and GELS.

Besides the "ANTICIPATION" rubric among the mental symptoms, there are other rubrics, anticipation, or what amounts to that, in other parts of the Repertory. We may as well give the complete list—so far as we have been able to collect them. . . . ARG. N. Ars. Carb. veg. GELS. (Lyc.) (Med.) (Pb.) Phos. a., SIL.

Carbo veg. and SIL. appear under " TIMIDITY, appearing in public." And *Ars.*, under " ANXIETY when anything is expected of him." The rest, of course, under ANTICIPATION.

Besides ANTICIPATION, which includes exam. funk (ARG. NIT.), *Gels.* combats the bad effects from great fright or fear; threatening abortion from fear. Guernsey says, " This *Gels.* fright is an awe-stricken feeling, a deep-seated fright or fear, that has made a deep impression." He also says, " All exciting news causes diarrhœa. . . . Fevers, where muscular power is affected ; patient feels so utterly without power."

Kent says, " A *Gels.* cold develops its symptoms several days after the exposure, while the *Acon.* cold comes only a few hours after exposure." He calls it " only a short-acting remedy, though slow in its beginnings". He says "running through its febrile complaints, and even in a cold, when the patient has hot face and red eyes, there is one grand feature, viz. a feeling of great weight and tiredness in the entire body and limbs. The head cannot be lifted from the pillow, so tired and so heavy is it, and there is great weight in the limbs—whereas the *Bry.* patient lies quietly and does not move, because if he moves the pains are worse."

In *Gels.* the heart is feeble, and the pulse soft and irregular. One of the peculiar sensations of the *Gels.* heart is, that " *it will stop if he does not move*". It is so enfeebled that it has to be voluntarily jerked into action—that is the feeling, anyway.

> *Feels, " if she moves her heart will fail", is*
> *A pretty strong plea for* DIGITALIS ;
> *" Must keep on moving, or heart will stop,"*—
> GELSEMIUM *here comes out easily top ;*
> *While with* LOBELIA, *you'll hear her say,*
> *That " it's going to stop, whichever way".*
> *With a* CACTUS *heart, iron-band constriction*
> *(Chest, uterus, rectum, all share the fiction).*
> *Then* LACH. *has constriction on waking ;* ARS. A.
> *Gets constriction—oppression, on walking ; you'll play*
> TIGER LILY *to splendidly comfort her woe,*
> *Whose heart is alternately grasped and let go.*
> IODUM *has a heart simply squeezed and no more :*
> *The most violent hearts for* SPIGELIA *roar.*

By the way, it is well to get your Homœopathic Remedies from a Homœopathic Chemist, and a first-class one, at that. This applies especially to GELSEMIUM. A homœopathic chemist was explaining this to me years ago. Cheap homœopathic medicines are apt to be made from dried herbs, instead of the fresh plant at its best. He said, with *Gelsemium* the inferior tincture of the dried plant was almost inert, whereas, if you got a good preparation in the ϕ, a drop or two would make you collapse on the floor. Some of the involuntary provings of *Gels.* are most illuminating, as to its paralysing properties. Here is one, from Clarke's *Dictionary*. " J. H. Nankivell drank two ounces of tincture of *Gelsemium* instead of a glass of sherry. He walked a few feet with assistance and in another minute his legs were paralysed. He dragged himself to the bedside with his arms, but they were unable to help him to bed, into which he had to be lifted. As long as he lay quiet there was no trouble, but on the least exertion there were excessive tremors. Vomiting occurred in the next twenty-four hours. Temp. rose to 101.5° F. Heart's action was very violent and intermittent. . . . All the muscles of the eyes were affected. . . ."

Another case of Clarke's emphasizes the double vision. A patient took a drachm of the tincture for headache. On going out he could not tell which side of the street he was on. He was near St. Paul's Cathedral and saw two Cathedrals instead of one. It would appear to be not wise to take *Gels.* in the ϕ in these days, before facing the dangers of London's traffic !

Allen's black letter and characteristic symptoms :
*Dullness of mind, alleviated on profuse emission of watery urine.
Incapacity to think, or fix the attention.
Dizziness of head and blurred vision gradually increased, so that all objects appeared very indistinct. Head felt very light.
Heaviness of head alleviated on profuse emission of watery urine.
Sensitive bruised sensation of brain.*

*Drooping of the eyelids.
Difficulty in opening the eyelids, or in keeping them open.
Dimness of sight and vertigo.
Smoky appearance before the eyes, with pain above them.
Objects appeared double.*

*Heavy besotted face, flushed and hot to touch.
No control over lower jaw, it wagged sideways.
Numbness of tongue. Tongue so thick, he could hardly speak.
Tried to swallow, but he could not.*

Frequent emission of clear, limpid urine, with seeming relief to dullness and heaviness of head.

Severe, sharp labour-like pains in uterine region, extending to back and hips.

Irregular beating of heart. Palpitation of heart.
(Pulse markedly affected.)

Trembling in all the limbs.

Lost control of limbs, could not direct their movements with precision.

Fatigue of the lower limbs, after slight exercise.

Trembling and weakness (accompanying profuse urination).

Complete relaxation of the whole muscular system, with entire motor paralysis.

Listless and languid.

Easily fatigued, especially the lower limbs.

Weakness and trembling through the whole system.

Chilliness, especially along the spine.

GLONOINE—NITRO-GLYCERINE

GLONOINE—Nitro-glycerine—that highly explosive liquid, which, admixed with some porus earth forms the " deadly dynamite ",. to the shaking of earth and the blasting of rocks, lives up to its reputation, even when potentized and used in medicine ; retaining its alarming characters : its *suddenness*, its *bursting* sensations and pains, its *upward*-surgings which threaten to lift and shatter the cranium.

Chemistry is fascinating, if only for its psychology, if one may (mis)use the term. Of two deadly elements, in combination, she may form something quite harmless, even essential to life : whereas from such mild and kindly creatures as the *glycerine* of the toilet table so inert that it never even " goes bad ", and *nitrogen*, that colourless, tasteless, odourless gas, which, four-parts to one in mixture with the life-supporter, oxygen, modifies the properties of the latter in such sort that, instead of burning us out rapidly, we just get, with every breath, that happy admixture that supports life without hastening its destruction. That nitrogen and glycerine should combine to produce such a wildly intemperate blasting agent is incalculable—absolutely unforeseen till "discovered". But, as a great chemist once said, " no one could tell, *a priori*, how even a lump of sugar would behave when dropped into a cup of tea ". Science is the plodding daughter of Experiment : and, as such, Homœopathy is scientific.

Dr. HUGHES (*Pharmacodynamics*) points out that, though Old School uses *Glonoine*, having even adopted that name for it, yet medicine owes its introduction to Constantine Hering, Hahnemann's great disciple. But we notice that, as always, when using those violent medicinal substances, so often the most splendidly curative agents of Homœopathy, Old School has, perforce, to follow into the fantastic region of infinitesimals.

" *Nitro-glycerine was discovered by Sobrero in 1847, but none could be obtained for physiological experiment until Morris Davis, a Philadelphia chemist, in the same year, after long and laborious trials, under direction of Hering, succeeded to produce the substance in sufficient quantity for proving. It was extensively proven here and abroad (see Allen's "Encyclopedia") and the symptoms have received abundant clinical verification.*"—HERING'S "*Guiding Symptoms* "

A quaint little verification of the care and exactness with which the provings of homœopathic drugs have been observed and recorded comes to hand, most opportunely, even as we write. . . .

A certain physician, busy with rather urgent mental work, and worried by a sensation of fullness at the back of head and neck, —a miserable, incapacitating fullness—took a dose of *Glonoine*— a drug that, as we know, produces *such* fullness, and *there*. It was *Glonoine* 3, merely a couple of pilules, of the only preparation available, probably inert, discovered among a number of homœopathic medicines that had belonged to some one long since dead— (certainly 25 to 30·years).

Well, the headache soon went (*post or propter hoc ?*)—but a couple of days later, while busy with out-patient work, the doctor became suddenly conscious of an unpleasant numbness of the *left* hand, never felt before, and rather disconcerting. Presently this disappeared, but only to be succeeded by numbness of the lower lip,—the exact sensation felt when cocaine has been injected for tooth extraction. This also went : but only to return again and again, and yet again, first to left hand and then to lower lip : nowhere else : always absolutely limited. Before night these rather alarming sensations sent him to Kent's *Repertory* to find the remedy—should it be needed. And there he discovered, under "Numbness, lower lip", two drugs only " (*Calc.*), and *Glon.*" Then he turned to " Numbness of left hand ", to find several remedies : *Glon.* among them ! The sensation was satisfactorily accounted for : and was the more interesting because *Glon.* is not down as producing numbness of right hand, or of upper lip.

Black Letter Symptoms

Well-known streets seem strange : way home too long.
Disinclined to speak ; would hardly answer.

A distinct feeling of pulse in HEAD.
Throbbing in front of head.
Immediately a sensation as if head were too large.
Head felt enormously large.
Pressure and throbbing in temples.
Pressure and pain from within out in both temples.
Fullness in head, and throbbing without pain.
Head very full : pulse full and quick.
As if the blood were mounting to head.
As if he were hanging with head downwards, and as if there were a great rush of blood into head in consequence.
As if skull were too small ; and brain attempting to burst it.
Afraid to shake his head lest it drop to pieces.
Holds head with both hands ; presses sinciput.
Shocks in brain, synchronous with every pulsation of arteries.

Undulating sensation in head.

Throbbing in head : in temples : in temporal arteries which were raised and felt like whipcords.

Sensation of fullness, vertex and forehead.

Shaking the head increases the headache.

Headache on damp, rainy days ; after taking cold ; after much sitting, and mental exertion.

Red injected hot EYES *during headache, with wild expression.*

Throbbing pain in all the TEETH.

Throbbing in whole BODY.

Intense congestion of brain induced in plethoric constitutions by sudden SUPPRESSION OF MENSES, *or appearing instead of menses.*

Headaches occurring after profuse uterine hæmorrhage.

Rush of blood to head in pregnant women, with pale face and loss of consciousness.

Violent palpitation of HEART, *with throbbing carotids, pulsating headache in forehead and between temples.*

Blood seems to rush to heart and mount rapidly into head.

Epileptic CONVULSIONS, *with congestion to head and heart.*

Bad effects from being exposed immediately to SUN'S *rays.*

(In fever) flushes of heat : waves of heat upwards.

OTHER, ITALIC, OR QUEER SYMPTOMS

Recognized no one. Raved ; screamed ; wishes to rush from house. Jumped out of bed, but legs gave way.

Fears : throat swollen ; chest as if screwed together ; of approaching death ; of having been poisoned.

Bad effects of fear, fright, mechanical contusions and their later consequences.

Could not allow head to be level with body.

Confusion of ideas : could not tell where he was.

Loss of location : (a cured case), began ten years ago ; loses himself in streets he has travelled in for years. All right in regard to everything else.

In familiar street everything strange. Had to look about him every few minutes to convince himself he was in the right street.

Houses not in their right places, on the route he had traversed at least four times a day for four years.

Convulsions, falls down frothing at mouth, after alternations of palpitation of heart and congestions to the head.

Congestion to head, causes sensation of coldness every time.

Tight and choky feeling throat, like strangulation.

Skull too small ; as if brain attempting to burst skull.

As if head and neck laced in : clothing too tight.

Pain in wens on scalp, as of a thimble pressed firmly on them.

Every motion, side to side, increased the pain (in head), but motions backward and forward did not.

Headache : ceases in sleep : better in open air : lessened by drinking coffee, after a few hours : tea lessens it better.

Feels as if ice-cold sweat were on forehead, which is not there.

Rays of sun on head were not to be borne, and head would not allow hat to touch it.

Frightful headache : runs about room with head pressed between hands. As if head would burst : knocks it against wall.

Hyperæmia of brain caused by excessive cold or heat.

Bad consequences of cutting hair.

SUNSTROKE.

Said her eyes were falling out : felt as if someone were pulling them from within outwards.

Letters seem smaller : flashes of lightning, sparks, mist or black spots, whirling and confused vision.

Wild, staring look : protrusion of eyes.

Supra-orbital neuralgia, from 6 a.m. to 11 or 12.

Cold sweat on face during congestion to head.

Lower lip feels swollen. Numbness lower lip.

Chin feel elongated to knees : obliged to put hand to chin repeatedly to be sure this was not the case. (Prover had injured chin by a fall twenty years before.)

Tongue numb as if burnt ; prickling, stinging.

Constriction in throat as if throttled.

Wine aggravates all symptoms : alcoholic stimulants cause delirium, congestion, stupor.

Seasickness.

Faint, warm sickening sensation in chest and stomach, like threatening seasickness Giddiness.

Disturbances in intercranial circulation at menopause.

Flushes, etc., during climacteric.

Violent palpitation : feeling she would die : numbness whole of left arm. Pressure at heart as if it were being contracted.

Alternate congestion to heart and to head.

" As an intercurrent in angina pectoris, to prevent organism from getting accustomed to influence of *Aur. mur.*"

Hot sensation down back ; burning between scapulæ.

Old contusions and jars (to head and spine).

Knees give way in headache. Unsteady gait.

Knees and thighs knock together during headache.

Convulsions, with clenching and jerking upwards of fists and legs. During spasms spreads fingers and toes apart.

Convulsions, with especially left fingers spread apart.

Cannot protrude tongue in a straight line.

Restless sleep : wakes with fear of apoplexy.

Congestions ; blood tends upwards : vessels pulsate ; veins, jugular, temporal, enlarged.

Rapid deviations in distribution of blood. Useful as a substitute for bleeding.

Bad effects from mental excitement, fright, fear, mechanical contusions and their later consequences, from having hair cut, and from exposure to rays of sun.

Antidoted by ACON., *Camph., Coffea, Nux.*

Compare AMYL NITR., *Bell., Ferr., Gels., Natrum carb., Potas. nitr., Sod. nitr., Stram.*

As seen from above, the action of *Glonoine*, so local, so sudden, so definite, so alarming and torturing, and therefore so remedial is, once grasped, impossible to forget. In fact, it seems hardly worth writing about !

However we will run through what some of our great prescribers and writers have to say about it. This one emphasizes one point coinciding with his experience, that one another ; and so one learns.

HUGHES writes : "The name *Glonoin* was formed by its introducer into medical practice, Dr. C. Hering, out of the chemical formula (Gl O NO5) denoting its composition. Dr. Hering proved it on himself and others in 1848. . . ."

Hughes says, "the action of *Glonoin* lies within a very small compass. If any one will touch his tongue with a 5 per cent. solution, he will pretty certainly find in a few minutes that his pulse has increased by twenty, forty or even sixty beats. He may feel a throbbing all over his body, but will almost always experience it in his head, which will go on beating until a pretty violent bursting headache has developed itself. With this, there will be probably some giddiness, a sense of fullness in the head and at the heart, and one of constriction about the throat. . . . All this reminds us of *Amyl nitrite :* . . . but the effects of the two drugs are not identical. *Amyl* causes a general flushing without marked sense of throbbing . . . nor is the pulse much affected by it. It seems to have been demonstrated that *Amyl* produces its dilating effects on the arteries by directly paralysing their muscular coats . . . while *Glonoin* affects the nervous centres of the circulation, and is limited to this sphere."

Then he distinguishes between the action of *Glon.* and *Belladonna*. "With *Bell.*, the circulation within the cranium is excited because the brain is irritated ; with *Glon.*, the brain is irritated because the circulation is excited. It would be indicated in such hyperæmia as can be produced by excessive heat or cold, by strong emotions, by mechanical jarring, by suppression of the menses or other hæmorrhages and excretions."

He evidences not only *sunstroke*, but the striking benefit he has obtained from the drug in the distressing after-effects of sunstroke.

He says, " perhaps the greatest boon which Dr. Hering has conferred upon patients in introducing *Glon.* to medicine is the relief it gives to menstrual disturbances of the cerebral circulation . . . as the intense congestion of brain induced in plethoric constitutions by sudden suppression of the menses. *Glonoin* is an exquisite similimum here : for in one of Dr. Dudgeon's provers, who took it while the catamenia were present, these immediately ceased, and the headache went on increasing in violence till night. . . . It does not, like *Lachesis* or *Amyl nitrite*, act on the flushings of the climacteric ; but is most valuable when these are localized in the head."

He says, "it was the statement of its discoverer, Sobrero, that 'even a very small quantity placed on the tongue causes a violent headache of several hours' duration ', which led Dr. Hering to investigate its action. . . ."

The kind of headache—fullness, tension, throbbing, bursting—these are the phrases used by the provers to describe it. . . . It acts as rapidly in disease as in health.

He discusses its striking power of relieving paroxysms of neuralgia, even in some cases, permanently curing.

GUERNSEY epitomizes *Glonoine*, and its uses. " Troubles from heat of the head in type-setters, in men who work under a gas-light steadily, so that heat falls on the head : bad results from sunstroke ; *can't bear any heat about the head ;* can't walk in the sun, must walk in the shade or carry an umbrella ; can't bear heat from a stove ; great vertigo from assuming an upright posture from rising up in bed, rising from a seat. Heat in head ; throbbing headache."

Patient feels lost, or strange even in familiar street or surroundings. Things look strange and unfamiliar.

NASH. One of our great head medicines. He says he used to carry *Glon.* 1 in his case, for those inclined to sneer at the young doctor and his sweet medicine. He seldom failed to convince, in five to ten minutes, that there was power here : for a drop on the tongue produced the characteristic throbbing headache. No one ever asked for more proof of the power of homœopathic medicine.

(One remembers a young woman doctor at the " New ", as the

Elizabeth Garrett Anderson Hospital was then called, who described the terrible headache from touching her tongue with some preparation of nitro-glycerine.)

The pains of *Belladonna* are sudden in onset, and suddenly gone : those of *Glonoine* are even more so.

Nash says that " *Glonoine* is better adapted to the first, congestive stage of inflammatory diseases of the brain : *Belladonna* goes farther, and may still be the remedy after the inflammatory stage is fully initiated." Neither can stand the least jar. But pain " waves " upsurging, are absolutely characteristic of *Glon.*

FARRINGTON emphasizes that the keynote to the whole symptomatology of the drug is expressed in this one sentence : " *a tendency to sudden and violent irregularities of the circulation.*" With that, he says, we can easily work out the other symptoms.

" *Glon.* is a drug that acts very quickly and very violently ; the throbbing (head) is not a mere sensation, it is an actual fact. It really seems that the blood vessels would burst, so violent is the action of the drug. . . . The blood seems to surge in one great current up the spine and into the head. The external jugulars look like tortuous cords, the carotids throb violently and are hard, tense and unyielding to pressure. The face is deep red. This throbbing is either associated with dull, distressing aching, or with sharp, violent pains."

" Sunstroke . . . also we find *Glon.* to be our best remedy for the effects of heat, whether the trouble arises from the direct rays of the sun, from hot weather, or from working in the intense heat of a furnace, as in the case of foundrymen and machinists. These effects are not confined to the head, but involve the whole body, and we note oppression of breathing, with palpitation of the heart and nausea and vomiting . . . the nausea not gastric, but cerebral . . . a horrible, sunken feeling in the epigastrium and often, too, diarrhœa. . . . Eyes too large and protrude as though bursting out of the head . . . eye diseases from exposure to very bright light . . . blood vessels of retina distended, or, in extreme cases, apoplexy of the retina. . . . Admirable remedy for puerperal convulsions : full, hard pulse, and albuminuria. . . ."

"Well-known streets seem strange to the patient (*Petroleum*). Suppose a person, subject to apoplectic congestions, is suddenly seized in the streets with one of these, and does not know where he is, then *Glonoin* is the remedy for him."

" Bad effects of fear (*Opium*). Horrible apprehension, and sometimes the fear of being poisoned."

"Then, trauma. An excellent ren .y for pains and other abnormal sensations, following late after local injuries : the part pains, or feels sore ; or an old scar breaks out again."

He, also, contrasts *Bell.* and *Glon.* " because they meet in the congestions and inflammations of the brain with children and old persons. They divide the honours here."

BELL.	GLON.
Cri encephalique.	Less marked.
Worse bending head backwards.	Better bending head backwards.
Head feels enormously large.	. . .
Better for uncovering head.	Better from covering head.
Better open air.	

We will end by extracting some of KENT'S most graphic little flashes; even where there is repetition, that merely serves to emphasize and drive the facts in.

"Surging of blood to heart and head. As if all the blood in the body were rushing round the heart : a surging in head ; a warm, glowing sensation in head ; or intense glowing from stomach or chest up to head, at times with loss of consciousness. . . . Wave-like sensations, as if skull were lifted and lowered ; expanded and contracted. Intense pain, therewith, as if head would burst. Great throbbing : beating of hammers ; every pulsation painful. Even fingers and toes pulsate. . . ."

"Head is relieved in open air: worse in warmth, often relieved by cold. Worse lying. Worse head low. Extremities cold, pale and perspiring, head hot, face flushed and purple or bright red. Mouth dry; eyelids dry, stick to eyeballs. All degrees of confusion to unconsciousness."

"Sunstroke . . . sudden congestions of head. . . . Cold feels good to head ; heat feels good to extremities. When lower limbs are covered with clothing in a cool room, and windows open, convulsions are relieved, and patient breathes more easily."

"In apoplexy, such medicines as *Opium* and *Glonoine* relieve the blood pressure when the symptoms agree. . . . They equalize the circulation, and the patient may not die."

"If sitting up, you will often see a *Glonoine* patient with both hands pressing upon the head with all the power possible until the arms are perfectly exhausted. Wants it bandaged, or a tight cap. . . . *Worse from wine, and worse from lying down.* You will be astonished to know how long a *Glonoine* patient will sit without moving a muscle, because motion is so painful. Whole crown of head feels as if covered by a hot iron, as if an oven were close by. . . . ."

GRAPHITES

(Black-lead)

HAHNEMANN gives us this valuable remedy ; in his *Chronic Diseases*, Vol. III. He says :

" Pulverize one grain of the purest black-lead taken from a fine English pencil, and prepare the triturations and dilutions in the usual fashion. One or two pellets of the 30th potency are sufficient for a dose.

" Pure *Graphites* is a sort of mineral carbon with a slight admixture of iron which cannot be regarded as one of the necessary constituents of that mineral." He calls it diamond transformed.

He tells us how a German doctor saw workmen in a looking-glass factory using *Graphites* externally for removing herpetic eruptions . . . " we go a little farther and employ *Graphites* as an anti-psoric, whether herpes be or be not one of the symptoms of the (non-venereal) disease."

It was proved, at first, by himself and three other provers.

Graphites affects especially the ears, the skin, the nails : and Guernsey says " it is especially useful for females with a tendency to unhealthy corpulence, with perhaps deformed nails, characteristic exudation, menstrual troubles, etc."

NASH gives one of his brilliant little pen-pictures of *Graph.* :

" Eruptions on skin, oozing out a thick, honey-like fluid.

" Mucous outlets : eyelids inflamed, with pustules : ears discharge : moist sore places behind ears : mouth cracked in corners : anus, eruptions, itching, fissured.

" Nails grow thick, cracked, out of shape.

" Constipation : stools knotty, large lumps united by mucous threads.

" Diarrhœa : stools brown liquid, mixed with undigested substances of an intolerably fœtid odour.

" Sad, despondent : weeps : thinks of nothing but death.

" Especially adapted to persons inclined to obesity, particularly females who delay menstruation.

" Hears better in a noise. . . .

" Sensation of cobweb on face : tries hard to brush it off."

He gives cases—eczema on legs of an old, obese woman :— *Sulphur cm.* brought out a rash all over body which exuded a glutinous, sticky fluid. A dose of *Graph. cm.* cured the eczema and " left skin as smooth as that of a child ". A child of three had eczema capitis, cured with local treatment, and followed by a very obstinate entero-colitis. The child was greatly emaciated, etc., and the stools were brown fluid mixed with undigested food, and of an intolerably fœtid odour. Nash cured it rapidly with *Graph. 6m.*

In eczema of lids he contrasts *Graph.* with *Sulph.* In *Graph.* the eruption is moist and the fissured margins of lids are covered with scales and crusts. *All the orifices under Sulph. are very red.* . . . Old, hard cicatrices soften up and go away under its action, especially those left by abscesses of the mammæ.

He says in conclusion, *Graphites* cures complaints of many *kinds*, when you have present two things.

First. *The peculiar tendency to obesity.*

Second. *The characteristic glutinous eruptions.*

In regard to the action of *Graphites* on *scar tissue*, which we have more than once verified, we would like to quote, rather at length, from KENT ; because in the latest edition of his *Lectures*, this paragraph seems to have unaccountably disappeared.

He says, speaking of *Graphites*, " In this low state of nutrition, and poor blood-making, the repairs of the economy are badly performed, and hence cicatrices are of a low grade and contract and indurate. Old scars cause much trouble in this remedy. They have a tendency to cause induration and knots. Think of *Graphites* when you come across women who have had abscesses in the breast several years before, and now the flow of milk is beginning for the new-born child, and there is a threatened abscess on the site of an old one, or there is an inflammation of the breast, at the site of an old cicatrice, with a nodular induration, sensitive and painful, while the rest of the breast is soft and normal. The cicatricial tissue was not good, it was of a low grade and it has steadily grown more indurated, and now those indurations are forming little strictures, as it were, and blocking up the flow of milk. *Graph.* will very often stop this induration, remove the hardness from the old cicatrice and make the patient comfortable. If you know a woman who is suffering from an old scar that has formed a lump, when she is about to go into confinement give a dose of *Graphites* as a general remedy, unless some other special remedy is called for . . ."

Kent notices that the eruptions of *Graphites*, besides being glutinous are apt to occur on flexor surfaces, in the bends (*Sepia*) of elbows—groins—popliteal spaces—behind ears, in corners of mouth, and in the canthi. But it has eruptions on other places— as *crusta lactea* : crusts ooze a liquid fluid that lifts them up : sometimes offensive (*Mez.*).

Kent says *Graphites* is a " very long-acting, useful and valuable remedy ".

In scar tissue, one remembers two cases in particular, where the effect of *Graphites* was dramatic : in each case it was the *cm.* that was given. A girl with a stiff elbow after inflammation (so far as I remember it had been rheumatic). She had had the adhesions broken down, but they recurred, and she again presented herself a year later. She got *Graphites*, and in a month's time the elbow was found to be freely movable. The other was the liberation of a little finger, contracted and immovable after inflammation.

We are told, " *Graphites is fat, chilly, costive.* It acts best where there is a tendency to obesity."

In our out-patient department one finds *Graphites* in high potency to have a remarkable effect upon obese elderly women. Farrington says, " This obesity is not the healthy solid flesh of the full-blooded, strong, hearty ; but the kind of fat of *Calc. c.*, showing improper nutrition."

He also gives these points, " Always cold, in and out of doors.

" With *Ferrum*, a rush of blood to head with flushing face. A shock about heart, and blood rushes to face.

" Patient anæmic.; mucous membranes pale, as in *Ferr.**

" Blepharitis, thickened lids, esp. edges, which are covered with scurf or scales.

"The blepharitis is worse in the angles of the eyes, in the canthi. There is a tendency for the lids to crack and bleed : if that is present you need not hesitate to use *Graphites*.

" Eyelashes become wild : turn inwards towards the ball of eye, and irritate the conjunctiva. Hardened styes. Double vision.

" Some symptoms like *Calcarea ;* but *Calc.* has sweat of head and cold damp feet (not prominent with *Graph.*).

" *Arsenicum* is provokingly like *Graph. :* only with *Ars.* the lids are spasmodically closed.

" *Sulph.* has edges of lids red : those of *Graphites* are pale."

And in regard to cicatrices he says, " It was long noticed that in workers on *Graphites*, wounds on hands healed and cicatrices disappeared very rapidly. In a case of cicatrices on eye which formed and contracted after operation *Graph.* relieved and the parts resumed their normal position."

---

* *These symptoms are interesting in view of the " admixture of iron " in the drug.* Graphites, *with* Ferr., *is " better walking in the open air "* (Puls.—*which also has iron in its make-up*).

We know of three " scar tissue " remedies—each according to its indications : *Drosera*, *Silica* and *Graphites*. No doubt other remedies will also do the trick, where indicated.

Graphites is one of the remedies for psoriasis palmaris.

Graphites has great value in gastric, or duodenal ulcer. As a matter of fact, it is here that we have most often employed the drug, and we have published case after case in back numbers of HOMŒOPATHY illustrating its successful use. Its indications here are very definite, and no other drug, so far as we know, has just that little complex of symptoms. . . .

Stomach pain relieved by food or drink.

Relieved by hot food or drink.

Relieved by lying down.

When one gets such little drug-complexes into one's head, prescribing becomes quick, easy, and sure. *Graphites* has even cured cancer ; and of the intestine.

One of the rivals of *Graphites* here is the little-proved remedy *Ornithogalum* (Star of Bethlehem—" allied to Garlic "). We have seen its great value in gastric ulcer, even with severe hæmoptysis : and it has cured cancer of the stomach (see Clarke's Dictionary).

The chief indications for *Ornithogalum* are great distension of stomach ; belching offensive flatus, must loosen clothes (*Lyc.*) : agonies of pain : relief (also) from warm food, but instead of the *Graph*, relief from lying, *Ornith*. is far worse at night. There may be a sensation " as if a bag of water turns, when she turns over in bed ". *Ornith*. has also " hateful depression and desire for suicide ".

BLACK LETTER SYMPTOMS

Sadness, with thoughts of nothing but death.

Despondent. Feels miserable, unhappy.

Apprehensiveness, with inclination to weep. Music makes her weep.

Pain as if HEAD *were numb and pithy.*

Pain as if constricted, esp. occiput.

Falling of hair of scalp. Itching on scalp.

Much scaliness of head, which causes distressing itching and becomes a scurf, which disappears on washing and then is humid.

Eruptions on vertex, painful to touch and humid.

Eczema capitis of entire scalp, forming massive dirty crusts which mat the hair. Painful and sore to touch.

Falling out of hair of scalp.

EYES : *Very inflamed margins of lids.*
Inflammation of the external canthi. Sore and fissured : bleed easily. Edges of lids much inflamed. Dry mucus on lashes.

Deafness : hears better in a noise, or riding in carriage.
Moist and sore places behind both EARS.

Soreness in NOSE *on blowing it.*
Nose painful internally. Dryness of nose. Nose stopped with badly smelling mucus.
Dry scabs in nose, with sore, cracked and ulcerated nostrils.
Smell abnormally acute : cannot tolerate flowers.

Constant sensation of cobweb on FACE.
Soreness and cracking of lips and nostrils, as from cold.

Burning blisters on lower side and tip of TONGUE.
Taste of rotten eggs which nauseates.

Constrictive pains in STOMACH *; better eating.*
Aversion to animal food : to fish : to cooked food.
Sweet things are disgusting and nauseous.

Burning pains radiate through ABDOMEN.   *Heaviness in abdomen.*
Great distension of abdomen.
Full abdomen as from accumulation and incarceration of flatus.
Pain in upper abdomen.
Hardness in region of liver.

Smarting sore pain in ANUS *on wiping it.*
Itching in anus.
Stools brown, fluid, with undigested substances : of intolerable odour.
Stool dark-coloured, half digested, of an intolerable odour.
Stool lumpy, conjoined with threads of mucus.
Sticking in anus (with hard stool and much urging).
Discharge of mucus from rectum.
Hæmorrhoids with burning rhagades at anus.

URINE *becomes turbid and deposits white sediment.*

Profuse leucorrhœa of very white mucus : acrid : excoriating.
Itching of pudenda before menstruation.
Menstruation delayed.

Hard cicatrices remaining after mammary abscess, retarding flow of milk.

Cancer of mammae, from old cicatrices, which had remained after repeated abscesses.

Constriction of CHEST *as if too narrow.*

Painful swollen GLANDS *at sides of neck.*

Soreness high up between the thighs.
Smarting soreness between the nates.

The SKIN *of hands is hard and cracked in several places.*
Finger nails become thick : become black.
Eruptions in the corner of the mouth.
Itching pimples on the face, become moist after scratching.
Itching eruptions full of corrosive water in many parts of the body.
Itching and moist eruptions on scrotum.
Cracks and fissures ends of fingers, nipples, labial commissures, of anus, between toes, etc.
Eruptions behind ears, oozes a sticky fluid.
Eczema, with profuse serous exudations ; in blondes inclined to obesity.

Numbness and deadness, with coldness of fingers, extending as far as middle of upper arm.
Weak exhaustion of whole body.
Cataleptic conditions : conscious but without power to move or speak.
Emaciation of suffering parts. (Plumb.)

HEPAR SULPHURIS

Hepar is a medicine that has its place in even the smallest of homœopathic domestic medicine cases : it is one of the nursery medicines for colds—coughs—croup—glands, etc.

Hahnemann's *Hepar Sulphuris Calcareum* is prepared according to his directions : " a mixture of equal parts of finely powdered oyster shells and quite pure flowers of sulphur, kept for ten minutes at a white heat." From this our potencies, are prepared.

Hepar is a powerful medicine, affecting both mind and body : a first-class irritant of temper—nerves and tissues : till the prover is distraught by a word—a touch—a breath of air—so hypersensitive is he to environment physical and mental. And, of course, it is just this touchiness and hypersensitiveness that provide a valuable clue to the employment of *Hepar* in many diseases.

Until the inwardness of the two drugs is grasped, there is a great tendency to use *Hepar* for *Silica*, and *Silica* for *Hepar* : they have so many points of resemblance. They both affect skin, glands, suppurations, till, in treating an abscess one is apt to think, " H'm ? *Silica* ? *Hepar* ? "—as if it were a mere toss-up between them.

They both have unhealthy skin, which festers instead of healing. One sees this so often in the children that come to the Out-Patient Department of our Hospital, where one or other according to symptoms, cures. They both have sticking pains— as the fish-bone or splinter sensation in throat, more especially *Hepar*. (*Arg. nit.*, *Kali carb.*, *Nit.-ac.* have this also.) In both, with the unhealthy skin every little injury suppurates. Both are chilly : but here they part company : because *Hepar* is *better in wet weather*—better in warm wet weather : while *Silica* suffers in wet weather—from wet feet, from *cold wet weather ;* and is better when it is *warm and dry*. Both perspire profusely : *Silica* (with *Calcarea*) has profuse head sweats at night, and its foot sweats are apt to be very offensive : the intolerable " smelly feet " that one comes across : also offensive axillary sweat : while *Hepar* has sour, profuse general sweats night and day which do not relieve.

So alike are these two remedies, *Silica* and *Hepar*, that the one may be used to antidote the other, as when a blunder in prescribing has been made, and *Silica* has been given after *Mercury* with alarming recrudescence of the bad symptoms : then *Hepar* comes in and " straightens things out ". We have seen this !*

Both have swellings, inflammations and suppuration of all the glands of the body : but the gland suppurations of *Hepar* are sudden and rapid : while those of *Silica* are slow, and very slow to heal—*till Silica is administered.*

The discharges of *Hepar* are offensive : smelling (characteristically) of old cheese ; ulcers very offensive, smelling like old cheese, and very sensitive. *Hepar* has horribly offensive leucorrhœa, " the odour can be detected when she enters the room " : while the *Silica* " smelly " feet leave their aroma in all the rooms and passages through which their unfortunate owner has passed.

" *Hepar* promotes and regulates suppuration in a remarkable manner (second only to *Silica*) but is generally required at an earlier stage than *Silica.*" (Farrington.)

But the genius of the two remedies is dissimilar, because their mentalities are as wide as the poles.

Silica, with its want of self-confidence ; its lack of " grit " ; its timidity ; its sufferings from anticipation—as when having to appear in public. . . .

Hepar—sensitive beyond all bounds of reason : Irritable— impetuous. Sensitive to draughts ; to air ; ulcers so sensitive that they cannot bear the lightest touch (*Lach.*) ; sensitive mentally—even to sudden murderous impulses.

Nash says of *Hepar:* "Its strongest characteristic is HYPER-SENSITIVENESS to *touch, pain* and *cold air.*

" The patient is so sensitive to pain, that she faints away, even when it is slight.

" If there is inflammation or swelling in any locality, or even eruptions on the skin, they are so sensitive that she cannot bear to have them touched, or even to have the cold air blow on them. . . . This supersensitiveness to pain runs all through the drug. It is mental as well as physical, for the slightest cause irritates, with hasty speech and vehemence.

"Next to this is the power of *Hepar sulph.* over the suppurative stage of local inflammations. It comes in only when pus is about to form, or is already formed. If it is given very high before pus is formed, and not repeated too soon or often, we may prevent suppuration and check the whole inflammatory process. But if pus is already formed, it will hasten the pointing

* " *It is well known to physicians that Merc. is not followed well by Silica. Sil. does not do useful work when Merc. is still acting, or has been acting. Sil. follows well after Hepar, and Hepar follows well after Merc. and thus Hepar becomes an intercurrent in that series of medicines.*" KENT.

and discharge and help along the healing of the ulcer afterwards.
. . . The most rapid pointing, opening and perfect healing
I ever saw was in the case of a large glandular swelling in the
neck of a child, under the action of the c.m. potency. *Hepar*
has a general tendency to suppuration, for even the eruptions on
the skin are liable to form matter, and slight injuries suppurate
(*Sil., Graph., Merc., Petrol.*)."

In regard to "skins" H. C. Allen (*Keynotes*) supplies a valuable tip. "The skin eruptions of *Sulphur* are dry, itching, and
not sensitive to touch; while in *Hepar* the skin is unhealthy,
suppurating, moist, and intensely sensitive to touch."

But *Hepar* also has its sphere in the respiratory system, and
in the nerves connected with the respiratory system.

It is one of the celebrated "Boenninghausen's Croup Powders",
sold for many years in our chemists' shops under that name :—
a packet of five powders, all in the 200th potency : they were
numbered, *Aconite, Spongia, Hepar, Spongia, Hepar* (should
so many be required to cut short the attack). Anyone acquainted
with these alarming attacks, a bolt from the blue in the middle
of the night, will see the appropriateness of the remedies. . . .
Aconite, sudden difficulty of breathing in the night, with the
Aconite fear and terror, after a chill from a cold, dry wind.
Spongia. Hoarseness : difficulty of drawing the breath, as if
a cork were sticking in the larynx, and the breath could not
penetrate through the narrowed orifice of the larynx. *Hepar*,
suffocative cough, excited not by tickling, but by tightness of the
breath ; dry, deep cough, from suffocation when breathing. Also
" Springing from bed, crying for help, felt that he could not get his
breath."

Hahnemann says that "Homœopathy has found the most
remarkable remedial employment of Roasted sponge" (*Spongia
tosta—Spongia*), "in that frightfully acute disease membranous
croup . . . The local inflammation, however, should first
be diminished or removed by the exhibition of an extremely
small dose of *Aconite*. The accessory administration of a small
dose of *Hepar sulphuris* will seldom be found necessary." And
in a footnote he adds, "The smaller the drug-doses in acute
and in the most acute diseases, the more quickly do they effect
their action." (*Mat. Med. Pura*—"*Spongia*".)

Hepar sweats with the cough. Weeps with, or before the
cough. Cough from the least exposure of any part of the person
to cold—to air—to draught. Breathing is rattling, anxious,
wheezing (in bronchitis) even to threatened suffocation—
almost asthmatic. In asthma, Nash contrasts *Hepar* with

Natrum sulph. with this diagnostic difference, which is very valuable : *Hepar* is worse in dry cold weather and better in damp : *Natrum sulph.* exactly the opposite of this :—extremely sensitive to damp. Nash says : " There is no other remedy that I know that has the amelioration so strongly in damp weather."

Hepar is a great remedy for ears and for threatening mastoid troubles. One remembers one's first acquaintance with *Hepar* in this connection. A child with offensive ear discharge . . . a hesitation—? *Merc.*—? *Puls.* ? But a doctor-woman who had learnt her Homœopathy in India under Dr. Younan, a great prescriber, suggested *Hepar*—which personally one would not have, *then*, thought of, and a dose of *Hepar* 200 had an amazing effect on the case. It is thus that one learns Materia Medica ! And one remembers another, later, ear case, during the war, when surgical persons were not " as common as pilchards at Loo ", as Kipling might put it. It was a girl with a very high temperature who came to Casualty one day, with ear trouble, and a tender—very tender, mastoid. She got *Hepar cm* and when she reported a day (or a couple of days) later it was no case of handing her over for surgery, because the whole thing had absolutely subsided in the most astonishing way.

Again, one does not usually think of *Hepar* for gastric ulcer. But one case, with a recent history of hæmatemesis, and a craving (surely unusual in that disease) for vinegar and pickles, cured up rapidly under *Hepar*, which has that craving. (The remedy had to be repeated once later, after an attack of flu.)

We will go to KENT for a few more hints in regard to *Hepar*.

" *Hepar* sometimes is bad for the occulist. When it is indicated, it cures eyes very quickly, so that the oculist does not have a very long case, and it does away with the necessity for washes in the hands of the specialist. . . . Offensive, purulent discharge " (*Arg. nit.*). " Inflammation with little ulcers " (*Tub.*, etc.) . . .

" A very important sphere for *Hepar* is after mercurialization. Syphilitic affection : ulcers of soft palate and osseous portions of roof of mouth . . . (*Nit. a.*). But everywhere the ' stick sensation ', the offensiveness, and the extreme tenderness.

" Sweating all night without relief belongs to a great many complaints of *Hepar*.

" Inspiring cold air will increase the cough and putting the hand out of bed will increase the pain in the larynx or cough. Putting the hand or foot out of bed is a general aggravation of all the complaints of *Hepar*."

" The mind takes part in this oversensitiveness, and manifests itself by a state of extreme irritability. Every little thing that disturbs the patient makes him intensely angry and abusive and impulsive. The impulses will overwhelm him and make him wish to kill his best friend in an instant. Impulses also that are without cause sometimes crop out in *Hepar* "—impulses to do violence . . . to burn, to . . . destroy . . . "

BLACK LETTER SYMPTOMS.

Constant pressive pain in one half of brain, as from a plug or nail (Thuja).

Epistaxis (Vipera, etc.).

Great swelling of the upper lip.

Sticking in throat as from a splinter on swallowing, and extending towards the ear on yawning.

Great desire for vinegar.

Nausea.

Abdomen distended, tense.

Buboes, abscesses of inguinal glands.

Stool soft, yet passed with great exertion.

Clay-coloured stool.

Urging to stool, but the large intestines are wanting in peristaltic action, and cannot expel the fæces which are not hard ; only a portion of which can be forced out by help of abdominal muscles.

Very difficult passage of scanty, not hard, fæces, with much urging.

Micturition impeded : obliged to wait before the urine passes, and then it flows slowly.

He is never able to finish urinating ; it seems as if some urine always remains behind in bladder.

Weakness of bladder ; urine drops vertically down, and he is obliged to wait awhile before any passes.

Paroxysms of cough, as from taking cold, with excessive sensitiveness of the nervous system, as soon as only the slightest portion of the body becomes cold.

Dyspnœa.

Abscess of axillary glands.

Bruised pain in anterior muscles of thigh.

Swelling of knee.

Drawing pain in limbs.

Cracked lines and chaps in hands and feet.

The ulcer bleeds on being merely gently wiped.

Eroding pain in ulcer.

Sensitiveness to open air.

At night the pains are worst.

Dreams of fire.

Night sweat.

Unhealthy, suppurating skin ; even slight injuries maturate and suppurate.

Soreness and moisture in folds between scrotum and thigh.

Perspires easily on every, even slight motion.

Catarrhal fever with great sensitiveness of skin to touch, and to the slightest cold.

Constant offensive exhalations from the body.

Among Hahnemann's symptoms are these other peculiar ones which may prove diagnostic :

The slightest thing put him into a violent passion, and he could have murdered anyone without hesitation.

Cross : and had such weakness of memory that he required three or four minutes to remember anything, and when at work thoughts often left him all at once.

In the evening frightful anxiety ; thought he must be ruined, and was sad to that degree that he could have killed himself.

In the morning after waking, he had the visionary appearance of a deceased person, which frightened him ; also imagined he saw a neighbouring house in flames, which terrified him.

When the smallest member becomes cool, there immediately occurs a cough, as from a chill and oversensitiveness of nervous system.

Suffocative cough, excited by tightness of breath.

At night, from 11 to 12, violent cough.

Before midnight he sprang out of sleep, full of anxiety, called for help, felt he could not get his breath. (Hepar is one of the great croup medicines.)

Even small wounds and slight injuries suppurate, will not heal, and become ulcers.

Hahnemann says : " *Belladonna* removes many of the sufferings caused by *Hepar*, where the symptoms correspond."

HERING (*Guiding Symptoms*) has put in black type a few more *Hepar* symptoms as being particularly diagnostic.

Purulent conjunctivitis, with profuse discharge and excessive sensitiveness to air and touch.

Gums and mouth very painful to touch, bleed easily.

Mercurio-syphilitic diseases of gums.

Hasty speech and hasty drinking.

Chronic tonsillitis, especially when accompanied by hardness of hearing.

Is never able to finish urinating, it seems as if some urine always remains behind in bladder.

Larynx sensitive to cold air.

Croup, after exposure to dry cold winds.

Croupy cough, with rattling in chest but no expectoration.

Paroxysms of cough, with excessive sensitiveness of nervous system, as soon as the slightest portion of body becomes cold.

Coughs when any part of the body is uncovered.

Tenacious mucus.

Habitual bronchial catarrhs, with loud rattling of mucus.

Pulmonary abscess, empyema, pyothorax.

Great chilliness in open air.

Ailments from cold, dry wind.

Cannot bear to be uncovered. Desires to be covered even in a warm room.

Sensitiveness to open air, with chilliness and frequent nausea.

Sweats easily by every, even slight motion.

Cold clammy, often sour, offensive sweat.

HYOSCYAMUS NIGER

(Henbane)

Hyoscyamus is said to be especially poisonous to fowls : hence its name. Some animals eat it, especially the young shoots, with impunity : but its effects even here are more or less purgative.

Hahnemann tells us that, when dried, the plant loses a great portion of its medicinal powers. But this is the case with many of the plant remedies : one needs to employ a competent homœo-pathic chemist always, in prescribing.

Old school uses *Hyoscyamus* and *Hyoscine* as " cerebral depressants, in acute mania, delirium tremens, febrile delirium and insomnia, sometimes with good results. They are mostly used in asylum practice ". The drug is also " put in to stop griping when Aloes, etc., are used for purgation ".

Poisonings, provings and experience of *Hyoscyamus* show its very definite range of action, also its striking resemblances to its natural relations, *Belladonna* and *Stramonium*. But it is, all through, easily distinguished from them.

In DELIRIUM it has its own peculiar features. Like *Bell.* it causes and cures cases with " increased cerebral activity ",. but with *Hyos.*, unlike *Bell.*, they are non-inflammatory in type. One peculiar symptom belongs pre-eminently to *Hyos.* : " desire to uncover." In INSANITY *Hyos.* may act as a mountebank, grimacing and making ridiculous gestures, and displaying a " comical alienation of mind "—or displaying a horrible " lasci-vious mania ", all its own. " In FEVERS the *Hyos.* patients throw the bedclothes off not because they are too warm, but because they will not remain covered." " A keynote for *Hyoscyamus* in fevers is, that the patient will not remain covered." (Later on we will quote KENT, who discusses this question.)

And here, in regard to *Hyos.* in fevers, we cannot do better than quote from Hahnemann's description of an epidemic of war typhus in Leipsic in 1813 (the year before Waterloo) where he treated 183 cases, " of which not one died ".

If the case had gone beyond *Bryonia* and *Rhus*, into its second period of delirium (" a metastasis of the whole disease upon the mental organs ") " the patient ceases to complain of his symptoms, he is hot, does not desire to drink, does not know whether to take this or that, does not know those about him, he abuses them, makes irrelevant answers, talks nonsense with open eyes, does foolish things, wishes to run away, cries aloud or whines, without being able to say why he does so, has a rattling in the throat, the countenance is distorted, the eyes squinting, he plays with his hands, behaves like a madman, passes the excrements unconsciously, etc. . . . Should the disease pass into that stage of delirium and mania, the *Hyoscyamus niger* meets all the indications of the case." A still later, third stage, of practical paralysis, mental and physical, may need the *Sweet Spirits of Nitre*, he tells us. N.B.—We reproduced in HOMŒOPATHY, July 1935, this most interesting description of Hahnemann's successful treatment of the terrible epidemic that followed the Wars of Napoleon. It is well worth studying.

*   *   *

The CHOREIC symptoms of *Hyoscyamus* are definite enough and unmistakable. " Every muscle of the body twitches, from the eyes to the toes." " Constant state of erethism : not a single part of the whole body, nor a solitary muscle in a quiet state for a moment. Convulsive motions. Spasms : spasms clonic."

The *Hyoscyamus* chorea, unlike " the gyratory motions of *Stram.*" has the coarse angular jerks that hurl the patient about, and make a pitiful little object look in danger of turning herself inside out with a jerk, when told to put out her tongue. Hughes speaks also of " *local chorea* "—squinting, stammering, twitchings of face.

*   *   *

In the EPILEPSY of *Hyos.* there is, before the fit, vertigo, ringing in ears, sparks before eyes, gnawing hunger : during the fit, face purple, eyes projecting, shrieks, grinding teeth and enuresis : followed by sopor and snoring. *Bell.* has *spasms of larynx and clutching of throat* during fit. In *Stram.* there is *risus sardonicus*, and quick thrustings of head to the right. *Stram.* has also " a stupid friendly look ".

Of course *Hyoscyamus* is " beautifully homœopathic " to DELIRIUM TREMENS, and to HYDROPHOBIA. We will quote at length a footnote of Hahnemann's (*Materia Medica Pura*— *Hyoscyamus*). He tells us that :—

For some cases of hydrophobia *Belladonna* is curative, for some *Stramonium*, while for others (according to the symptoms he enumerates), *Hyoscyamus*. " *Bell.*", he says, " has already effected some perfect cures, and would have done this more frequently, had not either other interposing remedies been administered at the same time, or, and especially, had it not been given in such enormous doses that the patients were killed by the remedy." He adds, what is interesting and important, in italics :

" Large doses of drugs, homœopathically suitable, are much more certainly injurious than such as are given without any similar (homœopathic) relation to the disease, or such as have an opposite (antipathic) relation to the case, that is to say, are quite unsuitable (allopathic). In the homœopathic employment of medicines, where the totality of the morbid symptoms has a great similarity to the action of a drug, it is really criminal not to give quite small doses, indeed as small as possible. In such cases the doses of the size prescribed in the routine practice become real poisons and murderous agents. Convinced by a thousand-fold experience, I assert this of the homœopathic employment of medicines universally and *invariably*, particularly when the disease is acute ; and this is especially true of the employment of *Belladonna, Stramonium*, and *Hyoscyamus* in hydrophobia. So let it not be said, ' One of these three medicines was given in the strongest doses, and not too seldom, but every two or three hours, and yet the patient died.' ' *That was precisely the reason* ', I reply with firm conviction, ' *that was precisely the reason why the patient died, and you killed him.*' Had you let him take the smallest portion of a drop of the quintillion-fold or decillion-fold attenuation of the juice of one of these plants for a dose (in rare cases repeating the dose after three or four days) then the patient would have been easily and *certainly saved.*"

Here is an accidental proving of *Hyoscyamus* :

A doctor tells how he once gave to a woman with hysterical paralysis, who had been in bed a month, an injection of Hyoscine $\frac{1}{50}$th of a grain. She got up in ten minutes, ran round and round the room as if intoxicated, shrieking with laughter ; jumped into bed, shrieking with laughter, and jumped out the other side : couldn't be kept in bed. Next day she could remember nothing—only knew that she had been doing something foolish. Then she went slowly back to her old state.

*   *   *

" *Hyoscyamus* is a drug of strikingly alternating symptoms. As,—The calls to stool and frequent evacuations of henbane are alternating actions with the delayed stool and absence of call thereto : but the former appears to be the principal primary action. Hahnemann indeed senses a two-fold alternating action : ' much urging with rare evacuations :—and more frequent evacuation with rarer calls :—with little or no evacuation, also with more frequent evacuations. But the frequent urging with the scanty and rare evacuations is the principal alternating action.' "*

Again,—" The excitation of the bladder to urinate and its loss of irritability—the scanty flow of urine and the copious diuresis are in henbane alternating actions, so that much urging to urinate with scanty and copious flow of urine—as also inactivity of the bladder with scanty and very copious secretion of urine may be present at the same time; but much urging to urinate with scanty flow seems to be the principal, more frequent primary action."*

And again,—" The overwakefulness is in henbane an alternating action with drowsiness and sleep, but the over-wakefulness seems to be the chief primary action."*

But the uses of *Hyoscyamus* are not confined to desperate conditions. For instance, it is a prompt and effective remedy in a not very serious, but very annoying form of COUGH. One has many times seen its success here, and been told by the grateful patient, " You are wonderful ! " But it is Homœopathy that is wonderful, *when drug-picture and disease-picture match.* The cough is a spasmodic, or a dry, tickling spasmodic cough, by night : especially by night. The patient lies down, and coughs, and coughs, and coughs ; sits up, and ceases to cough ; lies down again, and coughs and coughs and coughs ; sits up again, and again finds peace. This may go on all night, and night after night till *Hyoscyamus* is given, and that finishes it.

The most notable remedies of *suspicion* and *jealousy* are LACH., HYOS., PULS., *Nux* and *Stram.*

An interesting case of *Hyoscyamus* jealousy will bear repeating here, where it belongs.

A boy, mentally deficient, was, among other things, frightfully jealous, especially of the man his sister was engaged to. Whenever he came to the house the boy " was very naughty, and *passed his stool into his trousers* ". *Hyoscyamus* was found to have the symptom, *involuntary stool from excitement.* He got a dose of *Hyoscyamus cm*, and the next report was that " people remarked how much quieter he was, and that though the sister's fiance had been staying in the house, *he had not been jealous* ".

Among its fears and suspicions, is the fear of poison—suspicious of being poisoned. This fear of poison, it shares with *Lach.* and *Rhus. Bell.* and *Kali Brom.* have also a fear of poison.

A queer *Hyos.* symptom " thought he saw a policeman come in ", led to its successful prescription in a bad case of pneumonia. (*Kali brom.* has also that symptom.)

* * *

* Footnotes, *Materia Med. Pura.*

KENT says [we will condense and epitomize] : " *Hyoscyamus* is full of convulsions and contractions and trembling and quivering and jerking of muscles. . . . Choreic motions, but angular motions of the arms, etc. . . . The intermingling of jerkings and quiverings and tremblings and weakness and convulsive action of muscles are all striking features. . . .

" The mental state is really the greatest part of *Hyoscyamus* . . . delirium, and illusions and hallucinations all mingled together. Suspicious—of everybody ; of his wife that she is going to poison him : that she is untrue : refuses medicine, because it is poisoned. . . . He is pursued : people have all turned against him. Carries on conversations with imaginary people : really imagines that someone is sitting by his side, to whom he is talking. Talks to dead folk : calls up a dead sister or wife or husband, and enters into conversation as if they were here again on earth. . . . Another freak in this mental state :—lies and looks at a queer paper on the wall and tries to turn the figures into rows . . . imagines the things are worms, vermin, rats, cats, mice, and he is leading them as children lead round their toys . . . one patient had a string of bedbugs going up the wall, and he had them tied with a string, and was irritated because he could not make the last one keep up. . . . Lies and picks things."

Tongue " rattles in mouth, so dry ", looks like burnt leather. Muscles of throat—tongue—pharynx—œsophagus are stiff and paralysed so that swallowing is difficult. Fluids come out through nose (*Gels.*), or go down into larynx.

He compares *Bell.*, *Stram.*, *Hyos.* In order of fever, *Bell.* very hot : *Stram.* most violent and active, but usually only moderately hot : *Hyos.* fever, not very high with its insanity.

In regard to violence of conduct, the order would be, *Stram.*, *Bell.*, *Hyos.*—a more passive medicine : does not go into violence.

Then in regard to their reaction to water, and hydrophobia. Fear of water, of running water : all three. *Stram.* : fear of water : of anything that might look like water : shining objects : fire, looking-glass, or that have the sound of fluids (*Hydrophobinum*). *Hydrophobinum* has cured involuntary urination, or discharge from bowels on hearing running water.

Kent explains the " wants to go naked " of *Hyos.* thus :—He has such sensitive nerves all over the body in the skin that he cannot bear the clothing to touch the skin, and takes it off. He appears to be perfectly shameless : but has no thought of doing anything unusual : he does it from hyperæsthesia of the skin.

One wonders how "nudists" would react to *Hyoscyamus* in potency! But besides this, the insanity of *Hyoscyamus* has obscenity: with violent excitement and nymphomania, and exposure of the person. Lascivious mania. Especially where in the pure and good these things are merely a phase of sickness or insanity.

He is violent; beats people; strikes and bites; sings constantly and talks hastily. After convulsions, eye troubles, squinting, and disturbances of vision. "An object looked at jumps." . . . Both urine and stools are passed without his knowledge. . . . Many complaints come on during sleep:— "sleepless, or constant sleep". Suddenly sits up and lies down again:—keeps on doing that all night. Laughing during sleep. . . .

BLACK LETTER SYMPTOMS

Ravings: delirium: with restlessness: would not stay in bed.
Foolish laughter: talks more than usual: more animatedly: hurriedly.
Silly: smiling: laughs at everything: silly expression.
Comical alienation of mind: performs ludicrous actions like monkeys.
Makes ridiculous gestures like a dancing clown.
Strips himself naked: lies in bed and prattles.
Carphology. Picks at bedclothes: mutters and prattles.
Unable to think: cannot direct or control thoughts.
Answers no questions: cannot bear to be talked to.
Is violent, and beats people.
Jealousy with rage and delirium: with attempt to murder.
Lascivious mania: uncovers: sings amorous songs.
Suspicious. Fears: alone; of being poisoned (Lach., Rhus., etc.) ; *of being injured. Wants to run away. Fears being bitten.*
Wants to get up and attend to business, or go home (Bry.).
Delirium: talks of business: of imaginary wrongs.

Pupils dilated: insensible.
Small objects seem very large (reverse of Plat.).
Constant staring at surrounding objects. Self-forgetful.

Pressive squeezing on the root of the NOSE.
Deafness (from paralysis of auditory nerve).

Swallowing difficult: inability to swallow.

Tongue red or brown : dry, cracked, hard, looks like burnt leather.

Or clean, parched ; white, tremulous.   Foam at mouth.

Sordes teeth and mouth.   Grating the teeth.

Dread of water (Stram.).

Hiccough.

Inflammation of stomach, or peritonitis with hiccough.

Cutting low down in the abdomen.   Pinching in abdomen.

Urging to stool.   Stool passed involuntarily in bed.

No will to make water in childbed.

Puerperal spasms : shrieks : anguish : chest oppressed : unconscious.

Much mucus in larynx and air passages, which makes voice and speech not clear.

Almost incessant cough while lying down: disappears when sitting up.   Dry COUGH *at night.*

Cough at night : frequent cough at night, which always wakes him, after which he again falls asleep.

Angular motions : jerks of single muscles or sets of muscles.

Subsultus tendinum.

CONVULSIONS.

Suffocating spells and convulsions during labour.

Epilepsy : before attack, vertigo, sparks before eyes, ringing in ears, hungry gnawing : during attack, face purple, eyes projecting, shrieks, grinds teeth, urination.

Epileptoid spasms.   Epilepsy daily so violent it seemed as if spine or joints would be broken.

Very profound slumber.

Sleeplessness : long-continued sleeplessness : on account of quiet mental activity.

Unable to sleep the whole night : tried lying on one side and the other, yet unable to get quiet.   (Ars.)

Starts from sleep as if in a fright.

Intense sleeplessness of irritable, excitable persons, from business embarrassments—often imaginary.

Sleepless, or constant sleep, with muttering.

Long-continued sleeplessness.

Cannot bear to be talked to, or least noise during chill.

Curious, or Characteristic Symptoms

They babble out almost everything a sensible person would have kept quiet about all his life.

Fancies men are swine.

Ran against all objects that stood in their way, with wide-open wild eyes.

Ridiculously solemn acts in improper clothing, mixed with fury :

As " In a priest's cassock, put on over nothing but a shirt, and in fur boots, he wishes to go to church, in order to preach and to perform clerical offices there, and furiously attacks those who try to prevent him."

Rushes at people with knives : strikes and tries to murder those he meets.

Peculiar fear of being bitten by beasts.

Reproaches himself and others : complains of the injustice that he imagines has been done to him. (*Staph.*)

In despair wishes to take his life, and throw himself into water.

Serious illness from jealousy and grief about a faithless lover.

Desires to be naked (hyperæsthesia of cutaneous nerves).

After a fit of passion and sudden fear : so timorous as to hide himself in every corner, even to dread and run away from flies.

Continually counting.

Frequent looking at her hands because they seem too large.

Fingers feel too thick. Feels as if teeth would fall out.

Syphilomania.

Brain feels too loose : swashing, like water, in head.

Head shaken to and fro.

Objects look red (*Bell.*, black, *Stram.*).

Stupid expression. Muscles twitch, makes grimaces.

Bites the tongue when talking.

Paralysis of tongue.

After fright, loss of speech : motions of tongue impaired, with numbness and lameness.

Spasm ; or constriction of throat : inability to swallow liquids. ·

Involuntary stool while urinating.

Paralysis of sphincters : involuntary stool and urine.

Frequent emission of urine clear as water.

Every muscle of the body twitches, from the eyes to the toes (in chorea, etc.). Clonic spasms.

Patients with fever throw the bedclothes off, not because they are too warm, but *they will not remain covered*.

HYPERICUM

Hypericum—St. John's Wort—thrice blessed herb for the relief of pain : named through the centuries after the beloved disciple ; possibly, by analogy, from having been used by him for healing purposes ? (One could quote many herbs which had thus acquired their common names.) Had the name been merely of ecclesiastical bestowal, it would surely have been St. Luke's Wort, because it was Luke who was " the beloved physician ".

Among the Wound-worts and Bruise-worts of our land, none rivals *Hypericum* for its healing touch on *injured nerves*, and *for injuries—especially to parts rich in nerves.* Here we use it both externally and internally.

One remembers happy hours, roaming the Surrey woods and wastes with a certain herb-woman, whose mother had been maid to a Lady Shrewsbury, a great herbalist, from whom the lore had descended.

From this herb-woman one caught the habit of crushing herbs between thumb and fingers, to express and inhale their scents—fragrant or otherwise. According to her, health comes to those who so haunt the woods and taste their sweetness. The woman used to say, " There are two herbs of every kind ", i.e. the real (medicinal) herb and its counterfeit, which, to the un-initiated, looks curiously like it, but is valueless. But—crush them and see ! Crush *Hypericum*—flowers, stalk or leaves, and you will never forget the curious, almost resinous scent, which persists in the tinctures. Crush the small yellow flowers of *St. John's Wort*, and to your surprise, dark red smears stain your fingers. These are from glands at the base of the flowers ; and because of these the tinctures (" stinctures " mine were apt to be called !) are a beautiful red colour. But you will know for certain that you have found our medicinal *Hypericum perforatum* by holding up its narrow leaves to the light, and observing the pellucid dots with which they are studded. These " holes ", together with the " blood-stains ", suggested to the ancient searchers after " signatures " the uses of the plant—for *wounds*, and for *punctured* wounds.

That " Doctrine of Signatures ! "—one is not supposed to mention it in these materialistic days, because, you see, it is almost as absurd as Homœopathy. But it was really responsible for the discovery of many common medicines. The idea being, that the Almighty had set His seal on substances and plants useful for healing, so that they might be recognized by His suffering children in their need.

One remembers a poor old man who used to come and beg a few twigs of Barbery, to cure his " yaller jaunders". How did he use them ? Why, it was like this. He scraped off the yellow substance from just beneath the bark, steeped that in beer, and found it a sure cure for his malady. And indeed, most of the liver medicines *are* yellow—*Berberis*—*Chelidonium*, etc., while remedies that affect the blood especially are red—the salts of iron—*Hamamelis*—*Hypericum*, etc.

However, since the writer of the above is peculiarly sensitive to ridicule, may it be considered unwritten !

Among our indigenous wound-worts is the Daisy of the fields, *Bellis perennis :* of which Culpepper says, " This is another herb which nature has made common, because it may be useful." The Daisy is our English *Arnica*, and resembles it, even to the production and cure of boils. *Yarrow*, again, most difficult to get rid of !—Why, it had the impertinence, one year, to ruin the grass outside the National Gallery, right in the heart of London. But it has excuses for its ubiquity. It has been *Achillea millifolium* since the days when it was used by Achilles (as mentioned in the Iliad) to heal the wounds of his soldiers. *Millifolium* is a great remedy for bleeding wounds and for hæmorrhages.

Of course healing in the good old days was largely in the hands of wise women, who had learnt from wise women before them the use of the herbs of field and wood. But that was before the bad new days when a qualified doctor grows on every bush, his pockets bulging with aspirin—morphia—carbolic acid—iodine, to oust the simpler, and saner, and more beneficent herbs. For aspirin and morphia only blunt sensation ; they never *cure* the pain—which *Hypericum does*, as we shall see.

Culpepper thus describes *Hypericum*, whose uses he knew so well some 300 years ago. " The plant abides in the ground, shooting anew every spring . . . The two small leaves set one against the other at every place " (up the stems) " are of a deep green colour, narrow, and full of small holes in every leaf, which cannot be so well perceived as when they are held up to the light. At the tops of the stalks and branches stand yellow flowers of five petals, with many yellow heads in the middle, which being bruised do yield a reddish juice like blood . . .

" It is an excellent vulnerary plant . . . outwardly of great service in bruises, contusions and wounds, especially in the nervous parts. . . . The ointment opens obstructions, dissolves swellings, and closes up the lips of wounds . . . ."

And Kent gives one of his graphic pictures of *Hypericum* :
"When finger ends or toes have been bruised or lacerated, or a
nail torn off, or a nerve pinched between hammer and bone with
a blow, and that nerve becomes inflamed, and the pain can be
traced extending towards the body with stitching, darting pains,
or shooting up towards the body from the seat of injury, a dangerous condition is coming on.   Here *Hypericum* is above all remedies
the one to be thought of . . .   Lockjaw is threatening."

" Or," he says, " A vicious dog will take hold through thumb,
or hand, or wrist, and run his teeth through the radial nerve
or some of its branches in the hand, causing a lacerated wound
. . . .   or a wound may yawn, swell up, no tendency to heal,
look dry and shiny on its edges ; red, inflamed ; burning, stinging, tearing pains ; no healing process.   That wound needs
Hypericum.   It prevents tetanus.   A shoemaker may stick his
awl into the end of his thumb or a carpenter may stick his finger
with a brass tack, and he does not think much of it, but the next
night shooting pains extend up the arm with great violence.
The allopathic physician looks upon that as a serious matter, for
he sees lockjaw or tetanus ahead.   When these pains come on,
Hypericum will stop them, and from this stage to advanced states
of tetanus with opisthotonos and lockjaw, *Hypericum* is the
remedy.

" Punctured wounds, rat bites, cat bites, etc., are made safe
by *Ledum*, but if the pain shoots from the wound up the nerve
of the arm, it is more like *Hypericum* . . . .   Injuries to
spine . . .   Injuries to coccyx . . . ."

Kent's Lecture on *Hypericum*, where he compares it with
other such remedies, is a masterpiece.   We may reproduce it
in part later on.

Lockjaw . . .   One of the cases in which *Hypericum* was
curative in lockjaw, is given in *Clarke's Dictionary*.   It was in a
boy, bitten in the finger by a tame rat.   Some time afterwards
he became alarmingly ill : he could with difficulty speak ; jaws
firmly locked ; neck so stiff that it could hardly be moved.   Great
tenderness about the wound.   *Hypericum* 500th potency in water,
was given at 8 p.m., every 15 minutes at first, then every two
hours.   By 3 a.m. there was improvement and he fell asleep,
and next morning was practically convalescent.

Now for some homely illustrations in our own ken, briefly
told, but showing that *Hypericum* has not lost its healing power,
but that its ancient reputation is well-founded.

" *For injuries to nerves* . . ."   In the early days of
motor cars, coachman and groom were put under instruction,

learning to drive. The groom took his turn at the wheel. The coachman, a big Scotchman, stood up behind and leant over to watch. The groom swerved badly up on to the side of a hedge, and it was presently discovered that the coachman had been jerked out and left far behind on the road. He was in great pain ; though careful examination gave it that neither bones, nor joints had suffered. Two or three days later, the pain had become very severe (in spite of *Arnica*), with both legs powerless to support him, and as he lay in bed, every movement sent shooting pains down both legs to knees and ankles and feet. He cried out repeatedly as he was turned on to his side. There was swelling and tenderness over sacrum and over right sciatic nerve : and, because of the *shooting pains*, two drops of *Hyper. φ* were given.

Three hours later the prescriber met her father as he came in from his ride. " I'm frightened about F. We'd better get Dr. ——— to see him again. We don't want him paralysed ! " " Oh, he's all right," was the answer. " I went up to see him, and he's much better. He was up and dressed and walking about." A few more doses of *Hypericum φ* and *Hypericum* lotion externally, and he got up again that evening and walked the passage with sticks. *Next day*, went down stairs and across to the stables. Again, *next day*, was at work without a stick ; drove the carriage out, and cleaned it himself.

A month later, with the advent of cold weather, there were again shooting pains from sacrum up sides of neck, and shooting pains down both legs, with some numbness and difficulty in lifting feet. *Hypericum φ* and 30th potency improved matters quickly, and in a few days he was all right. This was in 1907, and *there has been no recurrence of the trouble*.

Here *Hypericum* justified its reputation for " shooting pains extending from the seat of injury ". Aspirin or morphia might have given temporary relief to pain. But it was only *Hypericum* that, in relieving, could *cure*. Which is scientific ?—to numb and dull ?—temporarily ! or to *cure ?*

And here, observe. *Arnica* is the remedy of injured " soft parts ". *Hypericum* the remedy for injured nerves.

" *For lacerated wounds* . . ." One of the carriage horses had come down on a bad patch of road, and had a beautiful pair of broken knees. The coachman said she was done for : they would heal, but the hair would never grow again as before. There would always be the tell-tale scars. However *Hypericum* was shaken up with water in a bottle with a spraying arrangement, and orders were given that the knees were not to be covered, but were to be constantly sprayed They healed rapidly, leaving nothing to show that the beast had ever come down. This was the cleanest and simplest way one could devise for treating such a patient in the stables.

" *To close the lips of wounds* . . ." A University professor was spending a couple of weeks at our hospital one Christmas time, and one thing he did take away with him was profound respect for the virtues of *Hypericum*. A girl had fallen through glass, and among other cuts had a nasty one on lip, a little bit of which was missing. Merely a compress of *Hypericum* that night left the lip healed by morning.

" *Instead of Arnica, where skin is broken, and where the injury is very painful.*" A case: He was down for his usual weekending at the farm, and on Saturday morning had climbed down from the dog cart to play with the horses in the field. They were rather restive today, because a stranger had been turned out with them. Suddenly a young cart horse lashed out and caught him on the outer side of the leg, just below the knee. He fell, and so mercifully escaped a second kick that appeared to the horrified onlooker in the dog-cart, to catch him in the abdomen. He managed to climb back into the high cart, and drove home in very great pain. The skin was broken, so it was no case for *Arnica*. There was a rush to find *St. John's Wort* in a certain hedge ; to pour boiling water on the herb ; and to apply it to the injury. The pain went by magic. He was nearly 80, and there was very little tissue between skin and bone, and healing ought to have been difficult and protracted ; but it was all healed by Monday, when he returned to work in London, albeit limping. One gauged the severity of the injury from the discoloration that gradually spread, like a huge bruise, up the thigh ;—the hurt having been below the knee.

" *For abscesses* . . ." During the war, a girl was sent to Hospital by a local doctor, with an abscess in the palm of hand, outer side, very tense and painful. He had incised it, but getting no pus, had sent her for further operation. She arrived in the morning, and merely got *Hypericum* internally and a compress of *Hypericum* for the whole hand. When seen in the afternoon, the pain was gone, the tension was gone, and it was pouring with pus. It rapidly healed. Is this what Culpepper means when he says, " *it opens obstructions and dissolves swellings*". It dissolved that one !

A certain theatre's carpenter was about to let off a gun for theatrical effect when it accidently went off with his hand on the top of the barrel—consequence, the wad was imbedded in his palm. He attended a hospital, week after week, where they did what they thought needful, and alternately soaked the wound, and then sent him away with a dry dressing. The man was suffering miserably and enduring sleepless nights of pain. Then someone sent him to see what the homœopaths could do for him. He got *Silica* internally, and a compress of *Hypericum*, with instant relief of pain, and restored sleep. Then, in a few days, the discharging wound began to smell so foully that a tentative compress of *Lysol* was applied ; but as this did *not* give relief, *Hypericum* was again used. Then, in a few days, when squeezing out pus, out came a burst of stinking wad, and next day another scrap, and then it healed beautifully. But one tendon had either sloughed, or been shot away, and a finger remains out of control—a memento of the time when he so nearly lost his hand.

A keen lay homœopath, long since dead, sent *Hypericum* to the Scotch sergeants at the Front. He published the following in the *Oban Times* of May 1st, 1915, and had it reprinted as a leaflet.

HYPERICUM ON THE BATTLEFIELD

LETTER FROM A HIGHLAND SERGEANT

Mr. Campbell of Barbreck has received the following letter :—

British Expeditionary Force,
April 19th, 1915.

DEAR MR. CAMPBELL,—I want to thank you for the box of splendid pellets you so kindly sent me. I would have written you long ago on this subject, but I wanted to test them thoroughly before I gave my opinion on them, and now I can state facts which must be very satisfactory to you. The result of my observation is this: About a week after I got your letter and pellets one of my Platoon was wounded by a sniper while he was on lookout in the trenches ; the wound was a bad one, through the shoulder, and he was suffering a lot with it. All the colour left his face, and I thought he was going to faint. I thought of the pellets which I had in my haversack, and I decided to give him two of them.

The effect of them I am sure I need not tell you, but it surprised me beyond words. To see a man badly wounded and in terrible pain to be transformed to laugh and joke, and lark with the men, by two little pellets is something wonderful.

This is only one case out of many which I could tell you about, and although I hope I shall never require them myself, I am pleased to have them to give to others.

I think I have said enough this time, but I will let you know about other cases later. I am, Sir, yours faithfully,

SERGEANT W. M.

———

Certified a true copy. J. A. CAMPBELL, Barbreck, Craignish.

April 23rd, 1915.

In the provings of *Hypericum* one finds nerve pains—stitching pains—and paralytic symptoms.

Hering in his *Guiding Symptoms* gives cases of cure by *Hypericum* of—*Concussion of spine :* man thrown from wagon who struck his back·violently against a kerb stone and had shooting pains down both legs, with partial paralysis. Boy with *traumatic meningitis* after a fall on the head. Woman with *headache after a fall on occiput*, with sensation of being lifted high into the air ; tormented by the greatest anxiety that the slightest touch or motion would make her fall down from this height ; and so on.

There are just a few persons very sensitive to *Hypericum*. One of these, the wife of one of our doctors, had a curious experience with *Hypericum* which, after producing symptoms, cured.

They were visiting the Battlefields after the war, when a piece of barbed wire penetrated her stocking, and made a rather deep puncture, with a large deep scratch on the skin. The wound was dressed and healed up.

Some time later it began to give acute pain at irregular intervals. The pain was severe—in the injured part. A number of remedies were tried, but nothing held. Then, because of the acuteness of the pain, as if the injury were fresh-inflicted, *Hypericum* 30 was given which she proceeded to " prove ".

In two hours there was faintness, paleness of face, she felt as if heart would stop : nausea ; legs trembled, couldn't walk, had to hold on to something. Exhausted, weak and faint. Had to lie down. This condition lasted till late evening. Appetite gone for two days. And the doctor concludes :—

" *Since she got the Hypericum* 30 *she has never had pain or ache in the part again.* No remedy had been given for a couple of months before the *Hypericum*, and nothing after it."

Another little known use of *Hypericum* is for PILES. Clarke (*Dictionary*) quotes " Roehrig ", who " considers *Hypericum* externally and internally, the nearest thing to a specific for bleeding piles." *It works !* and *should* work : because *Hypericum* is the remedy, *par excellence*, for parts rich in nerves—of which the anus is assuredly one ! And in the provings it markedly affected the rectum.

Besides *Hypericum perforatum*, there are other varieties with medicinal properties. One of these has the name " *Tutsan* " (all heal). Then the beautiful large-flowered variety, which clothes the railway embankments near Leatherhead. Some one used to send up a big packet of these flowers every year to the Hospital, and good old Sister Olive used to stir them over a fire in oil, to make a healing ointment for sores.

ED.

Black Letter Symptoms

Consequences of spinal concussion.

Effects of nervous shock.

Tetanus after traumatic injuries.

Injuries to nerves, attended by great pain.

Punctured, incised, contused or lacerated wounds, when pains are extremely severe, and particularly if they are of long duration ; pains like those of a severe toothache ; pains spread to neighbouring parts and extend up limb.

Punctured wounds feel very sore ; from treading on nails, needles, pins, splinters, rat bites, etc. ; prevents lockjaw.

Consequences of spinal concussion.

Piercing wounds ; from sharp instruments.

IGNATIA

Ignatia—great remedy of moods and contradictions : of mental stress and strain, connected with shock, bereavement, disappointment, or distress, which have spasmodically and completely unhinged judgment and self-control.

But, as Kent says, should the condition recur again and again, and threaten to become chronic, then *Natrum mur.*, the " chronic " of *Ignatia*, comes in.

Hahnemann speaks of the " directly opposite symptoms of this remarkable drug ". And says that, on account of these alternating actions, that follow one another very rapidly, it is particularly suitable for acute diseases, and for a considerable number of these—as may be seen by its symptoms, which correspond with morbid conditions so frequently met with in daily life. " It may be regarded as a medicine created for great usefulness (polycrest)."

Clarke says (Dictionary), " In order to obtain a proper understanding of the power and place of *Ignatia*, it is necessary to get rid of two prevalent erroneous ideas. The first of these is that *Ignatia* is a remedy for hysteria and nothing else ; and the second is that it is the only remedy ever required in cases of hysteria."

He says, " The seeds of *Ignatia* contain a larger proportion of *Strychnia* than those of *Nux vomica*, and the great difference in the characteristic features of the two medicines prove the wisdom of considering medicines apart from their so-called ' active ' principles."

Hahnemann, comparing the mentality of the two drugs, says, " Although the positive effects of *Ignatia* have a great resemblance to those of *Nux vomica* (as might be inferred from the botanical relationship between the two plants) yet the emotional disposition of patients for whom *Ignatia* is serviceable differs widely from that of the patients for whom *Nux* is of use."

He tells us that *Ignatia* is not suitable for persons in whom anger, eagerness, or violence is predominant, but for those who are subject to rapid alternations of gaiety and disposition to weep, or in whom we notice the emotional states indicated by its symptoms, provided that the other corporeal morbid symptoms resemble those that this drug can produce.

" Even in a high potency *Ignatia* is a main remedy in subjects who have no tendency to break out violently, or to revenge themselves, but who keep their annoyance to themselves : in whom the remembrance of the vexatious occurrence is wont to dwell in the mind, and so especially in morbid states which are produced by occurrences that cause grief."

And in regard to epilepsy he says, " Attacks of even chronic epilepsy, which only occur after mortification or some similar vexation (and not from any other cause) may always be prevented by timely administration of *Ignatia*. Epileptic attacks that come on in young persons after some great fright, before they become very numerous, may also be cured by a few doses of *Ignatia*. But it is very improbable that chronic epileptic fits of other kind can be cured, or have ever been cured by this medicine. . . . *Ignatia is only applicable and curative in sudden attacks· and in acute diseases.*"

And, in regard to *Ignatia*, he says," It is best to administer the (small) dose *in the morning*, if there is no occasion for hurry. When given shortly before bedtime it causes too much restlessness at night."

This is what GUERNSEY has to tell us about *Ignatia* :

" Anyone suffering from suppressed or deep grief, with long-drawn sighs, much sobbing, etc., also much unhappiness, can't sleep, entirely absorbed in grief ; for recent grief, as at the loss of a friend ; affections of the mind in general, particularly if actuated by grief ; sadness ; hopelessness ; hysterical variableness ; fantastic illusions."

" Catalepsy with bending backwards ; opisthotonos ; hysterical spasms, especially if accompanied with sighing . . . chilliness of single parts.

" Patient's face changes colour very often when at rest. . . .

" *Worse* : from mental affections ; from anger ; from anger with fright ; anger with silent grief ; from anxiety ; from anxiety with sorrow ; unhappy love ; mortifications caused by offence ; from exertion of the mind ; from sweets, coffee, tobacco ; from pressure on the painless side, can lie better on *painful* side ; from strong smells ; between swallowing ; from ascarides ; when yawning."

NASH calls *Ignatia* a " Remedy of paradoxicalities ! " Head better lying on painful side, goneness not better by eating, sore throat better by swallowing, thirst during chill, face red during chill, etc. . . . Relieved by profuse watery urination.

He says that *Ignatia*, like *Acon.*, *Cham.*, and *Nux*, seems to exalt the impressionability of all the senses, but unlike the others, it has in it a marked element of sadness, and disposition to *silent grieving*.

And another characteristic state of mind is a CHANGEABLE MOOD. No remedy can equal *Ignatia* for this . . . the patient is at one time full of glee and merriment, to be followed suddenly with the other extreme, of melancholy sadness and tears, and so these states of mind rapidly alternate.* *Ignatia* is easily frightened, and hence one of our best remedies for the effects of fright, vying with *Aconite, Opium* and *Verat. alb.* . . .

With *Nux*, it is a great nervous remedy, and acts on the spine, affecting both sensory and motor nerves. One of our best remedies for spasms or convulsions, especially when originating in mental causes, as after a *fright, punishment of children,* or other strong emotions. A physician while observing the patient in one of the spasms, noticed that she came out of it with a succession of long-drawn sighs. He inquired if the patient had had any recent mental trouble, and learned that she had lost her mother, of whom she was exceedingly fond, and for whom she mourned greatly, a few weeks before. *Ignatia* 30 quickly cured her. . . .

Ignatia has in a marked degree *twitchings* all over the body, hence it becomes one of our best remedies for chorea, especially if caused by fright or grief on the mental side, or teething or worms on the reflex irritation side. . . . Like *Aconite, Chamomilla* and *Coffea, Ignatia* is *over-sensitive to pain.* . . .

He says this remedy is very unique in its fever symptoms. There is no disease in which we are better able to show the power of the potentized remedy to cure, than intermittent fever. Chronic cases that have resisted the *Quinine* treatment for years are often quickly and permanently cured by the 200th and upwards. The following symptoms indicate *Ignatia* : 1st. *Thirst during chill and in no other stage.* 2nd. *Chill, relieved by external heat.* 3rd. *Heat aggravated by external covering.* 4th. *Red face during the chill.* No other remedy has thirst during the chill and at no other stage. (He points out that, in *Nux*, during the heat, the least uncovering brings back the chill.) He says, " the red face during the chill led me to the cure of an obstinate case, and after I noticed the red face I also noticed that the boy was behind the stove in the warmest place he could find. The 200th promptly cured."

KENT describes the *Ignatia* patient and condition : " A woman has undergone a controversy at home : . . . has had a great distress : . . . unrequited affections : . . . a nervous sensitive girl finds out that she has misplaced her affections : she has a weeping spell, headache, trembles, is nervous, sleepless.

---

* *Crocus here resembles Ignatia.*

. . . A woman loses her child or her husband : has headaches, trembles, is excited, weeps and is sleepless : unable to control herself ; is ashamed of herself. In spite of her best endeavours, her grief has simply torn her to pieces. She is unable to control her emotions and her excitement. *Ignatia* will quiet her. . . . If such troubles keep coming back, and the state keeps recurring, *Nat. mur.* will finish up the case. It is the natural chronic of *Ignatia*. . . . when the troubles keep coming back, and *Ignatia* comes to a place when it will not hold any longer." Or when a sensitive, overtired girl falls in love with an impossible person. "She lies awake at night, sobs. *Ignatia*, if very recent will balance up that girl's mind. If not, *Natrum mur.* comes in as a follower."

The *Ignatia* patient is not one that has been a simpleton, or of a sluggish mind or idiotic, but one that has become tired, and brought into such a state from over-doing it and from over-excitement. If rather feeble in body, from too much social excitement. Our present social state is well calculated to develop a hysterical mind. The typical social mind is one that is always in a state of confusion . . . dread, fear, anxiety, weeping run through the remedy. " Sensitive disposition ; hyper-acute." Overwrought ; intense.

Some of these overwrought girls that come back from Paris, overwrought in their music, will have violent pains in the face—hysterical pains : others with violent headaches ; others with the mental state and confusion ; others with all the hysterical mani-festations. Prolonged excitement. Musical excesses, etc."

And of the *Ignatia* patient Kent says : " You cannot depend on her being reasonable or rational. It is best to say as little as possible about anything. Make no promises, look wise, take up your travelling bag and go home after you have prescribed, because anything you will say will be distorted. There is not anything you can say that will please."

And *Ignatia* has another thing : " thinks she has neglected some duty."

Kent says again, " *Ignatia* is full of surprises . . . in *Ignatia* you find what is unnatural, and what is unexpected. You see an inflamed part where there is heat, and redness, and throbbing, and weakness ; you will handle it with great care for fear it will be painful . . . but you find it is not painful : sometimes not painful at all, and sometimes ameliorated by hard pressure. Is not that a surprise ?

" You look into the throat. It is tumid, inflamed, red ; the patient complains of a sore throat and pain. Naturally you do not touch it with your tongue-depressor for fear it will hurt.   You have every reason to suppose that the swallowing of solids will be painful.   But you ask the patient when the pain is present, and the patient will say, ' When I am not swallowing anything solid.' The pain is ameliorated by swallowing anything solid, by the pressure.   It pains all other times.

" Mentally the patient does the most unaccountable and most unexpected things.   Seems to have no rule to work by, no philosophy, no soundness of mind, and no judgment.   The opposite to what would be expected, then, will be found.   The patient is better lying on the painful side :   instead of its hurting the pain, it improves the pain.   ' Pain like a nail sticking into the side of the head,' and the only comfort that is felt is lying upon it, or pressing upon it, and that makes it go away."

And Kent says the stomach is just as strange in its indigestion. That gentle food, and the simplest possible things are given, because she has been vomiting for days, and she can keep nothing down.   " It is a hysterical stomach," and she eats some raw cabbage and some chopped onions, and from that time on she is well.

Again with cough.   He says, when people cough from irritation, from a sensation of fullness, or a desire to expel something, this is better by coughing.   But when such irritation comes in an *Ignatia* patient, you have the unexpected again :   because the more she coughs the more is the irritation to cough, till the irritation is so great that she goes into spasms.   You may be called to the bedside of a patient where the more she coughs the greater the irritation to cough and she is drenched with sweat, sitting up in bed with her night-clothes drenched ;   gagging, and coughing and retching, covered with sweat and exhausted.   Don't wait. You cannot get her to stop coughing long enough to say anything to you about it, only you will see that the cough has grown more violent.   *Ignatia* stops it at once.   Or spasm of the larynx from mental disturbance, fright or distress, a laryngismus that can be heard all over the house.   *Ignatia* stops it at once.

Thirst when you would not expect it.   Thirst during chill, but not during fever.

Ignatia will cure many " corporeal conditions " where the mental symptoms demand the remedy.

One of our doctors, late one night, was called to see a case of acute rheumatism, where the apparently indicated remedy had not helped.   He was now confronted by a perfect picture of the *Ignatia* mentality, and gave that remedy—which promptly cleared up the whole case, rheumatism and all.

Clarke had a similar case. He says, " In the early days of my homœopathic career I astonished myself once by curing rapidly with *Ignatia* (prescribed at first as an intercurrent remedy) a severe case of rheumatic fever, which had been making no progress under *Bryonia*, etc. The mental symptoms called for *Ignatia*, and along with these the inflammation of the joints, as well as the fever, disappeared under its action." One must never forget that the mental symptoms, if marked, and especially if indicating a change of disposition due to acute illness, are the most important in determining the choice of the remedy.

One remembers well an *Ignatia* case in early Dispensary practice. A youngish woman, who had been given *Sepia* for her goitre—a large, soft swelling of the thyroid—returned in a week in an alarming condition of distress and gasping for breath. The Hospital, rung up, had no bed to offer, and the only thing was to give her *Ignatia*, and to tell her to come back in a few days. When she reappeared, calm and happy, *the goitre had completely disappeared!* One wondered, which of the two remedies had done the trick ? *Ignatia* is the acute of *Sepia*, as well as of *Natrum mur*. Did *Sepia*, perhaps, cause an initial aggravation—a very severe one, and then cure ?—or was *Ignatia* really the curative remedy ?

But one thing is certain—if you have to treat a goitre in the acute stage with *Ignatia* mental symptoms, you cannot go far wrong if you prescribe *IGNATIA*.

Ignatia is the " sighing remedy ".

Ignatia yawns.

Ignatia cannot stand smoking, or tobacco smoke.

Ignatia is one of the very important remedies to be considered in troubles of rectum and anus.

BLACK LETTER SYMPTOMS (*Hahnemann and Allen*)

Uncommon tendency to be frightened.

Audacity.

Fickle, impatient, irresolute, quarrelsome, recurring every three to four hours.

Incredible changes of disposition, at one time he jokes and jests, at another he is lachrymose, alternately every three to four hours.

Whispering voice. He cannot speak loudly.

Delicate disposition, with very clear consciousness.

Finely sensitive mood, delicate conscientiousness.

Slight blame or contradiction excites him to anger, and this makes him angry with himself.

Incredible changes of mood.

Heat in the head.   Head is heavy.

He hangs the head forward.   Lays the head forward on the table.

Headache, increased by stooping forwards.

Aching pain in forehead above root of nose which compels him to bend forward the head, followed by inclination to vomit.

Headache like a pressure with something hard on the surface of the brain, recurring in fits.

Throbbing headache.   Headache at every beat of the arteries.

Itching in the auditory meatus.

Shooting in the lips.

Inner surface of lower lip painful, as if raw and excoriated.

Lips are cracked and bleed.

He is apt to bite on one side of the tongue posteriorly when speaking or chewing.

Stitches in palate extending into the external ear.

Sour taste in the mouth.

Aching pain in cervical glands.

Formication in the œsophagus.

Belches up a bitter fluid.

What he has ingested is belched up again into the mouth.

Retching (constrictive) sensation in the middle of the throat, as if there were a large morsel of food, or a plug sticking there, felt more when not swallowing than when swallowing.

Sore throat : sticking in it when not swallowing and even somewhat while swallowing ; the more he swallows, however, the more it disappears : if he swallows anything solid, like bread, it seems as though the sticking entirely disappeared.

After eating and drinking, hiccough.

Aching in scrobiculus cordis.

Extreme aversion to smoking tobacco.

A feeling in the stomach as from fasting.

Feeling of flabbiness in the stomach.

Peculiar sensation of weakness in upper abdomen and pit of stomach, and paleness of face.

Rumbling and rattling in the bowels.

On the left, above the navel, a sharp shooting.

Pinching and shooting pains in abdomen.

Prolapsus of the rectum during moderate straining at stool.

Violent urging to stool, more in the upper bowels and upper part of the abdomen ; he has great desire, yet the stool, though soft, does not pass in sufficient quantity.

Painless contraction of the anus.

A coarse stitch from anus deep into the rectum.

Pain one or two hours after stool, pain in rectum, as from blind piles, compounded of contraction and sore pain.

Blind piles, painful while sitting and standing, less while walking.

Prolapsus of the rectum, from moderate exertion at stool.

Sharp pressive pain in the rectum.

Sore pain in the anus, without reference to the stool.

Great urgency and desire for stool, in the evening, felt mostly in the middle of the abdomen, but no stool follows, only the rectum protrudes.

Frequent discharge of much watery urine.

Irritation and ulcerative pain—genitalia.

Complete absence of sexual desire, alternating with the reverse.

Provocation to cough in larynx, not relieved by cough, but only by suppressing cough.

Sensation of dry feathery dust in pit of throat, not relieved by coughing : but more excited the more he allows himself to cough. Inspiration is impeded as by a weight lying upon him : expiration is all the easier.

Single jerking of the limbs, on falling asleep.

Pain in sacrum, also when lying on the back in the morning in bed.

Pain in the joint of the humerus when bending the arm back, as from prolonged hard work, or as if bruised.

In the deltoid muscle a quivering twitching.

Hot knees with cold nose.

Creeping, gone-to-sleep feeling of the limbs.

In the joints of the shoulders, hip and knees, a pain as from a sprain or dislocation.

Simple violent pain, only felt when touched, here and there, on a small spot, e.g. on the ribs, etc.

Sleep so light that he hears everything in it.

Fixed idea in dream. Dreams all night of the same subject.

Snoring inspiration during sleep.

One ear and one cheek red and burning.

Sudden attack of flying heat all over the body.

External heat and redness, without internal heat.

External warmth is intolerable.

Feeling as if sweat would break out.

Shaking chill with redness of the face.

IODUM : Iodine the element

A VERY useful drug when used on its unique indications, viz. *Intolerance of heat : Inordinate hunger,* with *Emaciation : Emaciation* with glandular enlargement : *intense restlessness with apprehension.*

The drug was proved by Hahnemann who (*Chronic Diseases*) speaks of it as a heroic medicine, even when employed in the highest potencies ; but, he says, " its use requires all the discretion of a good homœopathic physician, lest he should abuse this substance . . . as allopathic physicians do. . . ."

He says the drug has rendered especial service in affections with the following symptoms : Dizziness in the morning : throbbing in the head : pain as from excoriation in eyes : buzzing in ears : hardness of hearing : coated tongue ; mercurial ptyalism : bad taste as of soap : sour eructations, with a sense of burning : heartburn after eating heavy food : *canine hunger :* nausea ; incarceration of flatulence : distension of abdomen : constipation : nightly micturition : delaying menses : cough : old morning cough : difficulty of breathing ; external swelling of neck : weakness of arms, early morning in bed : going to sleep of fingers : curvature of bones : dryness of skin : night sweats.

He quotes also from the provings of other doctors ; and then gives the schema of symptoms, in the usual order, from provings.

BLACK LETTER SYMPTOMS

Staring with wide, open EYES ; *lids seem to be retracted.*
NASAL *catarrh thin, excoriating.*
Increase of SALIVA ; *mercurial salivation.*

Suffers from HUNGER, *must eat every few hours ; gets anxious and worried if he does not eat : feels better after eating.*
Ravenous hunger, cannot be satisfied.
Most symptoms are better after eating.

Empty ERUCTATIONS *from morning till evening, as if every particle of food turned into " air ".*

Left hypochondriac region hard and acutely painful to pressure : SPLEEN *enlarged after intermittent.*

Chronic LEUCORRHŒA, *worse at M.P., makes thighs sore and corrodes linen.*

✝ *Dry* COUGH, *with stitches and burning in chest.*

Itching low down in lungs, behind sternum ; causing cough ; extends through bronchi to nasal cavity.

Sensation as if HEART *were squeezed together. As if heart were grasped by a hand (Lil. tig.).*

Palpitation of heart : worse least exertion : with faintness.

Chronic arthritic affections, with violent nightly pains in JOINTS, *no swelling.*

Great weakness and loss of breath on going up stairs.

Hypertrophy and induration of GLANDS.

Scrofulous diathesis.
Low cachectic condition, with profound debility and great emaciation.

Some of the Peculiar, or Italic Symptoms

" Has forgotten something, and doesn't know what."

Must keep in motion day and night : brain felt as if stirred up : and going crazy

Apprehends an accident from every trifle.

Fear of evil, with over-carefulness.

Excessive kind of impatience : is running about all the time : never sits down, nor sleeps at night.

Vertigo only on left side : worse stooping. With tremor at heart and fainting.

Goitre : hypertrophy of left ventricle : congestion to head and face ; hysteria and nervousness. Vertigo.

Headache left head and top : as if a tape tightly drawn round head : violent : makes him crazy : with paralytic feeling in arms.

Brain as if stirred round with a spoon : must keep in motion day and night.

As if a foreign substance were inside the brain.

Protrusion of eyeballs, or sensation of protrusion.

Sensation as if alæ nasi were spread wide open and nose dry.

Fluent coryza and continual tickling in middle of chest.

Convulsive twitching of facial muscles.

Tongue hypertrophied, painful, nodular or fissured.

Taste salty, sour, sweetish on tip of tongue : soapy taste.

Ulcers mouth, with putrid smell : profuse fœtid ptyalism.

Thick, brown exudation in mouth and fauces.

Thick grey-white exudate covers tonsils and palate. Diphtheria.

Eats too often and too much, and loses flesh all the while.

Alternate canine hunger and loss of appetite.

Desire for meat : for spirituous liquors.

Liver sore to pressure : jaundice.

Diarrhœa adiposa from pancreatic affections.

Atrophy of ovaries and mammary glands, with sterility.

As if a dull plug were driven into right ovary towards womb.

Heaviness of mammæ, as if they would fall off.

Bluish red nodosities both mammæ, size of hazel nuts ; dry, black points at tips.

Swelling and contraction of larynx. Spasm of glottis : cannot bear warmth.

Suffocating cough : can hardly get breath for it. Cough exhausts and chokes, and causes retching and pain in forehead.

Bitter taste of solid foods, not drinks.

Convulsive coughs in patients who are weak, sallow, short of breath, emaciated, with enormous appetites.

Expectoration : saltish, sweet, sour, putrid ; gray ; yellow ; blood-streaked.

Enlargement and induration of glands, cervical and mesenteric.

Gradual increase in size of neck, especially right side.

Marked increase of thyroid : acute pain in thyroid.

Hot, bright-red swelling of knees.

Acrid, corrosive sweating of feet.

Unendurable tickling through whole chest : in larynx : in throat.

Gradual or rapid emaciation, almost to a skeleton.

*   *   *

NASH sums up *Iodum* thus :

Always hungry ; eats or wants to eat all the time, yet emaciates. Better while eating.

Hypertrophy of all the glands except mammary, which dwindle. While body withers, glands enlarge.

Mentally anxious ; anguish ; wants to move, do something ; hurry, kill somebody, etc.

Warm blooded notwithstanding emaciation : wants a cool place to move, think, work in.

Pulsations all over, stomach, back, even arms, fingers and toes.

Especially suitable to the dark-haired, dark-eyed, dark-skinned.

Worse fasting : warm room. Better eating ; moving ; cold air.

.   .   .   Hard goitre in dark-haired persons : tumour in breast.

Heart squeezed : grasped.

Croup : child grasps larynx : face pale and cold.

Remarkable and unaccountable sense of weakness and loss of breath going upstairs. This relief from eating is not only of the sensation of hunger, but of his sufferings in general : *he only feels well while eating.* It makes no differençe whether it is phthisis pulmonalis, mesenteric, or general, this symptom, well developed, rules out everything but *Iodine* in almost every case, and it has made many remarkable cures. " I have cured many cases of goitre with *Iodine cm* when indicated, giving a powder every night for four nights, after the moon fulled and was waning."

* * *

FARRINGTON writes about *Iodine* : we abbreviate :—All the halogens may be remembered by this great characteristic : they act on larynx and bronchial tubes : on mucous membranes generally. They are decidedly irritating to mucous membranes, producing violent inflammation, rawness and excoriation, as anybody can testify who has once inhaled the fumes of *Chlorine*, *Iodine*, or *Bromine*. They all produce spasm of the glottis and this is most marked and characteristic in Chlorine. All tend to produce pseudo-membranous formations on mucous membranes.

Iodine causes absorption, especially of glandular structures, extending to other tissues, and involving finally even nervous structures. He is relieved while eating, yet emaciates despite the amount of food he eats. Sooner or later, nervous system becomes involved and he is afflicted with tremor. . . . Every little annoyance causes trembling. Longs for open air, as if cold fresh air gave him more health. . . .

Phthisis pulmonalis may call for *Iodine*. Indicated in young persons who grow too rapidly, are rather emaciated, with dry cough, excited by tickling all over the chest. Cannot bear a warm room. Expectoration tough and blood-streaked. Weakness in chest, especially going upstairs. The patient has a very good appetite and is relieved by eating.

Heart enlarged : palpitation after any manual labour. Heart sensation, as if squeezed by a firm hand. The patient can scarcely talk or breathe, so weak does he feel. In valvular disease, there is a feeling of vibration over heart, such as you get when stroking a purring cat. (*Spigelia*.)

Children cry for their dinner, feel better while eating, yet gain no flesh. Excessive mental irritability. . . .

Iodine may be indicated in cancer of uterus, particularly with profuse hæmorrhages. The leucorrhœa is characteristic, yellowish and very corrosive. . . .

* * *

KENT stresses the peculiar *anxiety* of *Iodine*, mental and physical : anxiety with a thrill that necessitates change of position, and makes it impossible to keep still. If he tries to keep still he is tormented with impulses to violence : " and so he walks day and night ! "—though exhausted with walking, and sweating profusely with slight exertion.

Hypertrophy, next : enlargement of glands ; liver, spleen, ovaries, testes, lymphatic glands : *of all the glands except the mammary glands : these dwindle ; while all the other glands become enlarged, nodular, and hard.* Enlargement especially of the lymphatic glands of abdomen and the mesenteric glands. ·

With *Iodine*, " while the body withers, the glands enlarge. The glands grow in proportion to the dwindling of the body and the emaciation of the limbs : as in marasmus. Muscles shrink : skin wrinkles, till a child looks like a little old person."

Iodine is always hungry : is relieved while eating, and relieved while in motion. In spite of hunger and much eating, he still emaciates.

He compares *Iodum* with *Arsenicum.* Restlessness with great anxiety : intense restlessness : must be doing something. " But if the patient is a hot-blooded patient we would never think of *Arsenicum :* if a cold-blooded and shivering patient, we would never think of *Iodine.*" He also contrasts *Iodum* with *Pulsatilla :* " they are both hot, both irritable, both full of notions : but here they part company : for *Puls.* is more whimsical, more tearful, and has a constant loss of appetite, while *Iodine* wants to eat much."

He also says : " *Iodine* has often cured a group of symptoms (in the constitution that I have named)—viz. enlargement of the heart, enlargement of the thyroid and protruding eyeballs, with cardiac disturbances, as in ' exophthalmic goitre '. But to cure such a case with *Iodine*, the patient must have the *Iodine* symptoms ; must suffer from heat, be emaciated and sallow, and suffer from enlarged glands."

IODUM

(for those to whom such things are helpful)

Ravenous *Iodine* howls for her dinner,
Eats much and eats often, but only grows thinner :
Her phenomenal meals she's for ever repeating,
Because all her symptoms are better by eating.
She is fidgety, fearful, unable to rest ;
While she eats, while she walks—in the cold, she feels best.
All her glands (save the mammæ) congested appear :
She's corrosive, destructive-to-clothes, leucorrhœa.

IPECACUANHA

OLD School studies and experiments with and teaches drugs for their physiological action, and lays down the maximum non-lethal doses for adults and for children. Homœopathy studies and employs, often, the same drugs, but for their exactly opposite effect, and in the fine dosage of vital stimulation.

Old School knowledge of drugs is therefore only half-knowledge, i.e. of their crude toxic and subversive action : and it is only in a few instances that it recognizes and employs them for their homœopathic action. *Ipecacuanha* is interesting as being one of the drugs that Allopathy uses to cure homœopathically : uses both ways, in fact, to provoke and to cure vomiting. It is especially in the vomiting of pregnancy that, forsaking the emetic dose of " grs. xv to xxx ", it is given in one-minim doses of *Ipecacuanha* wine. It works for us in the high and highest potencies. *Ipecac.* 200 is a mighty prescription.

But, in sensitives, as we shall demonstrate later, *Ipecac.* can cause, and therefore cure, the most terrible attacks of asthma and suffocation, and it is anything but a universally safe emetic. Its poisonings and provings are interesting, graphic, and instructive.

*　　*　　*

It will be seen that Asthma bulks largely in the poisonings and provings of *Ipecacuanha*, vide the following condensed quotations from the *Cyclopædia of Drug Pathogenesy*. Clinical confirmation in the use of the drug has laid special stress on its nauseating properties—provocative and curative :—and the " Nausea not relieved by vomiting ", and the " nausea, constant, with a clean tongue " have come to be the main suggestive symptoms for its exhibition. And yet—in its chest troubles, with agonies of dyspnœa and suffocation, there *may* be little or no nausea. Or, again, there may be nausea, with violent efforts *to vomit and to cough at the same time* producing indescribable terrors of suffocation ; seeming to threaten life.

HALE WHITE tells us that the drug affects not only the stomach, but the vomiting centre in the medulla, which may account for the clean tongue ?—in characteristic cases.

Recently we have seen a most interesting case :—asthma of years standing, combined with a skin disease ; the two, apparently, not alternating, but co-existing. A few doses of *Ipecac.* in highish potency, started almost immediate improvement in the skin condition—which one had not expected : but also greatly improved the asthma, which is " better than for years ". The prescription was consequent on this attempt to produce a Drug-Picture of *Ipecac*. By the way, a clever old homœopathic chemist used to say, " The young doctors make good prescriptions, because they are reading up Materia Medica." But—we should all do that—incessantly : and certainly writing up drugs, and teaching drugs, does, or ought to, teach oneself.

Who uses *Ipecacuanha* for " skins "?   Our books say, indeed, that it may be useful to bring out suppressed eruptions. As in scarlet fever, etc., " eruptions suppressed, or tardily appearing, with oppression of the chest ; vomiting and tickling cough ". In erysipelas, " where the redness disappears, with vomiting ". And it has " Itching of the skin, with nausea ; has to scratch till he vomits "   And Hale White says, that *Ipecac*. applied to the skin is a powerful irritant, produces redness, vesication and pustulation.

Now first, we will condense a few cases from *Cyclopædia of Drug Pathogenesy*, which show the effects of crude *Ipecacuanha* on sensitives, and thus point to the help it may give in the potencies to patients rendered *thus* sensitive by disease.

1.   Poisonings : from pulverizing *Ipecac*. root. Inhaled a quantity of the dust, which caused him to vomit three times and gave him oppression of the chest.   He left off pounding it, but one hour later had the most violent attack of suffocation, constriction of windpipe and throat, earthy cadaverous complexion, the most frightful anxiety during the suffocative attack.   These symptoms increased every minute . . .   after five hours he thought he would be suffocated.   Respiratory symptoms lasted for several days, though in a more moderate degree.

2.   Mrs. S., married to a doctor, had very troublesome short-ness of breath, with a remarkable stricture about throat and breast, with a particular kind of wheezing noise.   The fits were sudden ; often so violent as to threaten immediate suffocation ; generally went off in two or three days with spitting of a tough phlegm of disagreeable metallic taste.   It was at last discovered that these attacks occurred whenever *Ipecac*. was being powdered or put up.   For seven or eight years, by carefully keeping out of the way, she was clear of the attacks.   But one day her husband, without considering, opened a packet of a large quantity he had received, and put it into a bottle.   She, not far off, called out that she felt her throat affected, and was seized with stricture upon her chest, and difficulty of breathing.   She was exceedingly ill at night, and at three a.m. was seen, gasping for breath at a window, pale as death, pulse scarcely to be felt, in utmost danger of suffocation. Bleeding and laudanum had little effect.   About eleven a.m. she

got up after some sleep, and was less distressed till evening, when it returned in force and continued all night. This was repeated for eight days, and in a mitigated form for six days more. A slight return of menses, in the middle of the time :—coughed up at times small quantities of blood ; and there was some blood mixed with stools and urine.

3. A doctor, putting up a powdered dose of *Ipecac.*, was suddenly seized with a violent attack of asthma, attended with the most distressing dyspnœa and oppression at the precordia. In spite of bleeding and active cathartics it lasted five or six days. . . Much later, having occasion to take an emetic, he chose *Ipecac. wine.* The moment he had swallowed it, felt in throat and stomach as if he had drunk melted lead . . .   the distress settled into one of his worst attacks of asthma, and from that time was subject to them whenever exposed to the drug, or to the fumes of burning sulphur. . . . He observed in some of his attacks that when expectoration became free, in the mornings, mouthfuls would be thrown up, which any person might have pronounced to be a mass of small nearly transparent worms, but which were thickened mucus, which had collected in the small bronchia during sleep, now thrown off as casts of these tubes, often in such quantity as to surprise him that sufficient air could have passed through the lungs in sleep for the purposes of life.

4. Another sufferer, a doctor, supposing that it was only the powder inhaled which made him suffer, took some of the powdered root in tepid water, it having been weighed and mixed in a distant part of the house. In about the usual time for an emetic to work there seemed to be a simultaneous effort to breathe, cough and vomit, producing a state of suffocation totally indescribable by words. The whole muscles of chest and abdomen seemed in a state of violent irregular spasm, every effort to vomit being interrupted by an attempt to cough. Though a cold March wind was blowing he had to open the window, and support himself in the erect position for nearly an hour to prevent immediate suffocation —which was momentarily expected by his friends. The attack suddenly passed and at his request he was laid on the bed : breathing was free, but weakness was extreme, and the whole surface of the body was burning and covered with an erysipelatous eruption, covering every part. The patches were circular, from the size of sixpence to the palm of a hand, elevated with thick rounded edges, and of a fiery red colour. . . .

5. In another case, where a small quantity of *Ipecac.* powder had been scattered, " I " was instantly attacked by one of the most fearful paroxysms of asthma—extreme sense of suffocation,

oppression at the precordia, a most exhausting nausea, convulsive but ineffectual efforts to vomit with simultaneous spasms of the diaphragm and muscles of chest and abdomen, producing a state of suffering which defies description. . . . The quantity of *Ipecac.* inhaled must have been infinitesimally small.

6.   In some cases, pain in the eyes and loss of sight, with copious lachrymation was caused by pounding *Ipecac.* with, in one case, nausea and vomiting.   Saw flames before eyes, and woke later with violent pain in eyes, and pillow quite wet.   Right eye worst : quite blind ; with left saw iridescent rings of fire.   The pain was incessant and aggravated by a bright light.

*   *   *

Hahnemann says, " It will be seen from the following symptoms " (provings), " though they are not complete, that this powerful plant was not created merely for the purpose of causing a forcible evacuation of the stomach by vomiting (which in most cases is to be reckoned as one of the useless cruelties of ordinary practice), but that far higher and more important curative objects are attainable by its means.

"   .   .   .   We may learn from its symptoms that, as it can relieve some cases of tendency to vomit similar to its own, so it must, as experience has shown, exert a specific curative action more particularly in *hæmorrhages*, in *paroxysmal, spasmodic dyspnœa and suffocative spasms* and also in *some kinds of tetanus*—provided that in all these affections the other symptoms of the patient are met with of a similar character among those of *Ipecac.*

" Certain kinds of *ague* are so constituted that this root is their appropriate remedy, as is to be inferred from its own symptoms, in so far as they present a greater homœopathic similarity to those of the case of ague than do those of other medicines.   If the selection has not been quite suitable for this purpose it generally leaves the fever in a state in which *Arnica* (in other cases *China, Ignatia,* or *Cocculus*) is the remedy."

He gives it as an antidote after long-continued abuse of *Cinchona bark*, or to the unsuitable employment of *Arsenic*.

He says only very small doses are indicated : he used to use the millionth of a grain (the third centesimal) : but says that this dose should be still further diminished : and he tells us that it is a short acting remedy—from a couple of hours to hardly a couple of days.   [But *we* know what a magnificent remedy it is, in asthma cases, for example, in the 200th potency, when it " acts " for a long time.]

*   *   *

GUERNSEY (*Keynotes*), says, " One of the best guides to the use of this remedy, is a constant but unavailable desire to vomit ; or immediately after vomiting they wish to do so again ; constant nausea.

" Disgust at stomach for food. . . . No relief obtained by vomiting, the desire still remaining.

" Suffocative attacks of breathing . . . cough without expectoration ; with bloody expectoration ; without waking the patient.

" Threatened abortion ; often with sharp pinching pain about umbilicus, which runs down to uterus, with constant nausea and discharge of bright red blood . . . metrorrhagia, often after confinement, with low pulse, nausea, etc. There is a steady flow of bright, red blood, which may soak through the bed to floor, or run over foot of bed. *Where there is this steady flow of bright, red blood, give Ipecac. and don't resort to applications, manipulations, etc.*"

He gives it for dysmenorrhœa with the characteristic pain about umbilicus running to the uterus.

*   *   *

KENT is especially illuminating in regard to the uses of IPECACUANHA. We will quote—much abbreviating.

Most of its acute complaints commence with vomiting.

All the complaints in *Ipecac.* are attended more or less with *nausea :* every little pain and distress is attended with nausea.

The *cough* causes nausea and vomiting : coughs till face is red, and there is choking and gagging.

With every little gush of blood from any part of the body there is nausea, fainting and sinking.

Hence its value in uterine hæmorrhage : bright, red blood, with nausea.

The great overwhelming nausea runs through all the remedy with its symptoms.

Ipecac. does its work best where there is thirstlessness.

With the *Ipecac. fever* or chill, pain in back of head : congestive fullness : a crushed feeling in head and back of head : head full of pain.

It has symptoms that look like *tetanus.*

It has *opisthotonos :* useful in cerebro-spinal meningitis, where there is head-retraction, the whole body is inclined backwards, and there is vomiting of everything : tongue red and raw and constant nausea and vomiting of bile.

Gastritis, when nothing will stay down—not even a drop of water.

Dysentery, when patient is compelled to sit almost constantly upon the stool, and passes a little slime, or a little bright red blood : tenesmus awful : smarting, burning : with constant nausea. While straining at stool the pain is so great that nausea comes on, and he vomits bile.

Infants with cholera-like diarrhœa, ending in this dysenteric state, constant tenesmus, nausea, vomiting everything, prostration and great pallor.

Re *bronchitis of infancy* . . . how are you to distinguish from *Ant. tart.* ?   Both have rattling cough and breathing : both have vomiting.   *Ipecac.* corresponds to the stage of irritation, *tartar emetic*, to stage of relaxation.   *Ipecac.* symptoms come on hurriedly ; *Ant. tart.* slowly.   In *Ant. tart.*, when the lungs are too weak to expel the mucus, the coarse rattling comes on.

See its value in *Whooping cough :* the paroxysmal character ; the red face, thirstlessness, violent whooping, with convulsions, and vomiting of all that he eats.

Re *hæmorrhages*, KENT says, " I could not practise Medicine without *Ipecac.*, because of its importance in *hæmorrhages*.   I do not mean those from cut arteries, where surgery must come in : I mean such as uterine hæmorrhages, hæmorrhages from kidneys, bowels, stomach, lungs. . . .   In the severest form of uterine hæmorrhage the homœopathic physician is able to do without mechanical means, except where mechanical means are causing the hæmorrhage.   This does not relate to hour-glass contractions, it does not relate to conditions where the after-birth is retained,* or when the uterus has a foreign body in it, where manipulation is necessary . . . but when it is simply and purely a relaxed surface that is bleeding, the remedy is the only thing that will do the work properly.

" When the uterus is continuously oozing, but every little while the flow increases to a gush, and with every little gush she thinks she is going to faint, or gasps, and the quantity of the flow is not enough to account for such prostration, nausea, syncope, pallor, *Ipecac.* is the remedy."

But, he reminds us, when with the gushing of bright red blood there is overwhelming fear of death, *Aconite*.   Or *Phosphorus*, where there is a great thirst for ice-cold water, and though all has gone on in an orderly way, and you have no reason to expect such hæmorrhage.   Or in lean women, suffering from the heat : want covers off and to be cool ; with an alarming hæmorrhage with clots, or only an oozing of dark, liquid blood, you can hardly do without

* *Pyrogen has a great reputation in the U.S.A. for its power of expelling the retained placenta and one has seen it with cows also.*

Secale. " A single dose of one of these medicines," he says, " on the tongue, will check the hæmorrhage so speedily that, in your earlier experiences you will be surprised. You will wonder if it is not possible that it stopped itself.'

" *Ipecac. is full of hæmorrhages* " . . . and so on, in regard to colds, nose-bleed, asthma, and convulsions.

In regard to the latter, he says, " As a convulsive medicine, *Ipecac.* is not well enough known. Convulsions in pregnancy :— in whooping-cough ;—frightful spasms, affecting the whole left side . . ." *Bell.*, etc., are more often spoken of in the books and in treatises on spasms ; yet *Ipecac.* is just as important a remedy to be studied in relation to spasms, and its action upon the spine.

In *suppressed eruptions*, again, where acute manifestations of stomach and bowels follow, and colds settle in chest from suppressed eruptions. He says it will also cure *erysipelas*, where there is the *vomiting, the chill, the pain in the back, the thirstlessness and the overwhelming nausea.*

* * *

And now we will let NASH speak from his experience. Here is his summary. . .

Persistent nausea, *which nothing* relieves, in many complaints.

Headache as if bruised, all through the bones of the head, down to the root of the tongue, *with nausea.*

Stools as if fermented, or *green as grass*, with colic and *nausea.*

Hæmorrhages from uterus ; profuse, bright blood and heavy breathing, *with nausea.*

Spasmodic, or asthmatic cough ; great depression and wheezing ; child becomes rigid and turns blue.

Backache, short chill, long fever, heat usually with thirst ; raging headache, *nausea* ; and sweat last ; *nausea* during pyrexia.

Better than quinine, in intermittents, or after its abuse, the symptoms agreeing.

Ipecacuanha leads all the remedies for *nausea.* Any complaint, the patient being just as sick after vomiting as before :—persistent nausea. This should at once call attention to this remedy.

With *Ipecac.* the tongue may be perfectly clean. (*Cina.*)

He quotes Hering, " Nausea, distressing, constant, with almost all complaints, as if in the stomach, with empty eructations, accumulation of much saliva, qualmishness and efforts to vomit." NOTHING RELIEVES.

In regard to the dyspnœa, wheezing, and great weight and anxiety about the precordia ; and the threatened suffocation from accumulation of mucus, he says :

" This excessive accumulation of mucus in the air passages seems to excite spasm like a foreign body, and asthma, or spasmodic cough, or both together ensue. . . ." We may narrow down the respiratory troubles to two conditions : those with excessive accumulation of mucus : those in which spasm is the characteristic feature.

Then hæmorrhages . . . and in post-partem hæmorrhage, he says, it is not necessary to use it in large and poisonous doses, for it will stop them in the 200th potency, and is quicker in its action than *Secale*.

*   *   *

One notes also among its peculiar symptoms and modalities,—

Shuddering : malaise with shuddering, chilliness, yawning, flow of saliva and eructations.

Asthma that has to *stand for hours by the open window*.

Pain about the umbilicus, running down into uterus.

(As said) Nausea and vomiting, constant, unrelieved by vomiting : especially with a clean tongue.

Bright red hæmorrhages, especially with nausea.

Terrible spasms of respiration.

Simultaneous spasmodic attempts to cough and vomit causing unbelievable suffocative distress.

Black Letter Symptoms

Sulky humour, that despises everything, and he desires that others also should not esteem or care for anything.

Extreme impatience.

Ailments from vexation and reserved displeasure.

Headache as if brain and skull were bruised, which penetrates through all the bones of the head down to the root of the tongue, with nausea. Nausea : vomiting : better out of doors.

Headache as of a bruise of brain and skull, which pierces through all the cranial bones into roots of teeth ; with nausea.

Gastric headaches, occurring in nervous, sensitive persons, commencing with nausea and vomiting.

Pupils more readily dilatable ; dilatation of pupils.

Eye-gum in the outer canthi of the eyes.

Nose-bleed, blood bright red ; face pale.

Profuse accumulation of saliva.

Nausea as from the stomach, with empty eructations, and a great flow of saliva.

Nausea and vomiting. Distressing nausea.

Averse to all food, no appetite ; earthy taste ; stomach feels relaxed ; nausea.

Nausea ; distressing ; constant, with almost all complaints ; with empty eructations, accumulation of much saliva ; qualmishness, ar l efforts to vomit.

Nausea, with distension of abdomen and dryness in throat ; after vomiting inclines to sleep.

Indescribably sick feeling in stomach.

Sensation as if stomach hung down relaxed.

Pain most severe in front of abdomen, extending to left hypochondrium, to sides, to back, and base of chest, with swelling of stomach ; great agitation ; constant nausea proceeding from stomach, with empty eructations and accumulation of much saliva ; easy vomiting ; diarrhœa.

Pinching pain in both hypochondria, and in the region of pit of stomach.

Cutting pain about the navel with shivering.

Distressed feeling in abdomen, as though stomach were hanging down relaxed.

Griping, as from a hand, each finger sharply pressing into intestines ; better during rest ; much worse by motion.

Flatulent colic about navel, as though bowels were grasped by hand.

Cutting colic near umbilicus ; sometimes shivering.

Tenderness and pain about umbilicus, towards uterus.

Stools frequent : of greenish mucus.

Diarrhœic and as it were fermented stools.

Urine cloudy, with sediment like brick dust.

Dry cough from a tickle in upper part of larynx.

Cough which arises from a contractive tickling from upper part of larynx to the lowest extremities of the bronchial tubes.

Rattling in bronchi when drawing a long breath ; large accumulation of mucus in bronchi, difficult to raise.

Rattling noises in air passages during respiration.

Cough causing inclination to vomit without nausea.

Suffocating cough, whereby child becomes quite stiff and blue in the face.

Dyspnœa.

Difficulty of breathing from least exertion.

Violent degree of dyspnœa, with wheezing and a great weight and anxiety about precordia.

Spasmodic asthma with great constriction in throat and chest, with which a peculiar kind of wheezing noise is heard.

Loses breath with cough, turns pale and stiffens.

The body of the child is stretched out stiffly.

Whooping cough with nose-bleed ; bleeding from mouth; vomiting; loses breath, turns pale or blue, and becomes rigid.

Phlegm rattling on chest, sometimes vomited, in young children.

Hæmorrhage from lungs ; bright red ; coming up with slight effort ; < from least exertion ; frequent hacking with expectoration of blood-stained mucus ; with or without cough ; after disturbed catamenia ; after mechanical injuries ; after former bleedings have weakened lungs ; with dry cough in phthisis.

Pain in all the bones, as if bruised.

Pain in all the joints, as when limbs go to sleep.

Starts up in sleep.

Tetanic spasms from swallowing tobacco.

Fever : backache, short chill, long fever ; heat usually with thirst, headache, nausea and cough.

Paroxysms suppressed by quinine.

Hæmorrhages ; bright red, from all the orifices of the body ; after mechanical injuries.

* * *

The effects of *Ipecacuanha* in uterine hæmorrhages, with typical *Ipec.* symptoms, are so striking and so important that we will add the following cases by Dr. J. R. Haynes, U.S.A., accidentally come across in an old number of the *Homœopathic Physician*.

Mrs. T., (22), light complexion, brown hair, blue eyes, rather small in stature ; married ; the mother of a child about two and a half years old. Had had a miscarriage about a year before, and had made a poor recovery from it. Had been treated by a regular, and thoroughly dosed.

She had been feeling well ; was sitting with some light sewing in her hand, when she was taken suddenly with a severe uterine hæmorrhage. She was placed on the bed, and I was sent for—to come as soon as possible.

When I arrived, she had fainted two or three times. I found her pulseless, face pale, and so much exsanguinated that she could not speak. All the information I could get was from some member of the family, and that was very little.

The hæmorrhage had run through her clothing, through the bed, and a large pool had collected on the floor.

She was flowing very rapidly ; a large stream was gushing from the uterus, so that there was no time to wait. Whatever was done must be done at once, or death would take place in a few minutes.

The flow was of a bright red (purely arterial), the lower limbs were bathed in a cold perspiration ; hands cold and damp ; abdomen felt hot yet damp with perspiration ; the flow would come in large gushes, and life was ebbing out very rapidly.

The colour of the discharge was of a *bright red, and it did not coagulate easily*, but lay upon the floor in a liquid pool.

I considered that all the symptoms I could get pointed to *Ipecac*. A small dose of *Ipecac*. 10m was placed in a half-glass of water, and one teaspoonful was given as soon as possible.

It acted like magic, for in less than one minute there was a change for the better. It was repeated in fifteen minutes, when the active hæmorrhage ceased. I waited for an hour to see if there would be any return (which there was not) so I left placebo, and they promised that if any alarming symptoms should appear, I should be notified at once. I would not even allow her wet bloody clothing to be changed, but to slip some dry clothes under her, next to her skin to make her as comfortable as possible. There was a slight oozing for two days, then it entirely ceased.

She was very weak and prostrated after the tremendous flow ; and was given at intervals three doses of *China* 10m : and she made a good getting up. . . .

Mrs. K., (28), active, tall, slim, blue eyes. . . . Married : one child 7 years old : no pregnancy since. Was suddenly taken with active uterine hæmorrhage, *bright red* ; it would coagulate when cold : smelt of fresh blood. Had a heavy ache in lower abdomen : abdominal skin felt hot ; slight perspiration. Frequent urination, in small quantities. *The flow came in gushes*. She felt faint and nauseated ; had throbbing headache ; face pale and bloodless (? from loss of blood) a sallow look. Tongue coated white : . . . mouth clammy : cough with sticky mucous in larynx. . . . The flow was worse on motion, yet she was restless, and could not bear to keep quiet : thought she would never be well again, and what would become of her little girl. . .

Ipecac. 200 in water, one teaspoonful every hour, and as soon as flow began to cease, to throw it away, and take placebo. After the third dose the hæmorrhage was so much less that she did not continue the *Ipec*. By morning, there was merely a slight discharge which continued for a couple of days, then ceased entirely. No further trouble for many months :—I see her often.

Mrs. B., (24) dark : black hair and eyes : rather chubby. Married, one child two years old. Rather gloomy: goes half-way to meet trouble.

Taken suddenly ill with uterine hæmorrhage, *bright-red, which came away in gushes* ; began with a fainty nausea and some retching. Face bloodless ; pulse small and quick, 120 ; feet cold and clammy, abdomen hot; clammy sweat on face; sickening head-ache—whole head ; heavy ache in small of back, worse motion. Sore aching through front of chest ; spasmodic spells of coughing which aggravated the hæmorrhage, and brought it away in *gushes*. Heavy pressure lower abdomen, and, before the gush, considerable griping in uterine region. Gloomy and despondent " knew that she would bleed to death ". Best when perfectly quiet, but could not keep so. Flow worse when she moved, which would cause a gush, and make her more gloomy and restless.

Ipecac. 200 in water, a teaspoonful every hour for four doses, or as soon as the hæmorrhage " seemed to get low " to throw it away, and take placebo.

At the fourth dose, active hæmorrhage ceased ; next day a slight discharge, which grew gradually less but did not entirely cease till the third day. No further trouble.

The doctor adds, " A large number of remedies have a bright red discharge from the uterus ; but so far as I know, none of them have the peculiar characteristics of *Ipecac*. It seems to stand out very prominently in all its characteristics, and cannot be easily mistaken for any other remedy. One very peculiar characteristic is that the flow in active hæmorrhage is the peculiar gushing, which could be compared to that of a pump when the handle is vigorously worked ; the stream does not cease, but at every pulsation of the heart there is a peculiar gush, which is not credited to any other remedy, so far as I am aware. And then the blood does not easily coagulate, but remains fluid for some time, especially when active uterine hæmorrhage takes place."

IRIS VERSICOLOR
(Blue Flag)

Iris is not one of the great polycrests, drugs of " many "—
almost universal—" uses ", but it has a very definite place in our
Materia Medica which no other drug fills.   It is one of our greatest
remedies in bilious attacks and sick headaches ; in liver troubles ;
in some skin troubles ; is a remedy that affects the pancreas : but
everywhere it has very definite peculiarities of action, which should
make its prescribing easy.

It is one of the very precious drugs we have inherited from the
North American Indians.   What should we do without, for
example, *Baptisia, Gelsemium, Viburnum op., Caulophylum* ?

Iris affects the whole alimentary canal.   It has burning
distress in the stomach : the vomit is extremely sour and burns
stomach, mouth, fauces, œsophagus. Burning distress not only
in stomach but pancreas. In diarrhœa, the stools are watery, and
burn the anus, which feels on fire.   It affects the liver, increasing,
or tending towards deficiency of bile, with jaundice. From
regurgitation of bile, bilious attacks occur, with terrible headaches
and vomiting of bile—the typical recurrent bilious attacks which
make life a burden, and induce dread and uncertainty into the
daily routine.   Even the urine burns the whole length of the
urethra.   As BOGER succinctly expresses it, it stands for " rapid
elimination : with sour, burning, acrid excretions ".

The mouth is greasy, feels burnt or scalded : while profuse
ropy saliva may hang down from lips to floor, reminding one of
Kali bich.

With all these burning and acrid secretions, there is of course
pain : cramps, colics, spasms.   " Violent " pains : over eyes, in
epigastrium :   fearful cramps :—cuttings, shootings, burnings,
gripings.   It excites the secretion of glands, salivary, pancreatic,
intestinal, etc., and everywhere its abnormal secretions are
profuse, acrid, and cause the burning pains that are its
keynote.

It also affects skin : *tinea capitis* of babies : its eruptions
being typically eczematous or pustular.   It is in black type for
herpes zoster, and has been found useful in *psoriasis*.

Iris has marked periodicity : sick headaches every eighth day :
nightly colic, with diarrhœa 2-3 a.m., or every fortnight.

NASH writes, Burning mouth, tongue, throat, clear down to stomach : of anus, if there is diarrhœa.

Vomiting stringy, glairy, ropy mucus : hangs down in strings.

Gastric or hepatic sick headaches, with blur before eyes at beginning. Sour, or bitter vomiting.

Sometimes very serviceable in cholera infantum : substance vomited is very *sour*, so sour it excoriates the throat.

Burning of the alimentary canal is very characteristic of this drug. Or the vomiting may be bitter, or sweetish. There is a profuse flow of saliva.

One of our best remedies for sick headache. I used to give the remedy in the third potency, but of late years have given it in the 50*m* and am better pleased with the result, because it is more prompt and lasting.

He gives a case. " I once had a case of stomach trouble in a middle-aged lady. She had frequent attacks of vomiting of a stringy, glairy mucus which was very ropy, would hang in strings from her mouth to the receptacle on the floor. Then the vomit became dark-coloured ; like coffee grounds. Thinking she had cancer of the stomach, she made her will and set her house in order, to die. *Kali bi*. was given with no benefit whatever, but *Iris* cured her completely in a short time, and she remains well ten years since."

BLACK LETTER SYMPTOMS

Sick HEADACHE, *of gastric or hepatic origin, always beginning with a blur before eyes.*

Dull throbbing or shooting, right forehead : nausea :—
  Worse : evening, rest, cold air, coughing.
  Better from moderate motion.
  Sharp cutting pains of short duration, changing often.
  Mouth and tongue feel as though scalded.
  Profuse flow of SALIVA.

Nausea and VOMITING : *of sour food ; whole person smells sour ; of thin, watery fluid of exceedingly sour taste.*

Watery STOOL. *Anus feels on fire : disposition to strain and bear down : great burning in anus.*
  Anus feels sore : severe burning in anus after stool.
  Anus feels sore, or as if sharp points were sticking in it.

HERPES *zoster on right side of body.*

CURIOUS, OR ITALIC SYMPTOMS

Habitual headache ; violent throbbing on either side frontal protuberance : worse evening ; after exertion.

Chronic frontal headache : worse sitting down, studying, sewing.

Better standing up or working.

Headache with violent pains over eye, supra-orbital region, only on one side at a time.

Severe pain, through temples and over eyes, with vertigo, nausea and vomiting.

Violent stunning headache with facial neuralgia, followed by copious, limpid urine and vomiting.

Headache ; vomits sweetish mucus, occasionally with a trace of bile.

Headache reflex from acid stomach.

Tinea capitis : whole top of head one complete scab, yellow matter oozing from under crust which has matted hair : left ear covered with eruption. Gathers every two weeks and discharges a yellow-greenish pus. Numerous yellow pustules on scalp, each containing a hair.

Pustular eruptions, face, secreting a sanious, irritating matter.

Ropy saliva : drips from mouth during conversation.

Salivation : tongue and gums feel as though covered with a greasy substance.

Peculiar irritability of throat, palate and pharynx, coming on without appearance of inflammation, sometimes with cough.

Spasms of pharynx when swallowing food.

Chronic indigestion of milk : it sours and is vomited.

Nausea : from riding ; over exertion ; irregularities of diet : with retching.

Vomiting an extremely sour fluid which excoriates throat . with burning in mouth, fauces, œsophagus and stomach : of sweetish water ; of ingesta ; of soured milk in children ; of food an hour after eating : of bile, *with great heat and sweat.*

Periodical vomiting spells, every month or six weeks, last two or three days.

Vomits food, then sour fluid, at last bile, yellow and green : with great heat in head, some fever and great prostration : warm perspiration after straining and vomiting.

Violent epigastric pains at intervals : before breakfast : from drinking water.

Beating, throbbing, in and about heart and sternum, then fearful cramps or spasms from middle of sternum to pit of stomach, with repeated vomitings.

Burning distress in stomach and pancreas, with watery diarrhœa and great prostration.

Burning distress in pancreas, sweetish vomit.

Pain liver region : worse from motion.

Increase, then deficiency of bile, with jaundice.

Bilious colic.

Acute affections of the pancreas, inflammation or salivation.

Colicky, intermittent pains about navel, before vomiting.

Pain region of umbilicus, worse from motion.

Sharp, griping pains in bowels.

Urine scanty, red burning the length of urethra after passing it.

Or clear, copious watery in nervous headaches.

Protracted nausea and vomiting during pregnancy : profuse flow of saliva.

Pain left chest, as if ribs were pressing against lung.

Hering says, *Iris* will abort felon.

KALI BICHROMICUM

Kali bichromicum is a remedy with some very marked and characteristic features, all its own. It is a corrosive irritant poison, deeply destructive to the tissues it attacks. Therefore, acting gently and healingly in the potencies, it soothes and stimulates repair in certain, often terrible, conditions of mucous membrane and skin—i.e., where natural and drug-sickness match. . . . " Drugs are sick-making and sick-curing, and the sickness is the same."

*   *   *

One spots *Kali bich.* by its *stringiness*, its *spottiness*, its *yellowness*.

In *Crocus* the hæmorrhages, from whatever source, draw out into long black strings ; but with *Kali bich.* it is the purulent, or mucous discharges, from whatever source, that draw out into long strings—strings even " from mouth to floor ". Stringy discharges from nose, throat, ear, eye, chest, vulva, urethra—" urine alkaline and ropy " ; vomit of like character, even the milk looking like "stringy matter and water", suggest *Kali bich.* Though the drug also tends to produce " lumpy masses " (mucous), tough—and of all degrees from bland to very offensive ;—white—yellow —green.

Its most characteristic pains appear in spots. The characteristic pains of *Berberis* radiate from a centre : those that suggest *Kali bich.* occur in small spots which can be "covered with the tip of a finger ". Such pains occur in some of its headaches,— " semilateral headaches in small spots " ; "dull pain or stitches in right chest over a circumscribed spot "—in right hypochondrium : just to left of ensiform cartilage : in sacrum. Though it has also shooting and stitching pains.

Its ulcerations, also, are typically *round*—deep—looking as if punched out. They occur in mucous membranes, especially stomach : in skin : in eyes : even in bones. And the scars they leave are of like character—depressed, round, " as if punched out "

Then its *yellowness* :—yellow vision (*Cina*), yellow sclerotics (*Chel.*, etc.), yellow discharges, yellow vomit, yellow sputum. Yellow discharges from ear, nose, eye, while the tongue may be glazed, red, cracked, or " coated as with yellow felt " Clarke (*Dictionary*) makes a great point of its usefulness where large quantities of yellow watery fluid are vomited (these occur in the provings), and he gives cases.

HERING gives a case of the vomiting of pregnancy cured by *Kali bich.* " Sudden nausea ; yellow coated tongue ; inward coldness and heat of face ; constipation ; violent abdominal pains ; faintness. . . ." Again, " Long, and continued vomiting during pregnancy ; can retain no food in stomach ; great emaciation and debility."

KENT (*Lesser Writings*) details a stomach case cured by *Kali bich.*, where " There were no catarrhal symptoms of nose or chest, and no thick, ropy discharges, therefore *Kali bich.* was neglected. The stomach symptoms alone guided to its use, as he had no other symptoms of importance." " Here the patient looked over the provings, and underscored such symptoms as he had suffered from."

Among them, " Weak digestion ; stomach disordered by mildest food (as with chrome washers). Incarceration of flatulence in stomach and lower abdomen. Feeling of emptiness in stomach, with want of appetite at dinner. . . . Wakes in the night with great uneasiness in stomach, and soreness and tenderness *in a small spot to left of xiphoid appendix.* Sudden violent burning constrictive pain in anterior surface of stomach. Repletion after a mouthful of food, not helped by *Lycopodium.* Also, cutting as with knives : unable to digest potatoes or starchy foods."

*   *   *

Among other characteristics of *Kali bich.* are its rheumatism: wandering in type : or alternating with catarrh, or with stomach troubles.

Kali bich. has been found especially useful in diseases of mouth and throat, in tonsillitis, diphtheria, croup ; in asthma, bronchitis, whooping-cough, and in stomach troubles, especially in ulceration —the round variety. But everywhere it cures specifically mucous membranes affected in its own peculiar way, and finding them thus, proceeds to mend them.

*   *   *

Effect on the workers in chrome. " For the first few days there is discharge of clear water from the nose, with sneezing, chiefly on going into the open air ; then soreness and redness of nose with sensation of fetid smell. Then they have great pain and tenderness, most at the junction of the cartilage, and the septum ulcerates quite through, while the nose becomes obstructed by the repeated formation of hard, elastic plugs (called by the workmen clinkers). Finally, the membrane loses its sensibility and remains dry, with the septum gone, and frequently loss of smell for years." HUGHES (*Pharmacodynamics*).

HUGHES : A fully proved and largely tried medicine.

KENT (*Lectures*): Its principal use is in diseases of mucous membranes . . . catarrhal affections with its peculiar symptoms. It has been able to bring out in its provings symptoms from all the mucous membranes of the body. Slow, but intense inflammations of mucous membrane wherever it attacks. Of course he gives the thick, ropy or stringy, yellowish or yellow-green discharges . . . eye, ear, nose, throat, trachea, etc. . . .

Pains are aggravated by cough.

Mouth, often foul odour : teeth loose ; gums sore, oozing blood. Tongue ulcerated, becomes thick, dry, smooth, red, cracked, *shines like a glass bottle*. Tongue, thick, dry, bright-red. . . .

Pains wander, shoot, tear : wander from joint to joint and bone to bone, sometimes felt deep in the bones.

Worse beer : morning diarrhœa, worse beer.

Besides the round ulcers, Kent notices, ragged, eating ulcers : especially useful in old leg ulcers. The peculiar feature being that when the old ulcer heals it heals with a depressed surface, deep in, as if it had had a false healing.

Stomach like a leather bag. Digestion seems to have ceased. Food lies in stomach like a load.

Pains most violent in a spot you could put your finger on. Headache of that spot : patient says it is all there—at that spot— or that it begins there, or spreads from there.

Alternation of complaints, or complaints that move. When rheumatism is on, the other complaints cease. As the gouty state increases the catarrhal state or diarrhœa disappears.

FARRINGTON is especially illuminating in regard to *Kali bich.* We will extract and cull.

While there are evident general resemblances to the *Kalis*, there are decided differences arising from the acid combined with it. *Chromic acid* is a highly irritating acid : a powerful escharotic destroying animal tissues very rapidly, and penetrating quickly into the part, producing a deep ulcer.

Acts especially on fat persons, on fat, chubby children more than on adults.

Possesses great virtues in inflammations of mucous surfaces, with tendency to plastic exudation and pseudo-membrane. Causes on mucous membranes first violent inflammation with much redness and swelling, and produces an excessive amount of mucus rapidly turned into a fibrinous exudate : tending to formation of false membranes. This character of exudation gives us the well-known characteristic of *Kali bi.—discharges ropy and stringy*.

Ropy and stringy discharges, in pharyngitis, laryngitis, in coryza, in the vomited matters of gastric catarrh : in leucorrhœa and discharges from urethra. In the children it helps, where there are tenacious, stringy and purulent ear discharges, with stitching pains shooting into head and down into neck : glands, especially the parotid of that side swollen, while pains shoot down into that parotid gland.

Useful in diphtheria, with thick, yellow-looking membrane like wash-leather, and *stringy* discharges.

Specific ulcers on the fauces, which tend to perforate, surrounded by coppery-red colour.

Nasal catarrh : first dry with tickling and sneezing ; worse in open air : the secretion ropy and stringy, collects in posterior nares : may or may not be offensive.

Or in ozæna : with plugs, or " clinkers ". Lumps of hard green mucus are hawked from posterior nares especially in the morning. Or, ulcers which carry out the penetrating character of *Chromic acid*, and tend to perforate.

Croup in light-haired, fat and chubby children, with smothering spells which wake them from sleep, choking. Membrane forms thickly in larynx, narrowing it. Expectoration tough and stringy with pieces like boiled macaroni. Worse from 3 to 5 a.m. May extend down to bronchi : not common but very dangerous. Farrington says he remembers a patient who, after taking *Kali bich.* expectorated pieces looking like vermicelli and having numerous little branches—probably casts of the ramifications of the bronchial tubes. (*Ipec.*) See HOMŒOPATHY, 1937, p. 321.

Then the effect of *Kali bich.* on the mucous membrane of the stomach. The drug is so irritating as to produce gastritis. Its symptoms vary in severity from those of simple indigestion to those of malignant disease. Dyspepsia with supra-orbital headache, or with a peculiar headache. The patient is affected with blindness—objects becoming obscured and less distinct, and then the headache begins. It is violent : worse for light and noise, and sight returns as headache grows worse. He says, there are a number of remedies having blinding headache *Caust.* (but it does not diminish as headache increases), *Nat. mur., Iris. ver., Psor.,* and *Sil.* ; but with *Sil.* the blindness comes after the headache.

With this headache, Farrington says, the face is apt to get blotched and bloated and covered with pimples or acne. It is also sallow and yellowish, as if the patient were bilious. The stomach seems to swell up after a full meal, like *Lycopodium.* . . .

Gastritis : the vomited matter sour, mixed with clear mucus, or bitter, from admixture with bile. Renewed with every attempt at eating or drinking, with distress and burning rawness about the stomach. With this kind of vomit you may give *Kali bich.* in the vomiting of drunkards, and in the round, perforating ulcer of the stomach.

He notices the rash like measles, for which it has been used. May follow *Pulsatilla,* useful in the milder cases. "*Kali bich.* is one of the best remedies we have for measles " with the catarrhal symptoms of *Pulsatilla,* eyes, ears, mouth, with watery, yellowish-green secretions, only worse, and advancing to ulceration.

It produces papules, hard ; tend to develop into pustules, and even into ulcers.

*   *   *

Pulsatilla is indicated in measles. I think that it is often given in the wrong place. It is indicated when the catarrhal symptoms are prominent and we have coryza and profuse lacchrymation. . . .

Kali bich. is to be used when, instead of simple catarrh of the eyes, you have pustules developed on the cornea. The throat is swollen and pains go from the throat into the ears, the salivary glands are swollen, and there is catarrhal deafness.

BLACK LETTER SYMPTOMS

NOSE. *Septum narium completely ulcerated away.*

Entire cartilaginous septum destroyed, and the whole nasal mucus membrane in a state of purulent inflammation : the disease had been mistaken for syphilis.

Nose very dry with a feeling of pressure in the nasal bones.

Dryness of nose.

Formation of plug in nostrils.

Pressive pain in root of nose.

Expired air feels very hot in nose.

Nose stuffed up, especially upper part ; difficulty in detaching thick mucus, which more readily passes by posterior nares.

Clinkers in nose ; if allowed to remain a few days can be easily detached ; if pulled away too soon, leave soreness at root of nose and intolerance to light.

Discharge of tough green masses, or hard plugs.

Mucus tough, ropy, green, bloody ; in clear masses ; violent pain from occiput to forehead if discharge ceases.

Fetid smell from nose.

Chronic suppuration of EAR ; *membrana tympani perforated ; . . . secretion is often more mucus than pus ; discharge yellow,*

thick, tenacious, so that it may be drawn through perforation in strings;
lancinations, sticking sensations. . . .

Tongue smooth, red and cracked.
Dryness of MOUTH.
Syphilitic affections of mouth and fauces.
Hawking of thick gelatinous mucus in the morning.
Hawking of a considerable quantity of tenacious mucus in a.m.
On root of uvula, right side, an excavated sore, half the size of a
split pea, with a reddish areola, containing a yellow tenacious matter.
Deep-eating ulcers of fauces, often syphilitic.
Diphtheria : pseudo-membranous deposit, firm, pearly, fibrinous;
apt to extend downwards to larynx and trachea : bladder-like appear-
ance of uvula, much swelling, little redness.

STOMACH. Complete loss of appetite.
Vomiting.
Nausea and vomiting of drunkards.
Diarrhœa-like stool consisting of brown frothy water (with exces-
sively painful pressure), urging and tenesmus.
Bad effects of over-indulgence in beer ; great weight in pit of
stomach ; flatulence ; . . .
Prolapsus uteri, seemingly from hot weather.

Rough, hoarse voice.
COUGH (especially in a.m.) with expectoration of white mucus
" as tough as pitch ", which could be drawn out into strings.
Expectoration of very tough mucus, so viscid that it drew in
strings down to the feet.
Cough with pain, from mid-sternum through to back ; severe
stitching, or weight and soreness in chest.
Cough in a.m. on waking, with dyspnœa ; better by lying down.
Cough hoarse, metallic, in croup (membranous) or diphtheria ;
expectoration of tough mucus or fibro-elastic casts.
Expectoration is very glutinous and sticky ; adhering to fauces,
teeth, tongue and lips, finally leaving mouth in long, stringy and very
tenacious mass.

Sharp, stinging pain in region of kidneys.

Pain in coccyx while sitting.

Neuralgia every day at the same hour.
PAINS appear rapidly and disappear suddenly. (Comp. Bell.)
Pains in small spots which can be covered with the point of finger.
Pains attack first one part, then reappear in another.

Affections of any mucous membranes, with discharges of tough, stringy, adherent mucus, or can be drawn out into long strings.

Ulcers ; deep yellow, dry, oval, edges overhanging, bright red areola ; base hard, corroding ; becoming deeper ; blackish spot in centre ; cicatrix remaining depressed ; deep as if cut out with a punch, edges regular.

Complaints worse in hot weather.

SUGGESTIVE SYMPTOMS AND SENSATIONS

Milk, as it flows from breasts, has appearance of being composed of stringy masses and water.

As if head would burst : as if nose would burst.

Nose feels too heavy.

As if loose bones rubbed against each other in nose.

As of a hair high up in left nostril.

Insular large patches on tongue.

A hair on back of tongue.

Pains in spots, can be covered with finger tip.

Or, pains mostly stitching and shooting.

Burning headache with vertigo, during which all objects appeared to be enveloped in a yellow mist.

Pain in head at a point.

Periodic attacks of semilateral headaches on small spots that could be covered with point of finger.

Blindness followed by violent headache, must lie down ; aversion to light and noise. Sight returns with increasing headache.

Various colours and bright spots before eyes.

Objects seem to be covered with a yellow veil.

Corneal ulcers ; tend to bore in without spreading laterally.

Twanging like wires in left face and neck.

Tongue coated, as with thick yellow felt.

Plug in throat, not relieved by swallowing.

Ulcers in fauces—in pharynx : discharging cheesy lumps, often offensive.

Dislike to meat.

Longing for beer : for acid drinks.

Secondary bad effects from malt liquors ; especially lager beer.

Feeling of coldness, stomach and bowels.

Food lies in stomach like a load. Digestion suspended.

Pains and uneasiness in stomach alternate with pains in limbs.

Choking, as if something hard all down œsophagus : then jumping and shaking, as if stomach jumped up.

Round ulcer of stomach.

Nausea with burning pain in anus.

Nausea and vomiting of drunkards.

Gastric pains relieved by eating and rheumatic pains reappear ; when gastric pains reach to any height, rheumatic pains subside.

Curious sensation as if something eating in bowels.

Gulping up of food unchanged, not sour, with pain across middle of back.

Vomiting of greenish, watery mucus in morning.

Dull pain or stitches in right hypochondrium, especially when limited to a small spot.

Spasmodic attacks resembling those accompanying gall stones.

During emission of wind, sweat all over body, especially face, from which it runs in streams.

Urine alkaline and ropy.

Sensation of a drop of urine remaining behind in urethra.

Leucorrhœa yellow, ropy.

Tough mucus nearly strangles him.

Sensation of lump, upper part of trachea and hairs across base of tongue, which neither hawking, swallowing nor eating relieves.

Profuse yellow, stringy expectoration and much sweating.

Violent paroxysms of cough with scanty expectoration of stringy mucus : or much viscid expectoration in grey lumps.

Wakes with heaviness on chest, as from a weight.

Sensation of choking, on lying down.

Whooping-cough ; mucus so viscid that it stretched in long strings from mouth to ground.

Itching behind sternum, causing violent, racking paroxysmal cough.

Cold sensation about heart ; tightness chest ; dyspnœa.

When stooping, sensation as if something cracked across sacrum.

Cannot stoop or move from pain.

Violent aching ; pain in a small spot in sacrum. Worse at night.

Pain in coccyx.

Pustules on arms ; swelling on arm, turned into large ulcer with overhanging edges.

Dry eruption like measles.

Small pustules over body like small-pox disappear without bursting.

Pustules as large as a pea, with a small black scab in centre on inflamed parts of skin.

Suppurating, solitary skin tubercles, forming deep holes.

Itching, forearms and hands, then intolerable pain and formation of numerous ulcers, from which above a dozen nearly solid masses of matter fell on striking the arm firmly, leaving ulcers clean dry cavities.

Ulcer on wrist, oozed for several months, left a cicatrix depressed as if scooped out.

Hands completely covered with depressed cicatrices which look as if they had been punched out with a wadding cutter.

Small pustules on roots of nails. Fluid became thickened to a yellow tough mass.

Pains in shin bones (syphilitic periostitis).

Rheumatism alternating with gastric symptoms ; one appearing in the Fall, the other in the Spring.

Could hardly sit down : sensation of plug in anus. (*Anac.*)

Worse 2 a.m. : 2 to 3 a.m.

Pains fly rapidly from one place to another, not continuing long in any place, and intermittent.

SPECIAL LOCALITIES ATTACKED.

Diphtheritic formations in nose, mouth, fauces, pharynx, larynx, trachea, bronchi, uterus, vagina.

Affections of any mucous membranes with discharges of tough, stringy, adherent mucus, or can be drawn out into long strings.

Rheumatic pains, alternating with catarrh : with (above) gastric symptoms.

Bones : joints.

Eruption, covering nearly the entire scalp : consists of a number of minute vesicles, closely crowded, and filled with a transparent viscid fluid, which burst and form thick, laminated crusts of a dirty grey colour ; or swelling of skin between patches of eruption : much itching : agglutination of lids and discharge of purulent material from inner canthus : patches on face and thick crusts around nostrils : external ears greatly swollen, red and glazed, behind ears excoriated with profuse discharge . . . patches of eruption deeply fissured in folds of neck with sero-purulent discharge . . . fretful . . . sucks with difficulty, from stuffing of nostrils ; emaciation ; green, slimy diarrhœa.

Eruption began on ear and spread over half the head ; greenish crusts, with oozing of whitish, thick matter.

KALI BROMATUM

Bromide of potassium

"Bromides "—practically always " *Pot. brom.*", that powerful inhibiter, that grand suppresser, in almost universal use for the treatment of epilepsy, sleeplessness, " nerves ", and yet which, as commonly administered, has never cured the chronic conditions for which it is prescribed, *and never can.*

How do we know this ? Simply by the fact that the dose has to be always increased, as through the months or years the patient gradually asserts himself, and gets the better of the drug. You see there are two ways of prescribing. You may give a drug in order to *do something to a patient,* to " depress his nervous system and more or less paralyse the higher functions of his brain"; but this does not recommend itself as an ideal form of treatment to the homœopath, whose concern is, always, *the vital stimulation of the patient, according to definite laws, whereby he is roused to cure himself.* Drugs do not cure, popular opinion notwithstanding. Cure must come from within ; or there is no cure.

We will detail, presently, the joys, mental and physical, of the condition termed *Bromism,* from the pen of one of the best known teachers of Old School medicine in his textbook for the use of students. No wonder that one of them, years ago, preparing for her " finals " exclaimed, " Medicine is all pop. I shall *never* give medicine to *my* patients ! " We will also give extracts from the poisoning of men and animals by Potassium bromide ; our authority being the *Cyclopædia of Drug Pathogenesy.* We will also see how Homœopathy applies the drug, in non-poisonous but gently stimulating doses, to elevate and rouse latent qualities, inhibited by disease, and to relieve the sufferings of those whose health, or rather ill-health-picture resembles, but is not caused by, Bromide of potassium.

Personally, looking back, one has seldom, if ever, used this drug, or had occasion to use it. For " nerves " and sleeplessness, we have so many rapidly curative remedies which, given in regard to cause, and exact symptoms, act like a charm ; no need to " push " the remedy, or increase the dose. Take *sleeplessness*— caused, say, by over-exertion and extreme weariness of mind or body. Here *Arnica* never fails to summon " Tired nature's sweet restorer, balmy sleep". In sleeplessness from anxiety, restlessness, anguish, fear ; when man, woman, or child tosses feverishly, in despair of ever getting off to sleep, *Aconite* is simply scientific magic ; since it is *Aconite* that has thus tormented its provers, who, long ago, suffered for us, that we might cease to so suffer. Or, again, in the case of an elderly woman with a huge goitre— once,—who in one of the air raids of the last War was pinned down under a beam, while her house was burning over her head. (Some of the doctors who come to see what we are doing with our out-patients, know her.) When raids began again, last September, was it ? she turned up with the tale, " I cannot sleep ! I keep listening for them ! " and for this she, if anyone, had ample excuse. A dose or two of *Arsenicum* put her right ; and her next report was " Sleeping well ", and SHE HAD " LOST HER FEAR ". Who would, for this, substitute the stupefied sleep of bromide, which for a few hours would have made her unconscious of her terrors, but would have needed constant repetition, and would never, like *Arsenicum*, have simply, promptly, and entirely charmed them away. One sees her from time to time, and knows that during all these months of war, with houses falling around her, the healthy reaction from those few globules of milk-sugar, medicated with *Arsenicum* in potency, has sufficed to overcome even such great terror. With Hahnemann, one can only give thanks for " *God's good gift, Homœopathy* ", where it is no ques-tion of a few hours' inhibition and suppression, but of the one, most precious remedy that, causing a certain terror in those who are out to test its properties, can cure the same, when otherwise caused.

By the way, though the striking suppressions of *Pot. brom.* have never appealed to us, and we have never been tempted to shepherd our patients along that broad and easy path that can lead to a destruction of mind and body, yet, our drug picture of January last dealt with potentized *Bromium* the element, which, as we showed, was used to cure in the small doses of homœopathic preparation, the asthma of a sailor whose life was only tolerable when at sea. That is one of the precious tips of our school. It appears in the *Repertory* as, " *Asthma of sailors as soon as they go ashore,* BROM.", the only drug given, and in black type. Anyway it works ; and is, therefore, worth knowing, if only needed once in a medical life-time. We have also cured quite a number of cases of epilepsy, each with the special remedy demanded by the symptoms of the individual, and never by the remedy of the disease-name. One has also failed to cure—they are difficult cases, and this is the narrow way of those who seek to enter into life, and who regardless of difficulties and labour, and the necessity to use queer freaks of intuition and knowledge, aim sincerely at doing things that matter. There is no great merit in changing a beautiful and intelligent child into a " pimply idiot,"—even if, by doing so, the actual number of fits can be somewhat reduced . . . " *Ah, but a man's reach should exceed his grasp or what's a heaven for?* "

The price that may have to be paid, for a mere decrease, not cure, of epileptic fits, or for such sleep as bromides can offer, is, in our thinking, not worth having. Sedative drugs may be used with impunity, even with advantage, to tide over a difficult crisis ; but in chronic work—No !

Distrust any " cure " which never cures ; which can never be dispensed with, but which forms a habit, and in order to maintain a seeming alleviation must be ever increased Such a drug can never cure—such cases !

And yet, all these powerful drugs CAN be used to cure where prescribed for the symptoms they evoke : Such conditions as skin diseases, like those—five in number, we are told, that bromides can cause ; states of unconsciousness with bromide symptoms. Here, in the small and careful dosage of Homœopathy, they may prove curative, provided that the condition— ? cerebral hæmorrhage etc., has not gone too far ; for there are things that are incurable.

HALE WHITE, *Materia medica of Pharmacy, Pharmacology and Therapeutica*: (We will quote what Old School has to say in regard to this drug, so often abused by the profession and by the laity.)

" Bromides are powerful depressants to the nervous system. . . . In man at least, not only is the cortical area, but the brain as a whole is depressed, therefore these drugs are powerful HYPNOTICS. . . . the bromides are well worthy to be called powerful nerve depressants. . . . *Circulation.*—Large doses exert a direct paralysing influence on the heart, lessening the force and frequency of the beat and producing stoppage in diastole. . . .

" If bromides are taken for too long a period, a series of symptoms of poisoning, to which the name of BROMISM has been given may appear. The earliest of them is a rash, consisting of red papules, chiefly on face and back, exactly resembling some forms of acne. . . Next symptoms are general lowering of cutaneous sensibility, and also that of the pharynx; then there is a diminution of sexual power; the patient becomes lowspirited, easily fatigued, unfit for work and his intellect is dulled, . . . Potassium bromide in man, at least, the higher functions of the brain are depressed before the lower, and these again before the spinal. Thus the depression takes place in regular order from above downwards. In the reverse order of the physiological development of the function, and this is commonly the case with many drugs.

"Those who take bromides habitually find themselves unable to sleep without them. These bad effects are intensified by the fact that gradually larger doses are required to produce sleep, and thus the unfortunate sufferer becomes more and more a slave to the drug. . . . They are the most valuable drugs we have for the treatment of epilepsy. . . . They rarely cure, but often greatly diminish the number of fits. It is impossible to say of any given case, whether bromides will do good, therefore they must be tried in all. . . . insomnia of overwork, worry. . . ." And so on.

* * *

"Among the symptoms caused by the drug are some which have escaped the notice of previous observers, but which if not recognized, might lead to serious mistakes in diagnosis. I refer to cerebrospinal affections—characterized by general delirium, hallucinations, fancies about being persecuted, violent actions, ataxia of the limbs and of the tongue, and impeded articulation—which might be taken as indications of general paralysis. All these alarming symptoms disappear on leaving off the medicine."—ALLEN'S *Encyclopædia*.

In *The Cyclopædia of Drug Pathogenesy* we find :

A prover, after large crude doses of 1 oz. repeated in half an hour, found speech difficult. . . . painful sadness and indifference, almost disgust at life. Attempting to walk he experienced a strange vertigo: a sense of emptiness around and under his feet, which he was afraid of placing wrongly; the ground seemed at fault, the sense of resistance lost, his walk was staggering, and he was obliged to give it up. A profound obtuseness of sensibility, especially in regard to reflex actions. Tickling, pinching did not provoke their usual effects ; sense of touch was altered, so that there was inability to grasp with firmness. Pulse slower and compressible as if extinguished.

Symptoms of a toxic dose . . . nauseous breath ; œdema supervenes on congestion of uvula and fauces ; the whispering voice sinks into aphonia, sexual weakness degenerates into impotence ; muscular weakness becomes complete paralysis ; reflex, general and special sensibility disappears ; the ears do not hear, nor the eyes see, nor the tongue taste ; expression of hebetude becomes first that of imbecility, and then that of idiocy ; hallucinations of sight and sound, with or without mania, precede general cerebral indifference, apathy and paralysis. As the

16

bromism becomes more profound, the patient lies quietly in bed, unable to move or feel, or swallow or speak, with dilated and uncontractile pupils, and scarcely any change of colour. Extremities grow gradually colder and colder ; the action of the heart feebler and slower till it ceases.

In an epileptic who had taken large doses for a year, there was emaciation, yellowish · skin, face covered with acne ; she suffered from gastralgia, was harassed with dry cough and dryness of throat. Finally she died, delirious, oppressed in breathing, with small frequent pulse and acute abdominal pains.

There are five principal forms of eruption. Erythema, with fever, causing great pain ; acne, the most frequent form of " Pot. brom." eruption. A thickened, greasy skin, with comedones predisposes to this eruption of acne punctata and acne pustulosa. The number of the pustules are said to increase or diminish with increase or diminution of dose. The whole face is sometimes covered and disfigured by them. Another form is urticaria— erythema nodosum. The vesicular form—a moist eczema ; apparently rare. The furuncular form. Also warts have been seen on face and legs.

*   *   *

Remember : what a drug can cause, it can cure, *if properly administered*. One supposes that few drugs have been allowed to " cause " to the extent of potassium bromide ; the remedy that relieves and mitigates but never CURES sleeplessness, epilepsy, " nerves " in general, and therefore obtains such a wide application and gets so rudely " pushed ". But where you recognize, in any sickness, the *Pot. brom.* picture, and give that drug as a homœopathic remedy, it will act curatively. And in small dosage, discontinued when no longer demanded by symptoms, it is, of course, harmless.

BLACK LETTER SYMPTOMS

Loss of memory ; had to be told the word before he could speak it.

Hands constantly busy ; all sorts of fearful delusions ; walks the room groaning, bemoaning his fate ; full of fear. Unsteady.

Fits of uncontrollable weeping and profound melancholic delusions. Depressed ; low spirited. Nervous anxiety.

Night terrors of children (not from indigestion) with screaming. Unconsciousness of what is occurring around them. Cannot recognize or be comforted by their friends. Sometimes followed by squinting.

Seminal emissions, with depressed spirits, dull thought, backache, staggering gait and great weakness.

Nervous; restless; cannot sit still, but must move about, or otherwise occupy oneself; often suits nervous women.

Spasms: from fright, anger, or other emotional causes, occurring in plethoric, nervous persons, or in women at time of menses; during parturition; from sexual excitement. Too great reflex excitability; sleeplessness; during teething, whooping cough, or laryngismus stridulus; from Bright's disease.

Sleepless; restless; can only calm herself by incessant occupation.
Night terrors of children; grind teeth in sleep; moans; cries; horrible dreams.

Loss of sensibility; of body generally; of fauces, larynx, urethra, etc.

IMPORTANT ITALICS

Characteristic, or Queer Symptoms.

Memory absolutely destroyed; anæmia; emaciation.
Single words forgotten; syllables dropped.
Singled out as an object of divine wrath.
Imagines she is a devil; cannot sleep; fears to be alone.
A remedy of delirium tremens.
Frightful imaginings (in late pregnancy) have committed, or are about to commit some great crime or cruelty; such as murdering her child or husband.
Hallucinations of sight and sound, with or without mania, precede brain and paralytic symptoms. Delirium with *delusions*: is pursued; will be poisoned; is selected for divine vengeance; her child dead.
Dread of impending destruction to all near to her.
Acute mania, with fullness of blood vessels of brain.
Feels as if he will go out of his mind.
Melancholia; profound depression; feeling of moral deficiency; frequent weeping, low-spirited and childish; profound indifference, almost disgust for life.

Brain feels too tight; with a feeling of anæsthesia of brain.
Cholera infantum. Brain irritated, face flushed, pupils dilated, eyes sunken, rolls head, wakes shrieking, extremities cold.

KALI CARBONICUM

KENT says: " The *Kali carb*. patient is a hard one to study, and the remedy itself is a hard one to study."

And Farrington says that " *Kali carb*. is indicated in a great variety of diseases, but is a drug much neglected in practice ", perhaps because, except in a few of its uses, as in asthma and pneumonia, it does not appeal strongly enough to the imagination, and therefore is not—so to speak—" on the spot ".

To begin with, then, the *Kali carb*. patient is not one to arouse enthusiasm : a tiresome patient, irritable and sensitive to the last degree—especially when rendered so by ill-health and sickness. " Never at peace." Never wants to be alone. Full of imaginations and fears. " Fear of the future, of death, of ghosts ; fear that something is going to happen." " Does not seem to care for anything " . . . a drab, uninteresting, wearisome sort of person ; the " Here she comes again ! " with a groan, patient : especially if " she " happens to be " he ". Not the patient who fires your interest, or stirs your pity. Nevertheless one of a big crowd. Here there are no outstanding mental symptoms to catch the imagination ·and make prescribing easy : but *Kali carb*., so sensitive, so frightened, so unhappy and unflourishing, needs badly the help that the remedy can confer.

Nerves so sensitive—so on edge ! So easily frightened that, with *Kali carb*., " startled " means " frightened to death ". Peevish, nervous ; and, a curious symptom, very characteristic of *Kali carb*., any bang, shock, or bad news is felt in the stomach : fear is felt in the stomach. One remembers an aunt who, if you told her someone had cut his finger, would exclaim, " Oh, you gave me such a pain in my knee ! " With *Kali carb*. it is in the stomach. Kent says a patient of his expressed it thus, " Doctor, I don't have a fear like other people do, because I have it in my stomach. If a door slams I feel it right here " (epigastrium).

Kent talks of the " insidiousness of *Kali carb*." in the onset of its complaints, and " its nondescript appearance ".

Poor *Kali carb* !—not only nervous and on edge, but very chilly : " has not the normal resistance to temperature ". Catches cold from every exposure to open air : gets the " fish-bone in the throat sensation "* whenever he gets cold, and has in particular a " stubborn sensation of chilliness at noon ".

---

* Fish-bone, *or splinter sensation in throat*, ARG. NIT., DOL., HEP., KALI C., Nit. a., Sil., *etc*. " *From becoming cold*, Kali c." *only*.

Kent says : " *Kali carb.* is always cold : always shivering. If he covers up and warms the painful part, the pain goes to some other place : if he covers up one part, the pain goes to the part uncovered." And yet this is the one drug given in the Repertory for " perspiration of painful parts ".

And with all the coldness, *Kali carb.* has " burning pains which compare with those of *Arsenicum* ". . . . " Hæmorrhoids burn like fire : sensation of a red hot poker thrust into anus." But here you differentiate : the *Ars.* burnings are relieved by heat ; one doubts whether any other remedy has that ; whereas the burning hæmorrhoids of chilly *Kali carb.*, Kent says, are " temporarily relieved by sitting in cold water " ; so it is not difficult to diagnose between the two. One remembers a young prescriber so pleased because he had grandly relieved the hæmorrhoidal condition of a patient, where a fine prescriber of much experience had failed. It was *Ars.* that cured, when he once discovered that their pain was burning in character, and relieved by heat. People in these days love to inject, or remove piles : the older homœopaths used to cure them. . . .

But among the most notable characteristics of *Kali carb.*— indeed that which often first draws attention to the drug in many conditions, is its STITCHING PAINS. Pains STITCH, burn, CUT LIKE KNIVES—often extorting cries—in any part of the body. They resemble the pains of *Bryonia*, but here again, there need be no confusion between the drugs : for with *Kali carb.* the pains are worse during rest, worse from cold, from pressure, from lying on the affected side ; while, with *Bryonia* the contrary obtains : for *Bryonia* is better during rest, worse from the slightest movement, better from pressure and from lying on the affected side, and generally worse from heat. For instance, in pleurisy and pleuro-pneumonia, where they are both capable of rendering yeoman service, with *Bryonia* the pains are worse from movement, worse from respiration which means movement, while with *Kali carb.* they stitch independently of movement : pains that extort cries *between breaths*, and at any time. But, and one cannot say it too often, one remedy will not do for another, even where they both have stitching pains in excelsis ; the conditions—the " modalities "—must also agree. Homœopathy may be difficult because it demands careful differentiation where first-class work is to be done ; but is it not the more interesting ?—and truly its triumphs more than compensate for the time and care expended.

So, get it right ! Though the stabbing pains of *Kali carb.* and *Bryonia* affect often the self-same localities—pleura, pericardium, joints, etc.—it should never be difficult to distinguish between them, because in *Bry.* so long as the patient is still he is at comparative peace : whereas in *Kali carb.* they occur alike during motion and at rest, and especially when at rest : *Bryonia* is worse from motion and heat ; *Kali carb.* motion or no, but from cold. . . . And *Kali carb.*, unlike *Bry.*, is intensely sensitive to pressure and to touch.

Kali carb. shrieks when startled, and shrieks with its stitching and stabbing pains, which are everywhere: they transfix all tissues and organs—even eyeballs. One remembers trying to find the remedy for a patient with queer stitching pains in fingers and toes, and it came out *Kali carb.* Hahnemann tells us, that " STITCHES are the most characteristic symptoms of *Kali carb.*"

This remedy has a paroxysmal cough with gagging and vomiting, hence its value in whooping-cough. We quote (p. 78) from Boenninghausen (friend and disciple of Hahnemann) an account of an ancient epidemic of whooping-cough, where the symptoms were not those of *Drosera*, which failed, while *Kali carb.* proved curative : the curious symptom that suggested its use being a bag-like swelling between the upper lid and the brow. This swelling seems peculiar to *Kali carb.* " It is not a bulging and sagging of tissues as in old age, but a definite little sac, that looks as if filled with fluid."

Kali carb. affects the whole chest with its stitches and inflammations, heart, lungs, and the serous membranes that envelop them ; also the muscles of the chest wall. It chooses especially the right lower lobe in pneumonia, its rivals here being *Merc.* and *Phos.* But the indications for *Merc.* are the offensive mouth and sweat (we will give a little case), and those of *Phos.* are—thirst for cold drinks (not tolerated by *Kali carb.*) ; great constriction of the chest ; patient has to lie on the right side ; expectorates bright-red blood, or rust coloured, or purulent sputum which may have a sweetish taste. *Kali carb.* is useful also in peri- and endocarditis, with the characteristic stitching pains. One remembers one of those unforgettable cases, previously recounted, to which we shall again refer in a moment, because it belongs to the *Kali carb.* drug-picture and emphasizes it.

And now ASTHMA. *Kali carb.* is one of our very great asthma remedies. Here the patient cannot lie down : must sit up, bent forward. Must lean forward with head on knees. Terrible attacks of asthma *with aggravation at 3 a.m.* Wakes at 3 a.m. with difficult; wheezing breathing. By the way, the drug has a queer sensation of a lump rolling over and over on coughing, rising from right side of abdomen to throat, and back again.

How curative *Kali carb.* can be in asthma, the symptoms absolutely agreeing, we showed in a LITTLE CASE in HOMŒOPATHY, Vol. II, p. 24. Here a severe case of asthma was cured with one prescription of *Kali carb.* 6, 12, 30 on three consecutive days. Four years later (in sending another asthma patient), her report was that she "had never had another attack". We gave the working out of that case, to show how the drug may be " got at ".

The TIME AGGRAVATIONS of *Kali carb.* are very striking and definite, and have often led to the consideration of the drug. . . .

At 2 a.m. awakened with stomach pains or dry cough.

Between 2 and 4 a.m. awake with all ailments.

3 a.m. asthma : terrible attacks. Or dry cough. Or whooping cough. Or stitching pains awaken him : must get up and walk. Aggravation regularly. 3 a.m. is *the* bad hour for *Kali carb.*

3 to 4 a.m. the diarrhœa is worse.

5 a.m. suffocating and choking cough. (*Nat. sulph.*)

9 a.m. headache worst.

10 a.m. gets hungry and faint.

Noon, chilliness, " a stubborn sensation "

But one sees that the early morning hours are hours of especial suffering for *Kali carb.*

In the abdomen *Kali carb.* has repeated attacks of colic, which suggest *Colocynth*, the patient being doubled up with the pain.* *Colocynth* cures again and again : but Kent says where the attacks recur, the patient needs *Kali carb.* to end the trouble : in the same way as when *Bell.* has cured again and again, the finishing touch will come from its " chronic ", *Calcarea*. There is a poor little elderly woman who comes up to out-patients, and who from time to time gets these colicky diarrhœas which *Colocynth* cures, but which recur. She is a typical *Kali carb.* when one comes to think of it ! and at her next visit one will go over her symptoms again with a view to perhaps prescribing *Kali carb.* for a more all-round, and prolonged amelioration.

One must also mention,"anæmia with throbbing all through the body ". " Heart weakened with irregular and intermittent pulse." " *Kali carb.* is seldom indicated with a full, round pulse." ·" Dyspepsia in the aged, with empty weakness before food, and bloatedness after eating—and especially after soups and coffee." (Bloating is a strong feature of *Kali carb.*) " Nephritis with the *Kali carb.* stitching pains."

It is sometimes difficult to lay one's hand on illustrative and telling hospital cases—even to remember them : but some can

---

* *Here* " Kali carb. *is usually associated with gall bladder disturbances,* Colocynth *with bowel troubles and diarrhœa.*"

be traced. Here are three :—

Man of 65, admitted December 8th, 1917. Pleuro-pneumonia right base : prune-juice sputum. *Stabbing pains, especially right chest, extorting cries, with, and also independently of respiration.* Temperature to 104 ; Respiration to 40. Severe rigor on the 6th, and no sleep since, for the pains. *Shouts with them. Lies on left side.* Wants to be very warm. *Kali carb.* 30, *two-hourly.*

Pain stopped in two hours—" His first good night." Highest temperature on the 9th, 102 ; then down. Rapid recovery. The symptoms in italics are those of *Kali carb.*

(N.B.—*Bryonia* stabs occur with respiration, i.e. on movement.)

Kali carb. and *Carbo veg.* are " complementary " remedies : the one taking up the case where the other has done its part. We gave the following case under *Carbo veg.*, but will give it again here : A small girl practically in *articulo mortis*, with endocarditis, pericarditis with effusion and also pleuro-pneumonia with pleural effusion. *Carbo veg.* brought her back to life ; she was cold, unconscious, gasping her last gasps : then *Kali carb.* took up the case and pulled her through.

Case of rheumatic heart in a small boy. He got *Kali carb.* 200 and had a distressing aggravation for a few hours, screaming out with his pains, which nearly drove the Ward Sister out of her wits. However, it cleared up—heart and all : so the result was good. But Kent warns against *Kali carb.* in at all high potencies in gout, for instance—but he is speaking about old chronic cases, " where the remedy should have been given years before." But it is not a bad plan to start *Kali carb.* fairly low, say the 30th, or lower ; and then go up. The closer the prescribing, and the more a patient needs a drug, the more chance there is of an initial aggravation.

BLACK LETTER SYMPTOMS FROM VARIOUS SOURCES.

Puffiness, swellings between eyebrows and lids, like a sac.

Nose swollen, hard, red from tip to root.

Swelling of face, especially over eyes. Stitches in middle of eye.

Difficult swallowing : food descends œsophagus slowly and small particles of food easily get into windpipe.

Desire for sleep, during a meal.

Dyspepsia of aged persons rather inclined to obesity, or after great loss of vitality ; repugnance to all food ; constant chilliness, cold hands and feet, no sweat however great the heat.

Stitch pain in right abdomen, worse from motion.

Cutting pain left upper abdomen, extending from lower left chest, where there is a sticking at the same time.

Inflammation, soreness, stitches and tingling as from ascarides in varices of rectum.

Anal fistula.

Menses too early, scanty, of pungent odour, acrid, covering thighs with an itching eruption.

Violent colicky pain in abdomen before menses, constipation during.

Pressing and bearing down of pregnant females, as if a load were falling into the pelvis. (Sepia, Lil. tigr. etc.)

Violent pains in the small of the back in pregnant females.

Impending abortion with pains from back into buttocks and thighs ; discharge of coagula : habitual ; during the second or third month.

Labour pains insufficient. Violent backache : wants back pressed. (Sepia.) Bearing down from back into pelvis.

The pains are stitching and shooting, or they are in the back, shooting down into glutei muscles or pass off down thighs.

Difficult wheezing breathing.

Asthma : must lean forward with head on knees : worse in a.m.

Terrible attacks of asthma, worse at 3 a.m.

Cough at 3 a.m., repeated every half-hour.

Cutting pain in chest ; in evening ; after lying down ; does not know how she shall lie ; worse lying on right side ; in a.m. ; in lower part of chest, especially in left side : moving into epigastrium and leaving a stinging sensation in left chest.

Stitches in sides of chest on inspiration.

Sticking pressure in left chest on breathing.

Persons suffering from ulceration of lungs can scarcely get well without this antipsoric. Hahnemann.

Insufficiency mitral valves.

Tendency to fatty degeneration of heart.

Sharp pains in small of back, with very acute labour-like pains running through to front at intervals of a few minutes, occasionally shooting down to glutei muscles.

Backache while walking : feels must give up and lie down.

Back : sharp stitching pains awaken him at 3 a.m., he must get up and walk about ; pains shoot from loins into nates.

Stitching and shooting pains in back, shooting down into gluteal region or hips.

Great tendency to start—starts with a loud cry.

Cannot bear to be touched : starts when touched ever so lightly, especially on feet.

Sensation of lump rolling over and over on coughing, rising from right abdomen to throat and back again.

Liability to cold : inability to perspire : or great inclination to sweat : night sweats.

Frequent exhaustion : feels she must lie down, or sit.

Debility and desire to lie down.

Wakes about 1 or 2 a.m., cannot sleep again.

Awaking about 2 a.m. and 4 p.m. with nearly all ailments, but especially those of throat and chest.

Pains stitching, darting, worse during rest and lying on affected side. (The opposite to Bry., whose stitching pains are better from rest, and from lying on affected side.)

Oppression of breathing accompanies most complaints.

Anæmia with great debility, skin watery, milky-white.

KALI SULPHURICUM

(Potassium Sulphate)

We have been asked for a Drug Picture of *Kali sulphuricum*, and we are getting to work on it with all the more alacrity, since it is a valuable remedy about which we, and probably many of us, know very little.   It has always seemed to be almost a synonym for *Pulsatilla*, so identical are most of their interesting and more salient symptoms ; but this is explained by the fact that " a chemical analysis of *Pulsatilla* shows that one of its constituents is *Kali sulph.*, another is *Kali phos.*, and yet another is *Calc. phos.* Its mucous symptoms are probably due to the presence of *Kali sulph.*, and its mental and nervous symptoms to *Kali phos.*   But this is, of course, pure hypothesis, and only suggested for further study and observation ".   (Boericke and Dewey's *Schuessler's Twelve Tissue Remedies.*)

More than this, its modalities are mostly those of *Pulsatilla.* We read, " The grand characteristics of *Kali sulph.* are

THE EVENING AGGRAVATION.

THE AMELIORATION IN THE COOL OPEN AIR.

THE GREAT AGGRAVATION IN A HEATED ROOM.

Kali sulph. has also the bright yellow (or greenish) discharges from nose, etc., and the erratic pains characteristic of *Pulsatilla* when it comes to prescribing for " rheumatism ".

To again quote from the above edition of " Schuessler ", we find :

" The nearest analogue to *Kali sulph.* appears to be *Pulsatilla.* It is interesting to compare these two remedies, as they have many symptoms in common.   Thus both have :

" Aggravation of symptoms in a warm room.

" Amelioration in the cool open air.

" Discharges from mucous membranes are yellow, purulent in character ; sometimes yellowish-green.

" Coating of tongue yellow and slimy.

" Pressure and feeling of fullness in stomach.

" Gonorrhœa with yellow or yellowish-green, bland discharge.

" Yellow expectoration from the lungs on coughing.

" Hoarseness from a simple cold.

" Pains in the limbs, worse at night and from warmth : better in cool, open air.

" Palpitation of the heart.

" Migratory or shifting and wandering rheumatic pains."

Having shown the correspondences, it may be well to show the considerations that differentiate between the two drugs. They are vital.

MENTAL SYMPTOMS.

Kali sulph. " None of importance."

Pulsatilla is often prescribed on its mental symptoms alone. Mild, yielding, good-humoured ; yet apt to burst into tears when spoken to, or when they attempt to speak ; as when giving symptoms.

Very easily excited to tears.

Uneasiness and tears regarding their affairs and health.

Involuntary laughter and tears.

Changeable disposition ; caprice.

Desires and rejects things in the *Chamomilla* style.

Discouragement : indecision.

One of the drugs of suspicion and jealousy (*Hyos., Lach., Nux, Stram.*).

EYES. Both the drugs affects the eyes, and have a reputation for cataract.

EARS. Both affect the ears, with pains, deafness. In *Puls.* the pain may be almost insupportable, and accompanied by high fever. *Kali sulph.* is useful for polypi of meatus.

NOSE. In both, any distress and stoppage is worse in a warm room. *Puls.* has also epistaxis, and imaginary smells.

A characteristic of *Puls.* is no two stools alike.

Great rattling in chest is suggestive of *Kali sulph.* Rattling of mucus with cough.

Skin and nails are especially affected by *Kali sulph.*

Chilblains that turn blue suggest especially *Puls.*, and where they are unbearable when hot. (*Agar.* when cold.)

Kali sulph. is even suggested for epithelial cancer. " Soft polypi, epithelioma."

Again, thirstlessness, in fever, and in its preceding chill, are characteristic of *Pulsatilla.* Also one-sided chilliness, heat, or sweat—the last we have seen alarmingly produced in a young man who had been indulging too freely in *Pulsatilla.* People are apt to look on *Pulsatilla* as a sort of mild, inocuous nursery drug. But it is always useful, when symptoms arise during the exhibition of a remedy, to ascertain whether they are due to it— or in other words, are a partial proving. It is by spotting such provings that knowledge grows and is remembered.

CLARKE tells us that *Kali sulph.* is Schuessler's *Pulsatilla.* He says, " Therapeutically it answers to the process of desquamation which takes place after scarlatina, measles, erysipelas of the face, etc., to catarrh of the larynx, bronchi, nostrils, etc., where the secretion has the above-named characteristics " (the secretion of yellow mucus), " to catarrh of stomach, where the tongue has a yellowish mucous coating ; to catarrh of the middle ear and of the kidneys. . . . it facilitates the formation of new epithelium." He says, " it has had no proper proving ". He quotes a cured case of asthma, with *thick yellow expectoration*, much rattling in chest, laboured breathing, talking almost impossible. Also a case of psoriasis . . . eruption oval and annular with paler centres, covered with whitish scales, skin beneath red and smooth. The guiding symptom was " great desquamation of the epidermis."

KREOSOTUM

(A product of distillation of Wood Tar)

ANOTHER of the " offensive " drugs. Its vile odours are those of *putridity.* " Putrid odour from the mouth. Diphtheria with terrible fetor oris. Decomposition of mucous membrane, throat. Cadaverous smelling vomiting. Putrid stools. Urine fetid. Putrid state of the womb after childbirth. Leucorrhœa ; putrid, acrid. Lochia ; blackish, lumpy, very offensive ; excoriating. Septic pharyngitis, with softening and degeneration of mucous membrane of larynx, and especially of œsophagus. Gangrene of lungs. Putrid fever. Tendency to decomposition."

Putrid, then, and ACRID. Excoriation of mucous membranes generally.

Withal, rapid emaciation. One of the drugs of despairing conditions. But it alleviates, and when things have not gone too far (symptoms agreeing) may cure.

One has personally experienced the great value of *Kreosotum* in a few striking cases not easily forgotten. As, for example :

Some twenty years ago an old woman was brought into our hospital, dying of bronchitis, with fearful-smelling breath and sputum ; it was almost impossible to go near her screened bed. Two or three doses of *Kreosote* 200 entirely changed the picture— rapidly : and she made a good recovery.

Again, in cancer of the uterus, especially of cervix, with terrible offensiveness and bloody, fetid oozings, *Kreosotum* has at least palliated and made the neighbourhood of the patient bearable.

One has also used *Kreosotum* in potency for wee children on the indication ; " teeth decay as soon as erupted ".

BLACK LETTER SYMPTOMS

Chronic swelling of eyelids and their margins : agglutination of lids.

Lupus on NOSE *: left side.*

Bad odour from decayed TEETH.
Toothache ; extending to temple and left face : drawing, extending to inner ear and temples : caused by caries.
Teeth show dark specks and begin to decay as soon as they appear.

Gums : bluish-red, soft, spongy, easily bleeding, inflamed, ulcerated, scorbutic.

Putrid odour from MOUTH.

VOMITING : *of sweetish water : undigested food . . . with dimness of vision : of large quantities of sour, acrid fluid, or white, foamy mucus.*
Water, after it is swallowed, tastes bitter.
Painful hard spot at, or to left of stomach.

Frequent urging to URINATE, *with copious, pale discharge ; at night, cannot get out of bed quick enough.*
Urinates six or seven times a day, always with great haste, and always passing a great deal.
Smarting and burning in pudenda during and after micturition.

LEUCORRHŒA *of a yellow colour, also stains linen yellow, with great weakness of limbs.*
Leucorrhœa, if white, has odour of green corn.
Burning between pudenda after urinating.
Soreness between pudenda, with burning biting pains, as in little children.
Violent itching of vagina ; obliged to rub it. Posteriorly there is smarting : external genitalia swollen, hot and hard.
On urinating, vagina pains as if sore : in the evening.
Violent itching and biting between the labia : she could not refrain from rubbing.
Corrosive itching between pudenda and in vagina : so that she was obliged to rub them : with a feeling of burning and swelling in the pudenda.
Scirrhus of vagina, painful to touch.
Inveterate ulcers on neck of uterus.
Severe headache before and during menses.
Her hæmorrhage seems to pass into a corrosive, ichorus discharge, and then to freshen up again and go on.
During pregnancy, nausea and vomiting : ptyalism, vomiting of sweet water.
Lochia : blackish, lumpy, very offensive ; excoriating : almost ceasing, freshens up again ; persistent, brown and offensive.

Gangrene of LUNGS.

Left THUMB *pains as if sprained and stiff.*

SKIN : *itching : towards evening so violent as to drive one almost wild.*

HERE ARE SOME CURIOUS OR SUGGESTIVE SYMPTOMS OF *Kreosote.*

Protruding gums infiltrated with dark, watery fluid.

Absorbtion of gums and alveolar process.

Black softening and decomposition of mucous membrane of throat, with atony and extension of softening, especially towards œsophagus, in diphtheria.

Keen appetite, especially for meat : craves smoked meats.

Desire for spirituous drinks.

Stomach aches from acid food.

Deep and lasting disgust for food in convalescence.

Seasickness.

Cold feeling, epigastrium ; as if cold water or ice was there.

Malignant induration, fungus, and ulcers of stomach : ulcerative pain with hæmatemesis.

Painful sensation of coldness in abdomen ; icy coldness in epigastrium.

Colic, resembling labour pains.

Diarrhœa with vomiting : continued vomiting. Straining to vomit predominates : child resists tightening of anything round abdomen which increases restlessness and pain.

Wets bed at night : during first sleep. " Dreams he is urinating in a decent manner."

Mammæ : stitches ; dwindling away ; small, hard, painful lumps in them ; hard, bluish-red, covered with little scurfy protuberances, from which blood oozes when scurf is removed.

Shortness of breath : as if sternum crushes in.

Cough, with concussion of abdomen and escape of urine.

Cough, aggravated from exhaling.

Asthma : jars abdomen ; retching ; discharge of urine : chills and headache ; sleepiness.

Cough of old people : winter cough of old people ; spasmodic turns at night , pain or pressure referable to sternum. Better pressure.

Dreadful burning in chest : constriction.

Coughing spells with expectoration of greenish pus : of blood : of black blood.

Fever and inability to lie on one side.

Emaciation : intense hectic fever ; night sweats ; shortness of breath ; dry, teasing cough. Great debility.

Anxiety at heart.   Stitches.

Pulsation in all arteries when at rest.

Small of back will break : worse at rest : better motion.

Drawing pain along coccyx to rectum and vagina, where a spasmodic, contractive pain is felt.

Wants to be in motion all the time.

In turning quickly, danger of falling.

Child moans constantly, or dozes with half-open eyes (Dentition).

" Perfect depression of trophic nervous system."

Tosses all night without apparent cause.

Great drowsiness : frequent yawning.

Starts, when scarcely asleep : laughs in sleep.

Burning, as of red hot coals deep in pelvis.

BURNING PAINS are also a feature of *Kreos.* : eyes, ears, bowels, genitalia, back and lower abdomen, in chest, in small of back.

Heaviness : stiffness : numbness : tingling : crawling : itching.

*   *   *

As to the use of *Kreos.* in vomiting : HUGHES considers it is especially useful in sympathetic vomiting, where the irritation starts from some other organ than the stomach : i.e., in the vomiting of phthisis, of hepatic and uterine cancer, and of chronic kidney disease.

He says, *Kreos.* in children and adults is the chief remedy for odontalgia, when caused by caries of the teeth.

Also " when *dentition* is so badly performed as to become a disease, comprising general irritation and cachexia with degeneration of the teeth themselves, especially when the child is constipated. *Kreos.* is the specific remedy ".

And as to teething, he quotes Dr. Madden in regard to his first case—his own baby. " She had been extremely fretful and irritable and sleepless for three or four days, and *Chamomilla* had done no good.   I gave *Kreos.* 24, and in a quarter of an hour she was asleep, and slept eleven hours right off, and woke cheerful. The nurse was almost frightened, thinking I must have given an opiate."   And HUGHES quotes Teste, " The symptoms are usually worst from 6 p.m. to 6 a. m., so that the child (and nurse) gets little sleep."

Guiding Symptoms gives, " great restlessness, wants to be in motion all the time, and screams the whole night (Dentition)."

*   *   *

HERING gives, under TISSUES—

Hæmorrhages : small wounds bleed much.

Typhoid hæmorrhages with fetid stools, followed by much prostration.

Fetid evacuations and excoriation of mucous surfaces generally.

Skin wrinkled : restless and sleepless nights.

Profuse and offensive secretions of mucous membranes, and ulceration of the same ; with greatly depressed vitality.

Rheumatic pains   .   .   .   with numbness.

Rapid emaciation.

Spongy, burning ulcers : pus acrid, ichorous, fetid, yellow.

Gangrenous, cancerous and putrifying ulcers.

Epithelioma : carcinoma ventriculi or uteri.

Carbuncle.

Tendency to decomposition : great irritability : worse at rest.

Anthrax.

*   *   *

GUERNSEY'S chief indications for *Kreosotum* :—

Leucorrhœa putrid, with accompanying complaints. *Leucorrhœa* especially if very *fetid* and exhausting.

Putrid ulcers of any kind.   Putrid diarrhœa.

Yawning in general, complaints accompanying yawning.

Child suffering from *very* painful dentition—won't sleep at night unless caressed and fondled all the time.

*   *   *

NASH.   Cholera infantum : profuse vomiting : cadaverous smelling stools.

Hæmorrhagic diathesis ; small wounds bleed profusely (*Phos.*).

Acrid, fetid, decomposed mucous secretions : sometimes ulcerating, bleeding, malignant.

Sudden urging to urinate during first sleep, which is very profound   .   .   .   in some cases there is awful burning in the pelvis, as of red-hot coals, with discharge of clots of foul smelling blood.   .   .   .   I see that GUERNSEY recommends it in cancer of mammæ, saying it is hard, bluish-red and covered with scurfy protuberances.   I have never so used it, but in corrosive leucorrhœa and ulcerations I have used it with great satisfaction.   I generally use it in the 200th, with simply tepid water injections for cleanliness.

There is perhaps no remedy that has more decided action on the gums (not even *Mercury*), than this one.   It is not used often enough in painful dentition.   Gums *very painful*, swell, look dark-red or blue, and the teeth decay almost as soon as they are born.

A child that has its mouth full of decayed teeth, with spongy, painful gums, will find its best friend in *Kreosote*. Never forget *Kreosote* in cholera infantum which seems to arise from painful dentition, or in connection with it ; for I have seen some of the finest effects ever witnessed from any remedy from this one. (Here also is the 200th. . . .)

He recapitulates :—*Bad teeth and gums : fetid corrosive discharges ; great debility and hæmorrhagic tendency*, should always call to mind this remedy.

* * *

H. C. ALLEN (*Keynotes*) gives a few more hints for the use of *Kreosote*.

Especially for the dark complexioned, slight, lean, ill-developed, poorly nourished, overgrown :—" very tall for her age " (*Phos.*).

Children, old-looking, wrinkled. Rapid emaciation (*Iod.*) Post-climacteric diseases of women.

Then the hæmorrhagic condition . . . flow passive, in epistaxis, hæmoptysis, hematuria . . . dark oozing after extraction of teeth . . . Menses ; too early : profuse : protracted : pain during, but worse after it. FLOW ON LYING DOWN, ceases on sitting or walking about. . . Again, " can only urinate when lying ", is a curious symptom. . . (And the rest we have got.

But, generally, better from warmth. Worse in open air ; cold weather ; growing cold ; washing or bathing in cold water. Worse rest, especially when lying.

* * *

KENT, gives as the three characteristics of *Kreosotum*,

1. Excoriating discharges.
2. Pulsations all over the body.
3. Profuse bleeding from small wounds.

He says, when these things are associated in a high degree, *Kreosote* should be examined.

Lachrymation is excoriating : excoriates margins of lids and cheeks : they become red and raw. A purulent discharge is acrid. Saliva burns and smarts. Eyes smart and burn as if raw. Leucorrhœa causes smarting and burning, with mucous membranes sometimes inflamed, but always burning. Urine smarts and burns. *This tendency to excoriation from excretions and secretions applies to all the tissues of the body.*

Every emotion is attended with *throbbing* all over the body— and with tearfulness. Pathetic music will bring out acrid tears and palpitations and pulsations that are felt to the extremities.

With the *Kreosote* sore throat, the tongue depressor will establish oozing : little drops of blood will appear. Nosebleed. Inflamed eyes bleed easily. Pricked finger bleeds many drops.

KENT gives the typical *Kreosote* face : yellowish pallor ; sickly, semi-cachectic, with blotches that are reddish-looking : " it used to be called a scorbutic countenance ".

He also describes the *Kreosotum* infant, for whom most of us would think of *Chamomilla*—i.e., in regard to its trying mentality. " You see the child in its mother's arms. It wants a toy, and when given it slings it into the face of somebody : it wants this and that, and then something else, never satisfied. The lips are red and bleeding " (here we break away from *Cham., Cina*, etc.) " The corners of the mouth raw, eyelids red and skin excoriated. If it has, with this, loose motions, and you examine the fissure between nates you will find it red and raw. An older child will put his hand upon the sore genitals, and cry and scream in a most irritable way, because of the smarting and burning. Such is the *Kreosote* baby. It may be suffering from cholera infantum : may have wetting the bed ; may have spells of vomiting : it is a *Kreosote* baby.

" Wherever there is a mucous membrane, it is raw. The fluids that ooze continue to eat and cause ulceration. . . The fluids vomited from the stomach seem to take the skin off from the mouth, set the teeth on edge, make the lips raw. . . So, excoriation from acrid fluids, as well as throbbing all over the body, are features you must bear in mind with *Kreosote*."

*   *   *

It is well to realize these less frequently useful, yet indispensable drugs : drugs of extreme conditions, and with definite unusual complexes.

And now we will epitomize, for those who do not despise such aids to memory :

> This is the *Kreosotum* state . . .
> Discharges hot, excoriate :
> From mucous membrane—wound—or gum,
> Profuse and easy bleedings come :
> Sanguinous oozings, frightful stenches,
> Which *Kreosotum* only quenches.
> Leucorrhœa acrid, putrid, stains.
> Like red hot coals her pelvic pains.
> Dentitions painful, futile, too !
> The teeth decay as soon as through . . .
> For cholera infantum, note,
> With teething troubles—*Kreosote*.

LAC CANINUM
(*Dog's Milk*)

IN early medical days, unwilling to tie oneself down, even by
coming on the Hospital Staff, and being only desirous of " keeping
ones hand in ", and getting experience by helping in various out-
patient clinics (general medical, gynæcological, and the departments
for children's diseases and nerve diseases), one filled in half days
all the week round, and took the place of absentees, and worked
on in this desultory way from the day of qualification in 1903 till
1914, when one sought and was reluctantly given a Staff appointment :—reluctantly, because the, then, medical staff had an idea
of raising the status of the hospital by excluding any doctors who
could not boast the " highest qualifications ", M.D. Lond. being
the desideratum. Well, in those far-off days a certain woman
presented herself in the Gynæcology Department complaining of
ovarian pain ; which appeared first on one side, crossed to the
other, and then went back, always. The physician in charge was
horrified at the obvious prescription, *Lac can.* " Why give such
a drug ? "—to him most repulsive. However, when she next
turned up, a month later, the pain had, of course, disappeared.
It was quite a nice little introduction to *Lac can.* These are the
things that rivet a drug in the memory : and establish it as a
Power, and, as such, certainly not to be despised. By the way,
while we are telling tales out of school, the same doctor was
greatly disgusted at the idea of *Tuberculinum* as a medicine. " I
would not take it myself, and would not give it to my patients."
. . . Wee globules, mark you ! medicated with a highly
potentized alcoholic preparation, probably the 30th in those days,
that is to say, *one in a decillion*, and given by the mouth. Well
shortly afterwards, when the Koch excitement came along with
a perfect tornado of trumpets, and a little later, the Armbroth
Wright demonstrations, under the microscope, of tubercle bacilli
in the process of digestion, or elimination, safely ensconced in
white blood corpuscles, this same doctor began *injecting* his former
horror ; the dosage now crude, and the method far more questionable and perilous . . .

Ah, but !—we are told, such drugs are apt to get neutralized,
or digested, or something, and lost in mouth or stomach. Think
of the impurities of the buccal cavity ! Why risk delicate remedial

agents in—what is, after all, nature's own ordained way of absorption !

As a matter of fact, once potentized, remedies do *not* suffer the perils of neutralization. Hahnemann proved that to his own, most critical satisfaction 100 years ago : though we are still slow and reluctant to realize the true inwardness of his experiments and teachings. Among the unstable elements there is Phosphorus, which, if exposed to air, promptly changes its nature and properties. It must be kept under water in order to survive as Phosphorus, without metamorphosis into phosphoric acid. Yet Hahnemann proved that, when potentized, a few globules of phosphorus in a paper may remain for years in a desk, retaining their medicinal properties and without changing them for those of phosphoric acid. He says, " The medicinal chemical substances which have been thus prepared " (by potentization) " are no longer subject to chemical laws . . . A remedy which has been elevated to the highest potency, and by this means has become almost spiritualized, is no longer subject to the laws of neutralization : highly dynamized natrum, ammonium, baryta, magnesia, cannot, like their bases, be changed to neutral salts by acetic acid : their medicinal properties are neither changed nor destroyed." And he also says, " Besides the stomach, the tongue and the mouth are the parts most susceptible of · medicinal impressions." And Hahnemann was not only a most careful observer, but was accounted " one of the great analytical chemists " of his day. But of course all this has been of late physically demonstrated by Dr. Boyd of Glasgow.

Well : *Lac can.* is, as we must recognize, a very potent subversive and therefore remedial agent. If anyone doubt this, let him study the Provings : especially the mental symptoms, many of them detailed on page 438 ; which show that this remedy has as wide a range of imaginations and fantastic terrors as any drug in our pharmacopœa :—and it is the marked " mentals " that are, so Hahnemann teaches, of supreme importance in prescribing. And here, a point ! It is the drugs that have been proved in the higher potencies that reveal their delicate nervous and mental symptoms. The more crude dosages only evoke the more gross effects : the systemic lesions. Such drugs as *Lachesis*, and *Lac can.* are so very definite with their useful symptoms, because proved in the higher potencies.

But dog's milk, as a remedy, did not originate with the homœopaths ; but some among them, notably that pioneer in the Nosodes, the American, Dr. Swan, hearing of its extraordinary usefulness in an epidemic of malignant diphtheria, potentized it, and proved it, and thereby showed its exact sphere in medicine ; and demonstrated, moreover, that its ancient flame corresponded, as is so often the case, with its present, scientific uses as revealed by the provings.

All drugs of very special and unique action, are easily studied, and well worth learning up. The polychrests, " the common drugs of many uses ", will serve us ordinarily ; and when we have mastered *Sulphur*, *Sepia*, *Lycopodium*, *Calcarea*, *Nux*, etc., etc., we are a long way on towards running, fairly easily and success-fully, an ordinary out-patient clinic. But the less universally-useful drugs, of very peculiar and distinctive features, are less frequently, yet amazingly helpful. Once mastered, they romp in brilliantly every time, and make prescribing an excitement and a delight. Generally they do not " work out ", unless for one who has mastered the secret, that the best work is done with a few of the " strange, rare and peculiar symptoms ", fitting the case, rather than with a host of somewhat indefinite general symptoms, which, if politely given precedence, will often only suggest several remedies of the polychrest type, and perhaps completely miss the one brilliant and indispensable.

But, we must hark back to our subject, the peculiarities of *Lac can.* As said, it is the remedy, par excellence, of fears and terrifying imaginations : among them SNAKES loom tremendously. The tissues it can severely annoy and successfully comfort are, *skin* ; its ulcerations red and glistening :—*mucous membranes*, especially throat, as in diphtheria, where it has been found pro-phylactic as well as specifically curative :—*gland* troubles :—*nerve* troubles ; and as said, *mental* troubles.

The *Lac can.* throat is very sensitive to external touch (*Lach.*), sensitive also internally—terribly sensitive. It feels as if it were closing : he wants to keep the mouth open, lest he should choke. Swallowing is difficult—almost impossible, yet with constant inclination to swallow, when pains shoot up into ears (*Phyto.*). Feeling of a lump in throat which goes on swallowing, only to return (*Ign.*). The worst pain is when swallowing solids. Throat feels dry, husky, as if scalded. *Lac can.* is not only one of the great remedies of diphtheria, but of syphilis, when that attacks the throat, which has a shiny, glazed, red appearance, or characteristic patches, that " look like white china "

We have already pointed out the distinctive character of its pains : they fly about, or, characteristically, change from side to side and back again. These pains may be neuralgic, rheumatic, or ovarian. Boger (Synopsis) gives its special regions as " NERVES : THROAT : female generative organs." It not only affects the ovaries, but inflames and congests the uterus, whose hæmorrhages are bright and stringy. (Dark and stringy, *Croc.*) They come in gushes, but (unlike those of *Ipec.*) they clot easily. " Its sore throats are .apt to begin and end with menstruation." The mammæ are also affected : full, lumpy, sensitive to the least jar, very painful and must be supported when going up and down stairs. . . . And " *Lac can.* is serviceable in almost all cases where it is required to dry up milk." In this, and in its sensitiveness to jar, it reminds one of *Bell.*

Lac can. is an uneasy sleeper. Cannot get a comfortable position. " There is no way she can put her hands that they do not bother her : falls asleep, at last, on her face " (*Med., Cina.*).

*   *   *

Dr. H. C. ALLEN sums up more of its characteristics. *For nervous, restless, highly sensitive organisms.*

Very forgetful, *absentminded*, makes purchases and walks away without them.

In writing, uses too many words and not the right ones : omits letters or words : cannot concentrate to read or study.

Despondent, hopeless : nothing worth living for : her disease is hopeless ! has not a friend in the world. Could weep. Cross and irritable : child cries and screams all the time, especially at night. Attacks of rage ; cursing and swearing. Intense "ugliness".

Coryza : one nostril stopped up, the other free and discharging : these alternate. Discharge acrid : nose and upper lip raw.

Can't eat enough to satisfy ; as hungry after meals as before.

Sensation as if breath would leave her, when lying down : must get up and walk.

When walking, seems to be walking on air : when lying, does not seem to touch the bed.

Intense, unbearable aching of spine : aches from base of brain to coccyx. Very sensitive to touch and pressure.

His other important points, we have already indicated.

But in his *Materia Medica of the Nosodes* he writes, in regard to *Lac caninum,* " Like *Lachesis,* and many other well-known polychrests in the Materia Medica, this remedy met most violent opposition from ignorance and prejudice. It was for years looked upon as one of the novelties or delusions of those who believed in and used the dynamic remedy ; yet its wonderful therapeutic powers have slowly but surely overcome every obstacle.

It was successfully used by Dioscorides, Rhasis and Pliny in ancient times. Sammonicus and Sectus praise it in photophobia, otitis and other affections of the eye and ear. Pliny claimed that it cured ulceration of the internal os. It was then used as an antidote to many deadly poisons.

The use of the remedy was revived by Reisig, of New York, who, while travelling in Europe, heard it lauded as a remedy for throat diseases, and on his return used it successfully in an epidemic of malignant diphtheria. He called the attention of Bayard, Wells and Swan to the wonderful results he obtained during that epidemic, and induced them to give it a trial.

Reisig potentized it to the 17th cent. from which the potencies of Swan and Fincke were prepared. The profession is indebted to the indefatigable labour of Swan for its provings, which were made from the 30th, 200th and higher potencies . . . The provings of this remedy have placed it among the polychrests of our school and verified and confirmed the clinical accuracies of the observers of ancient times.

Dr. Allen gives striking cases of its power even in what we have called " Chronic Diphtheria ", i.e. " never well since diphtheria ".

* * *

NASH tells that he had thought it disgraceful to try to foist dog's milk on the profession, as a remedy, but after accumulated evidence, he tried it on a case of rheumatism, wandering from joint to joint, that had resisted *Puls.*, and where it not only wandered, but crossed to and fro, in the manner of *Lac can.* And the case cured very quickly. Then a case of scarlatina with side-to-side-and-back pains and throat trouble, and again *Lac can.* scored over *Rhus*, which had seemed indicated. Then a bad case of tonsillitis, choking and struggling in effort to swallow, where alternate sides were worse, and again *Lac can.* cured within thirty-six hours.

Then he got three clerks in a store to prove it:—in the 200th potency, taken two-hourly. They all got sore throats, one with patches on both tonsils.

Nash finds it especially useful not only for the inflammatory affections that alternate sides; but also for breasts and throats that get sore at every menstrual period: in mastitis, the great indication being. they cannot bear a jar; has to hold them up when stepping and going down stairs.

* * *

KENT, in his small Lecture on *Lac can.* says, All the milks should be potentized, they are our most excellent remedies, they are animal products and foods of early animal life, and therefore correspond to the beginnings of our innermost physical nature.

If we had provings of monkey's, cow's, mare's and human milk, they would be of great value. *Lac defloratum* has done excellent work and so has this remedy. *Lac can.* is in its beginnings yet, although it has made some marvellous cures . . . It is deep-acting and long-acting ; the provers felt its symptoms for years after the proving was made. It abounds in nervous symptoms . . . The mental symptoms are prolonged and distressing. It makes ulcers very red, and has cured such ulcers : ulcers are dry, glistening, as if covered with epithelium. An important remedy in complaints following badly treated diphtheria, in paralysis and other conditions dating back to diphtheria . . . oversensitive . . . hyperæsthesia of skin and all parts. It makes women violently hysterical, and causes all sorts of strange and apparently impossible symptoms. For example, a woman lay in bed with fingers abducted, and would go wild if they touched each other :—not worse from hard pressure, but she would scream if they touched . . . This state is difficult to cure outside *Lac can.* and *Lachesis.*

A strange and peculiar vertigo : as if floating in mid-air, or not touching the bed . . .

Then, the changing sides : in throats, rheumatic affections, headaches and neuralgias . . . Ambulating erysipelas attacks first one side, then the other, then back again . . . inflammatory sore throats do the same.

Full of imaginations, and harassing, tormenting thoughts. No reality in the things that be : thinks that everything she says is a lie. (Compare *Alumina.*) . . . she is not herself, and her properties not her own—as wears somebody else's nose. And so on :—we have already emphasized most of the points. Putrid mouth. Wherever there is mucous membrane, there will be exudate : a grey, fuzzy coating, like that piling up on the tongue . . . We have already given the characteristic symptoms of throat, mammæ, etc.

BLACK LETTER SYMPTOMS

Swallowing very difficult, painful, almost impossible.

Soreness of throat begins with a tickling sensation, which causes constant cough ; then sensation of lump on one side, causing constant deglutition ; this condition entirely ceases, only to commence on the opposite side, and often alternates, again returning to its first condition ; these sore throats are very apt to begin and end with the menses.

Tonsils inflamed and very sore, red and shining, almost closing throat; dryness of fauces and throat; swelling of submaxillary glands.

Diphtheritic membrane white like china ; mucous membrane of throat glistening as if varnished ; membranes leave one side and go to the other repeatedly. Desire for warm drinks, which may return through the nose. Post-diphtheritic paralysis.

Serviceable in almost all cases where it is required to dry up milk.

When walking seems to be walking on air : when lying does not seem to touch the bed.

Erratic disposition of symptoms : pains constantly flying from one part to another.

Great fear : of falling downstairs : of inability to perform duties. Fear of death, with anxious face.

Wakes distressed : must rise and occupy herself. Fear she will be crazy : that any symptom is some settled disease : that everything she says is a lie : that she is looked down upon by everyone : that she is of no importance : that she is dirty : that she wears someone else's nose : that she sees spiders.

That she is surrounded by myriads of *snakes*. Some running like lightning up and down inside skin ; some inside feel long and thin. Fears to step on floor lest she should tread on them, and make them squirm and wind round her legs. (Compare *Arg. nit., Sep.*) Fears to look behind her lest she should see snakes : *is seldom troubled with them after dark.*

On going to bed, afraid to shut her eyes lest a large snake should hit her in the face (compare *Bell.*). Has most horrid sights presented to her mental vision (not always snakes). Horribly afraid they will show themselves to her natural eye. Fear lest pimples would prove little snakes, and twine and twist round each other.

Feels that she is a loathsome, horrible mass of disease : could not bear to look at any part of her body, even hands, as it intensified the feeling of disgust and horror.

Could not bear any part of her body to touch another : could not bear one finger to touch another. If she could not get out of her body, she would soon become crazy.

Feels that heart or breathing would stop ; frightens herself, which makes heart palpitate. Fancies he is going out of his mind.

Looks under chairs, table, sofa, expecting some horrible monster to creep forth : feels that it would drive her mad. *Not afraid in the dark : only imagines she sees them in the light.*

Feels that she is going to become unconscious : wakes with sensation of bed in motion.

Dreamed of a large snake in her bed. (*Bell.*)

Dreams often that she is urinating : wakes to find herself on the point of doing so. (*Sep.*)

LACHESIS

THE greater the poison, the greater the remedy ; and some of the most rapidly-acting and heroic medicines in desperate diseases are the snake poisons. They cure, of course, just the conditions they produce : but, when used for healing purposes, these poisons must be given in small, innocuous doses ; and only to persons whose symptoms (physical, mental or moral) resemble the poison-symptoms. Where this is the case, the curative power is amazing.

We have quite a number of proved snake poisons, each valuable where its symptoms fit. We will consider one of the most impor-tant—LACHESIS.

Lachesis, the venom of the Surukuku snake of South America, was first obtained and proved by Dr. Constantine Hering, one of the most brilliant of Hahnemann's immediate followers. We have told the tale elsewhere, so will not repeat. But his handling of the live snake and its poison nearly cost him his life. He was rendered unconscious and delirious : but, on recovering, he demanded of his wife, " What have I been saying and doing ? " That, recorded, was the first crude proving of *Lachesis*.

Later provings (in many of them the higher potencies were used) have given us a very wonderful medicine. We must try to emphasize its more striking features—because it is indispensable in so many severe and desperate conditions. We shall borrow largely from Kent's illuminating Lecture, besides drawing on experience, and on the provings recorded in Allen's *Encyclopedia* and Hering's *Guiding Symptoms*.

Lachesis is very BLUE, OR PURPLE. In heart disease a purple, bloated face should make you think of *Lachesis*. One remembers a patient in hospital, dying of heart disease, with dropsy, a big liver, and a purple face—one of those pretty-hopeless cases ! Here, *Lachesis* so altered the seriousness of the condition that she was able, later, to be discharged, and to come up to the out-patient department for further treatment—when her face was seen to be no longer purple !

Another great *Lachesis* symptom is often found in those very bad cases of heart disease with failing heart, the *aggravation during, or after sleep*. This is *Lachesis*, pre-eminently. *Lachesis* is *afraid to go to sleep*, because of the increased sufferings—pain, suffocation—or whatever they may be. And yet these " bad " hearts need, above all things, sleep.

But BLUENESS anywhere points to *Lachesis*. Kent says, if there is an inflamed spot, it is purple. Ulcers eat in, have false granulations, are putrid, bleed easily—black blood, which coagulates and looks like charred straw. Parts turn black and slough. Enlargement of veins is also a prominent condition of *Lachesis*.

Lachesis affects supremely the THROAT and the MIND. We will take the throat first. Intense suffering in the throat, even when there is little, apparently, to account for it—though there may be very much ! Here, *Lachesis* is one of the out-of-proportion remedies. *Arsenicum* is another : for *Arsenicum* has a state of collapse quite out of proportion with the physical condition—so far as it can be diagnosed : and *Lachesis* has sufferings in the throat quite out of proportion to what can be observed there. Choking sensations. Feels as if grasped by the throat. Sensation of a lump in the throat : of constriction. *Lachesis* cannot bear a touch on the throat, and needs to loosen the clothing there. Cough excited by touching the throat. And all this is worse, since it is *Lachesis*, from sleep. Fulness of neck and throat : difficult breathing : choking when going to sleep : and the throat symptoms *worse from hot drinks*.

Everywhere, *Lachesis sleeps into an aggravation.* And *Lachesis* does not like heat : is worse from hot drinks : may faint in a hot bath.

But the throat sufferings of *Lachesis* are often serious, and of a destructive nature. Ulceration of the throat—red—grey—deep—spreading. Curiously, in the throat troubles of *Lachesis*, whether nervous or pathological, empty swallowing is far more painful than the swallowing of solids. When one thinks of the enormous masses a snake can " get outside " one can easily remember that the swallowing of solids does not worry *Lachesis* !

In *Lachesis*, again, we have a great remedy for diphtheria. This begins on the left side, though it may extend to the right : for *Lachesis* is pre-eminently a LEFT-SIDED remedy. It differs here from *Lycopodium*, which has many spheres of usefulness in common with *Lachesis*—even diphtheria : only *Lycopodium* is a RIGHT-SIDED remedy, and if it extends, it is to the left.

I came across an old *Lachesis* diphtheria case the other day. A wee boy of $5\frac{1}{2}$, in our Children's Ward, with a patch of diphtheria in throat, temperature 103.4, was given six doses of *Lachesis* 200. The K.-L. bacillus was found in swab and culture ; but the patch promptly disappeared : and a second culture twenty-four hours later, proved sterile. He was discharged, well, in six days.

And here one may as well quote a *Merc. cy.* case of diphtheria, with like happy result.

A few weeks ago, a nurse, with a patch on tonsil, proved, by swab and culture, to be diphtheria, was given six doses of *Merc. cy.* 10*m*, and sent off to a fever hospital, where, thirty-six hours later, her throat was found to be sterile. They 'phoned in surprise, questioning the diagnosis, and were told to come and see the slides, which had been kept. It is interesting to know further that, being a probationer, the girl's throat had been recently swabbed (before admission to work in the Wards) and had then been sterile.

Observe that, with the correct homœopathic remedy, this " swab negative " happens (with diphtheria) in 24 to 48 hours ; and the advantages of such homœopathic treatment must be patent to all. There is less risk of infection : there is the speedy cure of a most distressing and dangerous disease : and, as Hahnemann expresses it, here you have " *a gentle, rapid and permanent cure—the cure undisturbed by after-sufferings.*" This cannot be said of anti-toxin treatment—which, by the way, is not meeting with universal commendation in these days. In the *Lachesis* cases of diphtheria, the trouble not only is, or begins, on the left side, but the tongue is not the filthy tongue of the mercury salts.

We will take the mental and moral symptoms next : they are very interesting, and have led to beautiful cures.

Kent says, " self-consciousness, self-conceit, envy, hatred, and cruelty : an improper love of self. All sorts of impulsive insanity : with face purple and head hot : perhaps choking, and the collar feels tight." But short of the actual insanity which he describes, certain things stand out, as pointing to *Lachesis*. JEALOUSY ; SUSPICION ; " as when a girl never sees a whispered conversation going on, without thinking they are talking about her, to her detriment." *Lachesis* is an important remedy in states bordering on insanity ; as when " a person imagines her people are trying to damage her—suspects that people are contriving to put her into an asylum : that they are trying to poison her—or wonders if it is only a dream. Dreams of the dead : that she is dead, or about to die : that preparations are being made to lay her out".

Or; again, " thinks that she is under superhuman control : that there are commands—partly in dream—that she must obey. She may think she is commanded to steal—to murder ;—and she has no peace of mind till she confesses to something she has never done. Then, religious insanity : thinks she is full of wickedness, and has committed the unpardonable sin : that she is going to die, and go to hell." Kent says, " the physician must not make light of these things : they are very real to the patient, and must be treated with respect :—as if they were so."

Jealousy : Suspicion : and then LOQUACITY. With many of us, *Lachesis* stands for loquacity, and loquacity for *Lachesis.* " Makes speeches in select phrases, but jumping off to the most heterogeneous subjects." One word often leads into the midst of another story. Kent says also, so sensitive to surroundings, and so disturbed by noise, she can hear the flies walking on the walls, and distant clocks. In this *Lachesis* resembles one of the *Opium* states, and compares with *Lyssin.*

Here is an example of the jealousy of *Lachesis.*

A young man with a severe streptococcal infection of the back of tongue and throat—patchy and suggestive of diphtheria, got a few doses of *Lachesis* in high potency. His throat was quickly well ; but he proved *Lachesis* in an extraordinary and unexpected way. He " did not know what had happened to him " during that week-end in the country. He had become taciturn—suspicious—and " so frantically jealous that he had broken off his engagement "—perhaps a blessing in disguise, as it turned out. The proving soon wore off : but here one may say that, had not jealousy been latent in this youth, even *Lachesis* could not have evoked it. You cannot get out what is not there.

Here is a second case, that has been published, but is so illuminating as to the curative power of *Lachesis* in what was practically insanity, that it will be useful here.

A young woman suffering from insane jealousy of her husband. She was always looking at herself in the glass, because she said her face had changed. She was always peeping through the little window into their shop, to see what her husband was doing ; whether he was flirting with the shop girl. *Phos.* helped her a little, then not. She got pretty bad, was caught with a razor ; came down into the shop in her night-dress ; tried to do all sorts of extraordinary and mad things. They followed me about in despair about her : she was not safe. We discussed her case, and the doctor I was working with picked out the main symptoms, *jealousy* and *suspicion,* and of course she got *Lachesis.* I think she needed a second dose a month later. Then she bloomed into her old self, smiling and happy, all the trouble forgotten, and she had remained well seven years later, and was then lost sight of.

Here is another involuntary proving of *Lachesis* :—

A person had been taking *Lachesis* in the 30th potency for some old catarrhal symptoms, and later took a dose of *Lachesis* 200.

It had a most unpleasant effect. There was almost incessant urging for stool, with practically no result. This went on, most inconveniently, for days : till a dose of *Sepia* finished the trouble at once. In Kent's *Repertory* we find, " urging, but not for stool," with one drug only, LACH. in highest type. And elsewhere, *Sepia* is found, as antidoting this symptom in *Lach*. It is also interesting that the same person took *Lach*. 1*m* without any such inconvenience and misery. Certainly different potencies give very different results. And a German homœopathic physician, years ago, used to say that the 200th (of most remedies) was a *schlechter potenz*—a wicked potency—it had provided him with many cases of aggravation. He dreaded to use it. With some drugs, as *Lycopodium*, for instance, one prefers to start with a 30th, or a 1*m*, and to leave the 200th severely alone.

As to *loquacity* . . . There was a particular out-patient afternoon when one of the most trying of patients was pouring out her tale, with extraordinary volubility and a puzzling lack of sequence, while one " tried to get a note in sideways " for future reference. At last (to the missionaries who haunt our ways, and who were pretty on the spot with their medicines), " Well ?—what is the remedy ? " " *Lachesis !* " was the answering chorus. When that patient next turned up—*silence* and quiet answers, and then an irrepressible gurgle from the missionaries, who had recognized the patient—the erstwhile typical *Lachesis*.

But many drugs have opposite effects : and one finds with surprise, what few people seem to know, that *Lachesis* which has loquacity and hastiness of speech in the highest type, has also slowness of speech in the same black type. And *Lachesis*, as we saw just now in a case of involuntary proving, has TACITURNITY also. One must not be caught out by half-knowledge and pre-conceived ideas : it is always well to make sure.

Hyoscyamus vies with *Lachesis* in loquacity and jealousy ; and *Pulsatilla*, *Nux* and *Stramonium* can all be jealous and suspicious. But loquacity, jealousy and suspicion belong to *Lachesis* and *Hyoscyamus*, and in a lesser degree, *Opium* and *Stramonium*.

Lachesis is worse in Spring : in mild, rainy, and especially in cloudy weather.

In regard to " Worse from sleep—or in sleep." A small boy in Hospital was suffering from asthma, and he had attacks in sleep, which failed to wake him. Two drugs only have this, *Sulphur* and *Lachesis*. For some reason, *Sulphur* was given : but, later, *Lachesis* cured.

Here are some of the symptoms from the provings :—
As soon as she goes to sleep the breathing stops.

Afraid to go to sleep for fear he will die before he wakes.

Troubles come on during sleep, and patient wakes in distress or pain : as with cough—asthma—or spasm.

On waking, vertigo ; dry, hacking cough ; all symptoms worse. Some of the terrifying dreams we have already quoted.

In the headaches—the bursting headaches—it seems as if all the blood in the body had gone to head. Pulsating headache, with general pulsation from head to foot.

Hammering headaches : and " hammering ", Kent shows, is a strong feature of *Lachesis*. The inflamed ovary pulsates : and it may feel as if a little hammer were hammering on the inflamed part with every pulsation of the arteries. Fistula in ano has been cured, he says, when it feels as if a little hammer continually hammered the little fistulous pipe : and fissure, of long standing, when it felt as if the inflamed parts were being hammered. Hæmorrhoids also, with this sensation of hammering. *Bursting* and *hammering!* And, with the *Lachesis* headaches, probably purplish face, puffy eyes engorged and lids bloated. And always worse on waking : worse after sleep.

Other peculiar symptoms of *Lachesis* are disturbance of the time-sense, " an unusual confusion as to time ". Extraordinarily vivid imagination : but makes mistakes in writing (*Lyc.*). The raging pains in face and teeth, extend to ear. Pains in throat extend to ear. Eyes feel as if they had been taken out and squeezed, and then put back again. A thread drawn behind eye to eye. Feels as if, when throat was pressed, eyes were forced out. Enormous swelling of lips. Tongue difficult to protrude, *catches in teeth*. Fishbone sensation in throat (*Sil., Hepar.*).

I have always regretted, and never forgotten, a spoilt *Lachesis* case—spoilt for want of (then) knowledge. It was a huge cavity in a woman's calf : one of those big excavated ulcers one used to see so often in student days. *Lachesis* was her remedy, and was prescribed. The second time she appeared, there was most amazing healing in the ulcer. But instead of waiting to let the vital reaction carry on towards cure, it was interrupted, by repetition of the remedy. When she came again, it was much worse :— and then she came no more. It was a tragedy. " My people perish for lack of knowledge." Work is not always easy : but the spoiling of good work *is* easy, and deplorable. When things are going well, past all expectation, let them get on with it. Solomon says, " there is a time for everything ". But the time of rapid and extraordinary improvement is not the time to " butt in ".

17

Here are some of Allen's big black type symptoms, that is to say, symptoms repeatedly caused and cured by *Lachesis*.

" *Loquacity.*

Vertigo on waking. Vertigo on closing the eyes.

Headache extending to nose—or to root of nose.

Tearing, zygoma into ear.

Hawking of mucus, with rawness of throat, after a nap in the daytime.

Dry throat, in night, on waking.

Pains in throat, in connection with ears.

Throat and larynx painful, even bending head backwards.

Throat seems swollen, as if two lumps as large as fists came together ; on empty swallowing, not on eating, which seems to do good.

Sensation of a crumb of bread in throat.

Such a sore and ulcerated throat, that she could with difficulty swallow.

Sensitive throat, as if sore, with pain on left side.

Liquids can be more easily swallowed than solids.

Can endure nothing tight on the throat.

Throat very sensitive to external pressure . . .

Everything about the throat is distressing.

If in the evening on lying down anything touches the throat or larynx, it seems as if he would suffocate, and the pain is worse.

Throat sensitive, even to the touch of the linen.

Larynx painful to touch : whole throat painful to touch.

A feeling as if something were swollen in pit of throat and would suffocate him : it cannot be swallowed : with soreness of throat.

Cough worse after every sleep.

Cough caused by pressure on larynx.

Dry, hacking cough, caused by touching the throat : also occurring after sleep at night.

Constantly obliged to take a deep breath.

During heat, as of orgasm of blood, obliged to loosen the clothes about the neck, as though they hindered the circulation of the blood, with a suffocative feeling.

Beating in the anus, as with little hammers.

Diarrhœa followed by throbbing as with little hammers in the anus.

Cramp-like pain in precordial region, causing palpitation and anxiety.

Weakness of whole body, on rising in the morning.

Great physical and mental exhaustion.

Obliged to open the clothes, which affords relief (with faintness).
Obliged to wear the clothes very loose, especially about the
stomach ; even in bed is obliged to loosen and raise the nightdress
in order to avoid pressure ; she dares not even lay the arm across the
body on account of the pressure . . ."

*   *   *

OTHER NOTABLE SYMPTOMS (but in *Lachesis* they are endless !)

Quick comprehensions, mental activity with almost prophetic perception. Ecstasy : a kind of trance, or mind confused and wandering.

Thinks she is someone else and in the hands of a stronger power : that she is dead, or nearly dead, and wishes someone would help her off : is pursued by enemies. Fears ; medicine is a poison ; that there are robbers in house and wants to jump out of window. Is under superhuman control.

Fears she will be damned. Religious monomania.

Delirium, with most extraordinary loquacity. Makes speeches in very select phrases, but jumping off to most heterogenius subjects.

Extremely impatient at tedious and dry things.

Morbidly talkative : gives a rambling account of her ailments.

Talks, sings, whistles.

Wakes feeling friendless and forsaken. Hopeless.

Dread of death : fears to go to bed ; fears poison.

Fear of cholera : gets cramps in calves from fear.

Ailments from fright, disappointed love, or jealousy.

Stitches as from knives in eyes coming from head ; or from eyes to temples, vertex and occiput.

As if a thread drawn from behind, from eye to eye.

When throat pressed, feels as if eyes forced out.

Eyes feel as if they had been taken out and squeezed, then put back.

Headache frightfully severe : as if brain would burst skull.

Cutting headache, as if part of right side of head were cut off.

Weight and pressure vertex : weight like lead in occiput. Headache occiput to eyes.

Lips dry, black, cracked, bleeding.

Puts tongue out with difficulty : tongue trembles.

Tongue : blisters ; ulcers ; threatens suffocation. Gangrene of tongue.

Wants oysters, wine, coffee.

LEDUM PALUSTRE
(*Marsh Tea*)

WE have such a wealth of " wound-worts ", remedies for injuries
of different kinds, to different tissues, and of different seasons,
that we may always find one or other at our door all the world over;
and one prescriber learns to use, and swears by the one, one the
other : and indeed, their uses overlap : and yet the *one* called for,
if we know it and have it at hand, is always the ideal one for
rapid magic.

At the moment our Casualty Department is swearing by, and
discovering the transcendent virtues of *Ledum* : a remedy, as we
all know, of course ! for stings and punctures, and bites of angry
animals ; for the rusty nails that run dangerously into the sole of
the foot, or palm of the hand.   But we, most of us, have probably
a very small idea of its complete " inwardness ", and of its wider
ranges of usefulness.

A resident casualty officer, very keen at his work, and therefore
getting the dramatic results he deserves, gives us the following
experiences.

His indications are especially *punctured wounds*, or wounds
very sensitive to touch.   Abcesses, and septic conditions, very
tender, *relieved by cold*.   If the patient is not sure in regard to the
effect of heat and cold, he gets him to " put it under the cold
tap ", and if this is grateful, he is sure of his drug.

He cites a couple of recent cases : Finger ; scratch from
rusty nail ; had become septic.   Patient had put finger under
hot tap in the hotel, without relief.   It was early sepsis, not much
swelling, but it looked " angry ".   *Ledum* 12, six doses four-hourly
was prescribed, but patient was to stop the medicine if better.
Two hours after the first dose all pain went.   In twenty-four
hours there was nothing to show.

Case : crushed fingers ; badly lacerated.   Had been stitched
elsewhere.   Could not sleep.   The pain was throbbing, and shooting up arm: relieved by cold : could not bear touch.   After *Ledum*
was given there was no more pain.   .   .   .   And so on.

" *Relieved by cold*—of course ! "   Who does not remember
KENT's dramatic case, where he found a patient kicking ice about
in a tub, to relieve severe pain in his feet.   And perhaps we have
most of us come by the utterly erroneous idea that *Ledum* is therefore a " warm remedy ".   Go to Hahnemann and his provings to

find that the exact opposite is the case. And here you realize that in *Ledum* you have one of the remedies of priceless apparently-contradictory indications which make the choice of drug easy.

Ledum is really a *desperately chilly remedy, with its pains relieved by cold*. As GUERNSEY gives it, " For the complaints of persons who are cold all the time :—in bed, in the house, etc. they always feel cold and chilly."

But *Ledum* has also some other striking, often contradictory symptoms, as :—

Stiffness of all the joints : could only move them after applying cold water. Stiffness in joints is, surely, generally helped by soaking in *hot* water ?

Again, the wounded parts feel cold to touch and to the patient, and yet their pains are relieved by cold. Just as *Ars.* has *burnings, relieved by heat :* so *Ledum* has *coldness, relieved* by *cold*.

Ledum has also, general coldness without sensation of chilliness. Or, chilliness as if sprinkled with cold water on one part or another. (Contrast *Secale*, which has a sensation of burning coals falling on parts which are cold to touch). And the other way about. *Ledum* has shivering and chilliness and gooseflesh, *without* external coldness.

Or the chilly *Ledum* perspires, and cannot bear to be covered by bedclothes. Sweats all night.

Its rheumatism not only begins in the lower limbs and feet, and travels upwards (reverse of *Kalmia*) but it is also far more severe in the lower limbs.

Again, contrast *Lachesis*—puffy, purple and hot, with *Ledum*, puffy, purple and cold.

And, as said, *Ledum* wounds, abscesses and septic foci are tender, *cold, and relieved by cold*, while those of *Ars.* burn, and relieved by heat.

*　　*　　*

HAHNEMANN, who made a brief proving of the drug, says of *Ledum*. " The subjoined symptoms . . . are yet enough to show that this very powerful medicine is suitable for the most part only for chronic maladies in which there is a predominance of coldness and deficiency of animal heat.

He says also that in his day many intoxicating beers were adulterated to a hurtful extent and in a criminal manner with *Ledum* to which the police authorities should pay more attention."

*　　*　　*

CLARKE—*Dictionary*, has much to say about *Ledum* and quotes instructive cases.

He says that the leaves of *Ledum* are still used in Sweden to increase the intoxicating power of beer. . . . *Ledum* occupies the second place in Teste's *Arnica* Group, in which are also *Crot. h.*, *Ferr. magn.*, *Rhus* and *Spigelia* : but *Ledum* has a special action on the capillary system in parts where cellular tissue is wanting, and where a dry, resisting texture is present, as in the fingers and toes. " It is perhaps for that reason that it acts better on the small than on the large joints . . ." A sort of bluish or violet tuberosities, especially on the forehead, and an eczematous eruption, with tingling itching that spreads over the whole body, penetrating into the mouth, probably also into the air passages, and occasions a spasmodic cough, sometimes very violent, which might be mistaken for whooping-cough. . . . Especially useful in bronchitis with emphysema of the aged ; renders bronchial secretion less viscid, lessens dyspnœa, stimulates circulation and lessens cyanosis. Hæmoptysis alternating with rheumatism. . . . *Ledum* has often been given to horses when they go lame and draw up their legs. . . . In one case, sensation of feet held to earth as by a magnet when attempting to move : when moving felt as if pricked by needles ; pain rising from feet to head.

*　　　*　　　*

Scraps from Guernsey :

Punctured wounds from sharp pointed instruments—awls, rat bites, nails, particularly if the wounded parts are cold ; or, e.g. " Ten years ago I stepped on a nail, and ever since then, have had a pain running up to the thigh." Bad effects from recent or chronic injuries, especially from punctured wounds.

When striking the toe there is a coldness in the parts, and a gouty pain shoots through foot and limb. Cracking of joints.

Whitlows, felons, etc., often caused by needle pricks.

Sufferings are worse, or come on, after getting warm in bed. Must get out of bed, which affords relief.

For complaints of people who are cold all the time,—in bed, in the house, etc. ; they always feel cold and chilly.

Worse from moving, especially the joints ; while walking ; getting warm in bed.

Better while reposing.

*　　　*　　　*

Kent in his graphic and practical way, has a great deal to say about *Ledum*. We will cull, and condense.

He finds a good many features similar to those of *Lachesis* : mottled, puffy, bloated face. Therefore of course *Ledum* is antidotal to *Lachesis* : also to the poison of insects, to *Apis* and to animal poisons.

He calls it a great remedy for the surgeon, closely associated in traumatism with *Arnica* and *Hypericum* : especially for injuries from stepping on tacks, puncturing with needles : wounds that bleed scantily, but are followed by pain, puffiness and coldness of the part. Splinters : splinters under the nail : if such wounded part becomes cold, then pale, paralysed and mottled, think of *Ledum*. A horse steps on a nail, it goes through and strikes the margin of the coffin bone, with tetanus to follow and death : put *Ledum* on the tongue of that horse and there will not be any trouble. *Ledum* removes the tendency to such results.

If tetanus comes on after punctured wounds, think of *Hypericum* : but give *Ledum* at once, and prevent tetanus. Torn nails, or lacerated parts rich in nerves, and here *Hypericum* is the remedy. For bruising, however extensive, and sensation of bruising, the remedy is *Arnica*. Open lacerations and cuts, think of *Calendula*. He says, for local causes, use local remedies : for internal causes, treat with internal remedies.

(But, as we have seen, *Ledum* internally in potency is amazingly helpful and comforting to external injuries.) He says also, if a wound, carefully dressed, does not heal by first intention, look out for the constitutional cause, and ferret out its remedy.

The *Ledum* patient is very subject to constitutional coldness, coldness to touch : cold body and extremities, with hot head (*Arn.*). But also the other extreme : the body overheated, skin purple or highly coloured, throbbing and pulsating everywhere, and wants covers off at night. A *Ledum* headache,—she may want to put it out into the cold air (*Ars.*, *Phos.*), wants to bathe it in very cold water.

Bloated, swollen, mottled hands and feet : swollen as far as skin will allow : with excruciating pain : the only relief to be got is by sitting by the hour, with the feet in a tub of ice-cold water. He gives a case in a syphilitic drunkard : " When I first saw him he had a good-sized wash-tub, and he sat with the ice water two thirds up to his knees and pieces of ice floating around, which he liked to have coming in contact with the skin. He would go on putting in ice. He ' suffered agonies something dreadful '. Well, a dose of *Ledum* took his feet out of the ice water, so that he never used it afterwards. The purpleness disappeared, the swelling went down, the bloating went out of his feet and he quit drinking." *Ledum* even "cured him of very much of his syphilitic trouble" KENT says, " *Pulsatilla* and *Ledum* are the two principle remedies that want the feet in very cold water. But *Ledum* suited that man."

Ledum patients mostly are full blooded and plethoric: robust. Its inflamed surfaces tend to bleed, and the blood is black.

Hæmorrhages of eye—nose—cavities : bloody urine.

Ulcers—perhaps phagedenic and spreading : relieved by cold.

Rheumatic and gouty conditions : chalk stones : deposits in wrists, fingers and toes. Go from below upwards. Inflame, and are relieved by cold. Especially knees affected. " Such patients sit with joint exposed to the cold, fanning it, or putting on evaporating lotion."

Face, puffy, bloated, besotted, like that of an old drunkard. Takes away, to a great extent the crave for whisky, and counteracts its effects. He says " *Ledum* is to whisky what *Caladium* is to smokers : it will break off the smoking habit, so that they often got an aversion to it."

He talks of its kidney symptoms : its sand in the urine. " When the patient is feeling his best, there are great quantities of sandy deposits in the urine : when there is little sand, the deposits in joints become marked, and he feels less well."

Ledum tends to make complaints go away from the centre, because its complaints begin in the circumference and go towards the centre. *Lycopodium,* which often causes a return of red sand to the urine, also keeps conditions coming to the surface.

Emaciation of suffering parts, after infected injuries to nerves.

*   *   *

NASH has some extra things to emphasize in regard to *Ledum.*

Ecchymoses : *Ledum* sometimes comes in to finish up an *Arnica* case ; where *Arnica* was best at first, *Ledum* often removes the ecchymoses and discoloration more rapidly and perfectly.

" Black eye, from a blow or contusion : better than *Arnica.*" For this, he says, there is no remedy equal to *Ledum* in the 200th potency. But if there be great pain in the eyeball itself, *Symphytum* may have to be used. He adds, in all these affections I believe the 200th potency better than the lower preparations."

He talks of *Ledum* in *acute rheumatism :*—the joints are swollen and hot, but not red. The swellings are pale and the pains are *worse at night* and *from heat of the bed ;* wants them uncovered.

· In *chronic rheumatism* it is equally efficacious. Joints swollen and painful, especially in the heat of the bed ; with painful hard nodes and concretions first in joints of feet, then hands. Periosteum of phalanges painful on pressure. Ankles swollen and soles painful and sensitive ; can hardly step on them. And in these cases the *Ledum* patient is unnaturally cold : lack vital or animal heat. Under *Ledum* the relief from cold is so prominent that

sometimes the only amelioration is putting the feet into cold water.
He says, study *Ledum* in all cases of rheumatism of the feet.

BLACK LETTER SYMPTOMS

All day long, discontented with his fellow creatures, which at last amounted to misanthropy.
Vertigo. Head tends to sink backwards.

Considerable dilatation of pupils.
Contusions or wounds of eye or lids, especially with extravasation of blood.

A noise in the ears like ringing of bells, or like a storm of wind. Roaring in the ears, as from wind.

Hard pressure inwards in the lower jaw.

Sore throat, with fine shooting pain.
A sudden flow of watery saliva from mouth, with colic. Water-brash.

Tight, painful respiration.
Dyspnœic constriction of chest, worse movement and walking.
Chronic cough characterized by cold and deficiency of animal heat.
Expectoration of bright red blood with violent cough.

Pain in loins after sitting.

On raising arm, extremely painful shooting in shoulder.
Pressure in left shoulder joint, aggravated by movement.
Pressure in both shoulder joints, aggravated by movement.
Trembling of the hands when grasping or when moving them.
Whitlows, from punctured wounds, needle pricks, splinters.

Pressure in left thigh, posteriorly ; as if the muscles were not in their right places, like pain of dislocation ; in every position, but especially violent when touched and when walking.
Trembling of knees (and hands) when sitting and walking.
Weakness in knee joints, when walking, a tearing pressure in them. Tearing pressure in right knee joint and below it : worse by walking.
Swelling, and tensive, and shooting pain in knees, when walking.
Pressure above left ankle, worse by movement.

Very severe gnawing itching on dorsum of both feet : more violent after scratching : only allayed when he had scratched the feet raw : much aggravated by heat of bed.

Obstinate swelling of the feet.

Pressure on the inner ball of left foot.

Soles of feet painful when walking, as if filled with blood.

Ball of big toes is soft, swollen and painful when treading ; tendons stiff.

Gout, worse in feet : gouty nodosities on joints : fine tearing in toes.

Pain in ankles, as from strain, or false step.

Rheumatic pains going from below upwards ; joints pale, swollen, tense, hot ; stinging, drawing pains. Worse from warmth of bed, and bed covering ; worse motion and in evening.

Rheumatism and rheumatic gout ; begins in lower limbs and ascends ; especially if brought into a low, asthenic state by abuse of Colchicum ; joints become the seat of nodosities and " gout stones " which are painful.

Swelling of feet and legs up to knees, purple and mottled, pitting on pressure, with rending pains in periosteum ; comfortable only when holding feet in ice water.

Affects principally left shoulder and right hip joint.

Rheumatism begins in lower limbs and ascends.

Heat in the hands and the feet, in the evening.

Long continued warm sweat on hands and feet.

Cannot bear the heat of the bed, on account of heat and burning in the limbs.

Gone to sleep feeling of the limbs.

Uneasy dreams : he is sometimes in one place, sometimes in another, sometimes occupied with one subject, sometimes with another.

Sleeplessness with restlessness and tossing about.

On waking, slight sweat all over, with itching all over that compelled scratching.

Chilliness without subsequent heat : limbs extremely cold, while rest of body was warm.

Rigor over whole back, with rather hot cheeks and hot forehead, without redness of face, or thirst ; with cold hands.

Sprains of ankles and feet.

Punctured wounds, from sharp pointed instruments, as awls, rat bites, nails, etc. ; particularly if wounded parts feel cold to touch, and to patient.

Punctured wounds ; stings, of insects, especially of mosquitoes. Rheumatic, gouty diathesis ; constitutions abused by alcohol. Emaciation of suffering parts. (? Plumb.).

OTHER NOTABLE SYMPTOMS

One of its mental pictures is striking :—Cross, surly : everything is disagreeable. Restless ; cannot reflect steadily, or work quietly. Cross : he retired into solitude, and, almost weeping, longed for death.

Least covering of head is intolerable.

Mouldy taste in mouth every time she coughs, causing nausea.

Spasmodic, *double inspiration*, with sobbing, as after crying.

Child gets stiff before paroxysm ; bends himself backwards, followed by expectoration of clear frothy blood. (Whooping cough.)

Hæmoptysis, bright-red, profuse, with cough, rattling and hissing in air passages : burning pain in fixed spot in chest.

Great swelling of knees with rheumatic pain, comfortable only when applying cold.

Stiffness of all joints, could only move them after applying cold water.

General coldness, with heat and redness of face.

Parts cold to touch, but not subjectively cold to patient (*Arn.*).

Limbs and whole body painful, as if bruised and beaten (*Arn.*).

Purple spots over body like petechiæ (*Arn., Phos., Crot. h.*).

Bloodboils.

Eruption, only on covered parts. (*Thuja :* sweat only on uncovered parts.)

Sensation as if lice were crawling over surface : < from heat, motion, and at night.

LILIUM TIGRINUM

A precious remedy for most distressing conditions : well proved and of very definite and distinguishing symptoms, and yet not enough realized and understood, is *Lilium tigrinum*.

Tiger lily is a powerful poison, and therefore medicine. We read that a child put an anther of one of these lilies into her right nostril, and in spite of brandy, etc., given four hours later, she died after fifty-six hours.

Lilium is unknown to Old School practice : and perhaps it is just as well. It is a drug of such vehement action as to be only safe and useful in the hands of those who have learnt from Hahnemann how to prepare and prescribe such remedies.

Hahnemann directed that drugs should be proved by females as well as males, in order to discover what effect they produced in regard to sex.

And besides the symptoms produced on men, Tiger lily (proved for Carroll Dunham by a number of women doctors) manifested most terrific effects on women.

No one who has read Dunham's Lecture on *Lilium* will ever forget the startling features of that remedy.

Some of the provings were made with a tincture of the pollen alone ; others with a tincture of the fresh stalks, leaves and flowers. The drug was proved in the ϕ and in the 1st, 3rd, 5th and 30th and 500th potencies.

Lilium has many symptoms strikingly in common with *Sepia*, as we shall see. But it has very definite symptoms that distinguish it from *Sepia*. No one should have any difficulty in choosing between the two.

The mental and physical symptoms of *Lilium* are alike startling and intense : and except for the deep mental depression, and the intense physical " bearing-down " common to both drugs, they differ totally from those of *Sepia*.

Listen to *Lilium* ! . . . This is the answer of the drug, when pure science puts the question as to what it can cause and cure.

Depression. Constant inclination to weep, with fearfulness, and apprehension of suffering from some terrible internal disease.

Wild feeling in the head. Indescribable crazy feeling. Crazy feeling, her mind being in such a state that she could not even record her symptoms. Fear of insanity. Thoughts of suicide. Despair of salvation.

Can't read. Can't think. Keeps walking fast. Feels hurried: doesn't know why. Everything unreal. Makes mistakes in speaking. Dreads saying anything, lest she should say something wrong : yet wants to talk.

Sexual excitement, alternating with apprehension of moral obliquity : these alternating for months after the proving had ended. Aversion to being alone.

Constant hurried feeling, as of imperative duties and utter inability to perform them, during sexual excitement.

A sensation in the pelvis as though everything was coming into the world through the vagina. The dragging downwards towards the pelvis is felt as high as stomach—even shoulders. Worse standing, though not relieved by lying. Wants to place hand on hypogastrium and press upwards, to relieve the dragging sensation. (*Sanic.*) Wants to draw long breaths, in order to raise the abdominal contents.

Bearing down, with sensation of heavy weight and pressure in the region of the womb, as if the whole contents would press out through the vagina. A feeling, when on the feet, as if the whole pelvic contents would issue through the vagina, if not prevented by upward pressure of the hand on the vulva, or by sitting down. Burning and sharp ovarian pains. Unable to move, fearing her womb would drop from her.

Even this is not all ! *Severe pressure in rectum and at anus, and a constant desire to go to stool.* Diarrhœa, especially morning diarrhœa, with griping and smarting.

Even the bladder does not escape ! *Pressure on the bladder. She could pass water every quarter of an hour. Continual pressure on the bladder, wants to urinate all the time.* Passing little, with smarting and straining.

And then, the HEART. Sharp, quick pain, with fluttering of heart. Pressive pain in the heart, as if the heart were violently grasped, the grasp gradually relaxing. Palpitation. Every intermission followed by a violent throb.

Craving appetite for dinner. *Increased desire for meat.* Aversion to bread—coffee—to the usual cigar.

The above are the most important and characteristic symptoms of the drug ; in black type, most of them, which means that they have been again and again produced in provings, and been cured, again and again, by *Lilium.*

During the provings, actual displacements of the uterus were said to have occurred.

In one prover, the sufferings were such, that an end had to be put to the proving. *Platina* 200, in repeated doses, put matters right. (*Platina* was most like to her mental symptoms—her " superiority complex ".)

Now, to contrast *Lilium* with *Sepia*.

LILIUM.	SEPIA.
Bearing down.	*Bearing down.*
Everything forcing down, as if contents of pelvis were pushing down through a funnel, the outlet being the vagina.	Pressure from back to abdomen.
Must support vulva with hand, or cross legs.	Must cross legs to prevent protrusion of parts.
Feels the heat more.	Feels the cold more.
Intolerant of sympathy.	Intolerant of sympathy.
Hurried and worried (*Arg. nit.*) by imperative duties she is unable to perform.	INDIFFERENT.
SHE CRAVES MEAT.	Aversion to meat.
The terrible diarrhœa and straining (of *Merc. cor.* and *Lil.*).	are absent with Sepia.

Lilium is so very acute and intense. Her bearing-down is not the passive weight and distress of *Sepia*. *Lilium* feels she is being forcibly eviscerated.

Dunham says, the *Sepia* condition is more chronic.

There are a few poor creatures, like the writer, who can better grasp and remember things when rhymed. For such we append a Tiger-lily rhyme. Conscious superiority is warned to skip the following :

> TIGER LILY hurries about,
> Feels her inside's being all dragged out :
> Frequent urging to micturition,
> Almost approaching the *Cantharis* condition :
> Rectal distress (*Merc. cor.*) : a band
> Constricting the heart (just like *Cactus grand.*).
> *Pulsatilla*-like tears : her salvation's a worry :
> With *Silver nitrate*, she's " duties ", and " hurry ".

One has seen the beautiful action of *Lilium tigr.* in rapidly wiping out the distress after miscarriages.

Also a very striking case of the cure of " ulcerative colitis " of ten years' standing, and much treatment by " the heads of the profession ". In the early days of her illness she might have as many as thirty stools in a night. Even now, she was as white as a sheet of paper—a transparent whiteness. The distress, the straining and the number of stools in the morning made it impossible for her to appear till later on in the day : and she was ill enough to have a nurse with her.

She presented a few peculiar and characteristic symptoms—characteristic of herself, not of the disease labelled " colitis ". She had a big appetite : was hungry for the mid-day meal. She craved meat. And she had, not only the urging and bearing down at the anus, but also of the uterus. She got *Lilium tigr.* in high potency, responded promptly, and was presently a healthy young woman, with good colour, playing tennis and enjoying life : and, later on, she got married.

The power to deal gently, quickly and successfully with such conditions (denied to those who despise the teachings of Hahnemann) is a thing to bring joy—and thankfulness !

Kent says, " *Lilium tigrinum* has cured the most inveterate protuding piles, with burning."

There are quite a number of other drugs that have produced " bearing-down " sensations, and which are useful, each in its place, for such conditions : but there are none of such intensity as *Lilium* and *Sepia*. Two among them, but with quite different " modalities ", or conditions, are *Pulsatilla* and *Belladonna*.

It will be remembered that *Lilium* and *Sepia cannot stand* : must sit down, or cross the legs, or support the parts, in order to prevent protusion : that is the sensation. But the *Belladonna* bearing-down is *better standing* : while the *Pulsatilla* bearing-down is *worse lying*. These things are strange and unexpected, therefore important.

One remembers a poor woman, one of our " out-patients ", who came to hospital after a miscarriage, ill and with a disquieting temperature, who complained of distressing bearing-down sensations, worse sitting and lying, and only relieved when standing. She refused admission : was given *Pulsatilla* (evidently her remedy) and told to report next day : when the temperature was normal, and the distress gone.

The " modalities " or conditions accompanying such symptoms are enormously helpful for *correct* prescribing—without which, the beautiful results of Homœopathy are not seen. Such modalities help to diagnose between like remedies.

*   *   *

One may just mention here a little-used remedy, which comes down from antiquity, and which has produced and cured bearing-down pains, and even uterine prolapse—as one has seen. This is *Arctium Lappa*, or *Lappa Major*—Burdock. It is one of the unusual remedies with which the late Dr. Compton Burnett made such play. Its "virtues" have earned it the name of the "uterine magnet".

Black Letter Symptoms

Tormented about her salvation.   Uterine complaints.

Depression of spirits ; profound ; can hardly keep from crying ; DISPOSITION *to weep, with nausea and pain in back ; averse to food ; weeps much and is very timid : indifferent about anything being done for her.*

Dragging down of whole ABDOMINAL *contents, extending even to organs of chest ; must support abdomen ; as if whole contents were pushing down into a funnel ; is compelled to cross her legs for fear everything would be pressed out.*

Bearing down sensation in pelvis as though everything was coming into world through vagina.

Pressure in rectum, with almost constant desire to go to stool.

Continuous pressure in region of BLADDER, *constant desire to urinate, with scanty discharge, smarting in urethra and tenesmus.*

Frequent urination through day ; with dull headache moving from sinciput to occiput, finally settling in left temple.

If desire is not attended to, feeling of congestion of chest.

Sharp pain in OVARIAN *region ; burning ; stinging ; cutting ; grasping pain extends across hypogastrium to groin, down leg ; bearing down when standing ; sensitive to pressure ; ovary swollen to nearly size of a child's head.*

Severe neuralgic pains in UTERUS, *could not bear touch, not even weight of bedclothes or slightest jar ; anteversion.*

Anteversion and retroversion of uterus ; patients nearly all have constipation.

Sensation as if HEART *was grasped or squeezed in a vice ; as if blood had all gone to heart, producing a feeling as if he must bend double ; inability to walk straight.*

LYCOPODIUM

(Club Moss)

ONE of Hahnemann's precious gifts, and one that exhibits and justifies his teachings in regard to potentization.

Of *Lycopodium*, he writes : " This dust-like powder, which is yellowish, smooth to the touch, is obtained from the ears of a moss, *Lycopodium clavatum*, which grows in the forests of Russia and Finland" [also in this country.—ED.]. " Towards the end of Summer, the ears are dried, and afterwards beaten.

" When thrown into a flame, it flashes up, and has been used to cover pills which easily adhere to one another, and to protect sore places in folds against the friction occasioned by walking and otherwise. It floats upon liquids without being dissolved, has neither taste nor smell, and when in its natural crude condition, has almost no effect upon the health of man   .   .   .

" This drug has wonderful medicinal properties, which can only be disclosed by trituration and succussion   .   .   .

" A moderate dose acts from forty to fifty days. It may be repeated after the intermediate use of another antipsoric, but a second dose acts less favourably than the first.

" It acts with especial benefit, when homœopathically indicated, after the action of *Calc.* shall have passed over   .   .   ."

Kent says : " Though classed among inert substances, and thought to be useful only for rolling up allopathic pills, Hahnemann brought it into use and developed its power by attenuation. It is a monument to Hahnemann. It enters deep into the life.   .   .   . There is nothing about man that *Lycopodium* does not rouse into tumult   .   .   ."

This " unmoistenable powder "—inert, yet flashing brilliantly " when thrown into a flame " has been also used in the manufacture of fireworks. When the spores are crushed, an oily substance is liberated ; and it takes two solid hours of trituration with sugar of milk (we are told) to its initial preparation as a remedy at once potent and unique in its properties for good.

To start with, let us reproduce, more or less, one of those little old Drug Pictures, which boil down to their lowest dimensions what we know and find absolutely essential to the employment of a remedy   .   .   .

*   *   *

Lyc. is one of our most constantly used drugs. It does not always stare you in the face as the patient walks in ; but a few questions will generally have you hot on the trail.

Ask early as to *time of day*. This patient says, " worse afternoon, or worse 4 p.m., or worse 4 to 8 p.m.," and you look to see that he conforms to the *Lyc.* type, and enquire further.

Kent says : " Poor little Paul Dombey needed a dose of *Lyc.*, but Dombey did not know it, and lost his son."

In *Lyc.* the mind is better developed than the body. *Lyc.* is apt to look sickly and wrinkled—skinny, especially in the upper part of the body. The forehead may be frowning or wrinkled, and if it is after early dinner, the cheeks or nose are apt to be red, to the patient's great discomfort.

Anticipation is a very useful little rubric. Everybody knows that *Gels.* and *Arg. nit.* have it. But *Lyc.* has it too ; and *Ars.* and *Med.* ; and (though fewer people know this) *Carbo veg.*, *Phos. a.*, *Pb.*, *Sil.* and *Thuja*. These last have to be hunted in other parts of the repertory. It is well to add them to the rubric.

Years ago one of our very good prescribers made me understand a phase of the *Lyc.* mentality. He explained the terrors of anticipation as they affect *Lyc. Lyc.* has to meet his shareholders or his constituents with an important speech, and knows that he will flounder, and hesitate, and forget his points; is obsessed with the idea that he will make a mess of it. The dreaded moment arrives : he gets on to his legs, warms to his work, sails along in blissful self-forgetfulness, to sit down feeling that he has made the speech of his life. It was all joy and fluency ; he not only remembered all his points, but made new ones as he went along. But—he will have the same terror next time, unless he gets his stimulus, because he is *Lycopodium*.

Or again, *Lyc.* wants to be alone—*with someone in the next room*, because—he FEARS to be alone ! His desire for solitude is in italics ; his fear, when alone, is in black type. Drugs that have these opposite states in big type are most interesting. (*Lach.* has loquacity in the highest type, rapid speech and loquacity ; and, also in the highest type, slowness of speech ! This is not always realized.)

Lyc. has plenty of FEARS—fear alone, of crowds, of dark, of death, of ghosts, of people.

Lyc. has all the DYSPEPSIAS you can imagine. It competes with *Carbo veg.* and *China* for the distinction of being the most flatulent remedy. *Lyc.* will come and tell you that for days together she is distended like a drum, and has to loosen her clothing. After food she is distended and tense, almost to bursting, and cannot bear the pressure and constriction of her clothes. Or, she feels famishing, and after a couple of mouthfuls she is bloated and full, and can eat no more. Or, she may feel absolutely full up, yet hungry. For *Lyc.* has in black type the easy satiety, and also the opposite in black type, " hunger p.c." or " hunger p.c. with full and tense stomach ".

The *Lyc.* FOOD CRAVINGS are for sweet things—for hot drinks. *Lyc.* loves, but is made ill by oysters : Hates coffee and meat.

We all know the RIGHT-SIDEDNESS of *Lyc.*, and the direction of symptoms, from right to left, or from above downward.

URINARY symptoms are important. Red sand in the clear urine ; urine that is acrid and excoriates . . . thus you may spot a *Lyc.* baby by the red sand in the napkin, or by the rash where urine has inflamed the skin ; and you may cure its nephritis and dropsy—as one has seen.

Lyc. is AN INTELLECTUAL, as we said, with self-distrust. And *Lyc.* has intellectual sufferings and failures and confusions when ill. Loss of memory. Speaks wrong words and syllables. Makes mistakes in writing—mis-spells—omits words, or letters. May realize that " Z " is the last letter of the alphabet, and be unable to supply its name. To such a length may this go, that he may be unable to read—may be able to write what he wishes, yet unable to read what he has written.

Our doctors tell of great cures with *Lyc.* of literary persons unable, after an attack of 'FLU to get to work again. The intellectual sequelæ of 'flu often call for *Lyc.*, while the neurotic ones (to almost insanity) need *Scutellaria*, and those with long-lasting weakness and chilliness, find their rapid help in *China*.

There is no disease, acute or chronic, where *Lyc.* may not be the remedy—in a *Lycopodium* patient ! Toothache about 4 p.m. (one has seen this). Eruptions that wake up horribly at 4 p.m. (this also). Lingering pneumonias, where the temperature is found to rise at 4 p.m. and drop after 8 p.m. Diphtheria where the membrane starts on the right side and crosses to the left, the mouth and tongue not crying out for *Merc.* Or, post-nasal diphtherias that descend. *Lyc.* has also the post-diph. paralysis (its usual great remedy being *Gels.*) where food and drink regurgitate through the nose. Kidney troubles, as said, where the urine inflames and reddens the skin wherever it touches.

Two useful little rubrics may put you on to *Lyc.* Right foot cold, left normal. Burning pain like red-hot coals between scapulæ. (*Phos.* has this, and a very few other drugs.) These small rubrics are often very useful, if only to clinch the diagnosis of the remedy.

If you get < afternoon
            < 4 p.m.
            < 4—8 p.m.
            desires hot drinks
            craves sweets
            acidity and wind
            bloating

with its urinary troubles, you will not go far wrong if you scribble down LYCOPODIUM.

BLACK LETTER SYMPTOMS

(*Allen, Hering, with some of Hahnemann's italics*)

MENTALS. *Dread of men: of solitude: irritable and melancholy. Weeps all day, cannot calm herself. Worse 4 to 8 p.m.*
Sensitive: even cries when thanked.
Satiety of life, particularly mornings in bed.
Amativeness, and amorousness.
Sensitive, irritable: peevish and cross on waking. Easily excited to anger; cannot bear opposition, and is speedily beside herself.
Ailments from fright, anger, mortification or vexation, with reserved displeasure.
Oversensitive to pain. Patient is beside herself. (*Cham.*)
Speaks wrong words and syllables. Selects wrong words.
Becomes confused about everyday things.
Great apprehensiveness in the pit of the stomach. (*Kali c.*)

HEAD. *Vertigo in the morning when and after rising from bed, so that he reels back and forth.*
Throbbing in brain on leaning head back during the day.
Throbbing headache after every paroxysm of coughing.
With the cough, shattering in temples and in chest.
Pain in temples as if screwed together, worse during menses.
Rush of blood to head on waking.
Excessive falling of hair: hair becomes grey too soon.

EYES, *distressing pain, as if dry, with nightly-agglutination.*
Styes on lids, more towards inner canthi.
Ulceration and redness of eyelids.
Evening light blinds him very much: cannot see anything on the table.

Roaring, humming, rushing, etc., in EARS.
Loss of hearing in connection with otorrhœa.
Eczema of ears, with thick crusts and fissures.

Violent catarrh, with swelling of NOSE.
Stopped catarrh, so that he cannot get breath at night.
Complete stoppage of nose : child's breath stopped during sleep,
frequently for fifteen seconds, even while the mouth is open.
Fan-like motion of the alæ nasi.

FACE *yellowish grey.*
Spasmodic twitching of facial muscles.

TEETH *painful when chewing and when touched.*
Numerous blisters on the tongue. Ulcers on and under tongue.

Feeling as if a ball rose, from below, up into the THROAT.
Throat feels too tight on swallowing : nothing goes down : food
and drink regurgitate through the nose. (Gels., Diph.)

Excessive appetite, followed by distension of abdomen.
Hunger remains immediately after eating, though the STOMACH
and abdomen are full and tense.
She cannot eat at all : is constantly satiated and without appetite :
whatever she eats goes against her, even to vomiting.
Sudden satiety and great thirst.
Immediately after a meal, is full, bloated, distended.
Loss of appetite at first mouthful : weight in stomach after eating.
A sour eructation, the taste does not remain in mouth; but acid
gnaws in the stomach.
Incomplete burning eructations, which only rise to the pharynx,
where they cause burning, for several hours.
Epigastrium extremely sensitive to touch and tight clothing.
Digestion seems to proceed very slowly.
Discomfort in the stomach after eating a little.
Cramp in the stomach which is much distended.
Pressure in stomach, as if she had eaten too much.
Pressure in stomach, as if over-distended, in the evening, after
eating a little.
Pressure, heaviness in stomach, after eating a little in the afternoon.
Pain in epigastrium caused by coughing.

She dares not eat to satiety, because if she does, she has an unpleasant, distressed feeling in HEPATIC REGION.

Pressive pain, hepatic region, on breathing.

Sore pressive pain as from a blow in right hypochondriac region, aggravated by touch.

Liver is painful to touch.

Pain in left hypochondriac region, afternoon.

Violent gall-stone colic.

Ascites from liver affections, after abuse of alcohol.

Something heavy felt lying in left ABDOMEN, *not affecting the breathing, but constantly felt while walking, sitting and lying.*

Distension of the abdomen from gases. Relieved by emission of flatus.

Grunting and gurgling in abdomen.

Whole abdomen distended by flatulence after a stool.

Much flatus accumulates here and there in abdomen, in hypochondria, even in the back in region of ribs and chest, causing tension and bubbling, always relieved by empty eructations.

Immediately after eating the abdomen is constantly full, distended and tense. Tension with incarceration of flatus.

Sensation of something moving up and down in stomach and bowels. (Comp. Crocus, Thuja, Sanicula.)

Hernia right side.

ANUS *painfully closed.*

The rectum so frequently contracted that it protrudes during a hard stool.

Hæmorrhoids painful to touch.

Great tendency to excoriations about anus : bleed easily.

Itching and moist, tender eruption.

First part of stool lumpy, the second soft.

Aching in KIDNEY *before and after urination.*

Some red sediment in urine.

Red, or reddish yellow sand in urine.

Turbid, milky urine, with offensive purulent sediment. Disposition to calculi.

Renal colic, particularly right ureter to bladder.

Urging to urinate : must wait long before it will pass, or inability with constant bearing down : supports abdomen with hands.

Night COUGH *affecting stomach and diaphragm, mostly before sunset.*

Cough overpowering, evening before going to sleep, as if larynx tickled with a feather, with scanty expectoration.

Tickling cough as from sulphur fumes in larynx.
Difficult breathing, as if he had inhaled sulphur fumes.
Grey, salt-tasting expectoration.
Dyspnœa : during sleep ; from every exertion.
CHEST *feels oppressed and raw internally.*
Stitches left chest, and during inspiration.

Hering gives " Hydropericardium ". (Ars.)

BACK, *burning as from glowing coals between the scapulae*
(PHOS., KALI BICH., *etc.*).
Severe backache, better by passing urine.

One foot hot, the other cold.

Desire to go into the open air. (Puls., etc.)
Her symptoms are aggravated at 4 p.m. : at 8 p.m. she feels better,
but weak.
Headache, cough, fever, chill, EVERYTHING WORSE 4-8 P.M.
Nervous excitement : prostration of mind and body. Nervous
debility.

Hungry WHEN WAKING *at night.*
On waking, cross, kicks, scolds : or wakes terrified : **unrefreshed.**

Many years ago, one was asked to go to the " other end of
nowhere " to prescribe for a small boy—very small, yet already
a great cricketer at five years old. The trouble was recent :—
tormenting " frequency." One stood and watched him playing
cricket on the sands with the other little boys, and every few
minutes he had to rush away for relief. All this was very puzzling
to his parents. A few *Lycopodium* symptoms emerged, with *this*
one, also new to him—that he " woke up ugly " as the Americans
express it, " crying and cross ". *Lyc.* quickly cured ; and,
incidentally, hammered home a point which we will pass on . . .
Lyc. is, in almost everything, worse in the evening and better in
the morning, *except*, as one discovered over this case, that it is
(mentally) " *ugly on waking* ".

It is puzzle-cases that bite into the memory, and their triumphs
that teach one to know drugs.

Hughes quotes Dr. David Wilson in regard to the *fan-like*
movement of the alae nasi noted in the pathogenesis of *Lyc.* " When
this symptom is clearly marked, no matter through what organ
or tissue the symptoms of any attack of illness may manifest
themselves in children or young people, I venture to submit that
the whole group of the phenomena in such attacks will be found

under *Lycopodium.*" Dr. David Wilson was a great prescriber and, note! he does not say "when the alae nasi work, give *Lyc.*," but " *I submit that the whole group of the phenomena in such attacks will be found under Lycopodium.*"

It is in respiratory affections that this symptom is generally seen. This is the classical picture of a *Lycopodium* pneumonia, for instance.

Frowning forehead.

Working of the alae nasi.

Temperature rises each day at 4 p.m. till 8 p.m., and then declines. In a pneumonia that tends to hang fire, this last symptom puts one straight on to *Lyc.* which finishes the case.· Kent speaks of its use " in the advanced stage of pneumonia, in the period of hepatization, with the wrinkled face and brow, the flapping wings of the nose and the scanty expectoration. The right lung is most affected, or is affected first in double pneumonia ".

In a *Lyc.* diphtheria, as said, the trouble begins on the right side, and may spread to the left : we have seen such a case : but with none of the foulness of mouth and tongue that cries aloud for one of the *Mercuries.*

Lycopodium is one of the great polycrests—the Drugs of Many Uses. But the above black letter symptoms, the " caused and many times cured symptoms ", which are classical in our school, bring out its important points of attack for evil and for good.

The drug, as said, suits *intellectuals* ; (rather skinny and *old-looking* intellectuals) ; with more mental than bodily vigour. Hence it proves subversive, and especially curative of mentality ; affecting MEMORY, and restoring those who, after sickness or strain, are afflicted with confusion and mental tiredness and incompetence.

Again, its subversive effects and therefore its curative powers come strongly into play in the *digestive* and *urinary* regions.

One remembers one " new" patient in particular who for days had been almost bursting with flatulence and distension, and had had to loosen all her clothing ; and how quickly *Lyc.* put her right.

NASH says, " *Lycopodium* with *Sulphur* and *Calcarea* form the leading trio of Hahnemann's anti-psoric remedies. They all act very deeply. *Lycopodium* acts favourably in all ages, but particularly upon old people and children . . . on persons of keen intellect but feeble muscular development : lean people. . . . The *Lycopodium* subject is sallow, sunken, with premature lines in the face ; looks older than he is. Children are weak, with well-developed heads, but puny, sickly bodies. . . . This is one of the trio of flatulent remedies, *Carbo veg.* and *China* being the other two . . . remember, while *China* bloats the whole abdomen, *Carbo veg.* prefers the upper, and *Lycopodium* the lower parts. . . ." Guernsey points out here, " *China* has fulness after a full, normal meal ; *Lyc.* after eating a little." " Constipation predominates ; and like *Nux* there may be frequent and ineffectual desire for stool, but while that of *Nux* is caused by irregular peristaltic action, that of *Lyc.* seems to be caused by a spasmodic contraction of the anus, which prevents the stool and causes great pain. . . . *Lyc.* has often saved neglected, mal-treated or imperfectly cured cases of pneumonia from running into consumption. . . ." We have given its characteristic indications elsewhere :—the frowning forehead, the flapping alae nasi, the 4-8 p.m. aggravation of fever, etc.

Lyc. is down as a chilly remedy : yet it is one of the few remedies that appears in the Repertory in the rubric, *Better when cold*. (IOD., PULS., with *Lach.*, *Nat. mur.*, *Sulph.* and a few others.) But *Lyc.* is generally better from warm or hot things, drinks, etc., and even better warm in bed.

A few additional points from KENT, who reiterates, stresses and amplifies " *Lycopodium* emaciates above, while the extremities are fairly well-nourished. . . . The *Lyc.* patient cannot eat oysters. It does not seem to matter what is the matter with him, if he eats oysters he gets sick . . . headache, pain in the ovary, cough—*after eating oysters*. Oysters seem a poison to *Lyc.*, just as onions are a poison to the *Thuja* patient. The *Oxalic acid* patient cannot eat strawberries. If you are ever caught in a place where you have a patient get sick after eating strawberries, tomatoes or oysters, and you have no homœopathic remedies at hand, it is a good thing to remember that a piece of cheese will digest strawberries, or tomatoes, or oysters, in a few minutes."

" The eruptions of *Lyc.* and sometimes the ulcers and abscesses of *Lyc.* are better from something cool. The soothing thing to *Lyc.* is something cooling, while the soothing thing to *Ars.* is heat. . . . The old ladies of the house will want to do something, and put warm cloths or warm water on the suffering part, but these will make the *Lyc.* patient worse."

" *Lyc.* is tired. A tired mind, a chronic fatigue, forgetfulness, aversion to undertaking anything new, to appearing in any new role ; aversion to his own work.

" Taciturnity : desires to be alone. If there were two adjacent rooms in the house, the *Lyc.* patient would go into one and stay there, though very glad to have someone in the other. That is the state of the *Lyc.* mind. . . .

" *Lyc.* often breaks down and weeps when meeting a friend.
. . . An unusual sadness with weeping comes over this patient
on receiving a gift. At the slightest joy, *Lyc.* weeps . . . even
cries when thanked . . .

" Left foot cold, the other warm . . . red sand in urine,
red pepper deposit . . ."

In regard to throats and diphtheria, and the " right to left "
of *Lyc.* and the " left to right " of *Lach.* Kent points out that
" *Lach.* is better from cold, and has spasms of the throat from
attempting to drink warm drinks, while *Lyc.* is better from warm
drinks, though *sometimes better from cold drinks.*" It is important
to know this, or one is apt to discard *Lyc.*, when otherwise indicated.

To become a rapid and at all correct prescriber—for the bulk
of the patients that crowd in to a hospital out-patient clinic, or
for panel work, there are some dozen remedies that one needs to
make friends with, so as to be able to recognize them after a
minimum of glances and questionings. Such are SEPIA, SULPHUR,
LYCOPODIUM, CALCAREA, SILICA, NATRUM MUR., ARSENICUM,
BRYONIA—Hahnemann's anti-psorics all !—and for acute work,
ACONITE, BELLADONNA, again BRYONIA, RHUS, GELSEMIUM,
BAPTISIA, and a few other indispensables. These are all remedies
of distinct personality, and should not be confused—when once
their inwardness is grasped. It is to make these remedies easily
recognizable that in our little drug pictures we reiterate, and try
to produce a snapshot of one or another, with its various uses.
Such an assortment of drugs at one's fingertips should make
homœopathic prescribing, in a large proportion of the common
complaints, comparatively easy and sure.

LYCOPODIUM IN ANEURISM

DR. HUGHES (*Pharmacodynamics*) mentions a " curious point " in
regard to *Lycopodium*. He says : " *Lycopodium* has occasionally
been suggested for aneurism, but I had thought little of it, though
in a case treated by Dr. Madden and myself what *seemed* to be
an aortic aneurism ceased to be discoverable while we were giving
the medicine for the general health. But I have since seen most
striking results from it in an unmistakable carotid aneurism in an
old lady, for whose dyspeptic symptoms the remedy had often
proved serviceable. The shooting pains which accompanied
the swelling disappeared in the first three days of taking the
Lycopodium ; and in a fortnight the enlargement of the artery
was reduced to one-half, at which point it has since continued
stationary, giving her no pain or inconvenience."

MAGNESIA PHOSPHORICA

Mag. phos. is probably the most important and precious of the remedies derived from the bio-chemical studies of Dr. Schuessler. It is one of his twelve " Tissue Remedies ". It has been " fed in " in low potencies and frequent doses : but we can attest, from long and frequent experience, that it works magnificently in the high and highest potencies in very infrequent dosage : i.e. only repeated if, and when, the same symptoms recur, after perhaps months, to demand a repetition of the same remedy. But this, of course, only when it has been prescribed on similarity of *caused* and *cured* symptoms.

Mag. phos. is one of the greatest, if not the greatest, of the remedies of dysmenorrhœa : but only of dysmenorrhœa of its own kind : viz. where *the pains double the victim up ; are relieved by heat,* hot drinks, hot applications ; and *aggravated by cold.* In this relief from doubling up and from warmth, it is very like *Colocynth,* another great remedy for such forms of dysmenor-rhœa ; but *Mag. phos.* has a greater idiosyncrasy in regard to heat and cold ; and the mentalities of the two are not alike ; the pains of *Coloc.* being so often due to vexation. Anger and annoyance, with *Coloc.,* may produce pain in any part of the body—even in the spine. But it is no wonder that symptoms in *Mag. phos.* and *Coloc.* should present many points of resemblance, since *Coloc.,* which belongs to the vegetable kingdom, contains 3 per cent. of *Mag. phos.* " Among the " (other) " plants containing *Mag. phos.* are *Lobelia, Symphytum* and *Viburnum,* which explains the presence of similar symptoms." It is very interesting to trace, in vegetable remedies, the different elements or salts that occur in them, and which explain some of the symptoms they have in common. It makes them easier to remember.

In " THE TWELVE TISSUE REMEDIES OF SCHUESSLER " (Drs. Boericke and Dewey) we are told that Dr. Schuessler recommended the 6x trituration, and said that it acted best when given in hot water. . . . " But in view of the really surprising and apparently wholly trustworthy results obtained by the provers with the high and highest potencies, we would recommend these, should the lower fail." [We may add that our own results have been obtained, *always,* so far as we can remember, from single doses of the *cm* potency.]

One never-forgotten case, because of the unpleasant—even alarming reaction, was that of a child in the out-patient department many years ago, who got a dose of *Mag. phos. cm.*, for chorea. She was speedily brought back with an extension of the trouble, apparently, into the laryngeal region, i.e. with rather alarming respiratory spasms. She was promptly admitted ; got no other medicine ; and was well in a few days. The drug, prescribed in a lower potency, would probably not have evoked such an alarming aggravation—or proving : but the result was not too bad. One does not often completely cure a chorea within a fortnight ; which, so far as one remembers, was the case here.

Among the cases that assail one's memory in regard to *Mag. phos.* is that of a " very ill " baby, which was admitted to Hospital for diarrhœa with colicky pains causing it to draw up its legs. *Coloc.* was given, and the diarrhœa was relieved ; but the pains persisted, and the fear was that the baby would die. But it was noticed that a warm hand on the abdomen evidently comforted the babe : and *Mag. phos.*, thereupon, did the rest.

But one's chief use for *Mag. phos.* has been in the treatment of dysmenorrhœa. Single doses of the *cm.*, given just any time the patient happened to come up, not necessarily during the painful period, have cured for us quite a number of cases, the indications being *dysmenorrhœa, with violent abdominal pain, doubling the patient up, and only relieved by heat.*

BLACK LETTER SYMPTOMS

Neuralgia or rheumatic headache : better from external applications of warmth : very excruciating.

Tendency to spasmodic symptoms.

Shooting, stinging, shifting, intermittent or spasmodic pains : sparks before eyes.

More in young and strong persons. After mental labour.

Neuralgic pain, especially behind right ear : worse by going into cold air, and washing face and neck in cold water.

Otalgia, purely nervous.

Toothache, better by heat and hot liquids.

Severe pain in decayed or filled teeth : swelling of tongue.

Complaints of teething children.

Spasms during dentition, no fever.

Spasms or cramp in stomach, nipping, griping, pinching, with short belching of wind, giving no relief.

Spasms or cramp in stomach, with clean tongue : as if a band was tightly laced or drawn round body.

Enteralgia.

Flatulent colic forcing patient to bend double : (Coloc.) better from rubbing, warmth, pressure. Accompanied by belching of gas, which gives no relief.

Bloated, full sensation in abdomen ; must loosen clothes (Lyc.) and walk about.

Flatulent colic of children and the new born, with drawing up of legs : remittent colic ; crampy pain with acidity.

Radiating pain in abdomen.

Meteorism in cows (Colch.).

Nocturnal enuresis from nervous irritation.

Menstrual colic.

Membranous dysmenorrhœa.

Ovarian neuralgia, pain shooting and darting like lightning : worse on right side.

Spasmodic, nervous asthma.

Chorea.

Neuralgia at intervals, relieved by warmth.

Languid ; tired ; exhausted.

Chilliness : chills run up and down the back (Gels.) with shivering. Dread of uncovering (Nux).

Worse : right side ; from cold ; from touch : relieved by warmth ; by bending double.

*   *   *

Mag. phos. has been found useful in nystagmus : strabismus ; spasmodic squinting ; ptosis ; in spasmodic stammering : spasmodic constriction of throat with sensation of choking. In hiccough, day and night, with retching.

In vesical neuralgia after catheterization ; sensation as if muscles did not contract.

In laryngismus stridulus. In spasmodic coughs, and whooping cough. In angina pectoris. In intercostal neuralgia, constrictive kind. In 'shaking of hands and limbs ; sciatica ; cramps in calves ; even for violent pains in acute rheumatism of joints. All sorts of spasms with contractions of fingers and staring eyes. In convulsions, with stiffness of limbs, thumbs drawn in, and fingers clenched (*Cup.*). Cramps of piano or violin players : writer's cramp. In chorea . . . and when the muscular fibres of heart seemed to participate in the general spasm. In epilepsy. In palsy : paralysis agitans.

Violent pains ; maddening pains ; excruciating pains ; terrible pains ; great pain with retching.

Pains : sharp ; shooting ; lightning-like ; cutting ; stinging ; cramping ; boring ; griping ; drawing :—constricting :—pricking.

Said to be " a nutrition and functional remedy for nerve tissues."

* * *

NASH says, " Now we come to the prince of the *Magnesias*. It is comparatively new and has never been accorded a place in our Materia Medica according to its importance and merits.

" It takes first rank among our very best neuralgia or pain remedies : none has a greater variety of pains : " (he details them). " CRAMPING—this last in my opinion is most characteristic, and oftenest found in stomach, abdomen and pelvis. In dysmenorrhœa of the neuralgic variety, with the characteristic crampy pains, I have found no remedy equal to it." (N.B.— Nash gives it in high potency : 55*m* made on his own potentizer.)

" Alongside the cramping, is its characteristic modality— *relief from hot applications.*" Here, Nash makes a very important comparison—with *Arsenicum*. He says, " No remedy has this " (relief from hot applications) " more prominently than *Arsenicum alb.* But you will notice that among all the various pains we have mentioned as belonging to *Magnesia phos.* the one conspicuous for its absence is the one most characteristic of *Arsenicum*, viz.— *burning pains.* I watched this difference," he says, " and found that if burning pains were relieved by heat, *Arsenicum* was almost sure to relieve, while those pains not burning but also relieved by heat were cured by *Magnesia phos.* I think that this will be found a valuable diagnostic between the two remedies."

He says, " During painful menstruation *Magnesia phos.* is quicker in its action than *Pulsatilla*, *Caulophylum*, *Cimicifuga*, or any other remedy that I know." He thinks *Cimifuga* covers the rheumatic cases better, *Mag. phos.* those of a purely neuralgic character. " I have no faith in the Schuesslerian theory. *Similia similibus curentur* has stood the test with other remedies and will with the so-called tissue remedies, regardless of theories."

* * *

Now we will, at risk of some repetition, appeal for hints to the perspicacity and clarity of KENT ; condensing :

Best known for its spasmodic conditions and neuralgias. A pain localizes itself in a nerve and stays there, and becomes worse and worse, sometimes coming in paroxysms, but becoming so violent that the patient becomes frantic. *The pains are always ameliorated by heat and pressure* . . . pains are brought on when he becomes cold, or in a cold place. . . .

Pains are felt everywhere . . . stomach, bowels, with the same modalities . . . even pains in spinal cord, ameliorated by heat. . . . Cramps from prolonged exertion—writers, and players on piano and harp: they suddenly break down with stiffness and cramp after several hours' labour every day for years. . . . The labourer's, the carpenter's hand, cramp . . . this is a strong feature of the remedy, *in all sorts of over-exertion.*

Screams with the violent cramps in dysentery and cholera morbus. . . . " It was Schuessler's main remedy for chorea, but we can only use it by its proving. He prescribed it in all nervous conditions, but its proving justifies its use in neuralgia ameliorated by heat and pressure." Cramps and twitchings. . . . A tearing pain, as if the nerve were inflamed and put on a stretch. Shaking, as in paralysis agitans. Better from heat and pressure, and worse from cold, cold bathing, cold winds, cold weather, lack of clothing. Pains all over; but more likely pain located in one part.

" Mental symptoms not brought out. Used clinically when diarrhoeas have ceased suddenly and brain troubles have come on. Congestion of brain: but this is entirely clinical."

Headaches, with red face and throbbing, like *Bell.*, but relieved by tight bandaging and a warm room.

Spasms about the eyes: jerkings: squint. Neuralgias of face, violent supra and infra orbital neuralgias; especially of right side; better heat and pressure; worse from cold.

Pains in stomach with clean tongue. Colic ameliorated by doubling up, like *Coloc.*, and by heat. " The colic is not so markedly relieved by heat in *Coloc.*, but is relieved by pressure." Distension of abdomen with much pain. Radiating. Compelled to walk and groan. Meteorism. " It is said to cure cows of this condition. *Colchicum* will cure cows when they are distended with gas after being turned into clover patches." . . .

* * *

Nerve pains, then, with spasm, cramp, and colic, suggest *Mag. phos.* But one seems to notice that it is not indicated where there is fever :—except in some fevers where there is cramp. *The great sphere of the drug is to torture, and to soothe, nerve tissue.*

MEDORRHINUM

MEDORRHINUM is the sterilized and potentized product of one of those deadly acute diseases which Hahnemann recognized as basic to all chronic disease and therefore a life-sentence unless combatted and " annihilated " by their appropriate homœopathic remedies.   He put forward two of these, *Thuja* and *Nitric acid*, as producing symptoms " like " those of the acute gonorrheal manifestations, and therefore potently curative ; given, one or other, as most indicated.

Since his mundane work was accomplished, we have advanced yet further where he pointed ; proving and employing, with tremendous effect, the disease-product itself ; but tamed, after the the methods of preparation and administration he laid down, and so rendered absolutely harmless even to the new-born babe.   We saw that, once, when a mother brought her infant-of-days for advice, because it constantly struggled over to lie on its face (a *Medorrhinum* symptom).   She was in terror that it would suffocate.   But, after its tiny dose of *Medorrhinum* it became a reformed character, and slept peacefully and normally.

Homœopathy has, for the last 100 years employed the deadliest poisons with not only perfect safety, but with a maximum of success. But, Hahnemann's " Doctrines " in regard to their use must be observed or they would have gone the way of so many wonderful new drugs : vaunted to the skies : widely experimented with— *on the sick* : prescribed according to the individual fancy of the prescriber, or of someone who sponsored them :   discovered to be dangerous : exposed and decried in medical journals : abandoned in favour of something yet newer and more promising. And all the while Homœopathy may have been using them for a hundred years or more, and continue to employ them—in suitable cases, with the absolute foreknowledge of where and how they may be relied upon merely to stimulate vitality to curative reaction, and do no harm.

Medorrhinum was introduced as a homœopathic medicine 100-odd years ago, by Dr. Swan, U.S.A., the great pioneer in the use of disease-products for the prevention and cure of disease.   The drug was " proved " by a number of very eminent physicians, mostly Americans.   Its most notable symptoms, elicited by provings on the healthy, and confirmed by subsequent clinical experiences— i.e. its " pathogenic verified symptoms " are very many and very striking : especially those of the mental sphere.   We will endeavour to draw attention to them, as they are not easily got at by the student of Materia Medica, and as they reveal the genius of the drug.

But, first, let us say emphatically,—no one must think that because *Medorrhinum* is the remedy called for by the symptoms of any case, that therefore the patient must have had the disease. True, one *has* seen this nosode act brilliantly in some extreme and loathsome acute cases during the Great War. But far more commonly the taint may have filtered down through several generations ; and it may be impossible to obtain really satisfactory healthward progress and without a few intercurrent doses of *Medorrhinum,* suggested, of course, by symptoms "like" those of its provings. We may rest assured that, prepared after the methods of Hahnemann, and prescribed as he directed, it is impossible, as said, to do harm therewith. Moreover it can only affect curatively a patient rendered abnormally sensitive to its action by a sickness of "like" symptoms : these, possibly, only in the mental sphere—for *Medorrhinum* is one of the greatest of mental drugs.

Burnett, who had great experience of the nosodes, and by them largely won his enormous practice and the almost adoration of the patients who found in him a help nowhere else to be obtained, used to insist that "the vilest filth, prepared in the homœopathic manner, may be not only harmless, but the purest gold—homœopathically applied."

Among the symptoms of *Medorrhinum* are some peculiar to itself —so far as we know at present. Foremost among these is its "Better at the sea-side." It is the only drug given by Kent in his Repertory : though elsewhere we find *Bromium,* in black type, for the "*asthma of sailors as soon as they come ashore*". This we joyfully verified in the one case that presented itself for treatment. In regard to this "better at the sea-side" one of our keen young doctors is most enthusiastic, because it has helped him again and again to do very striking work. This "better at the sea",he says, "is acknowledged to be the great characteristic of the drug" and these are among his cured cases :

Man of 60, who complained of fear of death : worse when alone : worse at night ; and rheumatism which cleared up completely at the sea-side. Here *Medorrhinum* 30 gave practically instant relief of fears and the patient has been better altogether ever since some four months.

A woman of 38 : duodenal ulcer with the usual symptoms : pain two hours after food ; excessive flatulence ; already of eight years' duration. All her digestive troubles being better at the sea-side,

18

she was given *Medorrhinum cm*. This was followed by rapid improvement of all symptoms, which has held for three months.

Woman of 40, emaciated, with itching scalp, and hair falling out. She was better always at the sea-side. Coldness of breasts when the rest of the body was warm. A craving for salt—all *Medorrhinum* symptoms. She got *Medorrhinum* 10m. Itching and falling of hair ceased ; patient putting on weight ; with marked improvement in appearance also. He finds the indication, " physical complaints vanish at the seaside ", apart from the general tonic effect of a holiday, an extremely valuable one.

We also have seen its fine action in some rheumatoid cases, as well as in a diversity of difficult conditions ; prescribed on symptoms, or on history.

One remembers a fearful eye case, from gonorrheal infection in infancy, where an elderly woman gained much sight, and where the eyes became comparatively normal in appearance, under doses, at long intervals, of *Medorrhinum* and *Syphillinum*. One remembers a doctor friend, confronted with baffling mental symptoms in an elderly woman, most distressing to her people, who gave *Medorrhinum* with splendid results.

Medorrhinum as said : has a wealth of mental symptoms, strange clairvoyance : curious confusions of the time sense, " as though things done today occurred a week ago ". Loss of thought : difficulty in making right statements. Starts well, then does not know how to finish. Delusions of someone behind her, whispering. Faces peer at her from behind the furniture : persons come in, look at her, whisper, and say " come ! " Sees large people in the room : large rats running : feels a delicate hand smoothing her head from front to back. Sensation as if all life were *unreal*, like a dream. Is always anticipating : feels matters most sensitively before they occur and generally correctly. Is in a great hurry. Anticipates death. A tendency to suicide : gets up and takes his pistol, but is prevented. Everything startles her : news coming to her seems to touch her heart before she hears it. Fear of the dark. Had committed the unpardonable sin, and was going to hell, Desperate : not caring whether she went to heaven or hell. Very impatient, very selfish.

A feeling as if she stared at everything. Ptosis of lids.

Nearly total deafness of both ears. Partial or transient deafness. Sensation of being deaf from one ear to the other : as if a tube went through head. When whistling, sound is double, with vibration as if two people whistle thirds. Noises, frying and hissing, as if in mastoid cells. A worm crawls in right ear, and commences boring anterior wall of auditory canal.

Nose sore : bleeds : as if crawling of a centipede in left nostril.

Taste coppery : tongue coated. Tongue blistered : blisters on inner surface of lips and cheeks : skin peeling off in patches.

Throat as if scraped. Salivation. Stringy mucus comes out of mouth during sleep.

Ravenous hunger immediately after eating; or absolute loss of appetite. Enormously thirsty ; even dreams she is drinking. Insatiate craving for liquor, which she had hated.

Craving : for salt ; sweets ; green fruit ; ices ; sour things ; oranges.

The vomiting is of thick mucus, and black bile ; generally *without nausea.*

A paper of pins in stomach seem to force themselves through the flesh, making her double up and scream. Intense pain and tightness in stomach, with desire to tear something away.

Terrible pains in liver. Grasping pain in liver and spleen.

Throbbing and thumping in region of suprarenal capsule : drawing and relaxing; as if caused by icy-cold insects with claws.

Agonizing pain solar plexus. He applied right hand to stomach and left to lumbar region.

Beating of pulses in abdomen and in many regions.

Can only pass stool by leaning back. Oozing of moisture from anus, fetid like fish brine.

Bubbling sensation in kidney.

Medorrhinum is in black type in the Repertory, with *Sulphur,* *Pulsatilla* and *Chamomilla,* for burning soles, which are thrust out of bed at night.

One symptom which would make one consider *Medorrhinum* as the remedy, is the history of an acrid, offensive discharge from vagina ; perhaps greenish.

Medorrhinum affects the mammæ : as " Breasts cold as ice to touch, especially nipples, the rest of the body warm " and again, " nipples sore, sensitive and inflamed." " Peculiar tenderness of breasts ": even, " large, but not painful, swelling of left breast."

It is a remedy found useful in incipient consumption.

Hering gives cured cases : " Child of 15 months, brought on a pillow apparently dead : eyes glassy, set; could not find pulse but felt heart beat : running from anus greenish-yellow, thin, horribly offensive stool." " A baby of seven months, great emaciation, diarrhœa green, watery, slimy, yellow, curdled, smelling like rotten eggs ; stools involuntary : apparently lifeless, except that it rotates head on pillow." " Cholera infantum with opisthotonos, vomiting, and watery diarrhœa ; profuse discharge of blood and pus."

It has many urinary symptoms : pain in suprarenals : bubbling in kidneys : strong smelling urine ; colourless urine ; urine with greasy pellicle : is curative in some cases of nocturnal enuresis : even diabetes.

Among the symptoms of respiration we note, difficulty and oppression of breathing : has to fill lungs, but no power to eject air. Spasm of glottis, air expelled with difficulty, but inhaled with ease (*Chlorum*). In asthma, and for relief of cough, *Medorrhinum* lies on face. Burning heat in chest, is one of its lung symptoms: and it has a reputation for incipient phthisis. Pains in chest, in heart, in limbs. One has found it useful where joints are tense with fluid : that form of rheumatoid arthritis. One remembers a case where a woman, a cook, had had to give up work : all her small joints were so painful and puffed and full of fluid. A dose of " *gonorrhinum* " 30—and when next seen she had put on her shoes and walked Hampstead Heath, as a test : then she returned to work.

The burning of soles, we have noticed. Hering gives a case where, after suppressed gonorrhœa, the feet were so tender that the man had to walk on his knees.

In nerve diseases, judging by the provings, it were well to remember *Medorrhinum* :—tremblings : tongue trembling : numbness : loss of power.

The cardinal symptoms, therefore, of *Medorrhinum* are—
Better at the sea-side.
Better in wet weather.
Better lying on abdomen : bending backwards.
Worse daylight to sunset (rev. of *Syphillinum*), though some of its symptoms are worse at night.

It is a remedy of great power, of wide use—but on its very definite indications.

*　　*　　*

H. C. ALLEN, who, in his *Materia Medica of the Nosodes*, has made many of these drugs accessible to us, has a long article on *Medorrhinum*. He says there are two preparations : the acute and the chronic. He says, " Like every other nosode, it should be prescribed according to strict indications, just as we would prescribe *Arsenic*, *Opium* and *Sulphur*, irrespective of its origin or the diagnosis."

He gives a case of " obstinate acute articular rheumatism in a man of 60, from June to September ". He suffered excruciating agony from neuralgia. After a desperate battle for life in the first week of September, he was relieved, and rose from his bed a wreck. It was expected that time and out-door life and the best hygienic measures would restore him. But weeks and months passed without a change : he walked the streets leaning on a cane, bent over, muffled in wraps to his ears, and looking like an old man about to fall into the grave. Three months after my attendance I saw him pass my office, and considering his previous good health and robust frame the question arose : Why does he remain in this condition ? Is there any uncured miasm, hereditary or acquired, to explain the obstinacy of the case ? Could it be a gonorrhœal taint ? For reasons unnecessary to mention I could not ask him.

Dr. Swan's suggestion now occurred to me :

An obstinate case of rheumatism might be due to latent gonorrhœa, and *Medorrhinum* high will cure it : in many cases where improvement reaches a certain stage, and then stops, *Medorrhinum* has removed the obstruction and the case progressed to a cure ; and this, too, in cases where gonorrhœa appeared to be a most unlikely cause : teaching us, if anything, the universality of latent gonorrhœa and the curative power of the dynamic virus.

His wife consulted me on other matters, and said " her husband was as well as could be expected considering his age : she believed he would not do anything more, as he regarded his feeble state due to his age." However, he came next day, and I gave him three doses of *Medorrhinum*, to be taken every morning. Within ten days he returned feeling well, and looking well. I then gave him one dose to be taken after more time : this was the last prescription he has required. Within a month, after the *Medorrhinum*, he dropped his cane and muffler, walked the street with a firm step, a perfectly well man, having increased in weight from 140 to 212 pounds.

* * *

NASH says that " gonorrhœal virus is undoubtedly a great remedy. Anyone who has had to do with gonorrhœa well knows the severe form of rheumatism, which is often the consequence of the introduction of this disease product into the system. I have seen some remarkable results from the use of this remedy in chronic forms of rheumatism."

He gives telling cases. . . .

He says he has never found any history of gonorrhœa in the cases he has been able to benefit with this remedy. . . . " The question arises, is Swan's nosode theory true, or are disease products homœopathically curative only in those cases resembling them, not having a disease-product history ? . . .

" Since writing the above I have experimented more with the so-called nosodes and have had seemingly very good results from this remedy, as well as *Syphillinum* in intractable cases of chronic rheumatism. The most characteristic difference is that with *Medorrhinum* the pains are worse in the day-time, and with *Syphillinum* in the night.

" There are, no doubt, great curative powers residing in these two disease poisons, and they should not be discarded simply because they are the products of disease.

" In regard to the other nosodes, I have, within two years past, seen some remarkable effects from them."

BLACK LETTER SYMPTOMS

Time moves too slowly.

Dulness of memory: desire to procrastinate, because business seemed so lasting, or as if it could never be accomplished.

In conversation would stop, and remark he could not think what word he wanted to use.

Fears he is going to die.

Is in a great hurry: in such a hurry that he feels fatigued.

Epistaxis.

Continuous watering of eyes: sensation of sand under lids.

Impotence.

Incipient consumption.

Great pallor; yellowness of face, particularly around eyes, as if from a bruise. Yellow band across forehead close to hair.

Neuralgia right upper and lower jaws, extending to temple.

Hard swelling right upper jaw, as if in socket of a tooth gone years ago.

Pale gums.

Very sore mouth; ulcers on tongue and in mouth, like blisters.

Blisters inner surface cheeks and lips: skin peeling in patches.

Violent retching and vomiting for forty-eight hours, first glairy mucus, lastly coffee grounds, with intense headache, great despondency and sensation of impending death: during paroxysm was constantly praying.

Cramps in stomach, as from wind.

Sensation in pit of stomach as of a paper of pins, that seemed to force themselves through the flesh, causing her to rise and double up and scream: pins seem to come from each side.

Intense pain in stomach and upper abdomen, with sensation of tightness.

Congestion of liver.

Burning heat round back like a coal of fire.

Throbbing and thumping in region of suprarenal capsule, as if from abscess or sore spot just below fifth rib, right side. Creeping chills in region of right kidney, throbbing, contracting, drawing and relaxing as if caused by cold insects with claws.

Ascites : abdomen greatly distended, urine scanty and high-coloured.

Black stool.
White diarrhœa.
Can only pass stool by leaning far back; very painful; as if a lump on posterior surface of sphincter ; so painful as to cause tears.
Cholera infantum with opisthotonos, vomiting and watery diarrhœa : profuse discharge of blood and pus.
Painful attacks of piles, not bleeding : hot swelling left anus.
Pin worms.

GLINICUM 1000

" GLINICUM is none other than *Medorrhinum* ; then why multiply names ? Only because I obtained the matrix of this myself from a typical case, and macerated it myself in spirit of wine, so I *know* what it is, and how prepared, and anyone else can do the same at any time and anywhere in the whole world. . . .

" My indications for *Glinicum* are : roused in the small hours of the morning by pain, acidity, coated tongue, filthy taste and breath, uncleanably dirty tongue, weakness, pallor, chilliness, worse from cold wet ; and moreover *Glin.* is largely a left-sided remedy. *Glin.* wipes out half the cases of sciatica that pass my way. What a record ! "—BURNETT.

MERCURIUS

In order to obtain, by provings of the metal, an exact knowledge of its action on human health—to vitiate and therefore to cure—Hahnemann was at much pains to secure MERCURY in, at once, a pure and soluble state.

One of his preparations, " *Mercurius vivus* ", was quicksilver (purified from lead, etc.) and then made active by trituration and potentization. Because, as he says, " Mercury in its fluid metallic state has little dynamic action on man's health ; it is only its chemical compounds that cause great effects."

He discusses the various salts of mercury. He says that these, when carefully proved, " all display in their action a certain general similarity as mercurials ; whilst, on the other hand, they differ greatly from one another in their peculiarities, and very much in the intensity of their action on human health ".

So " this great analytical chemist "—for Hahnemann was known as such in his day—set to work " to obtain pure mercury in such a condition that it should be able to display its true, pure, peculiar effects on the human organism in a more powerfully curative manner than all other known preparations and saline combinations ".

The result was MERCURIUS SOLUBILIS HAHNEMANNII, the black oxide of mercury, which was quickly " preferred in almost all countries to all other mercurials hitherto in use, on account of its much milder, and more efficacious anti-syphilitic properties " ; and which still remains in general use in medicine, the world over, to-the present day.

Even this did not wholly content Hahnemann's desire " for the highest degree of purity " and he proceeded to prepare in the grey precipitate a perfectly pure oxide of mercury. However, its preparation requiring much care and labour,* and its effects being indistinguishable from the black oxide, it was the black oxide, *Mercurius solubilis* that was so drastically proved by Hahnemann and his band, and which we prescribe as *Merc. sol.*, or simply " *Merc.*" :—it being understood that all the other mercurials which we use will have their special designation attached—*Merc. vi.*, *Merc. cor.*, *Merc. cy.*, *Merc. bin-iodide*, etc., etc., to identify them.

* In *Materia Medica Pura*, he describes the processes of the various preparations.

HERING (*Guiding Symptoms*) says that " the symptoms of the *solubilis*, obtained by regular proving, and the effects of the *vivus*, gathered from toxicological reports carefully sifted and clinically verified, are sufficiently similar to be placed under one arrangement " ; though where possible, he places an " s " or a " v " to show to which especially the symptom belongs : and Clarke in his *Dictionary* follows Hering. While Allen's *Encyclopedia* gives symptoms under each preparation separately.

Mercurius is one of the " drugs of frequent use ", which we could ill do without. It finds its place, accordingly, in every little pocket case of a dozen domestic remedies : and no physician would sally forth on his rounds without " *Merc.*" in his portable armoury. It has its unique position in the treatment of alike the lightest and most serious diseases ; of colds and coughs ; toothaches and earaches ; headaches and eye troubles ; diseases of nose, mouth, gums, tongue, where its action is very marked ; of throat, liver, abdomen and stools—with constipation and diarrhœa ; of urinary organs, sexual organs, lungs, limbs, glands, nerves—with tremor ; skin with eruptions, and ulcerations, and sweat. But everywhere it has its marked peculiarities. Once fathom its " thus-ness " and it is difficult to miss.

Merc. is notable especially for its *foulness and offensiveness*— of breath—of its profuse saliva—of its drenching sweats : but, curiously enough, stool, urine, menses, leucorrhœa are not especially offensive :—excepting the stools in the case of *Merc. cor.*

Another great feature is " *Worse for the heat of the bed.*"

Another " *Worse at night.*"

Another *sliminess* of mucous membranes.

Now we will see how *Merc.* has appealed to, and been useful to, some of our great prescribers, and what tips they have to bestow on us, as regards its uses.

This is NASH's little summary. . . .

" Swollen, flabby tongue, taking imprint of the teeth : gums also swollen, spongy and bleeding ; breath very offensive.

" Sweats day and night without relief—in many complaints.

" Creeping chilliness in the beginning of a cold or threatened suppuration.

" Sliminess of mucous membranes.

" Moist tongue, with intense thirst.

" Glandular swellings, cold, inclined to suppurate. Ulcers with lardaceous base.

" Modalities : worse at night : in warmth of bed : while sweating : lying on the right side.

" Bone diseases ; pains worse at night.

" Dysentery : stools slimy, bloody ; with colic, fainting : with great tenesmus during and after, followed by chilliness, and a ' cannot finish sensation '. (More marked in *Merc. cor.*)

" The more blood and pain, the better indicated.

" Affects lower lobe of right lung : stitches through to back (*Chel.*, *Kali. c.*).

" Intense thirst, although the tongue looks moist, and saliva is profuse."

And Nash says, " in low potencies it hastens suppuration ; in high, aborts suppuration, as in quinsy."

Now we will let BOGER speak from his *Therapeutic Key*,

" Profuse sweat with nearly every complaint, which does not relieve.

" Catarrh. Nostrils raw, ulcerated (*Aur.*, *Sulph.*).

" Ptyalism—fetid. Metallic tasting.

" Tongue large, flabby, shows imprint of teeth (*Chel.*, *Pod.*, *Rhus.*).

" Thirst with a moist tongue and salivation. (*Puls.* dry, and no thirst.) (Also *Nux mosch.*)

" Dysentery. Stools slimy and bloody, with colic and *fainting*.

" No relief from stool (*Merc. cor.*). Never-get-done sensation (*Merc. cor.*).

" Salivation. Wets the pillow in sleep.

" *Trembling hands.*"

Nash further discusses and amplifies,—he writes,—

" The chill of *Mercurius* is peculiar, as I have observed it. It is not a shaking chill, but is simply a *creeping chilliness.*" (*Gels.*, big chills with heavy limbs : *Nux*, chills from every movement, from leaving the fire.) " Often when this creeping chilliness is felt it is the first symptom of a cold that has been taken, and, if left alone, the coryza, sore throat, bronchitis or even pneumonia may follow ; but if taken early, a dose of *Merc.* may prevent all such troubles. The chilliness is felt most generally in the evening and increases into the night if not removed by *Mercury*. . . . It is often felt in single parts. Then again it is felt in abscesses, and is the harbinger of pus formation."

(One remembers a case, where a surgeon was dressing several sinuses in a shoulder joint. The patient complained of this creeping chilliness in the wounds. *Merc.* was given, with (so one was told later) great benefit to the condition.

Compare *Sil.*, which has a sensation of coldness in ulcers.

" Now the *sweats*. They are very profuse and do not relieve like the sweats of inflammatory diseases generally do, but on the contrary the complaints *increase with the sweat*. (*Tilia*.) In what diseases is this condition found ? It may be found in almost every disease : in sore throat, bronchitis, pneumonia, pleuritis, abscesses, rheumatism, etc. . . . In short, *in any disease in which this profuse and persistent sweating without relief is present, Mercurius is the first remedy to be thought of.*

" *Worse at night*, and especially in the *warmth of the bed*, is another strong characteristic of *Mercurius*. (*Led.*) There is a long list of remedies that have aggravations at night, but not so many from warmth of the bed. I have cured many skin diseases of various names guided by this modality. . . ."

H. C. ALLEN points out that " *Merc*. is worse by heat of bed but is better for rest in bed : whereas *Ars*. is better for heat of bed, but worse for rest in bed."

It is knowledge of these little points that often makes successful prescribing quickly practicable in acute work : and Allen says, " Worse lying on right side—very few remedies have this."

And now a few quotations from KENT.

" *Merc*. has stinging pains like *Apis*. All routinists will give *Apis* for stinging pains, and yet it is often *Merc*. that the patient needs.

" Purulent, offensive otorrhœa . . . furuncles in external canal. Fungous excrescences and polypi.

" Taste and tongue : tongue flabby, mealy surface, often pale. The imprint of the teeth is observed all round the edge of the tongue. It is swollen and presses in around the teeth, and thus gets the imprint of the teeth. Old gouty constitutions ; the tongue will swell in the night and he will wake up with a mouthful of tongue (Comp. *Crot. h.*) . . . *copious flow of fetid saliva*.

" Milk in the breasts of the non-pregnant woman at the menstrual period. Milk in the breasts instead of the menstrual flow. I once had a freak in a sixteen-year-old boy who had milk in his breasts. I cured him with *Merc*.

" Urine burns and must be washed off. Itching from contact of urine.

" The complaints in general are worse while he sweats, and the more he sweats, the worse he is.

" . . . excoriating wherever two parts come together.

" *Merc*. especially affects the *joints ; inflammatory rheumatism* with much swelling, aggravated from the heat of the bed and from uncovering. It is difficult to get just the right weight of clothing. Rheumatic affections with sweat, aggravation at night, from the warmth of the bed and while sweating, with sickly countenance. It especially attacks the upper limbs, but is also found in the lower.

" *Merc.* is one of the best palliatives in cancer of the uterus and mammæ. It will restrain and sometimes cure epithelioma. I knew one case cured by the *proto-iodide*, an ulcerated, indurated lump in the breast, as large as a goose egg, with knots in the axilla, blueness of the part, and no hope. The 100*th* attenuation, given as often as the pains were very severe, took it away and she remained well.

" The loaded tongue and the bilious fevers fade out after *Merc.* It is wonderfully useful in hectic fever in the last stages of consumption, and in exhausting diseases with hectics, and in cancer, where there is aching, foul sweat, etc. . . . when the patient is icteric, low, prostrated, tremulous, with quivering muscles, great exhaustion and continued fever."

By the way : *Mercurius* and *Silica* are " inimicals ". One has seen the severe aggravations in abscess cases, when the one is administered after the other. Here *Hepar* will " straighten things out " and restore order.

Merc. besides its foulness of mouth and salivation, has salt taste ; sweet taste ; metallic taste ; taste of rotten eggs ; " slimy " taste.

" Troubles occurring in or on margin of eyelids ; forehead ; scalp ; bones of the head ; external top of head ; glands about the ears.

" Acrid nasal secretion, nose red and excoriated all the time ; ' dirty-nosed children' (*Sulph.*). Bridge of nose may swell up, very large on both sides and the top. . . . *Rarely give Merc. if the tongue is dry.*" (Guernsey's *Keynotes.*)

One cannot here discuss *Mercurius* in the treatment of venereal disease as laid down in Hahnemann's *Chronic Diseases* (which work seems to be coming into its own at last) : and yet one cannot pass it over without notice. For what we have to say on the subject doctors may like to glance through a little pamphlet, published by the British Homœopathic Association, entitled *Hahnemann's Conception of Chronic Disease as caused by Parasitic Micro-organisms.*

One remembers the rapid cure of a bad case of " 'Flu-pneumonia " just after the War, with a few doses of *Merc.* 30 : given because of the filthy mouth and breath, and profuse offensive sweat.

Black Letter Symptoms.

Hahnemann ; Allen's *Encyclopedia* ; Hering's *Guiding Symptoms.*

Hurried and rapid talking.
Memory weak : forgets things.
Itching on the hairy scalp.
The whole HEAD *is painful to touch.*
Tearing, drawing pains, in pereosteum, head and face : rheumatic headaches.
Congestion to head : feels it will burst : fullness of brain.
As if contracted by a band : as if in a vice.
External head painful to touch.

Black insects seem to be always flying before the sight.
Mist before one or both EYES. *Dimness of sight.*
The light of the fire dazzles the eyes greatly.
The eyes cannot bear the light of the fire, or daylight.
A fog before one or both eyes.
If she attempts to look at anything she cannot distinctly recognize it, and then the eyes are involuntarily drawn together : the more she tries to restrain the contraction, the less able is she to prevent it : she is obliged to lie down and close the eyes.
Lachrymation profuse, burning, excoriating.
Muco-purulent discharges, thin and acrid.
Blepharitis : lids red, thick, swollen. Worse open air : worse cold applications.
Aching in the eyes : itching in the eyeballs.

Roaring in the EARS.
Ear inflamed internally and externally, with cramp-like, sticking pain, and a feeling as if stopped by swelling.
Bloody and offensive matter flows from right ear, with tearing pain.

Epistaxis. Nose-bleed during sleep.
Offensive odour from the NOSE *as in violent coryza.*
Acrid matter flows from nose. Green fetid pus.
Nasal bone is painful when taken hold of.

Corners of MOUTH *ulcerated and painfully sore.*
Looseness of teeth, which are very painful when touched by tongue. A feeling as if all the teeth were loose.
Tongue white, as if covered with fur : great swelling of tongue.

A kind of aphthæ in mouth.

Violent toothache at night, followed by great chilliness over the whole body.

Jerking toothache at night. . . . Jerking from teeth of lower jaw into ear, and from upper jaw into head, with painfulness of gums.

Gums swollen ; separate from the teeth.

Bleeding of gum from slightest touch.

Gum painful when touched and on chewing.

Tongue coated white, with whitish swollen gums that bleed when touched.

Tongue swollen and so soft on the margin that it showed the imprint of the teeth in scallops, which looked ulcerated.

Corners of mouth ulcerated and sore.

Pain and swelling of salivary glands.

Constant ecptysis.

Sweetish taste in the mouth.

THROAT constantly dry : hurts as if too tight posteriorly : a pressure in it if he swallowed, yet constantly obliged to swallow because the mouth was always full of water.

Something hot rises to her throat.

When swallowing, shooting pain in tonsils.

Suppuration of the tonsils, with sharp, sticking pain in fauces when swallowing.

(Sensation of apple-core sticking in throat.)

Very salt TASTE on the lips. Salt taste on tongue.

Salt expectoration.

Taste of rotten eggs when he moves the tongue, and then involuntary swallowing.

Slimy taste in the mouth.

At night (1 a.m.) much water flows into the mouth, at the same time nausea, so that he wakes up from it and must vomit ; something very bitter comes up.

Frequent HICCOUGH.

Extremely violent THIRST. Extraordinarily intense thirst.

Burning pain in scorbiculus cordis.

Swelling of inguinal GLANDS, with circumscribed redness.

Inguinal gland becomes red and inflamed ; is painful when touched and walking.

Ineffectual urging to STOOL *every moment, with tenesmus in the rectum.*

Bloody stools with painful acrid sensation at anus.

Green slimy acrid stools, that excoriate the anus.

Along with soft stools, burning pain in anus.

Green diarrhœa : diarrhœa of green mucus, with burning and protrusion of anus.

Greenish, painless gonorrhœa, especially at night.

Burning in URETHRA.

Constant desire to URINATE *; indeed every ten minutes ; but only a little passed.*

Urine immediately after being passed very turbid and depositing a sediment.

He passes much more urine than the liquid he has drunk.

Too frequent and too profuse urination.

Nocturnal seminal emission, mixed with blood.

Catamenia too profuse.

Greenish biting leucorrhœa, with much scratching, especially evening and night, with violent burning after scratching.

Frequent sneezing without coryza.

Stitches in chest with sneezing or coughing.

A stitch in anterior upper chest, extending through to back.

During the cough, inclination to vomit.

Sticking in small of back on breathing.

Weakness and weariness of all limbs.

Trembling of the hands.

Ankle joint as if sprained.

As if bruised in the limbs.

Profuse PERSPIRATION *when walking.*

Perspiration on every movement.

Complaints increase during sweat.

Constant cold hands and feet.

Perspires day and night, though more at night.

Profuse perspiration at night. Very profuse.

Fatty and oily perspiration at night.

Profuse, offensive perspiration, soaking the bedclothes.

Large ULCERS *bleed, and when touched there is a pain affecting the whole body. Their margins everted like raw meat and their bases covered with a caseous coat.*

Bleeding of an ulcer that had previously existed.

Dropsical patients (so-called) very rapidly lost the swelling, and got instead fetid, rapidly decomposing ulcers on the legs.

Frequent waking from sleep.
Great weariness.
Very much exhausted after a stool.

As soon as he went to bed in the evening, the pains recommenced and banished sleep.

Among its queer sensations are
Head in a vice : growing larger.
Sparks from eyes.
A weight hanging from nose.
Feathers coming out of corners of eyes.
A wedge driven into ear.
Ice in ear : cold water running from ear.
Teeth loose, fixed in a mass of pap.
Worm rising in throat : apple core stuck in throat.

And among the mental symptoms, and dementiæ are :
Excessive fright at a small surprise : Cheek swells : feels bruised all over : cannot compose herself.
Indescribable sensation of internal, intolerable ill.
Imagines he is enduring the torments of hell.
Torment at night, as if he had committed some crime.
Desire to flee, with nightly anxiety and apprehension.
Extreme restlessness at night. Lies down, rises : nowhere rest.
Thinks, losing reason : about to die : illusions.
Cares for nothing. Extreme indifference.
Cross : irritable : suspicious : quarrelsome : disputatious.
Talks nonsense : acts the buffoon : does stupid, nonsensical things.
Mania : throws off clothes at night : tears and scolds. Leaps up high. Talks and scolds much to herself. Does not know her nearest relations. Frequently spits, spreads the saliva out with her feet ; licks some of it up again. Often licks cow-dung and the mud of ponds. (*Comp. Verat.*) Takes little stones in her mouth without swallowing them, yet complains they are cutting her bowels. Does no harm to anyone, but resists when touched :

does nothing she is told to do. . . . When taking a walk he felt a strong inclination to catch passing strangers by the nose. . . .

MERCURIUS VIVUS

BLACK LETTER SYMPTOMS

Slow in answering questions. Memory weak.

Face earthy-coloured, puffy.

Teeth black, loose.

Carious teeth. Decay of teeth, they become loose in succession. . . . blackened, laid bare, loose and carious.

Teeth become denuded of the gum and turn black, with nightly pain in teeth, jaws and head.

Violent toothache, with swelling of gum and salivary glands.

Gums red and bleeding at slightest contact, spontaneously.

Gums have a bright-red margin : small ulcers at intervals.

Gums spongy and bleeding. Sore.

Tongue black with red edges. Tongue red, swollen.

Coated tongue, showing impress of teeth upon the margin.

Tongue swollen and its movements difficult.

Bad odour from the mouth : fetid odour : sweetish.

Violent stomatitis and salivation.

Speech difficult on account of the trembling of the mouth and tongue. Speech stammering.

Tremor of hands. Trembling.

MERCURIUS CYANATUS

Almost specific for diphtheria.

MEZEREUM

(Daphne Mezereum)

ONE of Hahnemann's precious medicinal legacies. He says the juice, when touching the skin, produces a very painful burning, which lasts for a long time ; and he tells us that, since the medicinal power of this drug is not volatile, it is better to dry the plant and triturate it like all other dry substances. The bark, root and stem are used for making the tincture.

Mezereum is a hardy shrub, native of Great Britain and northern countries : flowers early in spring, sometimes in the snow. Was introduced by Stapf, and extensively proved by Hahnemann and his band. The proving appears in his *Chronic Diseases.*

It powerfully affects skin, bones, mucous membranes. Its action is characterized throughout by VIOLENCE. Violent pains : violent itching : sudden, violent pains in face during sleep ; violent sensations of hunger ; violent burning in mouth ; violent pains in stomach and œsophagus ; violent inclination to cough, lower down than can be reached by cough ; " violent acute fever ".

And all its violence is more violent *by night.* It is one of the remedies that may be needed in the treatment of syphilis ; also may be needed in a variety of skin conditions—very severe skin lesions, characterized by violent *itching,* and worse at night ; from heat of bed : the one drug that has got into the Repertory, as " eruptions itching, worse warmth of fire ".

It has annoying *twitchings* : twitching of eyelid ; twitchings and jerking of muscles of right cheek ; twitching of muscles in pit of stomach.

It is one of the few remedies that love and crave *fat ham* ; *Mez.* finds relief in drinking milk, and eating fat bacon. (Compare *Tuberculinum.*)

Some of its pains are violently *burning* : " peppery " burnings (compare *Caps.*) ; and it has fiery taste ; salty and peppery taste ; bitter and sour taste—especially *beer* tastes bitter (not water), and causes vomiting.

The stomach conditions (it has a reputation for gastric ulcer and even induration and carcinoma) are curious. Without hunger, there may be constant desire to eat and take something into stomach, whereby he has less pain. (Compare *Graph., Chel.,* etc.) Constant longing for food. Nausea disappears after eating. (Compare *Sepia.*)

In regard to its " skins ", one never forgets a recurrent experience with *Mezereum cm.*, when doing children's and casualty work at the hospital during the War : the children being ill-nourished, probably lent themselves to such miserable conditions. The experience was with the many cases of *kerion* (tinea kerion), thus described in text-books : " marked inflammatory symptoms with circumscribed boggy tumefaction of the scalp, which is covered with pustules, or with gaping orifices from which exudes viscid pus ". And one remembers vividly, how some of the cases were " running with lice ". One is told that kerion may fluctuate, and give the idea of abscess, but when incised, instead of a pocket of pus, a number of pus points merely exude, the individual hair cells being the seat of innumerable small abscesses. Anyway, *Mezereum* never failed to rapidly cure the condition. So much so, that when appealed to from the country in regard to some children thus affected, one sent *Mezereum cm.*, a few doses, which, as one was told, rapidly cured.

" *Specifics ?—how dare you teach specifics ? Is this the Homœo-pathy of Hahnemann, which you profess to teach ? "*

As a matter of fact, *it is.* Hahnemann tells us, if we would only heed, that for " miasmatic " diseases, acute or chronic, i.e. *for diseases caused by parasitic organisms, which have in each case the same origin, the same symptoms, the same course, " a specific should be found".* And doubtless kerion is a specific parasitic infection, caused by micro-organisms, and having the same origin, the same symptoms and the same course ; for which, so far as epidemic experience with a dozen or so cases is concerned, *Mezereum* is *the* specific ; and it proved itself so by acting magnificently in the single dose of the highest potency one had been able to lay hands on. Therefore let us once again quote Hahnemann, in regard to " Infectious diseases, caused by a peculiar contagium (a miasm of tolerably fixed character) such as small-pox, measles, true scarlet fever, etc. . . . These seem so fixed in their course as to be always recognized as old acquaintances. They can be named, and we can endeavour to lay down some fixed method of treatment suitable, as a rule, for each of them."

We may here, with advantage, give *in extenso* Dr. Carroll Dunham's classical case of the cure of an almost lifelong deafness, with *Mezereum.* He traced it back to a severe attack of just such *tinea capitis,* in childhood ; and, by treating that ancient condition—all those years later—he managed to restore hearing, utility and happiness to a boy whose life had, till then, been blasted. It was a case, evidently, of what we may venture to call, " chronic kerion ". It bears out our contention, fully explained in *No.* 12 *Post-graduate Correspondence Course*, that, *in ill-health dating from some acute illness, where the patient, apparently recovered, has never been well since*, we may be really dealing with *Chronic Measles, Chronic Diphtheria, Chronic Vaccinosis* (Burnett), *Chronic Pneumonia*, etc., and we may prove our case (to our own satisfaction, anyway) by seeing the rapid leap to better life and energy, after a dose or two of *Diphtherinum, Morbillinum, Pneumococcin, Scarlatinum* or *Streptococcin, Variolinum,* or *Thuja*, etc., according to the "past history" of the sufferer.

We make no apology for reproducing the case in full, together with the lessons deduced from it, by one of the past masters of homœopathic prescribing ; although it has been again and again alluded to by teachers of Homœopathy.

DEAFNESS CURED BY *MEZEREUM*, WITH REMARKS

From *Homœopathy the Science of Therapeutics*

By Dr. Carrol Dunham

G.W.W. (17), small but well proportioned and of good constitution, healthy since his ninth year, has been deaf since he was four years old. When three years of age, he had an eruptive disease of the whole scalp, which, after resisting for a year all the milder methods of allopathic treatment, was finally caused to disappear, in the following manner : A tar-cap was placed upon the head, and when firmly adherent to the scabs, was violently torn off. The scabs came with it, leaving the whole scalp raw. This raw surface was moistened with a saturated solution of nitrate of silver. The eruption did not reappear ; but from that time the child was deaf.

The condition of the youth now excites the earnest solicitude of his friends. His inability to move in society, or to get a situation in business, on account of his deafness, has produced a morbid state of mind. He broods over his infirmity, and secludes himself even from his own family.

Under these circumstances, he applied to me to be cured of his deafness. His present condition is as follows : He is quite unable to hear ordinary conversation, and has never heard a sermon in his life. A loud-ticking lever watch can be heard at a distance of three and a half inches from either ear. On application of the watch to his forehead, or to his teeth, he hears it distinctly. Occasional buzzing noises in front of the ears. A physical examination of his ears reveals the following conditions : The external meatus is abundantly supplied with soft, normal wax. The membrana tympani is white, opaque, and evidently thickened. When the patient attempts to inflate the middle ear (which he accomplishes with great difficulty, by closing both mouth and nose and making a forcible expiration) the membrana tympani becomes but very slightly convex, and it is impossible to distinguish its distended blood-vessels. There has evidently been a deposit in the substance of the membrane. On examination of the throat, it appears that the orifice of the eustachian tube is free.

Feb. 3rd, 1857. Patient received a powder containing three globules of *Mezereum* 30, to be taken on retiring.

Feb. 24th. Thinks he hears better—" every sound seems much louder than before ". Hears my watch at a distance of four and a half inches from the right ear, and four and a quarter from the left ear. (*No medicine.*)

March 1st. Has not improved during the last week. *Mezereum* 30, three globules.

March 27th. Hears my watch, with the right ear, six and a half inches, and with the left, seven inches. (*No medicine.*)

April 20th. Hears my watch, with the right ear, at a distance of ten inches, and with the left at a distance of fourteen inches. Hears ordinary conversation easily, with attention. (*No medicine.*)

Sept. 28th. Has been steadily improving until three weeks ago, when he became more deaf again, without apparent cause. *Mezereum* 30, three globules, on retiring.

June 26th, 1858. Hears my watch at a distance of fourteen inches from the right ear, and twenty-four inches from the left ear. Deafness returns when he takes cold, but disappears with the cold. *Mezereum* 30, three globules on retiring,

March 19th. To his surprise, on going to church, although seated at the extreme end of a very large building, he distinctly heard the whole sermon—for the first time in his life. On physical examination, the opacity of the membrana tympani is found to have disappeared, and its elasticity to have sensibly increased.

May 24th. Patient writes me that he has obtained, without difficulty, a situation in a store, and that he is no longer conscious of being deaf. His sole difficulty is that, as he has the reputation of being deaf, everybody shouts at him. His father writes that the son's hearing is " perfectly restored ".

REMARKS. The success of the treatment resorted to in this instance warrants a few remarks upon its rationale. Here was a case which presented to the practitioner apparently nothing on which to base a prescription. There was a thickened membrana tympani—nothing more. The work of thickening had probably been accomplished years ago. Here was a *pathologico-anatomical condition*, but no *pathological process* and, consequently, there were no abnormally performed functions—or in other words, no symptoms of disease—from which to draw indications for the treatment. The pathological-anatomical *condition* threw no certain light on the pathological process which had produced it —just as a knowledge of the town, at which a traveller has arrived, gives no certain clue to the road by which he reached it.

But, as Hahnemann advised his disciples, the *history of a case* is often of the utmost importance in determining the treatment. In the case before us the coincidence between the violent removal of the tinea capitis by nitrate of silver, and the appearance of the deafness, was too marked to escape notice. It could not fail to occur to the practitioner that the scalp disease was one phase of a *psoric* affection, as Hahnemann would have called it, or of a dyscrasia, as the modern school of German pathologists would say (for the doctrine of dyscrasias is but a rehash of Hahnemann's psoric theory), and that this affection, disturbed in its localization upon the scalp, had transferred itself to the tissues of the ear. It further occurred to me that, since in this latter localization there were no sufficient indications for a prescription, I might find such indications in the phenomena of the former localization upon the scalp. I accordingly addressed myself to the task of getting a complete picture of this affection, which had disappeared thirteen years before. By good fortune the mother of the patient was possessed of a good memory, and of very excellent powers of description, and from her I learnt that " thick, whitish scabs, hard and almost horny, covered the whole scalp. There were fissures in the scales, through which, on pressure, there exuded a thick, yellowish pus, often very offensive. There was great itching, and a disposition to tear off the scabs with the finger-nails —especially troublesome at night ".

The remedy which corresponds most closely, in its pathogenesis, with the above group of symptoms, is undoubtedly *Mezereum*. In the introduction to the proving of that drug, in the *Chronic Diseases*, Vol. IV, Hahnemann recommends it for moist eruptions of the scalp. In the proving, in the *Archiv.*, Vol. LV, many symptoms point to a similar eruption—itching, especially at night, but the conclusive group of pathogenetic symptoms is the following, from a new proving of *Mezereum*, by the late Dr. Wahle, of Rome, of which the manuscript was shown me by his son, the present Dr. Wahle :

" Head covered over with a thick leather-like crust, under which thick white pus collects here and there, and the hair is glued together ; on the head, great, elevated, irregular, white scabs, under which pus collects in quantity, and becomes offensive and breeds vermin. The child keeps scratching its face and head at night, and continuously tears off the scabs."

The resemblance between these groups of symptoms was so striking that *Mezereum* was at once selected as the remedy for this case of *deafness*, just as if the scalp affection had been still in its original form, and had been the immediate object of the prescription.

It not infrequently occurs that we are called upon to prescribe for what seem rather *results* of morbid actions, than active diseases. In such cases it would seem that we may often success-fully base a prescription upon the symptoms of a diseased condition which no longer exists, but which form, in reality, a part of the case. It may not be amiss to call attention to the complete-ness of the corroboration which this case affords (were any needed) of Hahnemann's *psora theory*. It is hardly necessary to say that Hahnemann had no idea of restricting psora to itch, as we under-stand that term, that is to the disease caused by the acarus. On the contrary, in his *Chronic Diseases*, Vol. IV, he expressly includes under it *various forms*, as " Itch, Tinea Capitis, Herpes, etc."

Black Letter Symptoms

Hypochondriac and despondent. Takes no pleasure in anything.
Everything seems to him dead, and nothing makes a vivid impres-sion upon his mind.

Very violent HEADACHE : *head painful to slightest touch (after a slight vexation).*
Bone pain in bones of skull, especially aggravated by contact.
Cranial bones pain, are swollen and sensitive to cold and contact : worse from motion and in the evening. Caries.
Itching and burning of SCALP.
Head covered with a thick leather-like crust, under which thick white pus collects here and there, and hair is glued together.
On the head, great elevated white scabs, under which ichor collects in quantity, and which begins to be offensive and to breed vermin.

EYES : sensation of dryness.
Obstinate jerking of the muscles of left upper lid.

EAR : Sensation of air distending the right external meatus. (Then the left.)

TEETH *feel blunt and elongated : painful on biting or from fresh air.*

Violent burning in mouth.

Heat and scraping in fauces.

Burning in THROAT *and pharynx : dryness in fauces, hacking cough ; anxious oppression of breath, loosening of scanty mucus on coughing.*

Vomits BEER, *which has a bitter taste (not water).*

Pain in periosteum of long BONES, *especially tibia : worse at night in bed ; least touch is intolerable. Worse in damp weather.*

Bones inflamed, swollen, especially shafts of cylindrical bones ; after abuse of Mercury and venereal disease.

Eczema, itching intolerably, copious serous exudation.

Neuralgia and burning after zona.

The SKIN *of face is of a deep inflammatory redness, and the eruption is " fat " and moist.*

The child scratches the face continually ; it becomes covered with blood.

In the night the child scratches its face so that the bed is covered with blood in the morning ; and the face is covered with a scab which the child keeps constantly tearing off anew, and on the spots thus left raw, large (fat) pustules form.

Ulcers covered with thick whitish-yellow scabs, under which thick, yellow pus collects.

Vesicles appear around the ulcers, itching, violently and burning like fire. After eight days these vesicles dry up, leaving scabs, the tearing off of which causes great pain and retards healing.

SOME QUEER, OR ITALIC SYMPTOMS

Irritable ; averse to everything ; desire to run away. (*Bell.,* etc.)

Apprehensiveness in pit of stomach (*K. carb.,* etc.) as when expecting some very unpleasant news.

Everything vexes him ; he wants to say all kinds of annoying and vexatious things.

Unable to recollect : or understand. Every intercurrent remark of others disturbed and confused his ideas.

Head dull. as if intoxicated : as of he had been up all night.

Headache from root of nose into forehead as if everything would press asunder.

On pressing frontal bone it pains and draws down to the feet.

Heat and perspiration on head ; chilliness and coldness in rest of body (morning).

Sensation upper part of head, as if pithy.

Pressing pains as if skull would split.

On head, great elevated white scabs : chalky scabs, extend to eyebrows and nape of neck.

Violent biting on head, as if from lice.

Pressure in eyeballs, as if too large.

Moist, itching eruption on head and behind ears. (*Graph.*)

Dry eruption on head, with intolerable itching, as if head was in an ant's nest. (*Favus.*) (A case of favus cured recently with *Puls.*—in a typical *Pulsatilla* child.—ED.)

Eczema of lids and head ; thick hard scabs, from which pus exudes on pressure.

Ears feel as if too open, and as if air was pouring into them ; or as if tympanum was exposed to cold air ; with desire to bore with finger into ear.

Oozing eruption behind ears.

Fluent coryza, scabs in nose—soreness. Constant excoriation of nose. (Compare *Aur.*, *Sulph.*)

Facial muscles drawn tense : troublesome twitching of muscles of right cheek.

Feeling as if eyes were drawn backward into head.

Wind blowing in the right ear.

Honey-like scabs about mouth.

Sensation as if tooth was being lifted out of socket.

Teeth decay suddenly above gums ; crowns remain intact.

Decaying roots.

Peppery sensation on palate and in fauces.

Canine hunger noon and evening. Loss of appetite.

Desire for ham fat, coffee, wine.

Beer tastes bitter and causes vomiting.

Burning in whole mouth as from pepper.

Ulcer of stomach.

Induration of stomach.

Burning, corroding pains in stomach, as if it were raw inside.

Stool contains glistening bodies. Small, white, shining grains in brown fæces.

Anus becomes painful and constricted about fallen rectum.

Stools hard as a stone and large ; as if they would split anus.

Sticking in kidney, and pain as if torn.

Corroding leucorrhœa.

Dyspnœa as if from adhesions or contraction of lungs.

Cough spasmodic : yellow viscid mucus : tastes saltish.

Cough : when eating or drinking anything hot must cough till he vomits : from beer.

Intercostal neuralgia, follows herpes zoster. (*Ran. bulb.*, *Ars.*) Limbs feel as if shortened.

Right hand cold, left warm ; or both cold.

Paralysis of flexors of fingers ; finger-ends powerless, cannot hold anything.

Violent pain in tibia as if beaten, or as if periosteum were torn off, after midnight.

Leg, from knee to instep, covered with thick yellow scab, from cracks of which thick, yellow matter oozes on pressure.

Scabs fall off in pieces, leaving skin deep-red, sore, itching violently and exuding a thin, clear, fluid, forming a thin scab under which pus again collects ; skin round scabs dark-red, tense, hot, itching. At night intolerable itching and burning in eruption. Foul odour. (Herpes crustaceus.)

Violent nightly pains in bones of feet.

Feeling of great lightness of body.

Especially indicated in January and February.

Worse from heat and cold.

Head especially worse cold : cranial bones, pains in scalp, etc.

Yet worse heat of bed : of fire : itching of scalp and feet. (Like *Puls.*), is chilly and drowsy in a warm room.

Hands and feet cold : nails blue. With hot spot on top of head.

Sensations : as if drunk. As if upper part of head were pithy. As if skull would split. As if top of head were gone.

Eyes drawn backward : ears open.

Teeth too long : ants running over chest.

As if skull would split : stools would split anus : kidneys as if torn. Periosteum torn.

Throat narrowing. Chest too tight : limbs too short.

Sticking like needles : Millions of insects crawling on him.

Twitching pains : in hollow teeth ; from hip joint to knee ; in cheek : in eyelid.

Like fire darting through muscles.

Constriction, throat, stomach, round prolapsed anus.

Bones feel distended.

HUGHES (*Pharmacodynamics*) tells us that *Mezereum* was one of the vegetable substances . . . with which it was attempted to replace mercury in the treatment of syphilis. He refers to its influence over nodes and nocturnal pains. He says, Hahnemann's pathogenesis in the *Fragmenta*, mentions such pains as caused by it in the cranium, clavicle and thighs, and several of the later provers report the same experience : in homœopathic practice we use it with much confidence in these affections, and in simple or rheumatic periostitis. " Whether it acts on the bones themselves, I hesitate to say." But he says there is on record a case in which it seemed to check the necrosis of jaw produced by phosphorus.

The Homœopathic method, he says, has added another valuable application of *Mezereum*—to cutaneous affections. The plant is a violent acrid, and irritates the skin when externally applied, and the throat, stomach and intestines when swallowed. He tells of intolerable itching over the whole body caused by the internal use of the drug ; and of the reputation of *Mez.* as " about the best medicine for shingles ; and not only for the eruption, but also for the consecutive neuralgia ". He also quotes Dunham : These symptoms suggest at once the applicability of *Mezereum* to crusta lactea, to various forms of pure impetigo ; and to some of those mercurial or mercurio-syphilitic ulcers on the lower extremities which are often so difficult to cure. I have frequently had occasion to witness the prompt curative action of *Mezereum* in these affections, in which I have generally used the 200th potency. This has proved efficacious in cases in which the lower dilutions have been inert. The characteristics of the *Mezereum* skin diseases are well defined in the above symptoms, viz. itching occurring in the evening in bed, aggravated and turned to burning by touch or by scratching ; sensitiveness to touch ; ulcers with an areola, sensitive and easily bleeding, painful at night ; the pus tends to form an adherent scab, under which a quantity of pus collects." Hughes also quotes Pareira, " The urinary organs are sometimes affected by it, an irritation similar to that of *Cantharides* being set up."

NASH gives, Pain in long bones, especially tibia. (*Dros.* and *Lach.*, *Asaf.*, etc. ED.)

Facial neuralgia or toothache, when pains are greatly worse by eating or motions of jaw : better by radiate heat.

Nose : vesicular eruption, with excoriations, formation of thick scabs, worse at night : Zona.

He says, " I once cured a very obstinate case of facial neuralgia with it : worse by eating : only relief was to hold face as near as he could to a hot stove : no other heat applied wet or dry, relieved. (This is interesting, because *Mez.* is, in "skins" anyway, markedly worse from heat of fire. ED.)

* * *

GUERNSEY, *Keynotes*, says :—Often useful in cases of very violent neuralgic pains about teeth or face, especially if pain be in left bone, running towards the ear. Also neuralgic pains at night in teeth : teeth left side. Shin bone.

Mouth waters.

Urine with red flakes which float on top of urine.

Subsultus tendinum. When fingers are put on wrist or on other parts of body, the tendons are felt to jump and jerk.

Burning ; darting in muscles, like fire darting through them.

* * *

Let us seek final enlightenment and emphasis from KENT, that graphic painter of symptomatology.

Eruptive complaints : eruptions and ulcerations.

The outer surfaces of the body are in a constant state of irritation : nervous feelings, biting, tingling, itching, changing from place to place on scratching. The part becomes cold after scratching.

As soon as he gets warm in bed, or into a warm room, itching begins.

Kent, of course, gives the thick, tough, leathery crusts ; with fluctuation beneath the crusts, where pressure causes the oozing of thick white pus . . . vermin often found among the crusts. Acrid pus, eats away the hair. . . . Cases with a history of suppressed eczema or syphilis. Eruptions, red cicatrices about face and eyes : fissures in corners of eyes.

Ear trouble from suppressed eruptions. . . . atrophic catarrh : degeneration of mucous membranes, ear, nose, throat. Has all the catarrhal states, the ulcerations and patches of copper-coloured eruptions found in syphilis.

It tends to manifest the sufferings of the body in the skin ; it throws the physical evils to the surface. The *Mezereum* patient is in fairly good health when the eruptions are out. When suppressed, catarrhal affections, nervous disorders, strange mental symptoms, constipation, rheumatism, joint-symptoms appear ; he becomes a mental wreck.

Religious or financial melancholy : melancholy in regard to his business : indifference to everybody and everything. . . . Insanity with melancholy, sadness, *and a history of eruptions that have called for Mezereum.* . . .

Sensation of goneness, fear, apprehension, faintness in stomach, as if something would happen. Every shock, pain, bad news, when the door bell rings, when he expects the postman, or a friend, or when introduced to someone, he experiences a thrill beginning in stomach : he is " frightened in the stomach ". (*Calc., Kali carb., Phos.,* and *Mez.*) Kent says also, "These *solar plexus* individuals have often a deep cracked tongue and are hard to cure."

MORBILLINUM

(*The Virus of Measles*)

WHAT we are trying to say here is merely tentative. But one has a feeling that the least one can do is to throw out suggestions, trusting that they may, if fertile, germinate in even unforseen quarters and bear fruit to the common good. This has happened e'er now, when one has joyfully discovered that it is not only " curses and chickens that come home to roost ". But—the seed must be good, and the soil on which it falls, propitious, or— " nothing doing ! "

In the past one has foolishly despised MEASLES ; scarcely troubling to record its occurrence in the patient's Past History : for has not nearly everyone had measles ? But now, at long last, *Morbillinum*, with like remedies of " childish diseases ", begins to loom up very big through the mists, in the treatment of Chronic Diseases. So much so, indeed, that one sets one's teeth and determines that, please God, one will not have any more Old Chronics. Sounds fantastic ?—extravagant ? We shall see !

Homœopathy has been taunted before now with its very moderate or non-success in the treatment of certain baffling diseases : and the fact that they are equally baffling everywhere else is no excuse. And now, it is just here that one is glimpsing a faint dawning of day, even in regard to the most terrible and baffling of them all. Hence this pointing finger, trembling with hope.

Let us emphasize once more the fact, that Hahnemann would have none of Old Chronics. When first he realized the stop-spot, in some cases, of the simple remedies of the present complex symptom-picture, he had to know WHY. And when he at length discovered (as he claimed and as would appear) the NATURE of Chronic Disease and its only possible treatment, he was so far ahead of his time as to provoke bitter animosity and scorn among outsiders, and neglect, because of the impossibility, in those days, of proving his contentions, among his own followers. Hence his greatest work (unfinished, as we are beginning to sense it) has been tacitly set aside and neglected.

To start with, let us try, once again, to enunciate and elucidate his later, all-important teachings : carrying them forward (as he *must* have done had he lived on) on his own lines.

And we will venture to reduce his dicta into terms of to-day. Anyone who desires to verify and explore farther is referred to

No. 12 of our *Correspondence Course,* published by the B.H.A. ; or, better still, to Hahnemann's own *Chronic Diseases, Vol. I.*

" *All chronic diseases* originate and are based upon fixed chronic infections, which enable their parasitical ramifications to spread through the human organism, and to grow without end."

" Certain diseases, such as small-pox, measles, true scarlet fever, the venereal diseases, the itch of workers in wool, canine rabies, whooping cough, etc., are caused by a peculiar contagium of tolerably fixed character. These are so fixed in their course as to be always recognized. They can be named, and we can endeavour to lay down some fixed method of treatment suitable, as a rule, for each of them."

In all these diseases, he tells us, " infection is instantaneous ".

And in all these, after infection, there is an incubation period of varying duration, before the disease comes to the surface with fever, and eruption or cutaneous manifestation capable of communicating the disease.

He asks, " Is there any parasitic disease in the world which, when it has infected from without, does not first make the organism sick, before its external signs manifest themselves ?—we can only answer, No : there is none."

" We find that all infectious diseases which form local affections on the skin, are *internal* diseases, the last result of which is the local cutaneous affection."

Some of the above mentioned acute infections are, for him, chronic diseases—syphilis, gonorrhœa, and psora (under which term he masses all non-venereal chronic diseases—epilepsy, asthma, melancholia and insanity, marasmus, diabetes, consumption, cancer, and a long list of inveterate conditions of viscera and special organs of sense. One observes that chronic diseases, for him, persist in varying forms and intensity so long as life lasts, *unless* cured by remedies homœopathic to the original disease. Whereas the others, seemingly acute merely, after running their course of about two or three weeks, end in a crisis by means of which the fever, together with the eruption, are annihilated in the system, and the patient either dies of these diseases, or else recovers. " They have the peculiar nature of becoming extinct in the body."

He reiterates, " The chronic infections are semi-vital infections of a parasitical nature, which can only be neutralized and antidoted by a more powerful remedy producing analogous effects."

He shows that everything, alike in the acute and chronic diseases, follows precisely the same course, the only difference being in their outcome : and it is only here that we, with later experience, part company with him, in order to travel a stage further in his wake.

Because we now know certain facts: that some of the apparently acute diseases may not be " annihilated ", but, only partially overcome: may become latent; modifying healthy reactions against sickness and injury, which thenceforward are *not* normally recovered from. For instance, a man, during his occupation, experiences frequent or constant pressure on bone. If he suffers from some latent, once acute, now chronic infection, such as syphilis, he develops a syphilitic necrosis. Another, in apparently perfect health, experiences a compound fracture ; the bone refuses to unite and the wound to heal. Pus is examined, and the organism of typhoid is found ; he having had enteric thirty or forty years previously.* A knock on the breast, or the pressure of a pipe stem, instead of being easily and speedily dealt with by the healthy organism, indurates, proliferates, results in a carcinoma. Why ? Probably, because of some latent chronic condition, once an acute disease, never wholly recovered from, which, as Hahnemann expresses it, "ultimates" there; and, not only prevents normal healing, but possibly, by supplying irritation, may determine an abnormal flow of blood to the part, and encourage irregular proliferation which entails pressure, and leads to atrophy of adjacent parts—the whole spelling malignancy. This theory suggests itself ; and is perhaps more plausible than most of the much-sought causes of cancer : where the only fact universally agreed upon is that cancer generally has trauma as a localizing agent. But—think ! that which healthy nature hastens most successfully to deal with, is trauma. " Healthy "—i.e. not subject to some once acute, now latent, chronic disease.

We have too long neglected the instructions and deductions of Hahnemann in this matter of chronic disease ; thus throwing away a very large portion of our heritage from that inspired Teacher and Healer. . . . " Inspired ? " . . . there are people who recoil from the word. And yet, it is noteworthy that, again and again, it is the scientists who claim inspiration for Hahnemann. How else, they demand, *could* he have enunciated, so unerringly, much of that which modern science is, bit by bit, elucidating ?

Inspiration ?—has wireless, then, nothing to teach us about inspiration—if only by analogy ? One remembers how, in childhood, it used to be so puzzling —the *Word* came to this one or that, who accepted, sometimes most unwillingly, the message ; constrained to pass it on, that those who had ears might hear. May

* *Op. cit., p.* 371.

it not be that the Word is always broadcast ?—and yet only clear to those—prophets—poets—musicians—scientists—who are *Receivers* ? This has again and again been apprehended; and yet generally missed.

Browning, for instance :—

> " *God has a few of us whom He whispers in the ear ;*
> *The rest may reason and welcome : 'tis we musicians know.*"

Kipling, again, in his marvellous *Explorer* :—

> " *Till a voice as bad as Conscience, rang interminable changes*
> *On one everlasting Whisper day and night repeated—so ;*
> ' *Something hidden. Go and find it. Go and look behind the Ranges*
> *Something lost behind the Ranges. Lost and* waiting for you.
> Go ! '

> . . . .

> " *God took care to hide that country till He judged His people ready,*
> *Then He chose me for his Whisper, and I've found it, and it's*
> *yours !*

> " *Yes, your ' Never-never country '—yes, your ' edge of cultivation '*
> *And ' no sense in going further '—till I crossed the range to see.*
> *God forgive me ! No, I didn't. It's God's present to our nation,*
> *Anybody might have found it, but—His Whisper came to Me ! "*

Rhodesia, probably ? :—but the same thing has happened again and again through the centuries, as we were reminded the other day in the *Evening Standard*, by Stephen Williams, in regard to " the beggar who found a new world ", *Christopher Columbus.*

" ' *Man is an instrument that must work until it breaks in the hands of providence, which uses it for its own purposes. As long as the body is able, the Spirit must be willing.*'

" These were the words of a humble and devout navigator, son of a Genoese wool-carder, who sailed into the setting sun on a voyage that was to change the map of the world and revolutionize the science of geography."

But does anyone ever discover anything without some other worker, unknown to him, hitting on the same thing ? Even in astronomy this has been so : rival synchronous claims everywhere ! You and I are deaf to the messages that fill the ether. In our ignorance we may say, " There is no sound—nothing ! "—*because we hear nothing.* Yet, bring a receiver, tuned to that we desire to hear, and lo ! the music of all the world is ours for the hearing.

And for those of us who desire with all our hearts and souls to heal, the heavens, at times, have seemed to open, and new light in regard to this or that remedial agent to flood in, never till now recognized and appreciated. As when, some sixty years ago, an American doctor, *Swan*, pioneer in the use of disease products for the cure of like disease, received the inspiration, and prepared from among many such substances, potentized *measles*, with which he did some astonishing work. (See HOMŒOPATHY, Vol. I, pp. 50, 461.)

And now, after all these years of dullness and neglect, we are receiving fresh impetus, and are already getting sudden astonishing results (some of which we hope to publish later on in detail—it is too soon as yet), but, already, in heart disease, in epilepsy (cases terrible and long treated with but a modicum of success) in rheumatoid cases ; even in one case of urgent, hopeless, inoperable carcinoma . . . It is not yet ready to be talked about :— but it *is* so suggestive, that we dare not refrain from passing the Whisper on.

Later, we may be in a position to dogmatize in regard to potency and dosage. Hitherto our tentative, yet effective method has been :—either the 200*th* potency, three doses on three successive mornings, or else (following Hahnemann's newer method, set forth in the sixth edition of the *Organon*, in order to hasten amelioration) in three doses of daily raised potency such as 12*th*, 30th, 200*th* or 30*th*, 200*th* and 1*m*. This we are doing not only with *Morbillinum*, but with many other nosodes. As a matter of fact, we have for years been making play with *Variolinum*, *Tuberculinum*, *Lueticum*, *Medorrhinum*, *Influenzinum :* only, as said, *Morbillinum* and several others have, till now, not entered into the picture, and *Morbillinum* threatens to become the most important of the lot. " Everybody has had measles ", and not everybody has managed to " annihilate the disease " so that nothing latent, and threatening, has remained. In future we shall do well to take notice when told of an old acute sickness, never, or very tardily recovered from. . . . ." Never well since diphtheria—scarlet fever—vaccination." " She lost one of her ears through measles." Tonsillitis, followed by chorea, then rheumatism :—heart damaged in childhood by rheumatic fever " these last put in a strong plea for that mighty remedy, *Streptococcin*.

Well, we have just attempted to pass on the Whisper, so that those with ears may hear, and those who catch on may pursue the matter to the advantage of humanity.

By the way, a word of warning. These disease-elements, used for healing of the like disease, are *homœopathic* remedies, and here also the Laws of Hahnemann obtain, if they are to do their best work, without possibility of danger or damage :—i.e., they must be prepared after the homœopathic manner ; must be potentized ; must be given by the mouth : in single dose, or single "divided" dose ; with due regard for possible initial aggravation, followed by ameliorative reaction—which must not be interfered with.

* * *

Yesterday two Out-patients appeared opportunely to emphasize the above last words. For each, the prescription had been *Streptococcin*, and the report was, " No better : worse ! " " In what way ? " " I've been having pains again in my fingers." " But how are you, yourself ? " " Oh, *I'm* better ! My heart " (in the one case) " my stomach " (in the other) " is *much* better." It is as well to ask, *in what way are you worse ?* because here the Homœopathic Philosophy comes in. " *Parts worse, yet patient better* " ; or again, the *direction of cure,* " *from within, out* ", demand always that we keep our hands off, and give the patient a chance.

MURIATIC ACID

Muriatic acid is not a remedy that one has often had to use except at times for anal conditions : therefore, to picture it, one must quote extensively, trying to bring out its peculiar features, which are quite distinctive and make appeal for this powerful remedy, when called for, even in alarming and threatening diseases, or phases of disease.

FARRINGTON has a most illuminating chapter on the ACIDS. He distinguishes between the mineral and the organic acids. The mineral acids, as a class, all produce an irritability of fibre together with weakness and prostration . . . whereas the vegetable acids produce weakness without irritability. . . . All the acids, too, produce a peculiar debility . . . a debility that arises from defective nutrition, particularly from blood disease. Thus we find them called for in very low types of disease, disease in which blood poisoning is a prominent feature, in typhoid states and in scarlatina, particularly when of a low type. . . .

CLARKE says : " Teste, who did much to define the powers of *Mur. ac.*, groups it with *Agnus cast.*, and *Hyosc.* ; he considers its action corresponds perfectly to a typical case of typhus." . . . " Like *Nit. ac.*, *Mur. ac.*, is a powerful antidote to *Merc.*, and it meets conditions caused by Mercury, and also similar conditions otherwise arising. Like other disinfectants, it causes as well as remedies rapid decomposition of tissues, and dynamically cures low putrid conditions met with in disease. . . . *Mur. ac.* not only corresponds to low febrile states, it also meets many of their sequelae. Deafness, otitis and glandular swellings about the ears often require *Mur. ac.* . . ."

HUGHES writes of *Muriatic acid :* " Its sphere of action may be said to be a low febrile condition of the blood with ulceration of mucous membranes and eczema of neighbouring cutaneous surfaces. . . . it is certain that *Muriatic acid* in doses too small to exert any chemical action, has a very high reputation in homœopathic practice as a remedy for low fever."

GUERNSEY : " Typhus or low grades of fever. Cannot bear sight or thought of meat. Urine too copious day and night ; it escapes when passing wind. Cannot urinate without bowels moving. Hæmorrhoids very tender. He slips to foot of bed, and must be often lifted."

FARRINGTON : " *Muriatic acid* is a very easy drug to study. This acid when abused produces two series of symptoms for study. We find its mental and nervous disturbances under two stages or classes. Patient is irritable, peevish ; senses all too acute. Light hurts his eyes ; distant noises cause buzzing or roaring in ears, aggravating headache ; smell and taste abnormally acute. . . . Sleepy but unable to sleep ; or tosses dreamy and restless all through the night. Irritability that comes under the head of irritable weakness.

" The next stage, of exhaustion : anxious about something real or imaginary. Brain feels torn or bruised. He becomes unconscious with muttering delirium, sighs and groans. Tongue grows more dry, seems actually shrunken, narrow and pointed : so dry that when he talks it rattles like a piece of leather in the mouth. And later is paralysed ; so that he can hardly move it at all. The characteristic pulse intermits at every third beat. Diarrhœa watery with prolapse of rectum. Stools involuntary when straining to urinate. Slides down in bed ; has actually not sufficient strength to keep head on pillow. Threatened paralysis of brain, indicated by vacant, staring eyes, dropping of lower jaw, coldness of extremities, which, if not checked, is followed by death. These are the symptoms that call for *Muriatic acid*, particularly in typhoid fever."

Black Letter Symptoms

Diarrhœa with protrusion of blue or dark purple hæmorrhoids, especially when occurring in feeble children suffering from gastric atony, muscular debility and threatened marasmus.

Hæmorrhoids swollen, blue ; painful to touch; appear suddenly in children ; protruding, reddish blue, burning, too sore to bear the least touch, even sheet is uncomfortable.

Slow emission of urine ; bladder weak ; must wait a long time ; has to press so that anus protrudes.

Leucorrhœa with backache ; sore anus from piles or fissures.

Great debility ; as soon as he sits down his eyes close ; lower jaw hangs ; slides down in bed.

Typhus. Constant restlessness or stupid sleep ; unconscious ; loud moaning or confused talking ; wishes to uncover ; lower jaw dropped ; aphthous ulcers in mouth, fetid, sour smelling ; tongue coated at edges, shrunken, dry like leather, paralysed. Thin, offensive smelling evacuations ; involuntary stools while passing urine ; rapid, weak, rattling respiration ; sliding down in bed ; urine dark, but clear ; bleeding from anus ; hæmorrhage of dark, liquid blood ; mouth full of dark bluish ulcers ; pulse omits every third beat ; legs flexed, feet drawn up, skin hot and dry. Typhoid fever also.

Scarlatina ; redness intense and rapidly spreading ; eruptions, scanty interspersed with petechiae ; skin purplish.

One of the greatest remedies of very bad cases of typhoid, diphtheria, scarlet fever, etc.

HAHNEMANN'S BLACK LETTER SYMPTOMS

Whirling in the open air and unsteady in walking.

Jerking, beating, tearing pain from the left half of the occiput to the forehead ; soon followed by a similar pain in the right half.

Heavy feeling in occiput, with drawing stitches there, more on the right side, close to the nape, with swelling of a gland in the nape, which is painful when touched ; at the same time heaviness and vertigo in the head, with dimness of the eyes, as when intoxicated.

Twitching pinching deep in left ear, which after frequent recurrence became cramp-like almost like earache.

Feeling of emptiness in the region of the stomach, especially in the œsophagus, which does not go off by eating, together with rumbling in the bowels.

Violent pinching from the umbilical region towards both sides, with grumbling.

Frequent urging to urinate with discharge of much urine.

In the right side of the chest a drawing sensation which commenced below the nipple, extended towards the throat, became weaker and then went off.

Cutting blows in the middle of the inside of the sternum, along with obtuse pressure at the back of the thoracic cavity, general oppression thereof, and impeded respiration, all day, occasionally.

When sitting, an aching pain in the middle of the back, and from prolonged stooping, which went off when standing or walking.

When sitting, an aching pain on the left side of the back, as from prolonged stooping, which did not go off by touching, walking, or standing.

When sitting and writing, in the muscles of the right upper arm a drawing and tearing, which went off on moving and extending the arm.

In the right elbow joint a drawing tensive pain, frequently.

In the left palm a voluptuous itching, which compels scratching.

In the right palm a voluptuous shooting tickling, which compels scratching, but is not immediately removed thereby.

When writing a spasmodic pain like cramp, on the ball of the right thumb, which went off on moving it.

When sitting a stitch-like pain, combined with aching and drawing in the muscles of the left thigh, close to the groin . . . which went off on standing or walking. . . .

Staggering when walking, from weakness of the thighs.

Persistent itching pricking in the dorsum of the left foot when moving, but worst when at rest.

When sitting her eyes closed from exhaustion, but if she stood up and moved about she immediately became lively.

Frequent waking from sleep.

Febrile shivering over the body, rigor with yawning and stretching of the limbs, but without thirst and without heat thereafter.

Sad disposition without assignable cause.

Hahnemann also gives some mental symptoms.

Laconic, silent and sullen.

Pusillanimous, desponding and cross about everything.

And the reaction, curative. Very tranquil, calm and free from care.

NATRUM MURIATICUM

(*Sodium Chloride : Common Salt, potentized*)

Natrum mur. is one of the drugs introduced and proved by
Hahnemann and five of his provers : reproved by the Austrian
provers, and by others : the provings being mostly made from the
1st to the 30th (centesimal) potencies.

HAHNEMANN says in regard to SALT . . . "If it be true
that substances which are capable of curing diseases are, on the
other hand, capable of producing similar diseases in .the healthy
organism, it is difficult to comprehend how all nations, even
savages and barbarians, should have used salt in large quantities
without experiencing any deleterious effects from that mineral
. . . Considering that salt, when ordinarily used, has no
pernicious effect upon the organism, we ought not to expect any
curative influence from that substance. *Nevertheless salt contains
the most marvellous curative powers in a latent state.*

"The transmutation, by means of the peculiar mode of preparation adopted in homœopathy, of a substance like salt, which
is apparently inert in its crude state, into a heroic medicine, the
use of which requires the greatest discrimination, is one of the
most convincing proofs, even to the most prejudiced, of the fact
that the peculiar processes of trituration and succussion resorted
to in homœopathy, bring to light a new world of powers which
Nature keeps latent in crude substances. These processes operate,
so to say, a new creation."

But in a footnote he alludes to the fact that even apparently
innocent substances, including salt, when taken to excess, may
become hurtful.

BURNETT, in one of his brilliant little monographs, takes
"*NATRUM MURIATICUM as test of the doctrine of Drug
Dynamization.*" He points out that many doctors accept Hahnemann's Law only, but regard potentization as irrational and
unscientific. But, he says, "our beliefs have nothing to do with
truth : . . . disbelieving a thing does not disprove it : . . .
in the same way that the presence of nothing but atheists in the
world would not do away with the Supreme Being." . . .
Again, "Drugs, as has been affirmed by many able practitioners,
by Hahnemann himself, and as daily and hourly re-affirmed by
men of sound science, DO act differently and better when dynamized. In fact many affirm, as did Hahnemann, that the doctrine"

(of potentization) " is of transcendental importance ; since many serious diseases can only be cured with dynamized drugs, being entirely incurable with the same drug in substantial doses, and therefore altogether incurable, unless with a highly potentized remedy."

Burnett, "had had no great respect for *Natrum mur.* as a remedy and had very seldom used it ; because how can any sensible man believe that the common condiment, which we ingest almost at every meal, can possibly be of any curative value : especially as some are known to eat salt in considerable quantities every day without any *apparent* deleterious effect . . ." While " to believe in salt as a remedy is almost synonymous with believing in the doctrine of drug dynamization, and a belief in this doctrine is extremely repulsive to one's common sense. Perhaps the proper spirit would be gratitude to a beneficent Creator", adds Burnett.

Burnett's " conversion " was thus. He had a patient with very obstinate neuralgia, on which he had exhausted all the neuralgic drugs, as set down for that disease. Being " at the end of his tether ", he sent her to the seaside, and—she came back worse ! The neuralgia had been *far worse at the sea.* He jumped at the idea that it might have been the salty air that had made her worse, and prescribed *Natrum mur.* 6—and cured her promptly. *Worse at the seaside* was thereafter one of his great indications for *Nat. mur.* But this also converted him as regards Hahnemann's claims for Potentization ; this and other cases : for had not this patient been eating salt, inhaling salt, with not only no cure, but with, on the contrary, aggravation of symptoms, and lo ! potentized salt immediately cured her. Burnett was no fool : with him, Prejudice bowed before Facts. In that little book—*Natrum muriaticum, the test of drug dynamization*, he gives a number of brilliant cures by potentized salt.

His idea was that, in the same way that an infant gets ample lime salts in its food, yet fails to assimilate enough for its needs till it gets the stimulus of potentized *Calcarea* ; so the hunger of *Natrum mur.* for salt is a very real hunger ; the patient is not assimilating enough to satisfy his tissue needs, till he gets the stimulus of the potentized drug.

In regard to this veritable transmutation of *Sodium chloride* from a common aliment into a powerful remedial agent by potentization, one remembers that the late Dr. Molson used to tell how he got the Coastguard at Brighton " because they had nothing to do " to go on triturating *Natrum mur.*, to produce higher and higher potencies. Instead of the usual three triturations which reduce a substance to one in a million, and by which the most intractable substances, becoming soluble in water and alcohol, are easily run up into the higher potencies, he found that by such repeated trituration his *Natrum mur.* became so intensely — almost explosively—active, that at last he was positively afraid to administer it.

Dr. Burnett, when first experimenting with *Nat. mur.* used to take frequent pinches of the potentized drug, to see what it could do. *Inter alia* it opened a crack in the middle of his lower lip !—a thing he had never had before, and never had again after discontinuing his pinches. It was his habit to thus crudely prove remedies that interested him, on himself.

Different persons realize, or visualize the self-same drug in different ways, according to their experiences of its different powers and uses. It is therefore wise to study drugs as described by different writers ; and for that reason we try to give the " cream of a whole library " in regard to any drug we are trying to picture. One finds one point emphasized by one exponent, one by another.

Burnett's *Natrum mur.* was a very chilly patient, with especial coldness of knees : coldness of legs, knees to feet. This chilliness over and over again disappeared after taking *Natrum mur.*

Worse at the seaside.

Deep crack centre of lower lip.

Unconquerable sleepiness after dinner in the evening.

Muddy urine, or urine very pale and limpid. He found that *Nat. mur.* would clear the urine ; or, in curing other troubles, would, in eliminating, cause the urine to become thick and cloudy.

Lachrymation with headache. Great lachrymation very characteristic.

MALARIA ; and ailments since malaria and quinine. With *Nat. mur.*, he cured fever and ague in a sailor, uncured by the salt provisions of those days, and by sea air. It needed the potentized drug to put him right.

I believe that it is to Dr. Compton Burnett that we owe this all-important use of *Natrum muriaticum* in malaria and quinine poisoning, even of years ago. It is one of the precious little tips that save the situation again and again for us.

Natrum mur. has "fiery zigzags" before headache (*Sep.*, etc.).

Emaciation, especially about the clavicles and upper parts of the body. (*Lyc.*)

Face shines greasily.

Nat. mur. has very marked periodicity. In malaria, the chill starts at 10 a.m. ; or 9—10 ; or 10—11 a.m., and the drug has other very definite hours for chill, headache, neuralgia, etc.

A Burnett tip which one has verified,—cases of apparent phthisis in patients who have had malaria and quinine, may clear up astonishingly on *Nat. mur.*

Mentally *Nat. mur.* is IRRITABLE :—hates fuss and consolation :—weeps :—weeps more, or flies into a passion if consoled.

Nat. mur. tries to remember old disagreeables—old insults—for the purpose of brooding over them and being miserable.

The *Lyc.* mentality gives way on the intellectual side, that of *Nat. mur.* on the emotional and sentimental side.   Kent says *Nat. mur.* is the chronic of *Ignatia*, and where the latter is too superficial, cures. " Falls in love with the wrong person, and breaks her heart.   Is absurdly obsessed by a foolish passion for a married man—falls in love with the coachman, and *Natrum mur.* brings order and sanity."

A little symptom-complex that means *Natrum mur.*, and *Natrum mur.* only is :

Hates sympathy, fuss and company.

Craves salt.

Loathes fat.

(Without the salt-craving it might be *Sepia*.)

But the late DR. BLUNT, a very keen and successful homœopathic prescriber, once wrote me :

" *Nat. mur.* is the last remedy I would part with.   I have more *Nat. mur.* cases than any two other drugs put together.   When I get < heat and cold, > in open air, then I ask early, ' How does wind affect you ? '   ' Eyes water.'   ' You say you weep ? from what ? '   *Nat. mur.* will answer ' from admonition and pity '. Is worse consolation.   These people hide their tears for fear of pity and consolation.   If asked, how are you ?   *Nat. mur.* will answer, ' Better thank you ', when he is *not*.   ' *Lachrymation with laughter* ' is pure gold.   As for ' Fond of salt ;   aversion to fats ; greasy skin ;   crack lower lip.'—I have found the remedy in *Nat. mur.* when all these are absent."

GUERNSEY, *Keynotes*, gives the fever symptoms of *Natrum mur.* thus: " The most characteristic and reliable symptoms are : intermittent fever with the mentioned sores (herpes) on the lips, the approach of fever being heralded by excessive thirst before the chill and during the chill, no thirst during the fever ;   during the fever, or at its close, the above hammering headache begins (*headache as though a thousand little hammers were knocking upon the brain*), which lasts for a long time after the fever and perspiration have passed away.   The attack comes on in the forepart of the day : after it passes off, the patient wishes to retain a recumbent position, does not ' feel able ' to get up, or go about anything.   Pulse intermitting, or irregular.   Chilliness with thirst."

So one sees how different prescribers find their leading symptoms differently ; and one can only learn from *all*.

One remembers an early out-patient case of severe asthma, unable ever to lie down in bed. Patient " worked out " to *Nat. mur.*, which was given, and rapidly cured. Then, on further enquiries it turned out that he had been in the habit of eating large quantities of salt. One wonders, was he poisoned thereby, and did the potentized remedy antidote, as so often it does, the crude drug ? or, was it a case of inability to assimilate salt, and therefore of salt famine ; and did the potentized drug stimulate him to take what he needed from his food ?

" *Dirty, unhealthy skin* " . . .

One remembers a malarial sailor, during the War, with a dreadful condition of the face, from blackheads and boils and abscesses, who cleared up astonishingly on *Natrum mur.*, and went out re-humanized.

. The following recent case shows the value of *Natrum mur.* even in epilepsy, the great indication being its curative power *in diseases that supervene on malaria and quinine.*

Middle-aged man, strong T.B. history : many vaccinations, the last unsuccessful : injections for enteric—plague :—many years in India, where he had dengue and malaria, and months of 30 grains of *Quinine.* Came for severe and frequent epileptic attacks ; bites tongue. *Thuja* did not help much : but, with *Nat. mur.*, the attacks lessened, and it is now a year and a half since he had an attack, while he has regained his old energy and power for full work.

Natrum mur. is one of the few remedies that has " mapped tongue ", "geographical tongue". Here it shares the honours with *Tarax.*, *Ranunc. sc.*, and one or two others.

And now we will dig for a few gems from KENT :

Natrum mur. is a remedy of many hysterical conditions. Weeping and laughing : rage with cursing and blaspheming. The remedy of unrequited affections, and the inability to control affections : knows they are unwise, but cannot help it. Of awful headaches, with no relief to the head till after sweat : or, on the other hand, headache, and the greater the pain, the greater the sweat, which does *not* relieve.

Nat. mur. is a deep-acting, long-lasting remedy. Kent says " it takes wonderful hold of the economy, making changes that are lasting." Like *Sepia*, it bears very seldom repetition in chronic cases. Kent says "it operates slowly, bringing about its results after a long time, as it corresponds to complaints that are slow and are long in action. This does not mean that it will not act rapidly :

all remedies act rapidly, but not all act slowly ; the longest-acting may act in acute disease, but the shortest acting cannot in chronic disease."

Black Letter Symptoms

i.e. those most often caused and cured by *Natrum muriaticum*.

Very much inclined to weep and be excited.
Depression. Hurriedness with anxiety and fluttering at heart.
Sad and weeping mood without cause. Involuntary weeping.
Sad and weeping : consolation aggravates.
Melancholy mood, preferred to be alone.
The more he was consoled, the more he was affected.
Hypochondriacal, tired of life.
Trifles provoke anger.
Indifferent.
Distraction : disinclined for mental work.

Head dull, heavy.
Pressing pain, as if head would burst.
When coughing, as if forehead would burst.

Redness of whites of eyes with lachrymation.
Eyes give out in reading ; writing.
Pressure in eyes, when looking intently.
Unsteadiness of vision. Letters and stitches run together.
Ophthalmia, after abuse of nitrate of silver.
Spasmodic closure of lids.

Upper lip swollen.
Great swelling lower lip followed by a large vesicle.
Crack in middle of lower lip.

Blisters on tongue.
Bitter taste in mouth.
Loss of taste : food has no taste.
Tongue coated, with insular patches.
Tongue heavy, difficult speech. Children slow in learning to talk. (One remembers one such very tardy child who started to talk the next day after a dose of *Nat. mur.*)

Very violent thirst. Unquenchable thirst.

Great longing for bitter things, beer ; for farinaceous food ; for sour things ; for salt, oysters, fish, milk.
Aversion to meat, bread, coffee.
Acid eructations and malaise after eating.

Chronic diarrhœa, watery: with fever, dry mouth: worse as soon as he moves about, and after farinaceous food. With much flatus. Sensation of contraction in rectum during stool: hard fæces evacuated with greatest exertion, so that anus is torn, bleeds, and is sore.

Constipation. Obstinate retention of stool. Seat worms.

An unusually hard, dry, crumbly stool.

Increased desire to urinate, with very light watery urine.

Involuntary escape of urine while walking, coughing, sneezing.

Intermittent heart beat.

Heart's pulsations shake the body.

Emaciation: great emaciation.

Easily fatigued.

Great weakness and relaxation of all physical and mental powers from exertion or after long talking.

Paralysis from intermittents, nervous exhaustion, sexual excesses, from diphtheria, from anger or emotions; from pain: of flexors.

Dreams: anxious: vivid: frightful. Of robbers in house, will not believe the contrary till search is made.

Eruptions especially margin of hair at nape of neck.

Herpes about mouth, arms and thighs.

White scales on scalp: dandruff.

Nettlerash; large red blotches with violent itching.

Tetter, bends of joints, oozing of an acrid fluid: crusts with deep cracks. Scaly eruptions on flexor surfaces.

Fever with headache: much heat in face: great thirst, drinks much and often; with nausea and vomiting: stitches in head: unconsciousness; blindness, blurred sight; faintishness; aversion to uncover; without chill, 10 to 11 a.m.

Or chill predominates, with thirst, yawning, severe headache . . . bursting headache; nausea and vomiting; tearing pains in bones; chattering of teeth; internal, as from want of animal warmth. . . .

*   *   *

A remedy of *periodicity* . . .

7 a.m. regularly, neuralgia of ophthalmic branch of trigeminus.

9 to 10 a.m. chill.

11 a.m. hard chill, lasting till 1 p.m.

Every morning wakes with headache. . . .

Every morning at 8 till 11 a.m. muscles of back and extremities stretched, while wrists and joints of feet are flexed.

After midnight, sweat.

Morning till noon, sick-headache : diarrhœa < chill.

From 1 to 3 p.m. quotidian.

2 a.m. wakened by heavy chill.

4 a.m. fever sets in.

5.30 p.m. chill begins and lasts an hour.

Daily, at regular time, lachrymation.

Attacks of sick headache, lasting 24 hours.

Neuralgia right eye, coming and going off with the sun.

Headache from sunrise to sunset, < at midday.

Every other day from 10 a.m. to 3 p.m. headache : tooth-ache ; every other day, constipation.

And so on : great periodicity : (*Ars.*—Clock-like periodicity, *Cedron.*)

Queer symptoms.

Cold wind blowing through head.

Throbbing in head as from little hammers. Bursting.

As if stepping on air.

Dazzling before eyes.

Fiery zigzags. Eyeballs as if too large.

Plug in throat.

Has to swallow over a lump.

Lungs too tight.

Feet filled with lead.

Back as if beaten : broken.

Water trickling into joints.

Terrible pain in head. Violent pain.

Numbness one side of nose ; of lips ; of tongue ; of arms and hands ; of fingers and toes.

Fluttering of heart.

Emptiness in head : in epigastrium.

Cold sensation : vertex : in stomach : about heart : in back.

*   *   *

By the way, a word of warning ! *Nat. mur.* may be needed to cure the most terrible headaches, but do not give it during a severe attack, at risk of a fearful aggravation. Give its " acute ", *Bryonia*, for the immediate pain, and to palliate ; and the curative drug later on, when the attack is over.

NATRUM PHOSPHORICUM

WE have been asked to paint a Drug-picture of *Natrum phos.*, and, as usual, have gone the round of writers on homœopathic Materia Medica, only to discover how little seems to have been written about it. Why?

For us, it happens to be one of the Twelve Tissue Remedies that has assumed a distinct individuality ;—which is not by any means the case with all of them.

This was the way of it. . . . On a well-remembered evening—late in the day—one was told that one of the house-maids had a "bad knee". In those days of early, keen enthusiasm, when the testing of power was more of a novelty and therefore eagerly grasped at, one hurried to the top of the house to find a joint, hot, swollen, very painful—acutely inflamed. One also happened to be interested in the Schuessler remedies—so simple —so delightful—only twelve of them !—to be applied ultra-scientifically for all the ills that flesh is heir to :—until, presently, the inevitable snag shot up, when it seemed, on attempting to assimilate his teachings, that quite a number of them would be probably needed for almost any case. Anyway, this girl got *Natrum phos.*—his great remedy for rheumatism and—*worms*.

It worked absolutely to schedule : for next morning the knee trouble had subsided, *and the patient had passed two round worms !*

That is the sort of case, you will allow, that impresses one's consciousness ineradicably. It has probably appeared already in the pages of HOMŒOPATHY ; it deserves to have done so, but its real place is here.

It was a happy introduction to *Natrum phos.*—thereafter no mere name, but a trusted friend, to be used again and again in rheumatic troubles, especially in children. One notes that an all-important claim is made for it as a remedy for that dangerous metastasis when pains quit joints or limbs for the heart . . . expressed in the provings thus :

" Pains base of heart, relieving pains in limbs and great toe.

" Heart feels uneasy and pains, when pains in limbs and great toe are better." One wonders how large a percentage of " heart disease " have some such origin ?

Natrum phos., as will be observed through all the records of its provings, is SOUR—ACID. As, for instance, " acid, exceedingly sour smelling sweats . . . acid taste . . . acid condition of stomach, with nausea and vomiting of acid fluids, sour eructations . . . vomiting of fluid as sour as vinegar . . . over-secretion of lactic acid . . . ulceration of stomach with sour risings . . . green, sour-smelling stools . . . leucorrhœa and discharges from uterus, sour-smelling, acid . . . eczema with symptoms of acidity."

What about that modern bogey, " acidosis ", supposed to need very careful dieting :—which does not commend itself to one's ideas of commonsense in growing children. There would be no possible danger, and much good to be anticipated from a few doses of *Natrum phos.* in potency.

Black Letter Symptoms

Thin, moist coating on tongue.

Soft palate has yellowish, creamy look.

Sour eructations, sour vomiting, greenish diarrhœa ; pains, spasms and fever with acid symptoms.

Gastric derangements with symptoms of acidity.

Yellow, creamy coating of back part of roof of mouth.

Italic, or important diagnostic symptoms.

☛—Intense pressure and heat on top of head, as if it would open.

Severe pain, head, as if skull too full ; frontal or occipital; with nausea and sour, slimy vomiting. Ejection of sour froth.

Squinting caused by intestinal irritation from worms.

Children grind teeth in sleep.

Tongue coated dirty white, with dark brown centre.

Heartburn and acidity : waterbrash.

Vomiting of acid fluids and curdled masses (not food).

Vomiting of fluid, sour as vinegar ; over-secretion of lactic acid.

Stomach ache when worms are present, accompanied by acid risings.

Ulceration of stomach : pain in one spot after food. Face red and blotched, yet not feverish.

Sclerosis of liver and hepatic form of diabetes, especially where there is a succession of boils.

Colic in children with symptoms of acidity, green sour-smelling stools, vomiting of curdled milk.

Diarrhœa from excess of acidity ; stools sour-smelling, green.

Itching, sore and raw anus.

Itching at anus from worms, especially at night when warm in bed.

Intestinal long, or thread worms, with picking at nose, occasional squinting, pain in bowels, restless sleep.

Polyuria. Diabetes.

Incontinence of urine in children, with acidity of stomach.

Feels as if a lump or a bubble started from heart and was forced through arteries.

Pains base of heart, relieving pains in limbs and great toe.

Heart feels uneasy and pains, when pains in limbs and great toe are better.

Pain lower third of sternum, as if torn in two.

Goitre (in thirteen cases) ; the feeling of pressure was relieved in three to five days ; in some cases a cure was affected.

Rheumatic pains . . . contractions : stiffness on rising. . . .
Synovial crepitation.

Crampy pains in hands when writing.

Worse thunderstorm : trembling and palpitation, and pains worse.

Diseases of infants suffering from excess of lactic acid, resulting from over-feeding of milk and sugar.

Ailments with excess of acidity.

Swelling of lymphatic glands before hardening.

Rheumatic arthritis.

Skin affections, with acidity. . . .

What about that modern bogey, " acidosis " ?

* * *

This is what Schuessler has to say about this great " tissue salt ", *Natrum phosphoricum*. (N.B.—It must be remembered that Schuessler was a homœopathic physician, whose ambition was to limit the number of remedies, and to make homœopathy easy by his " bio-chemical " studies.)

He says, this salt is found in blood, muscle, nerve and brain-cells, as well as in the intercellular fluids . . . useful in podagra, gout, as well as in the acute and chronic articular rheumatism, being thus a remedy for the so-called acid diathesis. ... . It is the remedy for conditions arising from excess of lactic acid. It prevents the inspissation of the bile and mucus with crystallization of cholesterin in the gall duct, and will thus remove the cause of many cases of jaundice, hepatic colic, bilious headache and imperfect assimilation of fats from lack of bile. Schuessler gives a lengthy paragraph on the rôle of this salt, in the course of which he says, the liver is the prime and master laboratory of the animal body. . . .

According to him, the great key-note for this remedy is the *moist, creamy, or golden-yellow coating at the back part of the tongue, also at the back part of the roof of mouth.* Blisters and sensation of hairs on tip of tongue.

Sour eructations, sour vomiting, greenish diarrhœa. He suggests " Possibly it is the remedy for diabetes, for, as is well known, sugar is changed into lactic acid. This, by the presence of *Nat. phos.*, is converted into carbonic acid and water ; while this salt thus lessens the quantity of lactic acid in the system, it furnishes room for a further supply of it from the sugar, and in this way reduces the amount of sugar to the normal degree.

Among the symptoms, as given by Schuessler : Mental ; imagines, on waking at night, that pieces of furniture are persons, that he hears footsteps in next room.

(In our copy of Schuessler, we have recorded in the margin, a suggestion from our lecturer as students, " *Exophthalmic goitre* ", but symptoms do not seem to warrant this.)

Vomiting of sour fluids, or of a dark substance like coffee grounds, sour risings, loss of appetite.

It has many urinary symptoms. Diabetes. Constant urging ; flow intermits, requires straining, and so on. We have given the most salient symptoms above.

Evidently *Nat. phos.* should be useful in the alarming metastasis where pains in extremities improve, while the heart suffers. This reminds one of one's old rhyme on *Benzoic acid* :

" Better when urine's thick and plus ;
When scant and clear his pains are wuss !
And when his limbs and joints find ease,
He takes a turn at heart-disease. . . ."

Schuessler suggests, as usual, the 6*x* or the 12*x* potencies ; but we are told the higher and highest potencies have also been employed with success. We have used 30's and 200's.

CLARKE (*Dictionary*) gives the experience of one of the provers, who developed " itching of ankles with an eczematous eruption ; fear, especially at night, that something would happen. Headache ; nausea ; some defect of vision, with one pupil dilated." Two years later he had a patient with visual disturbance and headache, with a sense of fear worse at night, and eruption about ankles : *Nat. phos.* cured promptly. This reminds one of what Hahnemann said in regard to provers :

" By making his own person the subject of experiments the physician will derive many invaluable advantages. . . . A self-prover knows with certainty what he has felt, and every experiment of the kind upon himself stimulates him to explore the powers of numerous other drugs. In this manner he will grow more and more expert in the art of observing, so indispensable to the physician, as long as he continues to make himself the infallible and undeceptive subject of his observations." And he shows (from his own experience) how the organism of the prover is " strengthened to repel injurious agencies from without, by means of these moderate experiments with drugs ".

And he lays it down that " Morbid disturbances called forth by drugs in the healthy are the only possible revelation of their inherent curative power."

Is it not true that one recognizes instantly that from which one has suffered !

NATRUM SULPHURICUM

Natrum sulphuricum, sodium sulphate, was discovered by Glauber in 1658, named by him *Sal mirabile*, and is commonly called "Glauber's salt". It occurs in many mineral springs, as Karlsbad, Marienbad, etc., and is used by old school as a laxative or purgative.

But Homœopathy has raised its status and established its great utility (*inter alia*) in pneumonia and asthma ; it is here that we, personally, have seen its great work ; but of course only in such cases as exhibit its peculiar characteristics, brought out by provings. We will speak of these later. With Grauvogel, that once great prescriber, it was his remedy *par excellence* of the " hydrogenoid " constitution, whose ailments arose from a chilly, damp environment. While Schuessler has laboriously explained the rôle it plays in the economy of life, where " by disturbance in the motion of its molecules, the elimination of superfluous water from the intercellular spaces takes place too slowly, and there arises *hydræmia*. . . . The state of health of persons suffering from hydræmia", he says, " is always worse in humid weather, near water, in damp, moist underground dwellings, and improved by contrary conditions ". So here keen observation, theory, organic chemistry, and the results of the provings absolutely agree, as will be seen later on.

Natrum sulph. is one of the remedies of marked PERIODICITY.

In chest troubles—pneumonia—asthma—even phthisis, there is the characteristic early morning aggravation—4 *to* 5 *a.m.* This has again and again drawn attention to the remedy and caused it to be studied with happy results.

Besides its 4 to 5 bad hour in pneumonia and asthma, *Nat.sul.* has a colic at 2 a.m., or 2 to 3 a.m. and a diarrhoea which comes on regularly in the morning, *after rising*, and returns quite regularly each day. There is excessive discharge of flatus with the stools. (N.B. *Sulph.* hurries the patient out of bed : the diarrhoea of *Nat. sulph.* occurs after rising.)

Then again, in regard to its periodicity, it is one of the remedies that has "*Worse every Spring*" (*Lach.*, *Rhus*, etc.),

It is notable as being one of the black-type remedies in that small group, " *Worse warm, wet weather* " (*Lach.*, *Carbo veg.*, and a few others ; among them, curiously enough, *Sil.* ; which is such a chilly remedy, and yet cannot stand warm, wet weather.

Then, in chests, it picks out especially *the base of the left lung*. A pneumonia of lower left lung, with a morning aggravation at 4 to 5 a.m. (rise of temperature, etc.) puts in a strong appeal for *Natrum sulph*. We have published some cases showing how rapidly and brilliantly it acts in these patients. For remember, it is no use whatever to say, " I find *Phos., Bry., Nat. sulph.*, or what not, simply wonderful in pneumonia ! " They are all *equally wonderful*, but each in his own case ; and they are all *equally failures* and " useless medicines " where not indicated by symptoms. The " splendid " the " wonderful " of the routinist depends on lucky hits, where the symptoms in patient and drug happened to match ; and his shrug " I've tried it—it's useless ! " where they did not happen to match. All the same, a very great number of pneumonias in their symptomatology correspond to *Bryonia*, and a great number of cured cases, therefore, are laid down to the account of that drug ; fewer to *Natrum sulph*. whose distinctions are less common.

And, as said, its distresses and ailments are apt to start from *damp cold*. *Nat. sul*. cannot stand wet weather, damp dwellings, living near water—even by the sea ; every change to damp weather. " Great dyspnœa with desire to take a deep breath during damp, cloudy weather."

It is one of the remedies for violent attacks of asthma : the sputum is apt to be greenish and copious, and always worse in damp, rainy weather.

We will extract from DR. KENT, who gives the most arresting and practical hints as to the choice and employment of this truly *Sal mirabile*.

He says : " It so disturbs the mind, as to fill it with direful impulses ; impulses to self-destruction, hatred and revenge . . . and disturbs the memory." (All these things come out in its provings and can be used to guide us to its uses.) He notes " a struggle between the desire to die, and the desire to live. The patient has to struggle with himself and with the impulse to destroy himself. Wants to die, and yet does not want to die, which means sleepless nights and fighting days. . . .

" The smallest noises drive her wild : even music. Worse from gentle music, mellow lights (*Aurum* ; but *Aurum* only *desires* to commit suicide, and has no desire to live)." Kent says that " Hahnemann always taught that the mental symptoms, in drug and patient, are the most important. And with the above, the morning aggravation, and the amelioration from cool air are most important. . . ."

" Eye troubles, with catarrhal discharges green and thick. Similar discharges from the nose, and from the posterior nares. Green discharges everywhere ; green leucorrhœa (*Thuja*). . . .

"Stomach troubles, with regurgitation of food (*Phos.*). 'Food always welling up.' Bitter taste; distension, weight, almost constant nausea. Patients who are always bilious, with disturbed livers. . . .

"Useful in cerebro-spinal meningitis (*Cic.*). Violent pains down neck and spine with opisthotonos. Must lie on the side; lying on the back impossible, in such cases: . . .

"Skin symptoms: (a great remedy for 'Barber's Itch'). And for warts. A gonorrhœal remedy, with *Thuja*; and it has many symptoms in common with *Thuja*."

Nat. sulph. with us is classical for after-effects of injuries to the head, concussion: headache, loss of memory, twitchings, even epileptiform convulsions. Kent says, "*Arnica* for the neuralgias, but *Nat. sul.* for the mental symptoms following a blow on the head." As he puts it, "A patient comes into the office, suddenly stops, breaks into a sweat, looks confused, embarrassed, comes to herself in a second and says, 'Doctor I have always had such spells since I got a blow on the head.' She must have *Nat. sulph.*" He says it has cured petit mal.

"*Nat. sulph.* pains are worse when quiet like *Rhus*, but worse from motion like *Bry.* Restless."

Asthmatic conditions in children of sycotic parents. Kent says "Asthma is sometimes a sycotic disease, when cured in such cases it has been by sycotic remedies." *Nat. sulph.* has also the *Thuja* warts about anus and genitalia.

* * *

Nat. sulph. cannot digest starchy foods, and milk and potatoes disagree (*Alum.*).

CLARKE draws attention to a peculiar symptom, "salivation with headache"; and he quotes several cases of asthma cured by *Nat. sulph.*, among them one that brings out its characteristics, "Violent, spasmodic asthma; greenish, purulent sputa; a *loose evacuation after rising the last two days.*" And among the symptoms of the provings we find (Hering): "Short breath with piercing pain left chest. Great dyspnœa, desire to take a deep breath during damp, cloudy weather. Violent attack of asthma; greenish, purulent expectoration; loose evacuation immediately on rising. Asthmatic attacks for years: expectoration greenish and remarkably copious." And so on.

But *Nat. sulph.* is also a remedy for chronic rheumatoid arthritis. Its arthritic conditions are always due to, or worse from damp and cold. They compel motion, but the relief from change of position does not last long.

Natrum sulph. has malarial symptoms ; alternate creeps and fever. Ague with bilious vomiting, brought on, or always made worse by damp weather, or moist atmosphere at the seaside. Greenish-yellow vomit, or brown or black.

* * *

NASH'S LEADERS for *Natrum sulph.* are : " Diarrhœa, acute or chronic ; < in a.m. and on beginning to move (*Bry.*) with much flatulence (*Aloe* and *Calc. phos.*) and rumbling in abdomen, especially right ileo-caecal region.

" Loose cough, with great *pain* in chest ; < lower left chest.

" Worse in cold, wet weather ; damp cellars " ; hydrogenoid (diarrhœa, rheumatism, asthma).

" Mental effects from injuries to head.

" Chronic effects of blows, falls . . ."

He says : " This aggravation in damp weather is not confined to diarrhœa in *Nat. sulph.*, but is especially present in cases of chronic asthma. I have seen very great benefit in such cases of this very troublesome and obstinate disease, and, as aggravation in damp weather very commonly occurs in cases of old asthma, this remedy is often indicated.

" *Loose cough, with soreness and pain through the left chest is very characteristic.* This is one of the chief diagnostic points of difference between *Bry.* and *Nat. sulph.*, that while with both there is great soreness of chest with the cough, with *Bry.* the cough is dry, while with *Nat. sulph.* it is loose. The patient springs right up in bed, the cough hurts him so."

He points out that " both spring up in bed with cough and hold the painful side . . ." and he says that he has " several times seen remarkably prompt relief and cure follow the administration of *Nat. sulph.* in pneumonia, when this symptom was present. . . . This pain running through the lower left chest is as characteristic for *Nat. sulph.*, as that of the pain running through right lower chest for *Kali carb.*"

* * *

In regard to the diarrhœa (from cold damp) of *Nat. sulph.* BOGER in his *Synoptic Key* gives in capitals, " RUMBLING, GURGLING IN BOWELS, THEN SUDDEN GUSHING, NOISY, SPLUTTERING STOOL ; *after rising, in a.m.*" and says *Nat. sulph.* is complementary to *Ars.* and *Thuja*. And, by the way, Kent, speaking of *Nat.sulph.* for asthmatic conditions in children, at puberty, etc., emphasizes that " sometimes the wheezing, the frequency of the attack, and the prostration would lead to *Ars.*, but *Ars.* will only palliate, and the case will come back more frequently for palliation ;

whereas the curative remedy will postpone the attacks until they are ultimately cured."

Observe that in the Repertory Glauber's *Sal mirabile* (*Nat. sulph.*) is one of the small group of remedies especially indicated for the *asthma of children*, viz. *Acon.*, CHAM., IPEC., *Mosch.*, NAT. SULPH., PULS., SAMB., with a few more in lowest type. Curious that Old School should know practically nothing of *Nat. sulph.*, save as a purgative !

NATRUM SULPH. would seem to need further provings in the potencies. But we will subjoin italicized symptoms from Allen and Hering.

— *Depressed. Irritable. Worse mornings : hates to speak or be spoken to.*

Satiety of life : must use all self-control to prevent shooting himself.

Pressure in forehead, worse p.e. ; as if forehead would burst. Better pressure of hand : *quiet : lying ; worse thinking.*

Hot feeling on top of HEAD.

Brain feels loose when stooping ; falls towards left " temple ".

Jerk in head : throwing it towards right side.

— *Violent pains in head, especially base of brain and back of neck: after injuries to head.*

— *Chronic effects from injuries to head ; simple concussions, and injuries without organic affections.*

— EYES, *large blisterlike granulations, with burning tears.*

Crawling in eyes.

Chronic conjunctivitis with granular lids, green pus, terrible photophobia. Lids heavy as if leaden.

Stuffing of NOSE, *with dryness and burning. Nose bleed before menses, after menses. Catarrhal discharge, green-yellow ; green.*

Dirty, greenish grey, or greenish brown coating on root of TONGUE. *Tongue burns as if covered with blisters. Tip burns.*

Blisters on tongue and palate. Palate so sensitive, could hardly eat. *Anything cold taken into mouth relieved it.*

Thirst for something very cold : desire for ice, or ice-cold water.

— *Disgust for bread, of which she was fond.*

— *Diarrhœa from vegetables, fruit, pastry, cold food and drinks and farinaceous food.*

Vomiting of bile ; of sour, then bitter fluid. Acidity.

Tension and sticking pains LIVER *region when walking.*

When taking a deep breath, a sharp, violent stitch right ABDOMEN, *as if in liver, as if it would burst open there : worse sitting. Unchanged by pressure, at* 4 *p.m.*

Great sensitiveness in liver ; very painful when touched.

Tearing pain round umbilicus, with flatulence.

Collection of flatus in abdomen, with pain, without evacuation of it. Grumbling and rolling around in whole abdomen, with sudden pinches ; then diarrhoea.

Loud grumbling in abdomen, with emission of very fetid flatus.

Flatulent colic : flatus passed with difficulty ; caused belly-ache, and bruised pain in small of back. Wakes her at 2 a.m.

Cannot bear tight clothing about waist.

Liver : swollen and tender. Engorged, worst lying on left side.

Bilious colic. Excruciating pains. Vomiting of bile. Bitter taste. Jaundice from vexation.

Diarrhoea in wet weather : in a.m. : after farinaceous food : in cold, evening air : from vegetables, pastry, cold food or drink. Alternating with constipation. Comes on regularly every morning and returns quite regularly each day.

Chronic DIARRHŒA. Tuberculosis abdominalis.

URINE burns, is less in quantity. Polyuria, esp. if diabetic.

Short breath, with piercing pain in l. side of CHEST.

Great dyspnoea, desire to take a deep breath during damp, cloudy weather.

Pressure on chest, as of a heavy load. Oppression in chest.

Stitches l. chest when sitting, yawning, during inspiration, running up from abdomen into l. chest.

Excruciating pain in rt. HIP joint, worse stooping and from some motions. When stretching or walking feels nothing. Most felt when rising from a seat, or moving in bed.

Plenty of pain in limbs, hand, fingers.

Panaritium, pain more bearable out of doors.

After striking head, FITS driving him to destruction, never knew when they were coming on : epileptiform. Very irritable ; wanted to die. Constant pain in head : photophobia.

TIME : Violent colic at 2 a.m. 2 to 3 a.m. flatulent colic. 4 to 5 a.m. asthma. 9 a.m. diarrhoea.

MALAŔIAL SYMPTOMS : alternate creeps and fever.

HYDROGENOID CONSTITUTION : feels every change from dry to wet ; cannot tolerate sea-air, or eat plants that thrive near water. Feels best on a dry day.

NITRIC ACID

HAHNEMANN points out that this medicine is more beneficial to individuals with a rigid fibre (brunette), than to those with a lax fibre (blonde). And, indeed, it is one of the drugs that, suggested by the appearance of the patient—brown eyed—makes one at once consider *Nitric acid* as a possible remedy : of course, *symptoms must agree*, but they so often do.

In out-patient work, where one has to " get along ", the symptom-complex, *desire for fat, desire for salt, chilliness, indifference*, puts you on to *Nit. a.* in Materia Medica ; to find, more often than not, that the rest of the symptoms fit the patient, and that you have got the curative remedy. In the desire for fat and salt, *Sulphur* only, in the Repertory, competes with *Nitric acid*, but in lower type. The Repertory gives us very few fat-cravers, *Nit. a.* being the one in black type : they are usefully memorized, viz. (Ars.), (Hep.), NIT. A., Nux and Sulph. But, among these, *Ars., Hep.* and *Nux* have not the salt craving : while the mentality of *Nitric a.*, as it seems to us, is more that of *Sepia* : but *Sepia* loathes fat, and does not crave salt. Here is the little *Nit. a.* symptom-complex which helps one to the drug, in rapid work : one cannot miss it !—

Nit. a., besides its craving for fat and salt, in its full development, is—

Chilly.
Depressed.
Indifferent.
Intolerant of sympathy.
Sensitive to noise—pain—touch—jar.
Irritable : suspicious : obstinate : restless.
Fears death.
Worse : wind ; thunder ; wet.
Has profuse sweat of hands and feet.

Some years ago, after one of our post-graduate lectures, a doctor from " the other end of nowhere " asked help of the lecturer in regard to a child-patient of his, with inveterate constipation. She was found to have the *Nitric acid* cravings for salt and fat, and the lecturer proceeded to read out to the astonished doctor, from Allen's *Keynotes*, the *Nitric acid* symptoms. " But—*do you know the child ?* " Of course he did not : but he knew *Nitric acid* ; and these symptoms suggesting the drug, the rest fell into line. That is how one gets through an overcrowded out-patient afternoon : a little symptom-complex suggests a drug, and you look it up, and are happy to find that you are " there ".

Hahnemann tells us that *Nitric acid* is more useful for persons who suffer from diarrhœa (*Puls.*) ; but Clarke says that it is one of the remedies that has been most useful to him for constipation. Clarke was always insistent about this :—that while positive symptoms are all-important, negative symptoms are less so. For instance, the fact that a person cannot kneel without faintness, or giddiness, or whatever it may be, suggests *Sepia*—the only drug that appears in the Repertory as " worse kneeling ". But the fact that she can kneel without suffering in such ways does not contra-indicate *Sepia*. You will find that symptom in very few *Sepia* cases : though I think you will find it under no other remedy. (By the way, this " worse kneeling " means *the patient* : not his inflamed and swollen knees. That would be a common symptom in arthritis and not helpful in the choice of the remedy.)

Another almost unmistakable feature of the *Nitric acid* sufferings, is the character of its pains :—not only *sticking*, but SPLINTER-LIKE. Wherever the pains occur, in bone, in mouth, in nose, in anus, the sensation is " a SPLINTER " : especially when the sore part is touched or pressed. Clarke, in his *Dictionary of Materia Medica*, has a brilliant little article on *Nitric acid*, introducing its provings. Here he points out, in regard to the *sticking pain as from splinters*—" This is a grand keynote of *Nitric acid*, and will serve to indicate it wherever it is found. It requires a touch or movement to elicit it. When it occurs in the throat it requires the act of swallowing to set it up ; in the anus, the passage of the stool ; in ulcers, the touch of a dressing. It may occur in any part of the body : in in-growing toenails." (*Magnetis Polus Australis*.)

Then, the localities affected by *Nitric acid*, to torture or to cure, are very striking and definite. It selects *orifices* : situations where mucous membranes are merging into skin—endothelium into epithelium. The eyes, the nose, and (especially) the mouth, with lips, tongue, gums, tonsils, extending down the throat. Then, passing by the digestive tract without much malice, it vents its spleen on the rectum and anus, the urethra and the genitalia, with, always, *ulceration, fissures, stitching, splinter-pains, bleedings* and *offensiveness*. As Guernsey says, " This remedy so closely resembles *Mercury* in many points, that it is often very difficult to distinguish between the two." And therefore, since we prescribe on symptoms, and since the antidote to any drug or to any disease is always the drug of most-like symptoms, *Nitric acid* is found to be the most useful remedy to counter poisonings and sicknesses from abuse of *Mercury*. And again, since the symptoms of *Mercury* and syphilis are almost indistinguishable, *Nit. a.* comes in also, as will be seen, for the treatment of that disease.

Nit. a. again, is like *Merc.* in *offensiveness*. It has offensive mouth and saliva : offensive sweat in axillæ and feet : offensive moisture about anus : offensive, strong-smelling urine (urine that smells like that of the horse is characteristic) : with (a peculiar symptom) " it feels cold as it passes ". Here the only other remedy is *Agar*, in lowest type.

Another painful symptom heads straight for *Nit. a.* :—not only painful stool, but *pain for hours after stool*. The anus suffers frightfully with *Nit. a.* There are not only hæmorrhoids— painful hæmorrhoids, but fissures, which gape and bleed and are exquisitely painful. To have to examine the rectum of a *Nit. a.* patient is a terror to doctor as well as to the victim. One remembers, years ago, being asked to go across Great Ormond Street to see a lady who was in agony with pain in anus, and who had applied to the Hospital to send one of its homœopathic doctors. The remedy was *Nit. a.*, which she got, with speedy relief, and on enquiry next day one heard that she was all right.

And here we will quote NASH. He says :—

" No remedy has a more decided action upon the anus, and one very characteristic symptom is, ' great pain after the passage of stool, even soft stool '. He walks the floor in agony of pain for an hour or two after a stool (*Ratanhia*). In dysentery this symptom distinguishes this remedy from *Nux vom.* which is relieved after stool and *Merc.* which has tenesmus *all the time*, or before, during and after stool."

Nitric acid helps in all Hahnemann's " Chronic Diseases ",— syphilis, gonorrhœa (sycosis) and that other one which he terms " psora ", as well as in *Mercury* poisonings and overdosings. In syphilis one has seen its magnificent work in acute and chronic cases. One was very interested in a patient who recently reappeared after some twenty years' absence from hospital. She had originally come for leucoplakia, which had been cured by *Nitric acid* in homœopathic dosage. She is now eighty, healthy-looking and robust : doctors sitting by guessed her age as sixty !— and, tell it not in Gath ! her " Wassermann " is still positive ! One recalls Hahnemann's contention that syphilis, untreated by the methods of the schools, is not such a deadly disease : and this woman, young looking and vigorous, complaining only of something trivial (one has failed at the moment to remember her name or discover her notes) has had no treatment all these years ! . . .

well, for the sake of our worried Old School brethren, we will put it at this, " The exception proves the rule."

Clarke says that *Nit. a.* is also an antidote to overdosing with *Potassium iodide* : and he says that Burnett cured brilliantly a case of actino mycosis, with *Nitric acid*, which, since it had been going the round of the schools, would doubtless have been much dosed with that drug.

For sycosis (? gonorrhœa) Hahnemann suggests that two remedies will be found useful—*Thuja* and *Nitric acid* : given according to symptoms, and each allowed to complete its work before—the symptoms changing—the other is made to follow. In this way only Hahnemann alternates. See HOMŒOPATHY, Vol. IV, pp. 202, 203, in regard to *Rhus* and *Bryonia* in war typhus.

Another use, to which Clarke alludes, for *Nitric acid*, is in lung troubles—pneumonia and phthisis. Inhaled, among all the acids it is the only one that produces a very rapid and fatal inflammation of the lungs—Clarke gives a case :—and in the provings quite a number of its symptoms suggest phthisis. Hence, wherever the key symptoms are those of *Nit. a.*, that drug should be considered in pneumonia and phthisis. One remembers a case, years ago, in dispensary days, where *Nit. a.* did surprisingly good work for a consumptive patient. But, somehow, it is not one of the drugs one readily remembers for lungs, acute or chronic : though Kent has it in italics for " inflammation of lungs ".

I do not know why, but one gets a sort of affection for *Nitric acid*. It is so dramatic and has such definite and intense characteristics and actions. One hopes that this little picture may help others to a closer acquaintance with " a very strong personality " among our drugs.

BLACK LETTER SYMPTOMS

Depressed and very anxious in the evening.

Anxiety, as if engaged in a lawsuit or quarrel exciting uneasiness. Anxiety about his disease, with fear of death. Morbid fear of cholera.

Anxious about his illness : constantly thinks about past troubles.

Mind weak and wandering.

Hopeless despair.

Nervous, excitable, especially after abuse of Mercury.

Vexed at least trifle.

No disposition to work, to perform any serious business.

Great weakness of memory.

After continued loss of sleep, long-lasting anxiety—over-exertion of mind or body from nursing the sick [Compare *Cocc.*]—*great anguish of mind from loss of dearest friend.*

VERTIGO *on rising in the morning : had to sit down.*
Heaviness, obtusion, fullness in HEAD. *Head as if surrounded with a tight bandage.*
Sensation, " head in a vice from ear to ear over vertex ".
Painful tension inside head extending to eyes : with nausea.
Head very sensitive to pressure of hat : < evening, and part lain on. As if contused all over, or in spots. Right side skull painful.
Profuse falling out of hair : especially vertex : from congestion of blood to scalp : from syphilis : nervous headaches, debility, emaciation.

Double vision.
Stitches in EYES *: smarting.*
In morning difficult to open eyes and to raise upper eyelids. [Compare *Sepia, Causticum.*]
Ophthalmia : neonatorium : scrofulous: gonorrhœal: syphilitic : from abuse of Potash and Mercury.
(Curious symptom, eyelashes of right side all point stiffly towards nose.)

Roaring in EARS. *Cracking when chewing.*
(*Deafness : > riding in carriage or train* [Compare *Graph.*] *: with induration tonsils : after abuse of Mercury : syphilitic.*)

Violent itching in NOSE. *Nose bleed.* (*When eating small pieces of food get into posterior nares ; are not got down till swallowed with saliva.*) [Compare *Gels.*]
Nasal catarrh ; acrid, watery at night, yellow, offensive ; corroding : with swelling upper lip. With scarlet fever, diphtheria ; or syphilitic.
(*Ozæna : green casts every a.m. with ulcers ; syphilitic, involving upper lip, which is swollen and honeycombed with ulcers.*)
Ulceration of nostrils, scurfy ; of inner nose with frequent bleedings.

Corners of MOUTH *ulcerated and scabby : with sticking pain.*
Cracking in articulation of jaw when chewing and eating.
Foul, cadaverous smell from mouth.

Ulcers, mouth, with sticking pains as from a splinter : within cheeks : edges of tongue ; deep eating : at first lardaceous, later discoloured, dark, dirty, putrid, destructive : syphilitic.

Mucous membrane gets between teeth, easily bitten : swollen, ulcerated : with pricking pains : especially after abuse of Mercury ; aphthous, covered with white or thin yellow-grey membrane.

Saliva ; profuse ; fetid, acrid, makes lips sore ; bloody.

Swelling of parotid and submaxillary glands with loose teeth and bleeding gums, after abuse of Mercury.

Looseness of teeth when chewing. [Compare *Merc.*]

Putrid smell from mouth.

Small painful pimples on sides of tongue.

THROAT. *A morsel sticks in pharynx when eating, as if pharynx constricted.*

Swallowing very difficult : distorts face and draws head down : cannot swallow even a teaspoonful of fluid : causes violent pain extending to ear.

Tonsils red, swollen, uneven, with small ulcers ; yellow streak ; white patches.

Stinging pains in swollen throat.

Sticking, painful sore throat.

Longing for fat : herring : chalk : lime : earth. (*Calc.*)

Bread disagrees.

Jaundice : pain, region of LIVER *; urine scanty and strong-smelling.*

Awakened at midnight with crampy pains in small intestines : chilly : pain worse if he moved.

Stitches, region of liver.

Abundant flatulence : rumbling in abdomen.

Nausea after a MEAL. *Sweat all over after a meal.*

Eructations before and after a meal.

Constant desire for STOOL *: unsuccessful.*

Colic, sometimes drawing, before stool.

Profuse discharge of blood during stool.

Burning of the varices of ANUS.

Itching of the rectum.

Burning : itching : of the anus. Moisture.

Sticking in rectum and spasmodic contraction in anus, during stool, lasts many hours.

With stool pain, as if something in rectum would be torn asunder.

Diarrhœa : great straining, but little passes : as if stayed in rectum and could not be expelled : with soreness and rawness of anus.

Constipation : painful, hard, difficult irregular stool : stool in hard masses : with every stool protrusion of hæmorrhoids with profuse bleeding : great pain during and after stool, as though there were fissures of anus. Piles bearing down on standing.

Hæmorrhoids : constant pressing out : painful or painless : prolapsing with every stool.

Needle-like stitches in orifice of URETHRA.
Ulcers in urethra : bloody mucous or purulent discharge.

SEXUAL ORGANS *much affected : with small itching vesicles : ulcers exuding an offensive moisture : bleeding when touched : sharp stitches.*

Condylomata : fetid : bleeding when touched : moist : resembling cauliflower : on thin pedicles : oozing : after abuse of Mercury.

Gonorrhœa : discharge yellowish or bloody : bloody mucus :— horrible pain. Condylomata about genitals and anus. [Thuja.]

Itching, swelling and burning.

Hæmoptysis. COUGH : *dry, barking ; tickling in larynx and pit of stomach with complete ptosis of both eyes from coughing.*

Chronic dry, laryngeal, with stinging smarting, as if small ulcers were in larynx, generally felt on one side.

Sputum seems to stick like glue : greenish-white casts as if from air cells : expectoration by day of dark blood mixed with coagula ; or yellow, acrid pus of offensive odour. Pain low down in lungs as if something were tearing away. . . .

HEART, *fourth beat intermits : alternate hard, rapid, and small beats.*

Want of breath, palpitation of heart and anguish when going upstairs. Sudden want of breath and palpitation when walking slowly. Panting breathing.

Stitches in and between scapulæ.
Neuralgic pains up back, especially left side.
Herpes between fingers.
Paronychia (applied in its incipiency).
Drawing all limbs, stretching being very agreeable.
Stitches in all parts of the body : drawing pains in all parts of body, suddenly appearing and disappearing.
Tearing in bones of lower extremities, especially at night.
Syphilitic nodes upon shin bones, with severe nightly pains.

o WEAK : *almost constantly obliged to lie down. Loss of breath and speech.*

Weakness : trembling : shocks on going to sleep. Depressed. Great debility, heaviness and trembling of limbs : < in a.m.

PERSPIRATION, *in the morning.*
Night sweats every other night ; or every night.
Profuse perspiration on the soles, causes soreness of toes and balls of feet, with sticking pain as if walking on pins.

Drowsiness by day.
Wakes at 2 o'clock every night and is unable to fall asleep again.

Among *queer sensations* are :—
Skull constricted by a tape, etc. (*Sulph.*).
Pain as from splinters in eruptions.
As of a splinter in nose.
Teeth as if elongated : would fall out : as if soft and spongy.
As if a splinter in ulcers in mouth.
As if food would not go down.
As if abdomen would burst : " a boiler working in bowels ".
As of a dry, hot cloth on abdomen.
As if stool stayed in rectum.
Splinters in rectum. Sharp sticks pressed into anus : jagging in ulcers of scrotum.
As if a splinter or piece of glass in finger (*Sil.*).
As if dogs gnawing flesh and bones.
Sharp splinter stuck in big toe.
Splinters running through carbuncles.

Hæmorrhages: bright, profuse; dark: from bowels : after miscarriage: post-partum: from over-exertion of body: uterine:— epistaxis : hæmoptysis : from rhagades.
Syphilitic *bone pains.*
Inflammatory swelling of inguinal or axillary *glands,* especially after abuse of *Mercury* or in syphilitic subjects.
Discharges thin, offensive and excoriating : if purulent, dirty yellow-green.
Diseases depending upon the presence of syphilitic, scrofulous, mercurial or gonorrhœal poison. Broken-down constitutions.
Warts, sticking and pricking : on upper lip smarts and bleeds on washing. Soft and moist. Large, jagged, often pedunculated : exuding moisture and bleeding readily. Syphilitic condylomata, elevated, exuberant, cauliflower-like.

20

NUX MOSCHATA
(*Nutmeg*)

OF nutmeg, Kent says : " A little remedy, but, when needed, nothing will take its place."

It so happens that one has come across this remedy several times, in rather dramatic circumstances, and has witnessed its rapid and wonderful action.   Therefore it is a drug one is greatly tempted to write about—probably little known—one of those remedies that will never " work out " unless one takes only its own *peculiar symptoms*—which are entirely distinctive.

A FIRST EXPERIENCE

Many years ago, in a state of greatest anxiety in regard to a patient of 80, with cerebral thrombosis, paralysed and comatose for nine weeks, where the coma had become so deep that it was almost impossible to get a mouthful of anything down, one went off late at night to ask advice of a certain homœopathic doctor in the south of London.

Absolutely the right man to go to ! for he had a curious tale to tell.   He had himself had bouts of indifference and automatic conduct after rather frequent attacks of influenza (and influenza was severe in those days !) in such sort that he would carry his letters about for days unopened ; took interest in nothing, and was pretty useless to his patients, who nevertheless trusted him greatly, and made allowance for his post-influenzal state, and waited for it to lift.   It was *Nux mosch.* that had proved the magic remedy and restored him to usefulness.   He was therefore able to point out its " virtues " and its applicability to the case in point.

And it worked—just a dose of the 200 (so far as one remembers) and all anxiety in regard to the patient was at an end.   She promptly woke up, and thereafter made a marvellous recovery, living on for another five years, in full possession of her faculties. Other remedies (notably *Zinc.* in very high potency) helped later ; but it was *Nux mosch.* that, humanly speaking, saved her life. After such an experience, one never forgets a remedy.

Here is another memory of nutmeg.   .   .   .

Some years ago a girl of 22 came, in a curious state, for help. Eight months previously, for boils, she had eaten a nutmeg ; had ground it up and eaten it on bread and butter.   This interesting experience had already cost them £100 in attempts at treatment, she said.

She described what had happened.

She became sleepy : eyes only half-open.

Felt she was losing consciousness : felt paralysed ; numb.

Took castor oil, and salts.

Repeated attacks of unconsciousness.

They tried to make her sick, and she vomited the castor oil. They thought she was " gone ".

Her heart was affected. Felt she was slipping down to one side.

Was in bed for one month, and never well since. Very nervous.

Now—if tired, feels frightened (? of what ?). Easily gets tired. Has had fear of death.

Dreams—nightmares : aeroplane crashes ; is chased.

Indigestion. Skin oily, all over head, face, back. Greasy.

She gave a number of symptoms, among them : Axillae pour with sweat. She had been vaccinated twice, first took slightly, second did not take.

One was tempted by *Thuja*, and by *Nux mosch*. high. But she got *Thuja* 1m, 10m, 50m on three following mornings.

In three weeks' time, " Distinctly better ; no more nightmares ; giddy attacks less frequent. It (the medicine) has put fresh life into me and I feel capable of doing anything now." And in another month, " I am a different person, and you'd hardly recognize me. . . . Playing tennis daily, and except for a qualm here and there, almost my old self." But some indigestion still for which she got *Nux mosch*. 200 and 1m on two succeeding mornings, and was not heard of again for eleven months.

Kent says, *It is better to do nothing than something wrong*. In this case, a dose or two of *Thuja* would have cured the boils, and she might have saved her £100.

Nux mosch. has been used to promote abortion. Its action is specific here, see symptoms. One remembers one or two such cases, long ago ; in all of them there had been the extreme sleepiness and comatose condition. But the effects have seemed to wear off quickly, in such cases.

CLARKE (*Dictionary*) gives one or two interesting instances of the effects of nutmeg : interesting and important because what nutmeg can cause, that, and that only, it can cure.

A young man ate two nutmegs one morning. In afternoon was exhilarated, able to do more than usual, to argue on any subject. At dinner mouth dry, great thirst, felt could not drink enough to quench it. After dinner head felt strange, as if in a dream ; but he joined a small musical party, as he had intended. *He seemed to be two persons, and his real conscious self seemed to be watching his other self playing*. He could not play well : had to desist : seemed lost, and when spoken to would come to himself with a start. Hearing for distant sounds much more acute than usual. . . A woman who ate two nutmegs with the idea of bringing on abortion had a hallucination that she had *two heads*. Another woman, when consciousness returned kept hands to her head "to prevent it falling off"; was obliged to move her head with her hands, it being " too large and heavy for her body ". Clarke also emphasizes three great keynotes of *Nux mosch.—Drowsiness* : *Chilliness* : and *Dryness*. " *The saliva seems thick, like cotton.*" Another keynote, *Tendency to fainting.* Clairvoyant state : answers questions accurately quite out of her sphere, and on returning to consciousness knows nothing about it.

For dual personality compare, *Bapt., Petrol., Pyrog.*

Black Letter Symptoms

MENTALLY : *Stupor and insensibility : unconquerable sleep.*
Vanishing of thoughts while talking, reading, or writing.
Weakness and loss of memory.
Uses wrong words (during headache).
Surroundings seem changed ; fanciful, dreamy images ; does not recognize the known street. (Opium.)
Inclination to laugh at everything, more in open air.

Sensation as if all vessels were pulsating, especially in HEAD ; *a throbbing, pressing pain, confined to small spots, principally to left supraorbital ridge.*
Severe tearing in occiput, towards nape of neck.

Dryness of EYES : *too dry to close lids.*

TONGUE *paralysed : difficult to move tongue : dry, feels as if gone to sleep or leather covered. At night dry, as if it would fall into powder ; sticks to roof of mouth : great complaint of its dryness ; in reality not very dry.*
Mouth so dry that tongue sticks to roof, yet no thirst (evening).
Greatly troubled with dryness of mouth and throat while sleeping : always wakes with a very dry tongue, but without thirst.

STOMACH : *No thirst, with dry mouth.*
Eating a little too much causes headache.
Vomiting : spasmodic ; during pregnancy ; from irritation of pessaries ; from acid stomach ; flatulence.
Fullness in stomach impeding breathing : during pregnancy.

STOOL : *soft but difficult ; rectum inactive ; slow ; undigested ; with great sleepiness.* . . .

MENSES *irregular in time and quantity : too early and profuse ; too late, preceded by pain in back. Flow generally dark, thick . . . pain in small of back, as if a piece of wood were lying cross-wise and being pressed out, . . . unconquerable drowsiness : mouth dry : hysteric laughter.* . . .
Threatened abortion ; hysterical females disposed to fainting : feel chilly and catch cold easily ; fears she will abort ; continued and obstinate flooding.

Hoarseness from walking against wind.
Difficult inhalation : hysteric asthma.
Dyspnœa with feeling of weight in CHEST.
Stitches in chest : tightness ; spitting of blood.

Pains now in BACK : *now in sacrum : knees very tired : worse during rest. Lumbago.*
Pain in sacrum when riding in a carriage.

HANDS *cold as if frozen : tingling under nails, on entering a warm room.*

NERVES. *Drowsiness : torpor : lethargy.*
Spasms : hysterical in inner parts : chronic hysteric fits : convulsive motions.
Hysteria : exhausted from least effort. . . .

Complaints cause sleepiness : irresistibly drowsy ; sleepy, muddled, as if intoxicated ; coma, lies silent, immovable : eyes closed : strange feeling on waking.

Want of sweat : skin cool and dry.

QUEER SENSATIONS

As if drunk : limbs floating in air ; head feels as large again.
As if brain struck against side of head.
As if all vessels were pulsating.
As if head would burst.
Brain as if loose.
Jaws as if paralysed.
Teeth as if held in a grip : teeth as if loose.

As if tongue would stick to palate.

As if she had eaten herring.

As if a piece of bacon were in throat.

Food forms lumps in stomach.

As if it were full of knots : a lump in abdomen.

As if a piece of wood stretched across small of back were pressing from within outwards.

As if heart would be squeezed off. (*Cact., Lil. tig.*) As if heart stopping. (*Gels., Dig.*)

Chest too narrow : a knife plunged into chest.

As if heart were stopping : blood rushing to heart, thence to head and all over body. Heart grasped. (*Cact., Dig.*)

Grasping sensations, heart, upper arm, knee.

Sensations of a blow from a fist : lumbar muscles, calves. . . .

Parts on which he lies feel sore. (*Arn.*)

As if bone from knee to ankle had been smashed from a blow.

Dryness of eyes, nose, lips, mouth, tongue, throat ; or at least a feeling of dryness.

Limbs as if floating in air.

*   *   *

Among the symptoms of poisonings by nutmeg given in the *Cyclopædia of Drug Pathogenesy* one notices also again and again its effects on the pelvic organs—ovaries and womb much swollen and tender to touch : many of the symptoms went on or recurred for months. The head is described by one after the other, as heavy : " would put hands to head to prevent it from dropping off " : it felt greatly enlarged : " obliged to use her hands to move her head, it being too large and heavy for the body." . . . " Head felt much too large, and drawn back." Everything too large : hands double their size . . . in one case objects grew smaller. Respirations were greatly affected, " the power of breathing was leaving me ". In one case, attempts to separate the hands brought on convulsions . . . " Dared not sleep, lest she should die." . . . " Hand red : covered with red spots, and enlarged. . . ." Floating sensations. " Heart seemed to beat in a vacuum : felt numb and cold : as if it dripped : as if it action were suspended," and so on.

*   *   *

Nux mosch. is " sleepy and COLD "—DROWSY, DRY, but with NO THIRST.

*   *   *

GUERNSEY'S summary of *Nux mosch.* : Drowsiness ; very sleepy ; stupor-like sleep. Complaints causing sleepiness.

Chilliness without thirst : heat without thirst : want of perspiration : no thirst.

Very dry mouth, so dry that tongue may adhere to roof of mouth, but no desire for water, rather an aversion to it. (*Merc.* on the contrary, has tongue very moist, perhaps dripping with saliva, and there is *great thirst*.) Headaches with very dry mouth and no desire for water.

Worse cold, wet weather ; in open air ; in cold air. When weather changes (dry to wet, or vice versa, until it becomes settled). Worse wet weather : windy weather.

* * *

FARRINGTON says: *Nux moschata* exerts a very novel influence upon the mind. The state varies from a bewilderment, in which the surroundings are strange, dreamy, or fanciful, to a condition of absent-mindedness, sleepiness, and finally deep stupor, with loss of motion and sensation. Mental states may alternate. At one time she laughs, as if everything partook of the ludicrous. She jests even about serious subjects. Suddenly her mood changes to sadness, with weeping and loud crying ; or her expression grows stupid, all ideas vanish, and she appears as if overwhelmed with sleep.

There are, likewise, errors of perception ; a momentary unconsciousness she regards as having been of long duration. Her hands look too large. Objects gradually diminish in size as she looks at them steadily.

The bodily functions come under the same influence ; great weakness and bruised feeling in small of back and legs ; knees feel as after a long journey ; prostration ; tendency to faint ; oppressed breathing, rush of blood to the heart, skin cold and dry. So relaxed that pulse and breath are scarcely discernible. Head drops forward, the chin resting on the breast. Head rolls about as if bulky. Bowels enormously distended with wind, as from weak digestion. Even soft stools are evacuated with difficulty.

It is this mental and bodily atony which has led to the excellent cures made with *Nux moschata*, not only in hysterical weakness, but in typhoid and cholera infantum. The hystero-spasmodic symptoms of the drug are intimately co-mingled with the above symptoms ; head jerked forward ; jaws clenched ; heart as if grasped ; sudden oppression of the heart, with choking sensation ; tonic, followed by clonic spasm ; unconsciousness or fainting.

Accompaniments are : Great dryness of mouth and throat, which, with her tendency to magnify, she complains of extremely. The least emotional excitement renews the symptoms, increases the distension of the abdomen, etc. Skin cool and dry, no disposition to sweat. . . .

* * *

KENT has a small article on *Nux mosch.* He says it is not a very great remedy, but is often overlooked when needed. We get into the habit of relying entirely on the polychrests. . . .

The root is much stronger than the nut in the same proportions, and contains the real medicinal qualities.

Dazed : automatic . . . a wonderful state of mind. Goes about performing her duties, but if interrupted forgets what she has done, forgets that she was in conversation with her son. Has no recollection of past events.

Lies with eyes closed : knows what is going on, but remembers nothing. Seems in a dream. Seems not to know her friends.

She is always ready to go to sleep . . . in season and out of season.

Useful, he says, in the coma of typhoid and intermittent fever. Answers slowly after a long interval, then looks confused again. The answer may have no relation to the question asked.

The sleepiness and the dazed state combined are difficult to cover with a medicine : this state is somewhat like *Opium.*

Faintness on long standing, as having a dress fitted.

Dry mouth : sleepiness and automatic conduct : has cured *petit mal.*

Especially suitable for lean women, who have lost flesh ; the breasts are flat. I remember a woman of thirty-five whose breasts once well-rounded, became perfectly flat. *Nux mosch.* restored the breasts.

A little remedy, but when wanted, nothing will take its place.

* * *

We will end with a quotation from *Neatby and Stonham's Manual :*

" As with all other medicines, when given according to the law of similars, *Nux mosch.* will give relief and effect cures in diseases, no matter how named and classified, if the correspondence between drug and disease is sufficiently close."

NUX VOMICA

No household should be without its little homœopathic medicine chest for common ailments, and no homœopathic medicine chest should be without *Nux*. The nursery medicine chest when we were children contained *Nux*, and the nurses were not far wrong when they dubbed it " temper medicine ".

Hahnemann, writing about *Nux*, tells us that there are just a few medicines whose symptoms are so similar to those of the common ailments, that they are very frequently found useful. These he terms the *Polychrests*—drugs of *many uses*.

It is the polycrests that should be at hand for common acute ailments, and pre-eminent among these is "the *Nux vomica* seed ". He says that formerly it was feared to employ it, because it used to be administered in enormously large doses (a whole grain, or several grains).* But that it proves the mildest and most efficacious remedy when administered in the small doses he indicates, where disease-symptoms correspond to those it is capable of producing in healthy human beings.

"From his careful experience of many years" he tells us that *Nux* is more frequently needed by persons of an anxious, zealous, fiery, hot temperament : or of a malicious, wicked, irascible disposition. (But this does not mean, of course, that *Nux* may not come in for any ailment, the symptoms agreeing.)

There seem to be remedies, always, to fit abnormal conditions, and that in the most extraordinary way. *Nux*, as you will see, should be an invaluable remedy in Paraguay, for the times when the natives run amok.

Sir John Weir, in his pamphlet " *Present-Day Attitude* ", quotes a Dr. Lindsay, of Paraguay, in regard to the powerful effect on the nervous system, in those parts, of the North wind. (It will be remembered that *Nux* is one of the few remedies worse in *dry* weather and worse in *windy* weather.)

Dr. Lindsay says,

"This is a dry, hot wind. It dries up everything it comes across. Its effects on animals of all kinds are most extraordinary.

" All domestic animals—horses, cattle, dogs, fowls, suffer in the same way as man does. . . . Everybody's nerves are on

---

* *Present-day official medicine gives the dose of Nux tincture as 5 to 15 m. But their Nux is standardized to 0.25 per cent. of strychnine, whereas ours is the strongest obtainable. From our " Nux φ " potencies are run up.*

edge.   The most trivial incident, a word in jest, misunderstood, may lead to murder.

" An older native, meeting a younger of a slightly better class, saluted him with, *Why, boy, you've got to look almost like a man*, and got a bullet from the boy and fell dead.

" During the north wind the number of woundings and murders is greater than at any other time.   When native dances are allowed during a north wind, we lie listening for the shots or for the footsteps of those running to fetch help for a knifing case.

" Now listen to the provings of *Nux vomica*.

Worse dry wind.

Exaggerated sensitiveness and irritability.

Excessive uneasiness.

Moral exaltation and excitability, with extreme sensitiveness to least pain, to least smell, noise or movement.

Insane desire to kill.

Takes everything amiss ; readily breaks out into scolding and abuse.

He is hasty.   Looks malignantly at anyone who asks him anything, without answering.

It seems as if he would like to strike anyone in the face who speaks a word to him, so irritable and uncontrollable is his disposition.

Every harmless word offends.   Peevish.   Malevolent.   Fiery, excited temperament.   Ill-humour, vexation and anger, breaking out in acts of violence.

Extravagant and frantic actions.

" Here you have some of the strange symptoms of the materia medica exemplified in a most astonishing manner."

The following are among the black type mental symptoms of *Nux* culled from Allen's *Encyclopedia* and from Hahnemann : symptoms repeatedly caused by the drug in provings or poisonings, and repeatedly cured thereby in homœopathic potencies.

Quarrelsome, even to violence.

Extraordinary anxiety.   Sadness.

She cannot get over the smallest evil.

Much disposed to scolding crossness.

Much given to reproach others for their faults.

He feels everything too strongly.

Oversensitive to impressions of the senses.

Cannot bear strong odours and bright light.

Cannot bear any noise or speaking.

Music and singing affect him strongly.

Irresolution.

Cannot endure the slightest ailment.

Very hypochondriac, and affected by the slightest thing, after eating.

Dread of literary work at which one must think and employ the ideas.

Nux affects body and soul, and that always in an extreme manner. Not only mind, head, brain, special senses, but the whole of the digestive system, mouth to anus ; the whole of the respiratory system ; the liver and portal system ; the urinary and genital systems. It affects nerves, muscles, skin, sleep. It is a great fever medicine—symptoms agreeing. No wonder that the homœopaths of what one may call the middle period of Homœopathy, who indulged in low potencies and got their best results in acute disease, made such great use of *Nux*. They had the polychrests at their finger tips.

In the head, *Nux's* black letter symptoms are :

Intoxication.

Drunken confusion in the head.

Dullness of head after dinner, which recurred twenty-four hours afterwards.

In the morning, drunken, giddy heaviness of the head.

Aching pain in the occiput in the morning immediately after rising from bed.

Squeezing headache.

Dullness, headache, felt even before opening the eyes.

Worse moving the eyes.

Morning headache, as if head had been beaten with an axe.

Headache, worse after eating, with nausea and very sour vomiting.

Attacks of vertigo, as if it turned round in the brain, with momentary loss of consciousness.

Drunken confusion of the head.

Here one may note that *Nux* is (as it should be !) a great medicine for drunkards. Even lay homœopaths used to know that. An aunt of ours, seeing the misery of a poor family where the father drank, sent some *Nux* : with the result, a happy family and no drink. And at out-patients in the Hospital, where a poor woman, sometimes, has confessed her trouble—a husband that drank, *Nux* has been sent, and changed everything. There was one, only the other day, where later, the report was—if the man drank still, he had ceased to be so sullen and impossible, for which she was grateful. (*Sulphur*, *Nux's* complimentary remedy, has also a reputation for persons " gifted for drink "—as one poor woman expressed it. One of the residents at Hospital, years ago, used to treat his " drunks ", at Casualty, with *Camphor* in potency.

And Burnett extolled *Spiritus glandium Quercus* (acorn tincture) as helpful for old drunkards who were paying the penalty.)

Nux, in addition to its hypersensitiveness to light, to noise, to odours, affects the organs of sense. The eyes, with smarting, especially the internal and external canthi," as from salt ". They are mattery, and weep.

But the nose, as part of the respiratory system, is especially affected by *Nux*. And here is one of the great spheres of action of *Nux* (in the common cold) where its indications are rather peculiar and very definite. We will again quote the black letter symptoms, running on down the whole respiratory tract.

Profuse discharge of mucus from one nostril, that seems obstructed by dry catarrh.

Frequent discharge from both nostrils, obstructed by dry catarrh.

Fluent coryza in the morning.

Coryza fluent during the day, and stopped at night.

Real coryza, with scraping in the throat, crawling and creeping in the nose, and sneezing.

Catarrh with headache, heat in the face, chilliness, and much mucus in throat.

Sneezing in bed : after rising, sudden fluent coryza.

Throat rough from catarrh. Painful, raw and sore, at the palate.

Rawness in throat that provokes cough.

Sore throat. Scraped throat.

Rawness and scraped feeling in larynx. Provokes cough.

Violent cough before rising in the morning, with expectoration of clotted blood, and soreness in chest.

Very early morning cough.

Dry cough, from midnight till daybreak.

Scraping in chest, causing hawking.

Cough which brings on headache as if the skull would burst.

Cough which causes bruised pain in epigastrium.

Asthmatic constrictive tightness transversely through the chest, when walking and going up hill.

Among the *feverish* symptoms of *Nux* are :

After drinking, immediately shivering and chilliness.

Hahnemann says, " serious ailments from catching cold are often removed by *Nux*. *Nux* has, *Chilliness on the slightest movement ; on the slightest exposure to open air. Chilled by the slightest draught. Cannot get warm. Great coldness, not removed by the heat of the stove, nor by bed coverings. He cannot get warm. Fever in the afternoon, chilliness and coldness, with blue nails, followed by general heat and burning hands, with thirst, first for water, afterwards for beer.*

And now to run down the digestive tract, from mouth to anus, as affected by *Nux*, giving only the black letter symptoms :

Putrid taste in the morning, but food and drink taste right.

Bitter taste.   Putrid taste on coughing.

Repugnance to food.   And to the accustomed tobacco and coffee.

Eructation of bitter and sour liquid.

Nausea—in the morning : after eating.

Smoking makes him nauseated and qualmish.

After a meal he is qualmish, anxious, nauseated and sick, as after a violent purge.

Inclination to vomit.   Vomiting of sour mucus.

Retching, as if to vomit, while hawking mucus from fauces.

Tension above stomach.

Pressure, as from a stone in epigastrium : worse walking.

Pressure in stomach, after eating a little, in the morning.

A metallic, herby taste returns.

Pressure as from overloading the stomach, immediately after eating.

Violent gastric symptoms.

Scraped sensation in stomach.

Flatulent distension of abdomen, after eating.

Colic, as if diarrhœa from taking cold would come on.

Cutting colic, with qualmishness.   Colic that causes nausea.

Colic speedily disappearing during rest—sitting or lying.

Pain in abdominal ring, as if a hernia would become incarcerated.

Sensation of weakness in abdominal ring, as if a hernia would occur.

Hahnemann has a number of black type symptoms in regard to the effect of *Nux* on intestines.

Pinching, tearing abdominal pain, as if diarrhoea from a chill would occur.

Needle-pricks—cutting pains—pinching pains.

After belly-ache evacuations of dark-coloured mucus, which caused smarting-burning at anus.

Sensation of weakness in the abdominal ring, as if a hernia would occur.

Forcing down towards the genitals in the lower abdomen.

Development of a tendency to inguinal hernia.

The rectum and anus are extremely affected by *Nux* :

Blind hæmorrhoids.

Sharp pressive pain in the rectum, after a stool and after a meal, especially on exerting the mind, and studying.

Tearing sticking and constricting pain, as from aggravated blind piles, in the rectum and anus, after a meal and after exerting the mind and reflecting.

After a stool it seemed as if some remained behind, and could not be evacuated, with a sense of constriction in the rectum, not in the anus.

Discharge of bright blood with fæces, with a sensation of constriction and contraction in the rectum, during stool.

With the stool it always seemed as if it were not enough, and as if the evacuation were incomplete.

Anxious desire for stool.

One has been told by the old Sisters at the Hospital, that in the older days of Homœopathy, no one dreamed of operating for piles : they used to cure them with *Nux* and *Sulphur*—low—and in alternation. (Pace shades of Hahnemann !) Sulphur has certainly produced piles ; and cured them.

Frequent ineffectual desire for stool, as if the evacuation were incomplete.

Diarrhœa of a dark colour, especially in the morning and immediately after dinner.

Obliged to go to stool three or four times a day : it was often ineffectual, and the stool when passed was soft.

Constipation, as from constriction and contraction of the intestines.

NASH elucidates this phase of the action of *Nux.* He says, " Frequent and ineffectual desire to defæcate, or passing but small quantities at each attempt. This symptom is pure gold. There are a few other remedies that have it, but none so positive and persistently.

" It is the guiding symptoms in the constipation to which *Nux* is homœopathic, and in my experience will then, and then only, cure."

He says, Carrol Dunham here contrasted *Nux* and *Bryonia.* That " there was never any reason for confounding them, or alternating them. The *Nux* constipation is caused by irregular peristaltic action of the intestines, hence the frequent ineffectual desire for stool : the *Bryonia* constipation is caused by lack of secretion in the intestines. With *Bryonia* there was no desire, and the stools were dry and hard, as if burnt." He adds :—

" This *Nux* symptom is found not in constipation only. It is present in dysentery ; where the stools (of slimy mucus and blood) are small and unsatisfactory. With *Nux* in dysentery, the pains are very greatly relieved for a short time with every stool : with *Mercury* (*Merc. cor.*) the pain and straining continue *after* every stool—*the never-get-done* sensation. . . . *But whether the patient has constipation, dysentery, diarrhœa or any other diseases, if there is this frequent, ineffectual desire for stool, we think first of Nux vomica,* and give it unless contraindicated by other symptoms."

What *Nux* really causes in the abdominal organs is irregular peristalsis: colicky pinchings here and there driving the intestinal contents at once forwards and back. Hence the character of defæcation. A little passed with relief, and then more to come: and always a sensation that there is more to come.

KENT says : "Another state running through *Nux* is that actions are turned in opposite directions. When the stomach is sick, it will empty its contents with no great effort ordinarily, but in *Nux* there is retching and straining as if the action were going the wrong way, as if it would force the abdomen open ; a reversed action ; retches, gags and strains, and after a prolonged effort he finally empties the stomach."

He describes, in the bowels, " a kind of anti-peristalsis. In constipation, the more he strains the harder it is to get a stool."

The urinary organs are also affected with the NUX spasmodic condition.

Urging to urinate.

Frequent desire to urinate : constantly called out that he would be better if he could pass water.

Painful, ineffectual desire to urinate.

Violent straining : the efforts to urinate were constant and most painful, without being able to pass a single drop.

Urine passed with difficulty.

Whilst urinating, a burning and tearing pain in the neck of the bladder.

Whilst urinating an itching in the urethra.

Menses three days early, with cramps in abdomen.

During the menses, nausea in the morning, with chilliness and attacks of fainting.

In the convulsions of *Nux*, one observes the strychnine element.

The slightest touch of the hand immediately brought on spasms.

Years ago, in the country, a wretched hen was cooped all alone, because "if one of the others touched her, she had a fit ". Tested, by shaking the coop, she was crumpled up, immediately, in convulsions. Some *Nux* was left for her, and when seen again a few days later, she was running about with the rest of the fowls.

"*Nux* has the most violent convulsions with opisthotonos ; convulsions of all the muscles of the body, with purple face and loss of breath from the movements ; conscious, or semi-conscious during the whole spasm, aware of the sufferings and contortions, which are horrible ; worse from the slightest draught of air ; tickling the feet ; the merest touch of the throat causes gagging." (*Kent.*)

Nux produces not only convulsions, but lockjaw. It has caused " contraction of the jaws, like lockjaw "—" closure of the jaws with complete consciousness." Lockjaw is very fatal to horses who have " picked up a nail ". One remembers, long ago, a paragraph in an evening paper. The owner of a horse with lockjaw called in a vet. to poison the beast, and the vet. administered a big dose of strychnine. Meeting the owner of the horse a few days later, he stopped him to ask after the horse. " *I'm driving him,*" was the reply. . . . One of the accidental homœopathic cures by a vet who knew no homœopathy. (Strychnine, of course, is one of the alkaloids of *Nux*.)

To write exhaustively on *Nux* " of many uses ", would be " to write a complete materia medica ".

But just a few more gleanings in regard to *Nux* :

NASH says, " Spasm, sensitiveness (nervous), and chilliness are three general characteristics of this remedy.

" Anxiety with irritability; and inclination to commit suicide, but afraid to die.

" For very particular, careful, zealous persons." (Kent gives only *Arsenicum* and *Nux* under the heading *fastidious* ; and *Nux* is again like *Arsenic* in its fear of knives for the impulses they suggest.)

" Twitchings, spasms, convulsions, worse the slightest touch. Convulsions with consciousness.

" Sleepy in the evening for hours before bedtime : then lies awake for an hour or two ; then wants to sleep late in the morning.

" When in sickness, or from abuse of coffee or alcohol *Nux* symptoms supervene, *Nux* will be curative.

" *Great heat, whole body burning hot, especially face red and hot, yet patient cannot move or uncover in the least without feeling chilly.* It matters not what the fever, inflammatory, remittent, the fever accompanying sore throat, rheumatism, influenza, with these indications give *Nux*, and you will not be disappointed in the result. It took me years to learn the value of this symptom," says Nash.

" The indigestion of *Nux* is an hour or two after eating—sour taste—heart-burn—bloating, must loosen clothes, with pressure like a stone in stomach—with the *Nux* mood and temper. The causes being, coffee, alcohol, debauchery, abuse of drugs, sedentary habits, broken rest from long night-watching, too high living. *Nux* is adapted to complaints from such causes."

One of the characteristics of *Nux* is a *scraped* sensation, throat —chest—stomach, in inflammatory conditions.

Nux dreams of lice, as a woman who had taken *Nux* for a month found to her cost. The dreams of *Nux* are angry, amorous, anxious, of disease, of misfortune, of quarrels.

Nux is one of the few drugs that crave fats; also alcohol and beer ; or, on the other hand, *Nux* may loathe ale, beer, coffee, food—even though hungry, and may hate meat, tobacco, and water.

KENT gives some vivid little *Nux* pictures. "*Nux* is an old dyspeptic, lean, hungry, withered ; bent forward ; premature age ; always selecting his food and digesting almost none ; aversion to meat, it makes him sick ; craves pungent, bitter things, tonics. Weak stomach ; after meals pain in stomach ; stomach sinks in ; withers and loses flesh."

And again: "A business man has been at his desk till he is tired out : he receives many letters, he has a great many little irons in the fire ; he is troubled with a thousand little things ; his mind is constantly hurried from one thing to another until he is tortured. It is not so much the heavy affairs, but the little things. He is compelled to stimulate his memory to attend to all the little details ; he goes home and thinks about it ; lies awake at night ; his mind is confused with the whirl of business, and the affairs of the day crowd upon him ; finally brain fag comes on. When the little details come to him he gets angry, and wants to go away, tears things up, scolds, goes home and takes it out of his family and children. Sleeps by fits and starts ; wakens at 3 a.m. and his business affairs crowd upon him so that he cannot sleep again till late in the morning, and wakens up tired and exhausted. He wants to sleep late in the morning. . . . Melancholy, sadness, but all the time feels as if he could fly to pieces, jerks things about, tears things up ; wants to force things his own way. Driven by impulses to commit acts that verge upon insanity—the destruction of others."

OPIUM

(*Papaver somniferum, the white poppy*)

ONE of the ancient saws of medicine has it : " *Sine papaveribus et sine medicamentis ex eis confectis manca et clauda esset medicina,*" which may be vernacularized, " Without poppy and its derivatives, medicine would be a wash-out."

Nothing better than *Opium* exemplifies the difference between the two ways of medical practice. *Opium* and its most important alkaloid, *Morphia*,* are a tremendous standby for the orthodox physician : and to the young and inexperienced doctor it may sometimes seem absolute cruelty to withhold them. True that, given in material doses they cure nothing. True that, the more they are given, the greater the need and the craving for the lying peace they bring. True, that one of the toughest problems of medicine is the cure of the Opium eater, and the rescue of the victim of morphia habit. At one period it was the fashion among the medicos of Paris to supply young girls with a morphia hypodermic, so that they might render themselves insensible to menstrual pain ; with shocking results. We used to be taught in our Insanity Course, that it might be worth while to attempt to break the morphia habit once, but that, if the patient relapsed it was more merciful to leave him to his fate : the sufferings were too terrible to be inflicted a second time.

The ultimate effect of these, at once seductive and tyrannical drugs, is to utterly destroy all sense of right and wrong. Lying and thieving are the characteristics of *Opium*. Nothing that the *Opium* victim says can be trusted : more especially so when the drug-need is imperative and the drug difficult to obtain. One remembers well the tragedy of a young naval officer ; this was many years ago. For a bad bout of sciatica he was doped with morphia till he acquired the craving, and unfortunately, with the ship's drugs in his care, he had only to help himself. He was at one time treated with a view to cure, and one heard of him, forcibly held down in bed at night, when he was raving for his dope. He was " cured ", only to relapse, and the last news that came through was his arrest for stealing a pair of boots.

Therefore *Opium* is a drug (in homœopathic preparation) to be thought of for those abnormal children whose moral sense has never been developed, who lie and steal, and are heading for a

* *We are told that " the action of Opium is due almost entirely to its Morphine ".*

Mental Institution. . . . But some children are merely late in growing a conscience, which seems to develop at different ages : and the " no conscience " child may turn out to have a very tender conscience later on.

But what to do about *Opium* or *Morphia* in the face of great pain ? We will let Nash answer that question for us. He says, " *Opium* in narcotic doses does not produce sleep, but stupor, and it only relieves pain by rendering the patient unconscious to it. How many cases have been so masked by such treatment, that the disease progressed until there was no chance of cure. Pain, fever, and all other symptoms are the voice of the disease, telling where is the trouble, and guiding to the remedy. The true curative often relieves pain even more quickly than *Opium*, and does so by curing the condition upon which it depends."

And here one remembers the warnings of one of our surgical lecturers in regard to the danger of these drugs in acute abdominal conditions that should call for emergency operation.

Even in the most hopeless cases of extensive, inoperable malignant disease, where *Morphia* would seem, in common humanity, to be not only indicated, but imperative, one sees again and again, that small doses of *Arsenicum*, or some other remedy to which the symptoms point, will abolish pain, improve health and spirits and add length to life, without the nausea and misery that dog such treatments by *Morphia*.

Hahnemann says, " *Opium is almost the only medicine that in its primary action does not produce a single pain.*" He tells us that every other known drug produces in the healthy human body pain, each after his kind, and is therefore able to remove such pains when they occur in disease ; but " *Opium* is alone unable to subdue permanently any one single pain, *because it does not cause in its primary action one single pain*, but the very reverse, namely, *insensibility*, whose inevitable consequence (secondary action) is greater sensitiveness than before, and hence a more acute sensation of pain."

And he quotes from Willis's *Pharmacia rationalis* : " Opiates generally allay the most excruciating pains and produce insensibility—for a certain time ; but when this time is passed the pains are *immediately* renewed, and soon attain their ordinary violence. . . . When the duration of the action of *Opium* is over, the abdominal pains return, having lost nothing of their excruciating character until we again employ the magic of *Opium*."

So, in the topsy-turvydom of curative medicine, *Opium* comes in for cases of painlessness where there should be distress and pain : for desperate sickness where the patient says, " I feel so

well !—so well ! '' or complains of nothing : for cases of insensibility—coma—as in apoplexy : for cases of painless, symptomless,
complete constipation ; and so on. But more of this anon.

Hahnemann tells us that it is far more difficult to estimate
the action of *Opium* than that of almost any other drug. The
primary action of small and moderate doses exalts the irritability
and activity of the voluntary muscles for a short time, but
diminishes those of the involuntary muscles for a longer period.
And while it exalts fancy and courage in its primary action, it
appears at the same time to dull and stupify the general sensibility
and consciousness. But thereafter the living organism, in active
counter-action, produces the opposite of all this (in the secondary
action), i.e. diminished irritability and inactivity of the voluntary,
with morbid exalted excitability of the involuntary muscles, and
loss of ideas and obtuseness of fancy, with faintheartedness, along
with oversensitiveness of general sensibility. And he says, " No
medicine in the world suppresses the complainings of patients
more rapidly than *Opium*.''

HALE WHITE tells us that in *Opium* the higher faculties are first
excited : intellectual power and mental vigour increased, especially
imagination : while reason and judgment are dulled. Then
follows sleep, wherein he responds to nothing, and feels no pain.
" This makes the drug invaluable,'' says Hale White.

And again, "*Opium* diminishes all secretions, except *sweat.*
It paralyses the peristaltic movements of stomach and intestines.''

Opium's drugged unconsciousness, with stertorous breathing,
jaw dropped, pupils generally contracted, face mottled, purple,
hot, with hot sweat, and cheeks blown out with every expiration,
gives a beautiful picture of apoplexy, and it is in just such cases of
cerebral hæmorrhage that *Opium* is so invaluable. As NASH
says " there is no response to light, touch, noise, or anything else,
except the indicated remedy, which is *Opium*.''

And KENT says : "*Opium* causes a flow of blood to the brain,
and when given homœopathically it checks this, and in six and a
half hours he will become rational, his skin cool, face normal
colour, pulse normal. We thus see the usefulness of the crude
effects of *Opium* in giving us a picture of apoplexy.''

Kent says, " among the striking features of *Opium* is a class of
complaints marked by painlessness, inactivity, and torpor
. . . deceptions in vision, taste, touch : deception of the state
he exists in : in his own realization : a perversion of all the senses
with much deception.''

He adds, following Hahnemann, " the general characteristic is
painlessness, but now and then the alternate state is produced, in

which a small dose of *Opium* will cause pain, sleeplessness, inquietude, nervous excitability. . . . The majority are constipated, but in some there is dysentery and tenesmus. The patient is sleepy, yet at times the drug is characterized by sleepless nights, anxiety, increased sensitiveness to noise, so that he says he can almost hear the flies walking on the wall, and hears the clock striking in the distant steeple."

We are told that few drugs have such different effects on different people.

And talking of *Opium*, as everywhere a producer of *insensibility* and partial or complete paralysis, Nash adds :

" Now we find an exactly opposite state of things under *Opium*. Delirious : eyes wide open, glistening ; face red, puffed up." " Vivid imagination, exaltation of the mind." "Nervous, irritable, easily frightened." " Twitching, trembling of head, arms and hands ; jerkings of the flexors, even convulsions." "Sleeplessness with acuteness of hearing, cocks crowing at a great distance keep her awake."

And CLARKE, commenting on Hahnemann's saying that, " It is more difficult to estimate the action of *Opium* than of almost any other drug," says, " That is true, if we conceive it necessary to divide the effects of the drug into primary and secondary. . . ." He finds that "whether the action is ' primary ' or ' secondary ' depends on the prover or the patient. I know some people who are made absolutely sleepless by *Opium* in all sorts of doses ; and *Opium* 30 has helped me in cases of sleeplessness as often as *Coffea*. *My experience goes to show that whether the drug-effect is primary or secondary, it is a drug-effect and is good for prescribing on. . . .*"

And again, " No doubt abnormal painlessness is a grand keynote for *Opium* ; but in the pathogenesis many acute pains will be found, and among them this, recorded by Hahnemann himself, ' Horrible labour-like pains in uterus, which compelled her to bend the abdomen double; with anxious, almost ineffectual urging to stool.' Whether this be primary or secondary I know not " ; and he records a case of severe dysmenorrhœa where *Opium* gave greater and more lasting relief than anything else, and another where *Opium* 30 given for constipation caused, with the onset of the next period, " sharp pain which caused vomiting and a desire to sit doubled up and keep warm ".

Among its contradictory things, *Opium* has twitchings, jerkings, even to convulsions. And here, Kent says : " an *Opium* patient with convulsions needs to be uncovered, and wants cool open air. Convulsions if the room is too warm." " If the mother puts such a child into a hot bath to relieve the convulsions, it will become unconscious and cold as death." (Compare *Apis*.)

Opium presents a vivid picture of extreme alcoholism—delirium tremens ; and is here, again, found useful.

Opium causes sensations of beatitude—physical and mental : great happiness, great confidence, in the first hours of the drug. As these wear off into the torments of the damned, the Opium eater must get back to that temporary state of delight, and he renews always the torment that is destroying him.

De Quincey's *Opium* visions were architectural, scenic; sensations of descent into chasms of sunless abysses, depths below depths, from which it seemed hopeless that he would ever re-ascend. He describes the gloom, the suicidal darkness. Space and time-senses were powerfully affected. Vastness of proportions—vast expansions of time, till he seemed to have lived 70 to 100 years in one night. . . . Dreams of lakes, silvery expanses of waters, . . . then " a tremendous change, which unfolding itself like a scroll through many months, promised an abiding torment. . . . For now that which I have called the tyranny of the human face began to unfold itself. Now it was that, upon the rocking waters of the ocean, the human face began to appear ; the sea appeared paved with innumerable faces, upturned to the heavens ; faces imploring, wrathful, despairing, surged upwards by thousands, by myriads, by generations, by centuries ; my agitation was infinite ; my mind tossed and swayed with the ocean."

Odd Symptoms and Tips

Painless. Complains of nothing. Wants nothing.

Thinks she is not at home. (*Bry*.)

Face expresses fear and fright.

Stool involuntary—after a fright (sphincter paralysed).

Bed feels so hot that she cannot lie in it. Moves for a cool place : must be uncovered. (*Sulph*.)

Retention with a full bladder (*Stram*. suppression) ; bladder full, but fullness unrecognized.

Lack of reaction to the properly selected homœopathic medicine.

Guernsey says : " In chest troubles, where there is continuous stertorous respiration, give *Opium*. Respiration deep, unequal." (Cheyne-Stokes.)

Among the symptoms that *Opium* can cause is awful fear or anxiety, . . . and it is useful in *complaints from fear, where the fear remains.* Shock, and the horrible thing cannot be recovered from : it comes back continually before the eyes.

Clarke remembers reading of the cure of an ulcer on the leg. There were *no sensations* on which a remedy could be diagnosed, but the *absence of sensation* indicated *Opium*, and *Opium* cured.

De Quincey writes that among his trials, as he gradually broke off the drug habit, was violent sneezing. He would sneeze for sometimes two hours at a time, and at least two or three times a day. He also had the *Opium* excessive perspiration, so violent that he was " obliged to use a bath five or six times a day ".

Kent says : " There is never any use for crude *Opium* in the sick room. In surgery at times it is admitted that something seems necessary, and we will not quarrel with the surgeon. But in disease in sick people it is not necessary. It performs no use and in the end is an injury ; it prevents finding the homœopathic remedy. It has masked the symptoms, and you cannot do anything for days."

Now look at *Opium* in the light of the Arndt-Schultz Law . . . *Large doses of a poisonous drug are lethal, smaller doses paralyse, while still smaller doses of the same poison stimulate the life-activities of the self-same cells.*

In largest doses, *Opium first produces excitement*, then drowsiness and incapacity for exertion—sleep—*finally coma.*

It is at first rousable : soon no stimulation is of the least use : pupils minutely contracted ; no reflexes.

It is cold, livid ; towards the end, bathed in cold sweat.

Pulse weak and slow : respiration slower and more irregular : at last stertorous, and patient dies from asphyxia.

In material doses (non-lethal), it diminishes all secretions except sweat. Mouth dry : stomach and intestines dry, and paralysed,—from paralysis of muscular structure in the wall of the intestines. Almost always constipation therefore : the most complete constipation.

Vessels dilate in the medulla and cord.

It is a direct poison to the respiratory system : produces slow, stertorous respiration.

And just what *Opium* can do—short of death—it can cure.

In minimal doses it cures its own kind of constipation : rouses consciousness in the comatose : and in those who are stunned by shock : can give sleep, to the abnormally wakeful with exaltation of senses, and so on. It is not the drug of universal " usefulness " of the old school, but it can do, *permanently*, far more wonderful things, when given after the manner of Hahnemann.

Black Letter Symptoms

Fear of impending death. Expression of fright and terror.

Complete insensibility. Impossible to excite any sign of uneasiness by pulling the hair, or pinching the skin, or sudden affusion of cold water.

Insensibility with complete apoplectic respiration.

Unconscious : eyes glassy, half-closed, face pale, deep coma.

Mania a potu : senses dull ; sopor with snoring. Sees animals coming towards him. People want to hurt him : creeps under covers : wants to jump out of bed. Believe themselves murderers or criminals, to be executed. Want to run away.

Staring look : facial muscles twitch. Lockjaw. Tremor.

Ailments from excessive joy, fright, anger, shame.

Ailments after fright, the fear of the fright remaining.

Trembling limbs after a fright. Spasms from emotion, fright, etc.

Face pale. Face flushed.

PUPILS *dilated, insensible to light : or contracted and sluggish. Paralysis of tongue with difficult articulation.*

Great thirst : unquenchable thirst.

Colic : transient : very violent : griping, with constipation, as if intestines cut to pieces. Painters' colic.

Stools : involuntary after fright ; fluid, frothy ; burning in anus ; tenesmus. Hard, round, dry, black balls : like sheep dung : feels as if rectum were closed ; come down and recede. (Sil.)

Almost unconquerable chronic constipation.

Cholera infantum: stupor, snoring, convulsions, contracted pupils.

Well selected remedy refuses to act. Want of susceptibility to drugs. Want of vital reaction.

Painlessness in all ailments. Complains of nothing ; wants nothing.

Paralysis : insensibility : after apoplexy—in drunkards—old people.

Weakens expulsive power of bladder : which is unable to expel its contents : retention of urine.

Frequent involuntary deep breathing. Respirations long, sighing ! or stertorous respirations.

Pulse show, with slow stertorous respirations : exceedingly red face : extremely profuse perspiration. Convulsions.

Whining in sleep. Drowsy, difficult to keep awake : at night, restless with much perspiration.

Sleepless with acute hearing ; clocks striking and cocks crowing at a distance, keep her awake.

ORNITHOGALUM UMBELLATUM
(Star of Bethlehem)

IN the days of the *Cooper Club*, which met in Dr. Clarke's house, and where the moving spirits were Dr. Robert Cooper, with his genius for the discovery of useful remedies, Dr. James Compton Burnett, who had a genius for grasping their idiosyncracies and possibilities and employing them with success for the patients who beseiged him and Dr. Clarke who noted them with the carefulness of genius and recorded them for the permanent help of humanity in his *Dictionary of Materia Medica* : working, as he used to say, in order to save himself work, because he MUST know where to lay his hand on any drug he might need :. one of the very important, but, so far, poorly proved remedies that emerged from their discoveries and deliberations was

ORNITHOGALUM,

a member of the onion, leek, and garlic tribe, with many of the peculiarities of action, in sensitives, of these comestibles.

Boericke has, now, a brief mention of *Ornithogalum* in his comprehensive *Pocket Book*. But all he says is :

" To be considered in chronic gastric and other abdominal indurations, possibly cancer of intestinal tract, especially of stomach and cæcum. Center (*sic*) of action is the pylorus causing painful contraction with abdominal distension.

"Depression of spirits. Complete prostration. Feeling of sickness keeps the patient awake at night."

Years ago one obtained a permit from Kew to pick specimens of medicinal plants. Dr. Cooper's way of obtaining his plant remedies, was seeking them out at their best, as regards not only season, but time of day or night. Armed with a small bottle three parts filled with spirit of wine, he would secure his choice specimen and bottle it forthwith. He thus provided himself with the purest and most uncontaminated " mother tincture " possible. In many cases he would give one drop of this, at long intervals, as required, waiting, always, till its stimulating action was spent before repeating. And, for remedies so prepared he had a name of his own " Arborivital remedies ". He evidently got astonishing reactions of healing. But, of course, for this purpose, and for such administration, he could not use a drug of virulently poisonous properties : this would have to be toned down to a " 3x " in order to be useful without endangering life.

But to return to Kew. . . . One was stooping, one day, over a bed of Stars of Bethlehem, choosing the ideal one for bottling *à la* Cooper, when, from behind, came a reproachful voice, " What are you doing ? " Of course it was a keeper, whose duty it was to prevent such depredations : and, equally of course, it was the first time that one had failed to bring along the never-used permit.

The only course was that of humble explanation, and one succeeded in so interesting and appeasing the keeper as to be hailed along to one of the big sub-tropical houses, and given a specimen of some other unknown, but very precious medicinal plant—or so the keeper said.

All this by the way. . . . The question is : What do we know of practical importance, from the prescribing point of view, about *Ornithogalum* ?

In one of Dr. Cooper's booklets entitled *Cancer and Cancer Symptoms*, he writes under

ORNITHOGALUM UMBELLATUM

quoting first from the *Treasury of Botany*, as follows :

" A common weed in many parts of England and Scotland. It is known as the Star of Bethlehem from its being abundant in Palestine and having star-like flowers. It is also supposed to be the Dove's Dung of Scripture (2 Kings ch. vi.); and its bulbs which are wholesome and nutritious when cooked are to this day eaten in Palestine. The genus is closely allied to Scilla, from which it is distinguished only by its flowers being persistent instead of deciduous, and white-greenish or yellow instead of blue. All the species are bulbous plants, with radical and not stem-sheathing leaves, and terminal racemes of flowers, each flower with a withered bract beneath it. Their perianth has six distinct segments, spread out star-fashion ; and their six stamens have flattened filaments, and are almost free from the perianth."

Cooper continues : " Belonging to the natural order *Liliaciæ* it is botanically allied to *Asparagus officinalis, Paris quadrifolia, Convalaria majalis, Scilla naritima, Agraphis nutans, Colchicum autumnale, Allium sativum, Allium cepa,* and *Polygonatum officinale,* besides, of course, many other less known but valuable remedies.

" My acquaintance with it in cancer cases was due to the very distinctive disturbance it produced in a woman very sensitive to all alliaceous flavouring substances in food. *The dose was taken at mid-day, and the same evening distension of the stomach and duodenum came on, with frequent belching of mouthfuls of offensive flatus obliging her to loosen her clothes, and this was accompanied by*

*the most hateful depression of spirits and desire for suicide, a feeling
of complete prostration and painful sinking across the pit of the chest,
and a feeling of sickness that kept her awake the greater part of the
night, and that did not pass off for several days.*

" The subject of this disturbance was about 54 years of age, of
quite a sanguine temperament, inclined to enfeebled digestion, and
with a history of pleuritic seizures, and possible phthisical
tendencies, but otherwise not subject to any settled form of
disease.

" Since the medical thrill above recorded, her general strength,
digestion and capacity for enjoyment of life have manifestly
improved.

" *The Ornithogalum umb. in those sensitive to it, goes at once
to the pylorus, causes painful spasmodic contraction of it, and distends
the duodenum with flatus, its pains being invariably increased when
the food attempts to pass the pyloric outlet of the stomach.*" (The
italics are ours.)

And elsewhere he says : " The *Ornithogalum umb.* is a species
of garlic (*Allium sativum*), and, like it and *Allium cepa*, produces
indigestion with excessive eructations of wind."

Dr. Cooper gives wonderful cases of apparently malignant
ulceration of the stomach, cured by *Ornithogalum*, and one actually
proved malignant by operation at one of the London Cancer
Hospitals, where the patient was afterwards informed that
" adhesions had been found between the stomach and the thoracic
wall with a cancerous growth and thickening of the pyloric
extremity of the duodenum, and that it had been impossible to
remove all the diseased tissue ". He was later readmitted to the
cancer hospital on account of his agonizing pains, but when sent
home six weeks later, was informed by his own doctor that
*everything possible had been done for him ; that he could not possibly
live long, and that he must bear the pain while life lasted.*

Cooper found him writhing in agony on his bed. He could
keep nothing long on his stomach ; warm foods relieved, cold
drinks aggravated. Pains were worse at night ; they spread from
stomach to heart and between shoulders, as if an iron brick were
being forced through the stomach and chest. The growth was
rapidly enlarging, with visible bulging underneath the attachment
of the diaphragm; with marked dullness on percussion; the bulging extending to scorbiculus cordis. Tongue red, coated towards
the back ; bowels confined, with sometimes diarrhœa.

In this case the effect of Dr. Cooper's unit dose of *Ornithogalum*
was, first, intensified pain, then bowels acted, and a frothy
substance came up which gave great relief. After a second unit

dose, he began bringing up a black jelly-like substance, with great relief to pain, and general improvement in his condition.

During a couple of following months legs and feet would go to sleep and he was unable to keep still. Then feet and ankles began to swell ; right leg felt bruised and got painful and angry ; then swollen and tense, and pitted on pressure. He had also a feeling as if food choked him, with some flatus. . . . These symptoms confirmed Cooper in his belief that this swelling of the absorbents shown by the condition of the right leg and the previous swelling of feet and ankles, resulted from the high pressure put upon the emunctories owing to the setting free of the poison in the system. Some few weeks later he came to show the terrible condition of his legs—swollen, with great red streaks and patches coursing down the limbs. Cooper insisted upon his walking away without another dose, believing that this was due to the rapid elimination of the cancer poison. After that his recovery was uninterrupted. He received no other medicine except at the very first, when greatly suffering, a few doses of *Carbo veg.* 3*x*, which seemed to increase the pain, and was discontinued, and at the last a unit dose of *Alliaria officinalis.* Cooper's treatment began in July 1898, and in May 1899 the man wrote that he was " in almost perfect health, appetite good : eating almost any kind of food, able to enjoy meals, which he had not done for many years ; able to get about well, and carry on his business without fatigue". "I have rejoined the Volunteer Force and have done two or three good stiff marches, besides firing in competitions, and feel no ill effects. I have never felt so well for nearly twenty years. I feel wonderfully well now, and have gained two stone odd which I lost during my illness."

We have quoted at some length, but condensing, in order that we may take heart, and learn to do, and to hope. It may be well to reproduce these booklets of Dr. Cooper's ; since the experiences of such men of originality and success should not be forgotten and lost.

We remember to have seen about half a dozen cases of gastric or duodenal ulceration clear up under this drug. They were all about the same time, at the end of the last Great War. so far as one remembers, when one saw a great deal of Ward work, and when only one of the lot resisted *Ornithogalum* and needed, one remembers, *Phosphorus.* In the worst of these cases, the patient was absolutely blanched from loss of blood, and had to be hurried into a bed in hospital, to brilliantly clear up on *Ornithogalum.* And that she *did* clear up one knows, since she still comes up for trifling ailments, all these years afterwards, and reports that she has never had a return of that trouble. Therefore one realizes that Dr. Cooper was correct in claiming that *Ornithogalum* can CURE, in suitable cases, gastric or duodenal ulcerations.

But we need definite symptoms if we are to prescribe the drug with any degree of assurance. Its locality and mode of attack are important, yet we need more, for, after all, other drugs have caused, and therefore cured, such ulcerations:—what about *Kali bichrom., Arsenicum, Phosphorus* ?—how are we to choose between them ? Try them one by one ?—or give the one that has helped with some previous case, and stands therefore first in our estimation ? . . . NOT GOOD ENOUGH ! We must know more, in order to make fit choice of the proper remedy, and so establish healing contact.

Like all the onions, as Dr. Cooper tells us, it is capable of evoking really terrible flatulence—in sensitives. And we must remember that it is only from sensitives that one can obtain useful provings, and it is only sensitives that will respond curatively to a remedy, i.e. be stimulated, thereby, to curative reactions.

We have turned up three of Dr. Cooper's original pamphlets published in 1897, 1898 and 1899. In one of these, in regard to his " Arborivital remedies ", he tells us :

"*An Arborivital Remedy is one whose action can only be explained, by supposing a hidden force to exist in plants that is not demonstrable to the senses, and that is independent of any special mode of preparation.*" And as to What is an Arborivital Dose ? he says :

" *It is simply a single drop of the preserved juice of a fresh plant that is allowed to expend its action till no evidence is forthcoming of this action.*"

One may say that Dr. Cooper had the reputation (as one learnt accidentally from a stranger at a garden party years ago) of " the one doctor who cures cancer ". Have we even *one* in these days ?

PÆONIA

(Peony)

ONE of our minor, partly proved remedies, which we have found most useful in its special sphere—hæmorrhoids and sufferings of rectum and anus. But besides its great province in fistulae, fissures and piles, it is said to be generally curative in varicose conditions.

Its chief action is shown in its black letter and italicized symptoms, which we will proceed to quote :

Biting itching in the anus that provokes scratching ; the orifice seems somewhat swollen.

A small ulcer on the perineum, near the anus, that constantly oozes moisture of offensive odour.

Hæmorrhoids with fissures in anus, intolerable pains during and after stool.

Very painful and sensitive ulcers and rhagades in rectum.

Very painful ulcer partly in integument ; round, sharp-cut edges, exuding much moisture.

Fissures of anus. Atrocious pains, with and after stool, recurring after an hour or two, and lasting twelve hours, preventing sleep ; must walk the floor nearly all night ; exudation of offensive moisture.

NIGHTMARE.

OTHER NOTABLE SYMPTOMS

Sleep : very much disturbed by anxious dreams that amount to real nightmare, even with a dream of a distinct figure sitting on the chest, and making respiration very anxious.

The prover adds in a footnote : " At the time I was ignorant of the fact that both Dioscorides and Plinius had stated that nightmare could be cured by this drug. . . ."

Dream of a ghost who was sitting upon his chest and oppressing his breath, so that he frequently woke groaning.

Anxious : afraid to talk with anyone ; much affected by bad news.

Vertigo ; on every motion, with constant reeling and staggering.

Burning heat ; in eyes, face, throat, anus.

Pressure in pit of stomach, as from great anxiety.

Complete loss of voice.

Violent shootings from collar bone down through heart to diaphragm.

We are told that *Pæonia* compares with *Hamamelis* in varicosis, *Silica* in ulcers, and *Sulphur* in diarrhœa.

Pæonia has proved very curative in chronic non-syphilitic ulcerations, as evidenced by cases quoted. Here is one :

Eighteen years of hæmorrhoids and ulcerations of rectum, after several operations. Patient constipated, nervous and emaciated ; disagreeable smell from body. Anus and surroundings purple and covered with a thick crust. At verge and entrance of rectum several fissured ulcers with elevated and indurated edges, exquisitely painful. Whole mucous membrane at verge and higher up studded with ulcers, cracks and rhagades. Rectum purple and congested.

* * *

CULPEPPER (1610-1644), in my " old " copy—it is only dated 1819, but it is large and square, solidly leather-bound and looks ancient—talks of MALE and Female Pæony. He tells us that physicians say, Male Pæony roots are best : " but Dr. Reason told me Male Pæony was best for men, and Female Pæony for women, and he desires to be judged by his brother, Dr. Experience."

Culpepper asserts (we will condense) : " The roots are held to be of more virtue than the seed ; next the flowers, and, last of all, the leaves. The roots of the Male Pæony, fresh gathered, having been found by experience to cure the falling sickness (epilepsy) ; but the surest way is, besides hanging it about the neck, by which children have been cured, to take the root of the Male Pæony, washed clean, and stamped somewhat small, and laid to infuse in sack for 24 hours at the least, afterwards strain it, and take it first and last, morning and evening, a good draught for sundry days together, before and after a full moon ; and this will also cure old persons, if the disease be not grown too old, and past cure. . . . He says it helps women after childbirth, and such as are troubled with the mother (the womb). . . . The black seed also taken before bedtime, is very effectual for such as in their sleep are troubled with the disease called Ephialtes, or Incubus, but we do commonly call it the Nightmare : a disease which melancholy persons are subject unto. It is good against melancholy dreams. . . ."

(Quaint and nice ! Modern renderings of " Culpepper " do not give all this. They boil him down. They give his clinical tips, but extract the man's soul.)

* * *

PARKINSON : a still earlier London Herbalist (1567-1650). In my copy of Clarke's *Dictionary*, above " Pæony ", I once wrote a quotation from his great old folio, which I no longer possess :

" The male pæony root is far above all the rest ; a most singular approved remedy for all epileptical (*sic*) diseases. . . . Green root better than the dry."

So we see that Pæony, besides its common uses with us, had a very ancient reputation for the cure of *epilepsy* : but this seems to have dropped out.

* * *

DR. OSCAR HANSON, of Copenhagen, in his *Rare Homœopathic Remedies*, gives us *Pæonia officinalis*, with its anal symptoms and painful ulceration in that region. Also its therapeutics, so concisely told that, with our restricted space, they are worth quoting.

Pasty diarrhœa, followed by burning in anus and internal chilliness.

Hæmorrhoids with ulceration ; the anus and surrounding parts purple, covered with crusts ; painful ulcers in ano ; fissures of anus.

Stool followed by burning and biting ; exudation of offensive moisture. (*Ratanhia*). Abscess below the coccyx. Nightmare.

* * *

CLARKE tells us that *Pæonia* belongs to the great order of the Ranunculaceæ (the Buttercups), which includes the *Aconites*, *Actæas* and *Hellebores*. " Its proving brings out many symptoms of congestions, rush of blood to head, face, chest ; burning, itching and swelling of anus. Ulcers in general ; ulcers from pressure, as bedsores, and from ill-fitting boots. It has intolerable pain during and after stool.

PALLADIUM

WE were proposing to take *Palladium* for our Drug Picture this month, so like in some of its rare and peculiar symptoms to *Platinum* : but Dr. Patrick, of Bexhill, has kindly sent us an interesting resumé of this little-known remedy, and we will gratefully produce his paper, only prefacing it with a few remarks and comparisons.

Palladium, as the Dictionary has it, is " A statue of Pallas, on the preservation of which the safety of ancient Troy depended. Any safeguard. A rare metal in colour and ductility resembling *Platinum*."

Palladium was introduced as a drug, and proved in 1850, by Constantine Hering and his band of provers. It had been proposed as a remedy previously as early as 1833. We are told that *Platina* and *Palladium*, both proved in dust form, showed such similarity in their effects that the question arose whether corresponding *differences* might be found.

A very striking mental symptom common to the two drugs is the sensation of *tallness*. Both are proud and haughty : and with both this extends into the physical sphere, and they *feel tall*, while things around them look small and insignificant. STRAMONIUM also imagines he is large and tall, and surrounding objects small. (*Cop.*)

Palladium, with *Platina*, has much uterine bearing down. With *Plat.* the sensation may be, as if the uterus would come out. Apparently *Plat.* affects the uterus more, *Pall.* the ovaries, especially the right ovary. But, in prescribing these remedies, it is the peculiar mentality—the haughtiness, the overbearing ; the sensation of tallness, etc., which distinguishes these rarer drugs from *Sepia*, with its dull indifference, or *Lilium tigr.* with its aimless hurry, and its worries, mental and even spiritual. A symptom, a locality, do not make up a prescription ! They may suggest it : but it needs the whole picture, especially the mental picture, to match, if the magic is to work.

Besides *Palladium*, *Crocus*, *Thuja* and *Theridion* have a sensation of *something alive bounding about inside the body*, but *Palladium* goes one better : it has, " as if an animal were snapping and tearing off small portions inside the abdomen ".

Palladium has " crawling as from fleas ",—on back, arms, abdomen, thighs and ankles ; and actual spots like fleabites

21

appear on various places, lips, nostrils, etc. It has also violent itchings.

*   *   *

CLARKE says: "The chief characteristic of *Palladium* is affections of the right ovary, attended with pains which are relieved by pressure. Skinner cured with *Palladium* a young lady who had excessive pain in the right ovary during the menses. The only relief she could get was by inducing her sister to sit on that region. This relief by pressure distinguishes the pain of *Pall.* from the similar ovarian pain of *Plat.*"

•

PALLADIUM

A REMEDY OF WOUNDED PRIDE

By DR. W. S. PATRICK

WOUNDED PRIDE ! How sharp the sting and how humiliating the mortification ! And yet the first step towards knowledge is the realization of how little one really knows. Pride, conceit, egotism—these self-made tyrants are just as much our enemies as any despot or dictator in human form ; and must be vanquished before one may progress along the path that leads to liberation. And yet we have remedies to heal the wounds of mental conflict and of the lesser known of these is *Palladium*, rich in mental symptoms and worthy of deeper study. *Palladium* is one of the remedies often overlooked in favour of her sister *Platina*. Those who care to personify their remedies may think of the Greek goddess Pallas Athene, neglected by her votaries.

Let us see how the thread of mental conflict runs through the whole remedy, including rubrics in block letters and italics only.

From KENT'S *Repertory*—"DELUSION THAT (S)HE IS NEGLECTED. MORTIFICATION. WEEPING—Tearful Mood. And, in italics— Anger (irascibility). Ailments from bad news.

Desire for company. < alone.

Delusion—that (s)he is insulted.

Discontented. Discontented with everything.

Egotism. Ailments from egotism.

Fear of evil.

Haughty. Hysteria.

Irritability. Obstinate. Easily offended."

From CLARKE'S *Materia Medica*—" As if he had grown taller." " As if something terrible would happen." " As if intestines strangulated." " As if an animal were snapping and biting off small portions of intestines."

From BOERICKE'S *Materia Medica*—(Italic symptoms)—
" Love of approbation.

Easily offended. Keeps up brightly when in company (much exhausted afterwards and pains worse).

Pains across top of head from ear to ear.

Pain and swelling in region of right ovary.

Outstanding particulars—The symptom-complex of chronic oophoritis (right). *Pain in right ovarian region ameliorated by pressure.*

AGGRAVATION in general—Cold. Motion. After exertion. After social excitement.

AMELIORATION in general—Touch (headache). Pressure (pain in ovary). Rubbing. Rest. Open air. Sleep."

From the Supplement of ALLEN'S *Encyclopædia*—" Mental symptoms—Strong inclination to use forcible language and violent expressions.

Time seems longer to him. . . . The child was irritable. Ill-humoured in the evening.

She is in a disagreeable mood ; feels as if she could not bear or put up with anything, without anything having occurred. The child is the only one with whom she is not impatient.

Though usually tired in the evening, feels mentally " gone " ; is very awkward in speaking English, it is too much trouble, he is tired of it."

And to conclude, a few rubrics " worked out " :
" HAUGHTY—*Caust. Hyos. Ip. Lach.* LYC. *Pall.* PLAT. *Staph. Stram.* SULPH. VERAT.

MORTIFICATION—*Arg. n. Aur. Aur. m. Bry. Cham.* COLOC. IGN. LYC. *Lyss.* NAT. M. *Op.* PALL. PH. AC. *Puls. Seneg.* STAPH. *Sulph.*

AILMENTS FROM BAD NEWS—*Apis* CALC. GELS. *Ign. Med. Pall. Nat. m. Sulph.*

DELUSION—that (s)he is neglected—*Arg. n.* PALL.

EGOTISM—*Calc. Lach. Pall.* PLAT. *Sil. Sulph.*

AILMENTS FROM EGOTISM—*Calc. Lyc. Pall. Sulph.*"

" *Palladium* is the only remedy running through the above six rubrics. The careful study of our *Repertories* is well worth while— there are other hidden precious metals besides gold ! "

PETROLEUM—OLEUM PETRE

HAHNEMANN says this product of the interior of the earth ought to be fluid and light yellow if it is to be used as a remedial agent. He tells how it may be purified, by treating it with sulphuric acid, " which acts on the foreign oily matters, leaving the petroleum untouched. If pure, a drop of petroleum deposited on paper, will evaporate in air, without leaving a trace behind."

Among the curious symptoms given by Hahnemann is, " Stitches in the heel, as if a splinter were lodged in it." One remembers a case. A doctor who had been taking the Compton Burnett Lectures, coming, week by week from Yorkshire, wrote to the Lecturer, later on : " I have a sticking pain in my heel. Hurts to walk." The answer was, " Take *Petroleum* . . ." Back came the report, soon after, " Damn you, W——, it's gone." Recently, at Out-patients, one had such a case, and remembered, and made a ready and successful prescription.

One is apt to remember any case, over which one first made contact with a real useful remedy, not previously realized. The introduction to *Petroleum* came in a case of deeply cracked palms, which had previously benefited by *Petroleum* in low potencies of frequent administration. It was most interesting and instructive, because a dose of *Petrol.* 10m was found to carry her through a whole winter with comfortable palms. This might have to be repeated, for *slight* threatenings, when winter sets in—not always. She would come up at very long intervals, year after year, always rejoicing : which glow of rejoicing was shared.

Another case, one remembers, of large and very painful lipomata on the outer surface of both thighs, just about the hip-joint, which made lying a problem. So far as one remembers, she got *Baryta carb.*—which is classical, but, in one's experience, disappointing, for lipomata. Then her hands were found to be badly cracked, especially the palms, and she got *Petroleum* ; whereupon the " lumps " became softer, and painless, and ceased to trouble her, and presently she came no more, so one cannot tell the absolute outcome, i.e. whether they " went " completely. BUT—and here is what makes Homœopathy such an annoying, almost intolerable amusement—one began to wonder whether one had found a specific for lipomata ; only to find that one had *not*. That particular patient needed *Petroleum*, and her palms betrayed the fact ; and it could act curatively even on her fatty tumours.

But the others, who did not need the drug, were not in the same way amenable to its action.

Among *bleeding eruptions, Petroleum* stands high.

*   *   *

ALLEN'S *Guiding Symptoms* puts it very tersely and delightfully. We will quote a few of his emphasized points.

Irritable : quarrelsome : vexed at everything.

Ailments from riding in carriage, car, or ship.

Symptoms appear and disappear rapidly (*Bell.*).

Ailments before and during thunderstorm (*Nat. c., Phos., Psor., Rhodo.*).

In sleep, or delirium : imagines one leg double : that another person lies by him in bed : that there are two babies in bed (*Val.*). (Compare *Bapt., Pyrog.*)

Vertigo, on rising : in occiput ; as if intoxicated (*Cocc.*). *Like seasickness.*

Headache in occiput : which is heavy as lead. As if everything in head were alive. . . .

Gastralgia : of pregnancy : *whenever the stomach is empty : relieved by constant eating.*

Diarrhœa . . . *gushing*: after cabbage; in stormy weather : *always in the day time.* . . .

Skin, hands, rough, cracked ; tips of fingers rough, cracked, fissured, *every winter.* Tender feet, bathed in foul-smelling sweat.

Painful, itching chilblains and chapped hands, worse in cold weather : decubitus. . . .

*   *   *

GUERNSEY, *Keynotes :*

Affections in general of any kind, appearing on the right eye ; internal or external occiput ; behind the ears ; inner surface of the thighs ; ball, or under part of the toes ; knee joint.

Eruptions or itching at night (affecting scrotum especially), eruption being dry or moist ; chilblains, particularly where they itch a good deal and are moist. Exanthema corroding and spreading ; very difficult to heal ; sensibility of skin in general ; sores produced from lying in bed.

Strong aversion to fat food ; to meat ; to open air. Worse from eating cabbage.

Catalepsy ; tonic spasms ; cracking of joints ; inflexibility of joints. Sprains : chronic sprains.

*   *   *

NASH sums up *Petrol.* thus :

Eczemas, on scalp, behind ears, scrotum, anus, hands, feet, legs. Hands chap and bleed. All *worse in winter* : get better in summer.

Diarrhœa preceded by colic, *only in the day time.*

Headache, or heaviness like lead in occiput ; sometimes with nausea or vomiting : worse by motion, as in riding in boat or carriage.

He calls it one of our best psoric remedies . . . its eruptions are very similar to those of *Graphites.*

" There is one very marked characteristic symptom that guides to this remedy, out of a large number having similar eruptions, and that is that the eruption is *worse during the winter*. There is no other remedy that has this so prominently.   The hands chap, crack and bleed, and are all covered with *eczema during the winter and get well in summer.*"   He says, " I have cured a case of eczema of the lower legs of twenty years' standing, always worse in winter, with one prescription of the 200th.   I have cured chapped hands the same way.   A case of obstinate, chronic diarrhœa, and as soon as the fact that he had eczema of the hands in winter came to light, I cured him quickly of the whole trouble, with *Petrol.* 200th." He says, chilblains which are moist and itch and burn much in cold weather, are cured by it. . . .   The slightest scratch or abrasion suppurates (*Hep.*). . . .

Petrol. is also one of our best remedies for seasickness (*Cocc.*). Another curious symptom is cracking of the joints (*Caust.*).   Both are valuable in chronic rheumatism, especially with this cracking. *Petrol.* has, with *Chel.* and *Anac.*, pain in stomach relieved by eating. . . .   Dysentery and diarrhœa, *worse by day.*

*   *   *

KENT. *Petroleum* is one of the abused remedies : when used in rheumatism and bruises, externally, it acts, by counter-irritation, by establishing a disease on the surface : this is not homœopathic action.

One of the early things it does to a prover, is to put him in a state of confusion and dizziness : so dazed that he loses his way in the street.   Imagines that there are persons near, who are not present.   That the atmosphere is full of strange forms : that her limbs are double : that another person is in bed with her : another child in the bed.   Dreams that he is two or more.

Eruptions, herpetic, vesicular, tend to form thick yellow crusts : or break early and ulcerate : may become phagedenic. *Petrol.* builds up eruptions on the site of old eruptions, with increasing hardness in the base of the old eruption.   Crusts dry, indurate ; and the induration cracks, bleeds, looks purple.   Cracks about the ends of fingers, and the backs of hands.   Skin rough, ragged, exfoliates, cracks, bleeds : the tissues are hardened : this also about the palms and nails.

All eruptions itch violently : can't rest till he scratched the skin off, when the part became moist, bloody, raw and inflamed, . . . keeps on scratching till skin bleeds (even without eruption) and the part becomes *cold.*

Coldness in spots is a feature of this remedy : in stomach, abdomen, uterus ; cold spot between scapulæ : sensation as if heart were cold.

Mucous membrane (internal skin) has little patches of ulcers, with induration about patch : useful in syphilitic ulcers. Nose, posterior nares and pharynx thicken. Larynx involved with loss of voice. Dry, hacking cough, alternating with copious expectoration.

A striking feature of the drug is that the cough is worse during the night, and the diarrhœa is worse during the day. *Diarrhœa during the day : better at night.* Constant hunger with diarrhœa, yet can't eat without pain. Hungry, all-gone sensation after stool, drives him to eat.

" *Emaciation : skin eruptions ; unhealthy, ragged fingers which never look clean : he can't wash them, as this causes them to chap.*"

Offensive foot sweat (*Sil.*), offensive sweats all over, especially in axillæ, where it is so pungent that it can be observed as the patient enters the room.

Occipital headache :—" All carbonaceous products (as *Graphites, Carbo veg.*), affect the back of the head more or less."

Then the peculiar vertigo of *Petroleum*, when on shipboard, riding in the cars or carriage, with nausea like seasickness. He says, "occipital headache, with vertigo from focusing eyes on the waves, or on passing objects, with relief in a dark place, and with the all-gone, hunger or pain in stomach driving him to eat, may be helped by *Petrol.* ; whereas, the awful, deadly nausea, with pallor, cold sweat, exhaustion, better in open air, in dark quietness, and worse from warmth, suggests *Tabac.*"

Then the eye symptoms : fissures in the corners of eyes, with much itching. All *Petrol.* congestions of mucous membranes itch . . . as eustachian tubes. Itching deep in ear, too deep to scratch. Itching in pharynx.

Skin hot in places : with coldness in spots. Parts that burn and itch much. Can tell when it will thaw, by the itching in chilblains. Chilblains which itch, burn and become purple.

The eruption and state of induration are like *Graphites : but the oozing in Petrol. is thin and watery, and in Graph. it is gluey, honey-like, sticky, viscid.*

He says, *Petrol*. and *Rhus* are of wonderful use in eruptions on genitalia, male or female.   But *Petrol*. produces small vesicles, *Rhus large* blebs.   Sweat and moisture of external genitalia.

Sensitive to change of weather, like *Rhod*. and *Phos*.   Worse before thunderstorms.

Hands and feet burn : wants palms and soles out of bed.   He warns us : " Don't be too sure of *Sulphur*, because the soles burn ; or too sure of *Silica*, because the feet sweat."

He shows *Petroleum* to be *a remedy of single parts* :. sweating of single parts :—coldness in parts :—eruptions in patches.

*   *   *

Many strange sensations which are peculiar and striking.

Did not know where she was in the street.

Melancholy mood, imagines but little time is left him to make his will.

Great anxiety about his family, when going on a short journey. The anxiety increases till he becomes inconsolable.

Sensation as if everything in head were alive.

Hair glued together by crusts and exudation—eczematous.

Easily dislocated jaw.

Sense of coldness, or numbness in teeth.

Tongue white : white in centre with dark streak along edges.

Hunger immediately after stool.

Violent thirst for beer.

Note well, the extraordinary accumulation of water in mouth.

Canine hunger after stool ; with much urging, as if large quantities were yet to be expelled.

Itching in meatus urinarius, during micturition : itching deep in ears : in eustachian tubes.

Imagines she has two babies : very concerned as to how she is to take care of them : imagines another baby in bed which requires attention.

Coldness : as if a cold stone in heart.

Psoriasis of palms : thick scales of epidermis, through which run moist fissures.   Hands completely raw from wrists to fingers, with constant watery oozing.

Offensive smelling ulcers tips of fingers.   Nails feel bruised.

Cold spot on knee, whence a cold current pervades limb.

Chilblains on *heel* : stitches splinter-like in heel : blisters.

Must stoop on account of nausea.

Cracking in joints, neck, etc.

Imagines another child is sleeping in bed with her : talks about it and becomes angry when contradicted.

Head made of wood : tight stiff skin over bridge of nose.
Extremities stiff, as without joints.

BLACK LETTER SYMPTOMS

Delirium : thinks another person lies alongside of him, or that one limb is double.
Out of humour and angry ; becomes vehement easily.
Forgetful, and not disposed to think.

Heaviness like lead in occiput : pinching in occiput.

Great pressure in eyes.
Conjunctivitis pustulosa, with acute inflammation of lids. Lids red, inflamed, covered with scabs or scurfs. Surrounding skin rough : blennorrhœa of lachrymal sac : pain in occiput.
Inflammation of lachrymal sac, when suppuration has commenced and a fistula has formed.

Eustachian tubes affected, causing whizzing, roaring and cracking noises, with hardness of hearing.
Redness, soreness and humour behind the ears.

Pustule in nose. Bleeding nose.

Nausea and qualmishness all day : every a.m. after waking. Could not eat breakfast.
In morning accumulation of water in mouth : sudden on walking : from riding in carriage : often so violent that it takes away the breath, without vomiting : violent, with cold sweat, incessant : with vertigo and vomiting.
Seasickness.
After a slight meal, feels giddy and head swims.
Heartburn towards evening.
Nausea and qualmish the whole day.

Obstinate, itching herpes on perineum : itching, redness and moisture, scrotum. Skin cracked, rough and bleeding.

Hoarseness : cough from dryness in throat.

Sharp pains, shooting up dorsal spine into occiput.

Painful chilblains on hands.
Tips of fingers rough, cracked and fissured.

PHOSPHORIC ACID

ANOTHER of Hahnemann's legacies in *Materia Medica Pura*. He gives directions for its preparation and for its potentization up to the " trillion-fold dilution ". Of *Phos. acid* he writes,

" The following remarkable, pure, artificial morbid symptoms produced by *Phosphoric acid* on the healthy body indicate of themselves the natural morbid states in which it is specially curative by reason of its homœopathic similarity."

Some drugs exhilarate, others depress : but among the depressants there may be an active depressant condition, *Aurum* being an extreme instance, where the depression is so great as to drive the victim towards suicide. Not so with *Phosphoric acid*. Here the depression takes the form of extreme indifference. " Listless, apathetic ; remarkable indifference to everything in life : especially if there be emaciation and debility."

It is " the remedy of ailments from care, grief, sorrow, chagrin, homesickness, disappointed love : particularly when accompanied by night-sweats towards morning, and emaciation ". Bodily, as well as mental functions share in its depression and debility.

And then Hahnemann's joyful experience, in return for his well-placed dose, " He became very cheerful and well disposed " ; the curative effect of a drug that has caused and can therefore cure. It is these things that make life worth living !

Phosphoric acid is a drug of rather narrow, yet very definite and great utility. Look at the types that need its help. The weedy, over-grown, over-wrought schoolchildren, with growing pains that may spell heart-destruction. The tired and apathetic from unequal struggling with adverse circumstances, mental and physical. The " neurasthenics " that plague us; those, at least, who are worn out, indifferent, apathetic and emaciated. Those for whom life—civilization—has been too strenuous : and its burdens and disappointments have proved the breaking strain.

" Deterioration of health from nursing." Here one considers *China* : which is also apathetic, indifferent, taciturn, but *from loss of vital fluids,*—hæmorrhages, excessive lactation, suppurations. One has probably aften prescribed *China*, when *Phos. ac.* would have been the better prescription, with its breaking down *from, especially, nerve strain*. Mental enfeeblement, as KENT has it : mind tired : perfectly exhausted.

Consider further :—" Ailments from care, grief " : here one thinks of *Ignatia*. But *Ign* is the remedy of the sensitive, the easily excited : with incredibly rapid changes of mood ; very un-like the apathy and indifference of *Phos. ac.*

" Ailments from chagrin." One thinks at once of *Staphisagria*, also apathetic, indifferent, low spirited, but with its ailments from pride, envy or chagrin. KENT tells us that when *Staph.* has to control himself, he goes all to pieces, trembles from head to foot, loses his voice, his ability to work, etc. *Staph.* is far more intense and energetic in suffering than *Phos. ac.*

" Ailments from disappointed love " : one is tempted to prescribe *Natrum mur.* or *Hyos.* or *Ignatia.* But *Hyos.* has marked jealousy, and is far more intense mentally : quite a different drug picture, and *Nat. mur.* with, possibly, the emaciation of *Phos. ac.*, is passionate, intense : weeps, hates sympathy : has none of the dull apathy that cries aloud for *Phos. ac.*

KENT contrasts *Phos. ac.* and *Muriatic ac.* In *Phos. ac.* he says, the mental symptoms are the first to develop : the remedy runs from the mental to the physical, from the brain to the muscles : the muscles may remain strong after the mind has given out. In *Mur. ac.* the muscular prostration comes first, and the mind seems clear until long after the muscles are prostrated.

KENT says, the *Phos. ac.* patient pines and emaciates, grows weaker and weaker, withered in the face ; night sweats ; cold sweats down the back ; cold sweats on arms and hands more than on feet : cold extremities : feeble heart and circulation ; catches cold easily and it settles on the chest . . . and so on to tuberculosis. Pallor with increasing weakness and emaciation.

Most writers on *Phos. ac.* give prominence to the curious fact, that with all its prostration, its diarrhœa, acute or chronic, does *not* cause prostration, and they point to *Calcarea*, which " feels better, every way, when constipated ". In *Phos. ac.* there may be " amelioration of complaints by their ending in a diarrhœa ". Kent talks, under *Phos. ac.* of the child with copious, watery stools in summer : so copious that the napkin seems no use : the stool runs all over the mother's dress and forms great puddles on the floor : the stool is almost odourless, thin and watery, and the little one smiles as if nothing were the matter. The mother wonders where it all came from, yet the child seems well." " The *Phos. ac.* diarrhœa often ameliorates many of the symptoms, and the patient feels better. Some patients say they are never comfortable unless they have diarrhœa."

N.B.—*Phos. acid* has pinching and squeezing pains.

GUERNSEY's great indication for *Phos. ac.* is a condition of *complete indifference* to everything : not a soporous, delirious or irritable condition, but simply an *indifferent state of mind to all things*. He does not want anything, nor to speak : shows no interest in the outside world. In fevers, difficulty of comprehension : will think about a question, perhaps answer it, then forget all about it. He calls it " dizziness of the mind ".

Besides ailments from mental affections, he gives :—" after suppression of cutaneous eruptions : i.e. any bad effect that comes from such suppressions ; from loss of fluids, especially seminal. . . ."

NASH's Leaders :—Drowsy apathetic : unconscious of all surroundings, but can be roused to full consciousness.

Chronic effects of grief : hair turns gray : hopeless, haggard look.

Grows too fast and too tall : young persons with growing pains in bones . . . and so on.

Phos. ac. is one of the drugs that are *better after a short sleep*. (Camph., *Phos.*, *Sepia*, etc.)

Salty expectoration. (Again, *Phos.* and *Ars.*, *Sepia*, *Lyc.*, *Puls.*, etc.)

Stupified with grief : a settled despair.

In regard to growth : " with *Calc. carb.*, they grow too fat, with *Phos. ac.* too fast and tall."

In regard to hard study, Nash says, " While it is true that youth is a time to get education, it is also true that it is the time when too great a strain in that direction may wreck and for ever incapacitate a mind which might, with more time and care, have been a blessing to the world. *Phos. ac.* properly exhibited, may be of incalculable benefit in such cases."

He says, also, " it seems very singular that, after so much talk about the general depression or weakness of this remedy we should be obliged to record that profuse and sometimes long-continued diarrhœa should *not* debilitate, as a characteristic symptom. Well there are a good many unaccountable things in both disease and therapeutics, and this is one of them, but the *fact* remains and we act upon it. . . . The profound weakness and depression of *Phos. ac.* is upon the *sensorium* and *nervous* system. . . . He points out that *China* debilitates by its diarrhœa or loss of fluids : *Phos. ac.* attacks the nervous system primarily . . . and its effects or results are not so much the loss of vital fluids, as in *China*.

In regard to the profuse watery urine of *Ign.* and *Phos. ac.* he points out that in the first case it is hysterical, the latter not at all so.

Black Letter Symptoms

Quiet.   Indifferent.

Loss of ideas, and weakness of mind.

He cannot collect his thoughts in proper manner.

He speaks unwillingly ; talking is irksome.

Speaks little and answers questions unwillingly.

Listless, apathetic : remarkable indifference to everything in life, especially if there be emaciation and debility.

Ailments from care, grief, chagrin, homesickness, or disappointed love : particularly with drowsiness, night sweats towards morning ; emaciation.

He looks very ill humoured and sullen.

Sad humour, on account of concern for the future.

He became very cheerful and well disposed : (secondary, curative reaction).

Schoolgirls' headaches, from over-use of eyes.

Occipital headaches and pain nape of neck from exhausted nerve power or excessive grief.

Confusion of whole head.   Headache like stupidity; buzzing in head.

Constant headache.

On the slightest shock or noise, the pains in the head become extremely violent.

Hard pressure on left side forehead.

Squeezing pressure right temple, more violent on moving.

Squeezing pressure in both parietal bones ; worse on moving.

Pain as if temples were pressed towards one another, as if violently pinched by forceps.

Drawing pressure in right parietal and occipital bones, more violent when moving.

Tearing and squeezing pain in brain, here and there.

Tearing pressure in occiput, worse noise and slightest movement.

Violent shooting pain, right temporal, extending into right eye.

Burning, sore pain on the side of nape.

Vertigo towards evening, when standing and walking.

Vertigo in the morning, making him fall when standing.

Transient burning left eye, as if something pungent had been smelt.

Pain as if eyeballs were forcibly pressed together and into head.

Itching in the point of nose : must scratch.

Violent burning pain in right lower lip, persisting when moved.

Bleeding gums.

Dry feeling, palate. Nausea, palate.

When swallowing food, shooting in throat.

An almost insatiable thirst for cold milk.

After eating, pressing down weight in stomach and aching.

In navel a periodical aching squeezing.

Loud rumbling in abdomen, especially upper part.

Extremely violent pinching contraction of bowels from both sides of the umbilical region.

Pressure on several parts of hypogastrium. Distress in the abdomen.

Thin, whitish-grey stools.

White or yellow watery diarrhœa, chronic or acute, without pain or marked debility or exhaustion.

Stools involuntary.

Urging to urinate, with scanty discharge of urine.

Quite pale urine which immediately forms a thick whitish cloud.

Very profuse emissions.

Onanism, with distress at its culpability.

Great hoarseness.

Difficult inspiration, from pressure and oppression behind the sternum. Pain in chest from weakness.

Pressive pain in middle of the chest, most severe when expiring.

Felt as if sternum would be pressed out : pain more violent on pressing hand on sternum, stooping, coughing, etc.

Dry cough from tickling low down just above pit of stomach.

Feels bruised in hips, thighs, arms, and nape : like growing pains : with single tearing stitches in all these parts at once.

Exhaustion in legs when walking. Formication right leg.

Squeezing pressure in soles (one or other).

Here and there, a creeping, like ants running about.

Itching creeping in body and hands, evening, lying down.

Drowsy in the morning : can hardly be roused from sleep.

Deterioration of health from nursing.

Weak and prostrated : weak and apathetic in the morning.

Neurasthenia : cerebrospinal exhaustion from overwork : least attempt causes heaviness in head and limbs.

Interstitial inflammation of bones : scrofulous, syphilitic or mercurial.

Periosteal inflammation, with burning, gnawing, tearing pains.

Scrofulous affections of children : hip disease, curvature of spine, rickets, FEELING AS IF BONES WERE SCRAPED WITH A KNIFE.

Children and young people who have grown too rapidly : tall, slender, slim : pains in back and limbs as if beaten : growing pains.

HUGHES (*Pharmacodynamics*) says, " Failure in memory is reputed a special indication for it in cerebral depression : the emotional condition is one of apathy and indifference. It is to ' nervous debility ' what iron is to anæmia."

It is in diabetes that *Phosphoric acid* has won its greenest laurels. Not only in the " insipid " form . . . but in true glycosuria cure has repeatedly followed administration of this acid.

In low fevers it is indicated when the nervous system rather than the blood is affected by the poison. . . . It has more than once proved curative in purpura and passive hæmorrhages.

*   *   *

HERE is typical *Phos. ac.* in typhoid : we quote from HERING.

TYPHOID : complete apathy and indifference ; takes no notice, even when pinched ; utterly regardless of surroundings : face pale ; nose pinched ; eyes sunken ; staring, stupid, vacant gaze ; eyes glassy ; desires nothing, asks for nothing ; grasps about him with hands as if he wished to seize something ; answers questions not at all or unwillingly ; gives short unintelligible answers, which at times are inappropriate, as of one slumbering ; sopor ; falls asleep while talking ; when awake complains of great and very annoying confusion and cloudiness in head, with great anxiety ; when slumbering sees many visions ; great roaring in ears ; hardness of hearing ; lies with eyes half-closed, indifferent to all around her, reflects long, then answers correctly, but slowly ; vertigo ; pointed nose ; dark blue rings around eyes ; rapid sinking of strength ; nose bleeds, which, however, gives no relief to symptoms in early stages ; bores fingers into nose ; itching of nose from irritation of Peyer's patches ; crusty lips ; sordes on teeth ; fetor oris ; thirst ; abdomen distended and bloated, with much gurgling and rumbling ; left side abdomen sensitive to touch ; stools watery, sometimes involuntary, and contain undigested food ; milk passes more or less undigested ; copious escape of flatus with stool ; stool bloody and slimy ; tongue dry, may have a dark red streak down centre, but is apt to be pale and clammy and sometimes covered with slimy mucus ; bites tongue involuntarily while asleep ; urine highly albuminous, milky, decomposing rapidly, loaded with earthy phosphates ; petechiæ ; ecchymosis ; decubitus ; enlargement of spleen.

PHOSPHORUS

BECAUSE everything that can hurt can heal, Homœopathic Materia Medica is really illimitable. It is only by constant reading and study that one can get an idea of the promise it already offers us in our fight with sickness and suffering.

As we have previously said, even diligent repertory work may to some extent cramp our style. It can never supersede Materia Medica, to which it is merely, and only up to a point, an INDEX ; and for this reason, that it is impossible that all drugs, not only those of daily use and utility, but those of only occasional need, should be equally well represented in any repertory that it would be possible to handle, far less to compile.

But most of the known drugs of unique and definite action do get a mention, if only in striking black type in some solitary rubric, and when we see an unfamiliar black type drug standing for the symptom or condition for which we are hunting, we shall do well to turn it up in Materia Medica, to see whether it does not *in toto* fit the case.

But PHOSPHORUS is not a drug of unproved, or unrepresented symptoms : on the contrary it is one of the best proved and recorded of drugs, a polycrest—a drug of many uses. In Allen's *Encyclopedia* it has no less than 3,920 recorded symptoms, each with its tiny reference number that refers to the beginning of the *Phosphorus* section, where, not only the authority for every single symptom is to be found, but how it occurred, whether in a child who had sucked matches (in the good old days when matches were anything but " safety "), or to workmen in match factories here or abroad, or to persons who ended their lives horribly, with rat poison, or again to the provers of more or less potentized *Phosphorus* from Hahnemann down ; and here the very potency that evoked the symptoms is given.

The Homœopathic Materia Medica is no fancy compilation, no haphazard collection of questionable drug symptoms. It is all so orderly, so carefully investigated, so tersely set forth, so scientific. One can only marvel at the enormous labour of the men who with patient purpose built up for us such a veritable temple of healing—not only Hahnemann and his band of provers, mostly doctors, but Lippe, Hering, Dudgeon, Hughes, Carrol Dunham, and all the rest down to Kent, who have made our work not only comparatively easy but safe, and have bequeathed to humanity a science—so unique and ordered, so simple, and accessible—and so practical that "the wayfaring men, though fools, may not err therein "

Phosphorus, then, is among our best-proved—our most constantly useful drugs, and besides this, a remedy of very definite characteristic symptoms. For practical purposes of prescribing, it may be useful to compare and to contrast it with *Sepia* and *Natrum mur.*, because *Sepia* (cuttle-fish ink) must get some of its symptoms from the phosphorus and some from the salt that go towards its make-up. But, as with *Ferrum, Pulsatilla* and *Kali sul.* with *Calcarea, Calc. phos.* and *Calc. sulph.*, or with *Colocynth, Elaterium* and *Mag. phos.*, even when certain chemical substances are common to their elaborate make-up, and though some of the symptoms *must* resemble one another, the totality is not the same, and *one remedy will not do for another.*

Phosphorus, in its poisonings and provings, and in the conditions it can cure, is markedly INDIFFERENT (*Sepia*; and *Natrum mur.* less so) : is indifferent to relations and loved ones (*Sepia*). Is apathetic : answers slowly, has a great sense of fatigue with disinclination to work. It is a great headache medicine, with *Natrum mur.* and *Sepia.* But the head pains of *Phos.* are worse in a warm room and from heat, and better from cold applications, quite unlike *Sepia*.

Phosphorus is sympathetic, craves company, and touch, and rubbing, and help. *Sepia* and *Natrum mur.* are better alone, and *Sepia* " only wants to get away and be quiet ". And *Sepia* and *Natrum mur.* hate, or are irritated by, sympathy—can't stand it—weep. *Natrum mur.* and *Phos.* crave salt : not so *Sepia* : while *Sepia* and *Natrum mur.* are recorded as loathing fat, which is not the case with *Phos. Phos.* and *Sepia* are chilly drugs, i.e. suit chilly persons, while *Natrum mur.* is one of the drugs recorded as being better when cold. Again, it is *Phos.* and *Sepia* that fear thunder, and suffer in a thunderstorm—or even on approach of thunder—and so on.

Sympathetic	Phos.	—	—
Hates sympathy	—	Nat. mur.	Sep.
Wants company	Phos.	—	—
Better alone	—	Nat. mur.	Sep.
Craves salt	Phos.	Nat. mur.	—
Loathes fat	—	Nat. mur.	Sep.
Worse cold	Phos.	—	Sep.
Chilly, but better cold	—	Nat. mur.	—
Fear thunder	Phos.	—	Sep.

Groupings of symptoms with contrasts and likenesses are a great helps to rapid and correct prescribing.

HAHNEMANN tells us in regard to *Phosphorus* that it acts most beneficially in persons who suffer from chronic loose stools and diarrhœa. He also draws attention to the favourable reaction of the *Phos.* patient to mesmerism. *Phos.* is one of the drugs that loves to be rubbed.

Hahnemann also uses *Phosphorus* to prove that potentized medicines "are no longer subject to chemical laws". We all know that phosphorus when exposed to air oxidizes : that indeed when dissolved in disulphide of carbon, and deposited in finest subdivision as the latter evaporates, it spontaneously combusts. This is supposed by some to have been the ancient "Greek fire", used for incendiary purposes, and more recently, one imagines, by militant suffragettes, when, to annoy, they burnt the letters in pillar boxes. And yet, as Hahnemann points out, a powder of *Phos.* in highest potency may remain for years in its paper in a desk, without losing its medicinal properties, or even changing them for those of Phosphoric acid. He gives other instances also to show that "A remedy which has been elevated to the highest potency . . . is no longer subject to the laws of neutralization." If this were not the case how could we carry about our little phials of medicated globules, secure in the knowledge that they would not interfere with one another, or neutralize one another, but would be always ready for use, and never fail us—provided they were correctly prescribed.

GUERNSEY, that man of " Key Notes to the Materia Medica ", says " *Phos.* is particularly adapted for the complaints of tall, thin persons having dark hair." He draws attention to the characteristic stool, long, slim, hard and dry, evacuated with great difficulty. He calls attention to the WEAK, EMPTY, or GONE SENSATION, felt in the whole abdomen, especially when accompanied with a burning sensation between the shoulder blades. And a striking stomach symptom, when cold drinks are tolerated till they become warm in the stomach, when they are vomited. (Opp. to *Ars.* *Ars.* has burning pain in stomach, relieved by hot drinks. With *Phos.* the burning pain is relieved by cold.) Also, he emphasizes the hard, dry, tight cough, which racks the patient, and the saltish sputum.

To *Lach.* belongs the worse on waking : worse from sleep : fear to go to sleep for the aggravation of symptoms. The exactly opposite belongs to *Phos.* and *Sepia* : they have great relief from sleep, even a short sleep : headaches cured by sleep.

" In *Phos.* wounds bleed very much, even if very small: wounds that appear to have healed break out again." *Phos.* is a bleeder, and bruises easily.

* * *

NASH paints his vivid little miniature of the *Phos.* patient, i.e. the person who needs *Phosphorus.*

" Tall, slender, narrow-chested, phthisical persons, delicate eyelashes, soft hair ; or nervous weak persons who like to be magnetized. Waxy, anæmic, jaundiced persons.

" Anxious ; universal restlessness, can't stand or sit still : worse in the dark, or when left alone, or before a thunderstorm.

" BURNINGS everywhere, mouth, stomach, intestines, anus, between scapulæ, intense, running up spine, palms of hands.

" Craves cold things, ice-cream which agrees, cold water, which may be vomited when it gets warm in stomach. Must eat often, or is faint. Gets up to eat in the night.

" Sinking, faint, empty feelings—everywhere.

" Diarrhœa, profuse, pouring out as from a hydrant ; with wide-open anus.

" Cough, worse lying on left side. . . . In lungs, right lower lobe most affected. Cough worse going from warm to cold room. Worse inhaling cold air " (*Rumex*), etc.

He says, " *Zincum* has fidgety feet, *Phos.* is fidgety all over."

He says, " *Phosphorus* is bound to bleed " and " *Phos.* attacks the bones in the form of necrosis." What about " phossy jaw " ?

GUERNSEY's typical *Phos.* is dark-haired : NASH has " tall, slender persons of sanguine temperament, fair skin, blonde or red hair, quick, lively, sensitive." Both are right.

Abnormal craving for salt (*Nat. mur.*, *Nit. a.*, *Arg. nit.*, but *Nat. mur.* craves salt with a loathing for fats. *Nit. a.* with a craving for fats, and *Arg. nit.* with a craving for sweets and sugar).

And now we will turn to KENT, that fine observer and great teacher, to help us to see *Phosphorus* in the patients that need the help of that remedy. We will merely run through his lecture on *Phosphorus*, just picking and choosing, and taking and leaving, as seems good.

" The complaints of *Phosphorus* are most likely to arise in the feeble constitutions—born sick, grown up slender, and grown too rapidly—persons emaciating, rapidly emaciating—who have the seeds of consumption fairly well laid." " Violent pulsations and palpitations : hæmorrhagic constitutions : small wounds bleed much bright blood. Hæmorrhages from all organs and tissues. Petechiæ and bruisings."

Phos. complaints are worse from cold and cold weather, better from heat and warm applications, except the complaints of head and stomach, which are ameliorated from cold.

In *Phos.* the symptoms of chest and limbs are relieved by heat, those of the stomach and head by cold. (It is such symptoms, contradictory in regard to the patient in general, and his parts in particular, that are of great value as pointers to the remedy that exhibits them.)

He gives the fears of *Phos.*, one of the hypersensitive remedies. " Fear something will happen : anxious at twilight : fear of thunderstorms : trembling : attacks of indigestion from fear. Fear in the evening : fear of death : fear of strange faces looking at him from the corner. Full of strange, insane imaginations."

Apathy, indifference, to friends and surroundings, even to his children (*Sepia*). Will not answer, or answers slowly, thinks slowly. Vertigo and staggering. Worse from mental exertion, from noise : worse in the dark : worse alone.

Phos. may come in for fatty degenerations, and for softening of the brain.

The deafness of *Phos.* is especially for the human voice.

Better for eating : better for sleeping. Nausea and vomiting from putting hands into hot water, from warm room, from taking warm things into stomach. Regurgitation of mouthfuls of food are very characteristic of *Phos.* " *Phos.* is the surgeon's friend— the great remedy for vomiting after chloroform."

ALLEN (*Keynotes*) gives a curious *Phos.* symptom during pregnancy. She is unable to drink water. The sight of water makes her vomit : must close her eyes while bathing.

He says the perspiration of *Phos.* smells of sulphur.

And, remember, *Phos.* has not only burnings in stomach, etc., but also burning in lungs. A symptom that might be helpful in some cases of pneumonia.

Phos. affects the liver (one remembers the acute yellow atrophy of phosphorus poisoning) and is one of the remedies of hepatitis and jaundice (*Chel.*). In some of its symptoms *Phos.* reminds one of *Crotalus hor.*, rattle-snake poison.

Phosphorus affects all the organs and tissues, but its great spheres of action, for hurting and for curing, are lungs and bone— and liver. We will give a selection of the black letter symptoms of *Phos.*—somewhat condensed. They afford a key to its most useful possibilities, and to the organs it most markedly affects.

By the way, in regard to the relation of *Phosphorus* to hæmorrhages. . . . One has seen a case of cancer of tongue where pretty severe bleeding stopped quickly after a dose of *Phos.* 200 and did not recur. On the other hand we are warned that it is dangerous to give *Phos.* in high potencies to persons with advanced phthisis, as it may start a hæmorrhage that may endanger life. Here keep to the lower potencies, 12 or 30.

One remembers a youngish woman suffering from purpura hæmorrhagica. She had numerous big blood blisters, and bruises. She had been warned that she must not become pregnant, and she *was* pregnant. *Phos.* cured the condition, and she went through a normal confinement.

A SELECTION OF THE BLACK LETTER SYMPTOMS OF PHOSPHORUS

Respiration very difficult.
Great apathy : unwilling to talk.
Answers slowly and sluggishly.
Fatigue, disinclination to work, without cause.
Disinclination to study, or work, or converse, or think.
Slow ideas.
Vertigo : as soon as he made any effort to rise, the vertigo returned (Bry.).
Could see better when pupils were dilated by shading the eyes.
(*Phos.* has great photophobia.)
Nose-bleed. Nose swollen and dry.

During the prostration (of *Phos.* poisoning) *tuberculosis frequently develops ; at times also lobar pneumonia, terminating in gangrene of lung and pyæmia.* (Here one sees the great use of *Phos.* in severe pneumonias.)

Vomiting of food. Pressure, as from a hard substance, in stomach.
Emptiness and sensation of weakness in abdomen.
Diarrhœa. Evacuations as if involuntary the moment anything entered the rectum. Stool grey—whitish grey.
Menses earlier and scantier.

Rawness larynx and trachea, with frequent hacking cough and hawking.
With suffocative pressure in upper part of chest.
Voice rough—husky—can hardly speak above a whisper.

Cough with oppression of chest.
Violent dry cough when reading aloud.

Frequent dry cough, with slight dullness in right lower portion posteriorly, with diminished respiratory murmurs and fine vesicular râles. (Both lungs, especially right side.)

Tenacious, purulent mucus.

Violent oppression of chest.

Cough from constant tickling in throat. Cough with difficult respiration.

Bloody expectoration, with mucus.

Bloody expectoration from the lungs.

Mucous râles both lungs, more noticeable in lower lobes.

Respiration anxious, panting, oppressed. Very laboured.

Difficult. Respiration is impeded by rapid walking.

Great dyspnœa.

Tubercles of the lungs develop, with hectic fever.

Great oppression of chest, so that the patient, during attack of cough, must sit up in bed, when she experiences great pain, with a constrictive sensation under sternum.

Heaviness of the chest, as if a weight were lying on it.

Distressing anxiety and pressure in chest amounting to real suffocation, so that deep inspiration was difficult, but not impossible.

(If *Phos.* can cause all this, what wonder that it is one of our greatest remedies for pneumonias, and phthisis.)

Anxiety about heart and a peculiar sensation of hunger, somewhat relieved by eating, distressing her even in bed.

Violent palpitation.

Burning pain between scapulæ.

The spinous processes of the dorsal vertebræ between the scapulæ became extremely sensitive to pressure.

Weakness of all limbs.

" Fingers all thumbs."

Extensive gangrenous periostitis of tibia, with severe febrile disturbance, periosteum peeled off from a large area upwards, as far as knee-joint ; the bone was rough.

Emaciation.

Lay constantly on the right side. He lay only on the right side at night.

Mucous membranes pale.

The blood from the hæmorrhages was very fluid and difficult to coagulate.

Sense of suffocation.

Small wounds bleed very much.

Lax muscular system.
Great weariness.   Weakness.   Weak and oppressed.   Weak and prostrate.   Excessive exhaustion.
Heaviness of whole body.
Lying on left side causes anxiety.
Ulcers bleed.
Constant sleepiness.   Great sleepiness, even by day.
Cannot fall asleep before midnight.
Flushed cheeks (in fever) especially the left one.
Evening chilliness.
Cold knees constantly, at night, in bed.
Heat at night without thirst.
Febrile heat and sweat at night with ravenous hunger.
Profuse perspiration over whole body.
Profuse sweats on slight exertion.
Exhausting profuse sweats every morning.
Perspiration in the morning in bed—with feeling of anxiety.

" *Of one hundred and seventy workers in match factories (mostly boys) one hundred and twenty were attacked with typhus, often complicated with pneumonia and bronchitis, that often developed into consumption* " (*Russian Med. Zeit.*, 1850).

PHYTOLACCA DECANDRA

(*Poke-weed*)

IT is always a red-letter day when one makes friends with a new drug. Instead of being merely a bowing acquaintance—not much more than a name, one suddenly discovers a new Power, always at hand, opportunely suggesting itself for the precise help it can afford in appropriate cases. And it is in order to act as an Introducer, or at least a Remembrancer between Drug and Doctor that these " pictures " are penned.

Have you not noticed that in any crowd (and our Homœopathic Materia Medica is, in all conscience, a dense crowd !) there are certain persons—and drugs—which catch from the first our attention and assert themselves vividly. As on board ship, from the moment of embarking there are persons who rivet attention and get watched, whether with approval or disapproval, throughout the voyage. One comes to know what they will say and do on all occasions, though one may never care to make their acquaintance. On the other hand, on the very last day of the voyage one may discover a stranger, never noticed before, though a fellow-voyager for weeks. So with drugs : quite a number of them—the majority—are to us merely a name and no more : when, lo ! presto ! they turn out to possess undreamed of characteristics and possibilities. . . . Some one once said, on the last day of a voyage, "Why did I waste this whole voyage? Why did we not make friends before ? " Thus with drugs, " Why did I not make friends with you years ago ? You would have helped me with that case and this, where, not knowing you, I miserably failed."

For drug-friendship also one needs to recognize character and possibilities, to be able to rely on reactions and response.

After which disquisition let us proceed to the study of PHYTOLACCA, on whose magnificent powers one has, perhaps, never drawn sufficiently in difficult conditions, *acute and urgent* as well as *chronic*. For *Phytolacca* fills a late but unique niche in the Temple of Hahnemann.

Phytolacca is one of our newer, very powerful and promptly-acting remedies.

We get the most useful data in regard to this drug from Hale's *New Remedies*. Like *Baptisia, Gelsemium, Caulophyllum* (Squaw-root) and others it comes to us from America, from domestic or native practice—but rendered useful on lines of precise indications, by provings.

Hale calls it " one of our most valuable and powerful indigenous remedies". But, he says, " until subjected to scientific experimentation by our school and its effects on the healthy discovered by means of provings, but little was known concerning its range of curative powers."

But *Phytolacca* is still in need of further provings, to complete its drug picture.

Hale says it has been used especially in chronic diseases, rheumatism—venereal disease—some severe cutaneous diseases . . . " but its curative powers are not limited to chronic diseases. It has proven one of our best remedies in many acute affections of the severest character."

For instance, one doctor, says Hale, " reported prompt and curative effects in diphtheria from a tincture made from the leaves gathered late in Autumn." While recently the prompt cure of a case of diphtheria *with Phytolacca symptoms*, endowed in perpetuity a bed in the London Homœopathic Hospital.

The ashes of *Phytolacca* are said to contain over 50 per cent. of caustic potash, which accounts for some of its drug relationships.

The officinal parts of the plant are the *roots—leaves—*and *berries.*

We are told that " Birds which feed on the berries lose all their adipose tissue ", and a tincture of the berries has been used for purposes of " slimming" and (?) as a remedy for fatty tumours.

Poisoning by the berries has caused " pinching agony in the stomach with nausea and violent vomiting, followed by purging and pain, when any pressure on the stomach extorted cries. There was also dimness of vision : the tongue was coated white : there were spasmodic jerkings of arms and legs : and *sore throat*, the fauces *congested and dark-coloured*, the throat dry, and tonsils a little swollen."

Hale further says, " it affects the *nervous system* powerfully, also the *fibrous* and *osseous tissues*."

Again—" The sphere of action of *Phytolacca* includes skin, mucous membranes, fibrous tissues, the periosteum, and the cerebro-spinal nerve centres."

" In its action on the skin it resembles *Arsenicum* and *Mercury* " (Kent says it should be called " *vegetable Mercury* "), " and it has cured psoriasis, pityriasis, tinea capitis, lupous and squamous eruptions in general "—i.e. with *Phytolacca* symptoms, which we will endeavour to give later on.

In the provings of *Phytolacca* we find, " A very peculiar tension and pressure in the parotids " ; which may be an important pointer to the use of the drug—even in cases of chronic rheumatism.

For among the cases of cured rheumatism which he recounts is a most interesting and suggestive one of rheumatism of joints with enlargement of the parotid and submaxillary glands, where there was " rapid subsidence of the glandular tumours also ". One gathers that *Phytolacca* might be more useful in the cases with peri-articular involvement than in the cases with extensive bony joint-changes.

But perhaps *Phytolacca* is best known for its amazing affinity for the MAMMARY GLANDS—whether for evil or good. For in medicine it is only the evil doers among drugs that can be trusted to cure, and, even so, only the precise evils that they can cause, in locality—tissue—and conditions of aggravation and amelioration. Hence the minutely-recorded provings of Homœopathy.

In the provings we find " Inflammation, swelling and suppuration of the mammæ." And KENT says, and this is so important that we will quote it in full—

" It seems that the whole of the remedy centres in the *mammary glands.* Soreness and lumps in the breasts from each cold, damp spell : becomes chilled and a sore breast results ; sore breast in connection with the menses ; a nursing woman is exposed to cold, and the breasts inflame and the milk becomes stringy and hangs down from the nipple ; coagulated milk. This comes out in the proving, but poke root has been extensively used by cattle raisers when the cows' milk became thick and there were lumps in the bag, and when the condition was brought on from the cow standing out in the rain.

" Almost any excitement centres in the mammary gland ; fear or an accident ; lumps form, pains, heat, swelling, tumefaction, even violent inflammation and suppuration. *No other remedy in the Materia Medica centres so in the mammary gland.* . . . If every tribulation makes the glands sore in a nursing woman, give her *Phytolacca.* When a mother says she has no milk, or that the milk is scanty, thick, unhealthy ; dries up soon ; *Phytolacca* becomes then a constitutional remedy if there are no contraindicating symptoms. A bloody watery discharge which continued five years after weaning the infant, was cured by *Phytolacca.* The breast is so sore that, when she nurses the child, she almost goes into spasms, with the pain extending down the back and limbs and all over the body."

As Kent says, in cows it has a big reputation for " caking " of the udders : for such cases as this, " swollen indurated udders intensely hot, painful and sensitive, where not a drop of milk could be drawn : here in a few hours the milk could be drawn, the gland softened and recovery was complete." (By the way, I was told the other day of a case on our farm. One of the cows was getting, every few weeks, attacks of stringy milk. This absolutely stopped after a dose of *Phytolacca*.)

But it is not only in early inflammatory troubles of the mammæ that *Phytolacca* is indicated and efficient. It has
" Nipples sore and fissured.

Pain starts from nipple and radiates all over body.

Breast feels like a brick, lumpy and nodular.

Breast stony-hard, painful. Caked breasts.

Mammary abscess : pus.

Large fistulous, gaping angry ulcers, discharging a watery, fetid pus.

Pain is unbearable. Irritable. Restless. Indifferent to life : or death : sure she will die."

(BORLAND, *Homœopathy for Mother and Infant*.)

Kent tells us that *Phytolacca* is a very imperfectly proved remedy, but that it has some striking features ; and that much of what he gives is from clinical experience.

And now we will give some of the distinguishing modalities of *Phytolacca*, so that one may be able to prescribe with assurance, and leave it alone where another remedy better fills the picture.

Phytolacca has :—Aggravation at night : on cold days : in cold damp weather ; in a cold room. Kent gives also worse from heat of bed, "so that there is a controversy between heat and cold " : and in diphtheria the throat is worse from hot drinks. Exposure to cold damp weather causes or aggravates the cough, the pains of intercostal, abdominal and lumbar muscles, the stiff neck, the rheumatism generally, and the pains in joints.

Pains like electric shocks—shoot, lancinate, rapidly shift : worse motion : worse night : with the *Rhus* "desire to move but worse motion ".

In SORE THROATS, where one has most used *Phytolacca*, the fauces and pharynx look dry, and congested, and of a dark-red colour, utterly different from the smooth bright-red swelling of *Belladonna*. The pharynx is dry, rough, " feels like a cavern ", or "throat feels full, as if choked". Hot feeling, as if a ball of red-hot iron had lodged in pharynx. Deglutition is painful, difficult : and with every attempt excruciating pain shoots through the ears. There may even be regurgitation from the nostrils ; inability to swallow even water—this almost impossible because the throat feels so rough and dry.

Then ulceration of mouth and throat : follicular sore throat : patches in throat : even diphtheria with these symptoms, i.e. the blueness, the dryness, the pain (root of tongue and throat) shooting into ears : the worse for hot drinks. All worse for cold, except the throat symptoms, which are worse for hot drinks.

Curious symptoms—not only may the throat feel " like an empty cavern ", but the chest may also feel " like a big empty cask ".

Among the symptoms of *Phytolacca* one finds, in a poisoning case, " Extremities stiff, hands clenched, feet extended, toes flexed, teeth clenched, lips everted, firm, chin drawn on sternum, opisthotonos, tetanic convulsions."

FARRINGTON (*Comparative Materia Medica*) says, " *Camphor* and *Phytolacca* are very similar to *Strychnia* in tetanic spasms. Both of these have showing of the teeth from drawing up of the corners of the mouth. *Camphor* is indicated in tetanus with the ever-present deathly coldness."

Phytolacca has been found useful in scirrhus, in cancer of lips, and in " cancerous ill-conditioned ulcers of face ". Punched-out ulcers (*Kali bich.*).

The periosteal pains (tibia) remind one of *Asaf., Dros., Lach.*

NASH draws attention to a queer symptom " that has been of great value to me : ' Irresistible inclination to bite the teeth or gums together.' On this indication I have often relieved the complaints of various kinds incident to the period of dentition.

" I once had a case that was sent up to the country from New York City. The child had been sick a long time with cholera infantum (entero-colitis) and its physicians said it must leave the city or die. But country air and change of diet brought no relief. The little fellow was greatly emaciated, having frequent loose stools of dark brown colour, mixed with slime or mucus of the same colour. After trying various remedies I discovered that the child wanted to bite its gums together, or to bite on everything that it could get into its mouth, and the mother then told me that this had been the case all through its sickness. *Phytolacca* produced immediate relief of the symptoms and rapid recovery followed. I have since verified this symptom several times."

Phytolacca has also a great reputation for stiff neck, so here is a little recent personal experience which suggested *Phytolacca* as our Drug Picture.

Of course one knew the wonderful action of *Phytolacca* on the mammary gland, and had again and again found it rapidly curative for acute, dull, blue-red throats, with the pillars of the fauces congested and stiff, and the throat distressingly painful, even, in one case, with the sides of the neck also swollen, sore, and stiff. But—*rheumatism*? It was always staring at one from text-books, and one felt that it would be well to look up its modalities here, in order to secure one more trusty weapon against this haunter of out-patient rooms : easily, with difficulty, or not, cured . . . which last is disgraceful for the homœopathic prescriber. But of course the cases vary. The patient comes in with a ready-made diagnosis of rheumatism, or more often the popular " neuritis ", which in many cases yields to a little manipulation—i.e. when the sciatica or pain is due to a subluxation. In some cases one has seen, under careful prescribing, severe and long-standing cases of rheumatoid arthritis improve beyond what would have seemed possible : in some NOT : which is vexatious.

Well, this personal experience was merely a " stiff neck ", but a real bad one, in which the whole of the trapezius was involved, and its attachments and actions beautifully demonstrated. For the pain, only *in* movement, read the Ancient Mariner :—

" Forthwith this frame of mine was wrenched

" With a woeful agony,

" Which forced me " [to remain at rest]

" And then it left me free."

Bry. (worse for movement), *Rhus* (worse on first movement, and with its reputation for stiff necks), and *Cimicif.* had been useless. It was as much as one could endure to slither down into bed ; the trapezius refused any sideways support to head without sharp protest ; and to wake in the night, and slightly turn the head, was an excruciating experience. One wondered how it would be possible to get up ! Next day, "What *is* that remedy ? " and Allen's Keynotes were consulted. " Ah ! here it is ! '*Phytolacca* occupies a middle place between *Rhus* and *Bry.*, and cures when these fail, though apparently well-indicated.' " And it did !—and oh, the joy, that night, to be able to lie down, and to move the head, and lift the head and turn over with never a twinge. By the way, not only was movement affecting the muscle so painful, but cold and draught were unbearable . . . and there was a slight temperature, and one was feeling *ill*.

That experience clinched one's friendship with Poke-weed, and is only recounted that it may appeal to, and be remembered, for future triumphs, by YOU.

BLACK LETTER SYMPTOMS

When rising from bed feels faint. (Opium.)

Painful pressure on forehead and upper part of both eyes.

Disposition to bite teeth together.

THROAT *sore ; the isthmus congested and of a dark red colour ; dryness of throat, with some swelling of tonsils.*

Diphtheria ; sick and dizzy when trying to sit up ; frontal headache ; pains shooting from throat into ears, especially on trying to swallow ; face flushed ; tongue much coated, protruded ; thickly coated at back, fiery red at tip, breath fetid, putrid ; vomiting, difficulty of swallowing ; tonsils swollen, covered with membrane, first upon left three or four patches, tonsils, uvula, and back part of throat covered with ash-coloured exudation ; tonsils covered with dirty white pseudo membrane ; small white or yellow spots on tonsils coalesce and form patches of membrane ; membrane has appearance of dirty wash-leather ; exudation pearly or greyish white ; great thirst ; < from hot drinks ; dyspnœa ; ropy, offensive mucus lining mouth and throat ; glands of neck very tender ; pain in neck and back, body sore as if bruised, groans with pain, especially when trying to move or turn in bed ; aching limbs ; great prostration ; violent chill, soon followed by high fever ; fever without chill ; pulse 120, 140, *weak ; rash on skin ; remarkably nervous phenomena ; consecutive paralysis ; leaves vision impaired, hearing dull ; in* ·*cold weather generally epidemic ; usually of catarrhal or rheumatic origin, brought on by exposure to damp and cold atmosphere or sleeping in damp, ill-ventilated rooms.*

ABSCESSES *or fistulous ulcers of mammœ.*

MAMMARY GLAND *full of hard, painful nodosities.*

Breast shows an early tendency to cake ; especially useful when suppuration is inevitable ; when child nurses pain goes from nipple all over body.

Caked breasts ; nipples cracked and excoriated.

Barber's itch (local application of tincture).

Ringworm : herpes circinatus.

Squamous eruptions, pityriasis ; psoriasis.

PICRIC ACID

Picric acid has taken its place as perhaps the greatest remedy of all for BRAIN FAG.

One of its queerest symptoms, is that *the least study causes burning along the spine.* Other remedies noted as having burnings of back or spine are *Arsenicum, Phosphorus, Lycopodium,* and *Zincum.* But, while the burning spine of *Ars.* is not qualified, except that the burnings of *Ars.* generally are relieved by heat, the *Lyc.* burnings are chiefly between the scapulæ (as are those of PHOS. and KALI BIC.) : but those of *Phos.* throb, and want to be rubbed. Those of *Picric acid,* only, are caused by mental exertion. *Phos.,* in poisonings, is like *Picric acid* in causing fatty degenerations ; *Phos.,* especially of liver : *Picric acid* especially of brain and spinal cord. Everything in *Picric acid* is worse from study, its great characteristic ; this applies not only to the pains of spine, but also those of joints. One may mention, while about it, that the spider poison *Theridian,* stands in black type for burning in lumbar region ; but *Theridian* is distinguished by extreme sensitiveness to noise and touch.

Picric acid was discovered by a doctor of observation and application, who noticed that the burns of *Picric acid* are painless : and its chief use has been as a dressing for burns. (*Urt., Canth.*)

We have always associated *Picric acid* with *Phosphoric acid* : their uses being so similar that one would wonder sometimes which to employ. Let us study, once for all, their distinctions, in order to prescribe one or other with a maximum of good result.

Phos. acid. Weakness and debility. *Slowness : apathy.*

Picric acid. Weak ; tired ; heavy, mind and body. Easy prostration.

Phos. acid. Affects especially MIND ; nerves ; spine, with paralytic weakness ; bones.

Picric acid. BRAIN ; spine ; nerves ; kidneys.

Both affect sexual organs : *Phos. acid* with weakness ; *Picric acid* with irritation.

Phos. acid is worse from fevers ; loss of fluids ; sexual excesses ; fatigue.

Picric acid. Worse exertion, physical or MENTAL ; wet weather.

Phos. acid is better from warmth ; short sleep ; stool.

Picric acid is better from rest, cold air, cold water ; the sun ; bandaging.

No two drugs are alike in their action on organs, tissues and, especially on mentality, however much they may seem to be required in like conditions. And here, in the matter of exhaustion and debility, there are quite a number of essentially differing drugs to choose from ; having regard, naturally, to the cause of the trouble, emotional, mental, physical ; so we are giving in this number some suggestive remedies with indications.

Patients are apt to demand a " tonic ". The only real tonic, remember, is the curative drug of like symptoms ; but taking into account, as we are finding more and more, the latent dyscrasia of a long-past acute sickness, which must be combated by its own remedy, never hitherto been used to cure.

Another use of *Picric acid* is for boils in the external ear. Here one thinks also of Merc. and Sulph. But recently in a bad case of recurrent boils in the external auditory meatus, with terrible, incapacitating pain, *Morbillinum* cleared them up ; prescribed on a history of ancient measles.

Black Letter Symptoms

Neurasthenia.

Tired feeling, on least exertion, all over body ; with heaviness ; excessive languor ; no desire to talk or do anything ; indifferent to everything ; is obliged to lie down ; it seems difficult to move limbs ; great muscular debility ; readily winded by walking up hill ; inclined to day sleepiness ; poor appetite ; general sense of torpidity.

Some of the Italic, or Curious Symptoms

Brain fag.

Disinclined for mental or physical work ; desire to sit still without taking any interest in surroundings.

Headaches ; dull throbbing ; heavy feeling, or sharp pains.

Worse study, or movement of eyes. Better rest, open air, binding head tightly.

After every severe mental effort, intense throbbing headache ; worse base of brain ; often with congestion of spine, sexual excitement, etc.

Headaches of overworked business men ; or when grief or depressing emotions have resulted in nervous exhaustion. Seat of pain, occipito-cervical region.

Brain fag of literary or business people ; slightest excitement. mental exertion or overwork brings on headache.

Ears. Furuncular or circumscribed inflammation of meatus: Chronic or sub-acute forms of otitis.

Furuncles in external auditory meatus.

Terrible erections ; priapism ; satyriasis, etc.

Burning along spine, and very great weakness of legs and back ; soreness of all muscles and joints, *worse from study.*

Heat in lower part spine ; aching and dragging (lumbar).

Great weakness of legs, especially left, which trembles; heavy like lead ; lifted from floor with difficulty.

Great weakness, hips.

Extremities cold. And heavy.

After severe mental shock from a death, languor, exhaustion ; so tired ; wants to lie down and sleep all the time, which she would do if not roused.

Weariness, progressing from slight fatigue on motion to complete paralysis.

Paralysis from softening of the cord.

Tingling of lips ; crawling as of ants over surface of head.

Pains worse wet weather ; better cold air and cold water.

Played out feeling of whole body.

Small furuncles in any part of body, especially in ears.

Coldness : of genitals ; down back ; of feet.

Restorative of a wasted and worn-out system.

In progressive, pernicious anæmia.

In spinal sclerosis.

PLATINUM

Platinum, or *Platina,* as some authors prefer to call it, is a great Black Letter medicine : by which we mean one which has repeatedly vindicated its place in our Pharmacopœa by causing (in provings) and by curing (in homœopathic preparation) diverse maladies, especially mental, or those connected with perverted mentality—such mentalities, moreover, as make life unbearable for the unfortunates doomed to contact with *Platina.*

Platinum wounds and bruises ; not, indeed, in the violent and malicious sense of *Nux* and *Hepar,* but by the assumption of superiority : the hurtful, pharasaical attitude that despises others, and goes about thanking God that he (or *she*) is not as other men are.

The curious thing is that, with *Platina,* this mental subconsciousness extends outwards into the physical sensorium ; so that *Platina* not only secretly dislikes her children, as too small, too insignificant ; but she feels tall and stately herself, while her surroundings seem to grow small, and mean, and contemptible. As Kent says, " *Platinum* provings represent the woman's mind perverted." And he says that " the remedy is especially suited to hysterical women who have undergone fright, prolonged excitement ; or for the after-effects of disappointment, shock, or prolonged hæmorrhages." *Platinum* therefore not only inflicts, but cures mental traumatism.

What exactly is traumatism ? It is defined as " an abnormal condition of the body caused by external injury ". Again, as " a wound : or other injury produced by wounds ".

Therefore by Mental Traumatism we would express wounds of mind—heart—soul. The very phraseology we apply to these is borrowed from physical traumatism . . . " feeling very hurt" . . . " deeply wounded " . . . " cut to the heart ". And we speak of " lacerated feelings " ; of being " broken-hearted ", while Shakespeare reminds us how " *sharper than a serpent's tooth it is, To have a thankless child* ".

In order to suggest remedies to counter such injuries and the damage, acute or chronic, inflicted by them, we must match them with drugs which, in the provers, have produced sensitivity to just such traumatic agents.

A physical wound may be a stab, scratch, tear, an acute abrasion, or chronic damaging pressure which, persisted in, may conduce to even malignant ulceration. Mentally one may experience all these wounds. And here *Platinum, Staphisagria, Colocynth, Ignatia, Natrum muriaticum, Phosphoric acid* may be found to have been not only causative, but curative—according to symptoms.

One remembers a typical *Platina* mentality, where one longed to administer the drug to someone who returned from a trying plague time in India. She was hardly recognizable : her once pretty young face had grown strained and waspish ; while her whole conversation was painful to listen to, reiterating the marvels she had wrought in keeping that terror out of her compound. There was a terrible display of at once self-glorification and contempt of everyone else. Of course all that was merely how anxiety and worry had affected *her* because she was *Platinum*. It is times of stress that bring out in us the characteristerics of remedial drugs ; and much suffering for the individual and her surroundings can be averted, where someone with a knowledge of the Law of Similars and the chance to employ it, happens to be at hand.

The *Platinum* patient may be skating on very thin ice, from the point of view of sanity. One recalls several " borderline cases " cured by *Platinum*. One, especially, many years ago, where *Platinum* restored to sanity and great usefulness a woman whose sensations of local physical enlargement had created suspicions of poisoning against her husband and a woman friend, an inmate in their house. It was a pretty case, and to one's knowledge she remained normal for many years afterwards. It is very difficult—one has tried it more than once, and has even now a case in hand—to get the certified out of grevious captivity : and it is one of the joys of life to restore the certifiable to normality, and thus to save them from the stigma attached to residence in a mental hospital. *Platina* is one of the remedies that comes up for consideration in *paranoia*.

Platina is said to be the remedy of prim old maids. *Platina* is better walking in the open air, and in the sunshine (reverse of *Natrum muriaticum*.) Among the physical symptoms, menstruation is very profuse. Intensely sensitive genitalia may lead one to the curative drug, *Platinum*, in which this symptom is very marked and characteristic.

The sensations and pains of *Platinum* are very suggestive, as regards the employment of the remedy. The patient may feel constricted, as if bandaged : numb and dead ; paralysed. She complains of trembling, numbness, crawling, cramping, shocks. Even the brain feels numb. There are also sensations of local coldness (here one remembers *Calcarea*).

A curious symptom, which one associates with *Plumbum*,

belongs also to *Platinum* : drawing pains in the naval, as if by a string, which causes a sensation of retraction. Kent says these are so much like *Plumbum* that *Platinum* has been used as an antidote. (*Plumbum* has " Navel seems to adhere to spine.")

* * *

Among other things, in regard to *Platinum*, GUERNSEY says : " Mental symptoms in general : amativeness ; state of madness ; hysteria. The patient is very haughty, looks with disdain upon everyone and everything. Sensations of dread and horror . . .

Menstruation : where the discharge is very abundant, thick and black like tar. . . .

Stool : discharged with difficulty ; seems to stick to anus and rectum like putty. . . .

Epistaxis with dark coagulated blood. . . Frequent changing colour of face. . . . Tape-worm, other symptoms agreeing.

BLACK LETTER SYMPTOMS

Illusions of fancy as if everything about her were very small, and all persons physically and mentally inferior, but she herself physically large and superior.

Arrogant, proud feeling.

Contemptuous, pitiful looking down on people usually venerated, with a kind of casting them off.

(She thought she had no place in the world, life was wearisome) but she had a great dread of death, which she believed near at hand.

Pride and overestimation of one's self : looking down with haughtiness on others.

The room seemed gloomy and unpleasant, with apprehensive and fretful mood.

A numb sensation in forehead, as if constricted.

Cramp-like drawing constriction in the head from time to time.

Tense, numb sensation in the zygomata and mastoid processes, as if the head were screwed together.

(Head-shocks) followed by a numb sensation, as if too tightly bound.

Crawling, like formication, on right temple, afterwards extending down along the lower jaw, with a feeling of coldness in it.

Headache gradually increasing till very severe, then decreasing as gradually.

Painful cramp-like sensation of numbness in the left malar bone.

Fermentation in the epigastric region.

Constipation : after lead poisoning ; while travelling ; frequent urging with expulsion of small portions after great straining, after failure of Nux.

Painful pressing downwards towards genitals, as during menstruation.

(Urging with scanty stool) with a painful sensation of weakness.

Voluptuous crawling in genitals and abdomen.
Painful sensitiveness and constant pressure in the mons veneris and genitals.
Emission of much clotted blood during first day of M.P.
Menses about fourteen days too early and very profuse.
Menses six days too early.

While sitting a sensation of numbness in coccyx.

Tightness of thighs as if too tightly wrapped.
Tremulous crawling and uneasiness in legs while sitting ; a sensation of numbness and rigidity.
Great numbness. Painful numb sensation, as from a blow, here and there.
The parts affected by cramp-like pain are painful to pressure, as if bruised.

Sensation of coldness, crawling and numbness in the whole right side of face. (In fever.)

Some Curious or Italic Symptoms

Indescribably happy especially in open air, so that she would embrace anything, and laugh at the saddest things.

Very restless, could remain nowhere ; sadness, so that the most joyful things distressed her.

Dislikes her children, calls them too little.

Any serious thought is terrifying.

Anxiety and trembling of hands with flushes of heat over whole body.

Deathly anxiety with trembling, oppressed breathing, violent palpitation.

Very peevish, would have beaten anyone without provocation.

Out of sorts with the whole world, everything seems too narrow.

Weeps with pains.

Physical symptoms disappear and mental symptoms appear, and *vice versa. The body suffers when the mind is cheerful ; and the body feels well when the mind is affected.*

It seems to her that she does not belong to her own family ; after a short absence everything seems entirely changed.

Disturbed state of mind ; religious, with taciturnity, haughtiness, voluptuousness and cruelty.

Mental disturbance after fright, grief or vexation.

Vertigo : she dare not move her eyes.

Feeling as if head were enlarged.

Sensation of coldness, crawling, numbness in eyes.

Sensation of water in forehead.

Numb feeling in brain.

Vertigo as if torn and pulled into threads.

Sensation of coldness in ears.

Coldness, crawling and numbness in whole right side of face.

Sensation as if tongue scalded.

Ravenous hunger and hasty eating, detests everything around him.

Painter's colic : umbilical pain goes through to back. He screams and tries to relieve pain, by trying all possible positions.

Ovaries inflamed, with burning pain in paroxysms.

Ovarian tumours and cysts.

Dreadful, excessive itching in uterus (in spinal irritation).

Indurated, prolapsed uterus : parts painfully sensitive to touch.

Painful sensitiveness with inward coldness of vulva.

*   *   *   *

CLARKE (*Dictionary*) explains that the original name of *Platinum* was *Platina*, from the Spanish meaning " like silver ", Hahnemann was the first to think of it as a medicine, and his proving (*Chronic Diseases*) is the basis of our knowledge of its action. One characteristic symptom, found alone or associated with other conditions, has led to many cures with *Plat.*—lost sense of proportion in both ocular and mental vision. Objects look small, and the patient thinks them small : this becomes pride and hauteur in the mental sphere, the patient (generally a woman), looks down on everything and everybody. . . . Another keynote is the occurrence of cramping pains and spasms, developing into convulsions. Another is the alternation of mental and physical symptoms. He says Nash cured an old case of insanity, where the mental symptoms alternated with pain the whole length of spine. He says, Jahr cured with *Plat.* a woman who had an inspiration to kill her child : and Jules Gaudy, a woman who was tormented with an almost irresistible impulse to kill her husband, whom she loved passionately, and with whom she was perfectly happy.

PLUMBUM

(*Lead*)

ONE very important indication for the use of *Plumbum* (we have
verified it) is *Hyperæsthesia with loss of power*. We got this tip
from *Nash* (*Leaders*). It may be well to quote. Nash writes:
" I cured one case of post-diphtheritic paralysis with it. It was
a very severe case in a middle-aged man. His lower limbs were
entirely paralysed, and there was at the same time a symptom
which I never met before, nor have I since, in such a case, viz.
excessive hyperæsthesia of the skin. He could not bear to be
touched anywhere, it hurt him so. After much hunting I found
this hyperæsthesia perfectly pictured in Allen's *Encyclopedia*,
and that, taken together with the paralysis, seemed to me good
reason for prescribing *Plumbum*, which I did in one dose of Fincke's
40m, with the result of bringing about rapid and continuous
improvement until a perfect cure was reached. . . . A repetition
was unnecessary."

We have already, somewhere, quoted a notable case, inspired
by Nash : but it will bear repeating. A strong, stoutish
woman of middle age, after a chill, developed a semi-paralytic
condition (one is writing from memory). She was admitted into
our hospital where, with the loss of power, hyperæsthesia was so
intense, that it was not only agony when her pulse was taken, but
that ceremony had to be omitted, because it gave her not only the
" ditherums ", as she expressed it, but her arm actually swelled
up. *Plumbum* restored her to active life, with normal sensation
and powers ; so much so that, during the Great War then waging,
she was able to get employment—writing—at the War Office.
For a long time afterwards, she used to come back for treatment, at
the least suggestion of recurrence—which never materialized. But
one never forgets that great indication for *Plumbum*, which Nash
discovered and emphasized, *Hyperæsthesia with loss of power*.

Another of its great indications is, *Emaciation of suffering parts*.
This would, of course, be at a later stage of the poisoning.

And yet another *Plumbum* feature : *Retraction of parts*. It has
not only the " boat-shaped abdomen ", where the sensation is,
the umbilicus drawn back to, or attached to the spine (*Plat.*), but,
with *Plumb.*, the abdomen is actually retracted ; hard, painful ;
and the patient may roll about on the ground, pressing the abdomen
with violence. The provings express it thus : " Navel seems to

adhere to the spine, and the pain also involves pectoral region."
. . . " Sensation as if abdominal walls were pulled inwards ; as
if abdomen and back were too close together." . . . " Excruciating, tearing pains, especially around navel, as if bowels were
twisted." . . . " Intense retraction of the integuments of
abdomen towards spine, and a hard, knotty feeling in the muscles
in various places over its surface." . . . " Violent colic ; abdomen
drawn in, as if by a string, to spine ;—better from rubbing or hard
pressure ; abdomen hard as a stone : anxiety, with cold sweat and
deathly faintness " . . . and so on. Such are some of the
features of " Painter's colic " and of lead poisoning.

Lead is a mighty and deep-acting poison, which causes
degeneration of all the tissues of the body. It interferes with the
blood corpuscles, with resulting anæmia. It affects nerves and
muscles, inducing cramps, indurations, softenings, wastings,
contractions :—" its phenomena being those of colic, paralysis,
arthralgia, and encephalopathy". And *Plumbum* is therefore a
powerful remedy, symptoms agreeing ; palliative even where
destruction has gone too far. Among other things, it has a
reputation for colic with paralysis of the lower extremities : incarcerated hernia ; intussusception with colic and fecal vomiting ;
strangulated hernia (only here one dare not wait too long on any
remedy, or on any attempt at replacement, lest nipped vessels of
the gut should have failed with their blood supply long enough to
have led to gangrene).

But other parts may also be retracted by *Plumbum*. As
we read of " intolerable pain, from spasms of rectum—a horrible
sense of constriction and spasmodic contraction ;—if the evacuation were not liquid, the torture was extreme. Anus violently
constricted and drawn up ".

Many of the symptoms of *Plumbum* are very similar to those
of *Platina*, which is the one other drug, so far as we know, that has
the *Plumbum* sensation of " drawing pains in the navel as if by a
string, which causes the sensation of retraction of the abdomen".
Platinum has been given as a remedy for painter's colic, because
of the similarity of its sensations and pains.

But in disposition the two drugs differ widely. Indifference,
depression, somnolence, melancholy are the characteristics of
Plumbum, with none of the arrogance, pride, and over-estimation
of self that call for *Platina*.

*　　　*　　　*

Of *Plumbum*, KENT points out, the general paralytic state of
this remedy. All activities of the body and the functions of the

organs are slowed down in pace. The nerves do not convey their messages with the usual lightning-like rapidity. The muscles are slow and sluggish. There is first paresis, then paralysis ; of parts first, and finally of the whole. . . . You will wonder what the patient is thinking about, when making up his mind to answer. Prick him, and you have to wait a second before he responds. *There is hyperæsthesia in the acute affections, but in the chronic, loss of sensation and ability to feel—anæsthesia of the skin.*

The skin withers : the painful part withers to the bone.

Slow, insidious, chronic conditions ; with no tendency to recover : progressive paralysis ; progressive muscular atrophy.

He gives a case of uræmic coma : in a doctor's wife. Catheter showed that there was no urine in the bladder : she had the pulling sensation at the navel. . . . In the middle of the night her husband came in great distress : she was pale as death, and breathing slowly : deeply comatose. " A single powder of *Plumbum* high was given, and she passed urine in a couple of hours, roused up, and never had such an attack again."

Such remedies are surely worth study and realization. Homœopathy is indeed a marvellous power. Get the right remedy and you can work seeming miracles—with, seemingly, nothing : —but miss the remedy, and you *have* nothing !

Kent also points out, in the mentality of *Plumbum*, a confirmed hysterical state ; with an inclination to deceive, to feign sickness : to exaggerate one's ills.

One is reminded of *Tarentula* when he says, " She would be in a hysterical condition for hours when anyone was looking at her. When she thought no one was near she would get up, walk about, look in the glass to see how handsome she was ; but when she heard a foot on the steps she would lie on the bed and appear to be unconscious. She would bear much pricking ; and you could scarcely tell she was breathing."

In colic the patient bends backwards. (*Diosc.* : reverse of *Colocynth.*) He points out the inclination of *Plumbum* to take strange attitudes and positions in bed.

Plumbum, he says, is *intensely emotional while the intellect is slowed down.*

* * *

HUGHES *Pharmacodynamics* says : The first symptoms of lead poisoning are *wrist-drop*, from paralysis of the extensor muscles of the forearm. More profound poisoning induces a kind of degeneration of all the tissues. The nerve centres are found indurated, or softened : headache, amaurosis, neuralgia, palsy, anaesthesia, epilepsy occur during life. The muscular tissue is wasted or contracted. The kidneys are small and granular. There is complete decay of the bodily and mental powers, with profound melancholia : and the impairment of nutrition shows itself in the anaemic and cachetic appearance, with a yellowish hue of the skin (*Icterus saturninus*).

He says, the abdominal phenomena of lead poisoning at once suggest the metal as a remedy for colic and constipation, occurring separately or together. " Indeed I know of no better instance of the truth of the law of similars than the beautiful action of *Plumbum* in such conditions. . . . We rely upon the medicine in any form of obstruction of the bowels that has not a mechanical cause, and in incarcerated and even strangulated hernia." He gives a striking case of Dr. Holland's. " The patient had been suffering from most agonizing abdominal spasms for two days, with vomiting and suppression of stool and urine. A grain of *Plumb. ac.* third decimal, was given, and in less than ten minutes the patient fell asleep, waking after many hours free from pain, and able to relieve his bowels of a mass of scybala. The next day he was well."

He says, " The association of colic with constipation, and of constipation with colic, always forms the special indication for *Plumbum* as a remedy for either. But the constipation may be quite painless : and a neuralgic enteralgia may be cured by it, where the bowels were regular enough. In such cases the sense of retraction in the abdomen, or the hard, tense condition observed by Bähr, may guide to its choice.

" The patient may resemble a walking skeleton : the muscles post mortem are wasted and very pale, with sometimes the appearance of white fibrous tissue." Here he mentions progressive muscular atrophy, and instances a patient, who presented the appearance of a living skeleton, where the presence of fibrillary contractions in the paralysed muscles led to the use of *Plumbum* . . . with results most gratifying. . . .

Hughes gives six aspects of lead poisoning. (1) the COLIC, to which we have drawn attention : " always relieved by pressure, and the more, the firmer this is made." (2) The PARALYSIS, beginning with wrist-drop. This is partial rather than general. He says it has been noted that muscles were paralysed, whose nerve supplied others that were not paralysed. There is always a marked atrophy of the affected muscles . . . sometimes this condition becomes so general that the patient resembles a walking skeleton. (3) The NEURALGIC and SPASMODIC pains : often lightning-like : suggesting the lightning pains of locomotor ataxy.

(4) The ENCEPHALOPATHY :—its cerebral symptoms :—sometimes uraemic, more commonly primary. They start with violent headache and amaurosis, then maniacal or melancholic conditions may supervene, but most frequently eclampsia : the convulsions are quite epileptiform in character, and coma or delirium may fill up their intervals. In regard to epilepsy Hughes says, " I agree with Bähr in ranking *Plumbum* with *Cuprum* as the remedy from which most is to be expected in confirmed cases of the disease."
(5) Its action on the URINARY ORGANS. There is increase of mucus in the urine, with irritation of the lining membrane of the bladder. *Plumbum* is claimed to have cured chronic affections of the urinary organs. Its action on the kidneys leads to the small, granular, contracted kidney which constitutes the most serious form of Bright's disease. During life, albuminuria is an evidence of the mischief being set up. (6) The AMAUROSES : " secondary to the renal mischief, or, apparently an optic neuritis, with its central scotoma."

* * *

Evidently, from the cases given, *Plumbum* may do its magnificent healing work whether prescribed in the single doses of high potency, or after the manner of the " low potency people ". It is *the remedy of similar symptoms that is imperative :* its exhibition is a matter to some extent of dispute. Both will work : but in our experience the highest potencies, when we dare to use them, are the greatest of miracle-workers. But an occasional contretemps has inspired one with a lively respect for what some would consider these fantastic nothingnesses. And it was Dr. H. C. Allen who was reported to have said, " Gentlemen, the potencies can kill."

* * *

Plumbum has, " Paralysis preceded by mental derangement, trembling, spasms, or shooting, darting, intense tearing pains in tracks of larger nerves ; the parts emaciate ; wrist drop, caused by apoplexy, sclerosis of brain, or muscular atrophy, alternating with colic ; after apoplexy rapid emaciation, atrophy and loss of sensation of affected part ; of arms, with pain, dryness, deathly paleness and coldness of hands.

* * *

DR. BOERICKE says of *Plumbum* : "The great drug for general sclerotic conditions. Lead paralysis is chiefly of extensors, forearm or upper limb, from centre to periphery, with partial anæsthesia or excessive hyperæsthesia, preceded by pain ; localized neuralgic pains ; neuritis. The blood, alimentary, and nervous systems are the special seats of action of *Plumbum*. Hæmatosis is interferred with, rapid reduction in number of red corpuscles ; hence pallor, icterus, anæmia. Constrictive sensation in internal organs."

BLACK LETTER SYMPTOMS

Slow of perception.

Loss of memory, so that while talking he was often unable to find the proper word.

Headache.

Complexion sallow. Sallow pale face.

Distinct blue line along the margins of gums. Dark blue line on the gums.

Gums pale, swollen ; show a lead-coloured line ; blue, purple or brown ; painful, with hard tubercles.

Breath fetid.

Constrictions of the throat.

Loss of appetite.

Nausea.

Vomiting. Frequent vomiting. Constant vomiting.

Vomiting of food.

Extremely violent pains in the umbilical region, that shoot to other parts of the abdomen, somewhat relieved by pressure.

The navel seems to adhere to the spine.

Violent colic.

Excessive pain in abdomen, radiating thence to all parts of the body.

Constipation : stools hard, lumpy, like sheeps' dung ; with urging and terrible pain from constriction or spasm of anus. . . .

Difficult micturition.

Urine albuminous.

Urine dark coloured and scanty, evacuated drop by drop.

Morbus Brightii ; contracted kidney.

Vaginismus.

Violent pains in the extremities : especially in the evening and night : especially in the muscular part of the thighs.

Neuralgic pains in the limbs.

The pains in the limbs are worse by paroxysms, which are so severe that he cries out.

Jerking, trembling, numbness of limbs.

Pains in the extremities.

Pains in the limbs aggravated at night.

Wrist-drop.

Very sharp neuralgic pains.

Extremely acute and paroxysmal pains.

Lightning-like pains in the lower limbs.

Emaciation.

Anæmia.

Convulsions.

Paralysis.

General prostration.

Lassitude.

Faintness.

Uneasiness.

Excessive hyperæsthesia.

Anæsthesia.

Arthralgia.

Pain in trunk and limbs.

Emaciation extreme, with anæmia and great weakness : of paralysed parts followed by swelling.

Muscular atrophy ; from sclerosis of spinal system.

Dry skin.

Yellow skin.

Sleeplessness (entire sleeplessness).

* * *

Some footnotes, *Allen's Eneyclopedia.*

"Microscopic examination of the brain showed granular fatty degeneration of the walls of the vessels and deposition of large quantities of amyloid corpuscles."

" The heart was fatty, the walls thicker and paler than normal. The capsule of the kidneys was found adherent to its substance : the kidney showed interstitial inflammation. The brain was softened."

Italics, or Queer, Noteworthy Symptoms

His delirium turned on the idea that his life was in danger from assassination or poisoning, and that everyone about him was a murderer.

As if something were working at top of head.

Eyelids as if paralysed.

A ball rises from throat into brain.

Eyes feel too large.

A plug in throat.

Everything weighted down.

As if abdominal walls pulled inwards : abdomen and back too close together.   As if abdomen were drawn to spine by a string. (*Plat.*).

A sensation in abdomen at night in bed, causes her to stretch violently for hours together.   Feels she must stretch in every direction : the will to do so alone cannot accomplish it ; as if from paralysis.

Sphincter ani feels drawn in.

As if not room enough in uterus for fœtus.   A bag not quite filled with fluid lay in bowels.

As if feet were made of wood.

Violent, loud motion of lower jaw and frightful grinding of teeth.

Paralysis of throat, with inability to swallow.

Sweet taste : gulping up of sweetish water.

Anæsthesia, or excessive hyperæsthesia.

Inclination to take the strangest attitudes and positions in bed. May be absolute absence of sweat.   Or cold sweat with pallor.

Fetid foot-sweat—on soles—smelling like old cheese.

*   *   *

Nash gives an interesting *Plumbum* case, which we will condense. Man, over seventy, was attacked with severe abdominal pain. Finally a large, hard swelling developed in the ileo-cæcal region, very sensitive to contact or to the least motion.   It began to assume a bluish colour, and on account of his age and extreme weakness it was thought that he must die.   In Raue's pathology, however, the indications for *Plumbum* were found, given as therapeutic hints for typhlitis.   It was administered in the 200th potency, which was followed by relief and perfect recovery.

PSORINUM

HAHNEMANN'S first " nosode ",—disease-product for the cure of disease.

Hahnemann's proving of *Psorinum* appears in *Stapf's Archiv*, 1833. He used the " sero-purulent matter contained in the scabies vesicle ". Some of the provings were the product of " *Psora sica* " (epidermoid efflorescence of pityriasis). (Hering's *Guiding Symptoms.*)

We say Hahnemann's *first* nosode advisedly, because evidence has been deduced from his writings that he had used others ; but " that their effects on the *healthy* organism had not yet been sufficiently ascertained " to justify their publication. He was most insistent on the provings, on healthy humans, of all drugs, before teaching or even suggesting their use on the sick.

But we will quote one passage (from *Chronic Diseases*, vol. 1, p. 195). Hahnemann had evidently been exercised in his mind as to whether disease products used for the cure of disease were *Isopathic* or *Homœopathic*—identical or similar. He decided, as we shall see, that by its preparation (triturations with milk-sugar, and then further potentization by repeated succussions, one minim to ninety-nine minims of alcohol each time), the material is no longer identical, but changed—" similar " only.

He says, " In the subsequent list of antipsoric remedies no *isopathic* remedies are mentioned, for the reason that their effects upon the healthy organism have not been sufficiently ascertained. Even the itch-miasm (psorin) in its various degrees of potency, comes under this objection. I call psorin a *homœopathic* anti-psoric, because if the preparation of psorin did not alter its nature to that of a homœopathic remedy it never could have any effect upon an organism tainted with that same identical virus. The psoric virus, by undergoing the processes of trituration and shaking, becomes just as much altered in its nature as gold does, the homœopathic preparations of which are not inert substances in the animal economy, but powerful acting agents.

" Psorin is a *similimum* of the itch virus. There is no inter-mediate degree between *idem* and *similimum* : in other words the thinking man sees that similimum is the medium between simile and idem. The only definite meaning which the terms isopathic and equalæ ' can convey, is that of similimum : they are not *idem*."

H. C. ALLEN, in his *Keynotes of Leading Remedies*, gives great prominence to *Psorinum*, and in his *Nosodes* gives sixty-four pages to this drug and its provings ; curiously enough, he fails to show, even by inverted commas, that the above quotation, with which he begins his list of provings, is from Hahnemann !

He emphasizes this, " *Psorinum should not be given for psora or psoric diathesis, but like every other remedy, upon a strict individualization—the totality of the symptoms—and then we realize its wonderful work.*"

In regard to its normalizing action on scalp and hair, Allen gives a curious case. A young man of dark complexion and brown hair had a " perfectly white " patch of hair and skin above the forehead. After *Psor.* hair and spot became natural colour.

And elswhere he quotes, " Whether derived from purest gold or purest filth, our gratitude for its excellent service forbids us to enquire or care."

* * *

CLARKE (*Dictionary*), says, " *Psorinum* has been proved entirely in the potencies, and I know of no more trustworthy proving in the Materia Medica." He gives a number of cases, showing its uses ; also cases where some of its symptoms have been evoked in patients under treatment by the drug.

His *Chief keynotes* are " *Lack of vital reaction*, prostration after acute disease ; depressed, hopeless ; night-sweats." He says, " Hopelessness, despair of perfect recovery, is part of the lack of reaction." " *Foulness* may be considered *its second keynote*," i.e. foulness of all discharges : as we shall see later on, from eruptions, from ears, from bowels ; and offensiveness of leucorrhœa, sweat, sputum, etc.

He points out some of its peculiar conditions, such as " Sick babies will not sleep day or night, but worry, fret, cry : or, good and play all day ; restless, troublesome, screaming all night." . . . " Feels unusually well before attack." . . . " Profuse sweat after acute diseases, with relief of all sufferings." He says, " *Psor.* has cured more cases of hay fever in my practice than any other remedy." Among the peculiar symptoms, to which he draws attention are, " Stupid in left half of head. As if brain would protrude : had not enough room in forehead. As if head separated from body. As if he heard with ears not his own. Teeth as if glued together. Hands and feet as if broken . . . *Psorinum* cannot bear the limbs to touch each other at night : or the weight of arms on chest." (*Lach.* on abdomen.)

* * *

GUERNSEY, *Keynotes*.—The symptoms of this drug are very closely allied to those of *Sulphur*. If the latter appears to be indicated, but fails to cure, study up *Psorinum*.

Dry, lustreless, rough head of hair. Eructations tasting like rotten eggs : stools (diarrhœic) smelling like rotten eggs. Debility remaining after acute diseases.

* * *

Now we will draw from the wisdom and knowledge of KENT ; condensing.

Psorinum is closely allied to *Sulphur*. He, also, dreads to be washed : looks dingy, dirty, foul, as if covered with dirt. Skin rough, cracks, bleeds ; rough and scaly. He cannot wash it clean. Always seems to have dirty hands. Skin complaints worse from bathing, and from warmth of bed. Itching when warm. (And yet *Psorinum* is the chilliest of mortals.) Rawness, itching, tingling, crawling, bleeding of skin.

In eczema, worse from warm applications, worse at night, worse from anything that will keep the air away. " This is the very opposite of the general *Psorinum* state, which is aggravated by the open air." (*The patient wants to get away from the open air ; " his skin needs it "*. It is these contradictory symptoms, contradictory as regards the patient and his parts, that make prescribing more easy : as in the chilly *Phos.* who wants ice for his suffering stomach, and icy cold drinks in plenty : or the typical *Ars.* who needs " blankets up to his chin, and his head out of the window ".) " The oozing of eruptions is offensive like carrion or decomposed meat : nauseating, sickening odour from the oozing fluid."

Offensiveness runs through *Psorinum*—stinking odours, fetid breath. Discharges and oozings—stool, perspiration, leucorrhœa, all abominably offensive. Stool, flatus, eructations smell like rotten eggs. *Psor.* is *offensive to sight and smell*.

And so through all the complaints of eyes, nose and other parts : discharges yellow green, horribly offensive.

" *Debility* : but worse in open air : can't breathe : wants to go home and lie down so that he can breathe. Wants a warm place to lie down and be let alone." Lies on his back, arms wide apart, thrown across bed, to relieve the breathing, in asthma, etc. Worse the nearer the arms are brought to the body.

In fevers the heat and sweat are intense : " covered with boiling sweat in fevers " : the heat as great as that of *Bell.*, but not the dry heat of *Bell.* : *hot steam* under the covers. (Or, as usual, the opposite. " In typhoids, after least exertion, sweats, and the sweat is cold.")

In regard to stool, Kent quotes, " In *Psorinum* we find the haste of *Sulphur*, the flatulence of *Olean.* and *Aloe*, and the difficulty of expelling a soft stool like *Alumina, China* and *Nux mosch.*"

Psorinum hates draughts : scalp cold : wears a fur cap in summer.

Mentally hopeless and sad : business will be a failure : has sinned away his day of grace : no joy in his family : these things are not for him !   Anxiety, to suicide : despair of recovery.

*   *   *

Psorinum, before treatment, is in no wise an ideal companion ; is not, like the Mr. Guppy made famous by Dickens," a nice young man for a small tea-party ".

One has not used *Psorinum* at all frequently, having, perhaps, failed to grasp its " inwardness " in other than *very* characteristic cases, where it has hit one in the eye, and refused to be missed. But one remembers just two or three striking instances of its employment.

A young girl, dying very rapidly of phthisis, came to out-patients years ago ; so offensive—breath a nightmare—that one was unable, almost, to breathe near her : sputum green and horribly fetid. *Psorinum* was prescribed, and we hurriedly got doors and windows open and a big draught to blow away her memory. Next time she appeared, there was nothing unpleasant to notice, the odour was gone.   What happened to her later, one cannot relate, she only appeared a few times and was seen no more.   That is the worst of the out-patient crowds.   They come and their condition and remedies are carefully studied and noted. Some of them continue to come ; some that one greets with an inward groan—like curses and chickens that come home to roost : while out of some of them great joy arises.   Or, again they cease to reappear, and others take their place : and it requires effort —a good deal—to follow them up later, when it would be most interesting and instructive to know what had happened.   One's best cases are often heard of only years later, when a new patient arrives with, " You cured Mrs. So-and-So, some ten years ago ; and now I have come to see if you can cure me too. I've got just the same that she had!"   In Hospital work, history repeats itself : " Where are the nine that have not returned to give thanks ? "   The ONE, is often a very precious and encouraging personage. But it is the case of Hahnemann's washer-woman, over again.   " So many weeks in great pain, and unable to work !

—*why* should the poor woman leave her job merely to tell the doctor that she is well ? "

Another *Psorinum* case, many years ago, was a wee boy, admitted into our Children's Ward with a T.B. abdomen and chest. The odour of that unfortunate—or, as it turned out, fortunate—child was so awful, one could hardly go near his bed. He got a dose of *Psor.* 30 and he was put out on the balcony for a few months ; and went out apparently well.

And yet another case, from early dispensary days, of a miserable, sickly little girl, with insufferably evil odour, and dry harsh skin—it was almost ichthyosis—who improved greatly on *Psorinum.* One quotes from memory : the cases are very long ago, and to look up the notes, not even knowing the names, would be a considerable task. But they may serve to impress on others also, two of the great characteristics of *Psorinum,—its insufferable mal-odour,* never to be forgotten—only to be compared to that of rotten eggs (and any one who has broken a rotten egg will realize how, having hurled it as far away as possible, one is impelled to flee in the opposite direction !) and the *harsh, dry skin,* which is, or may be, a great feature in the *Psorinum* picture.

Another drug of appalling odour is *Kreosotum.* A woman supposed to be dying of bronchitis (? bronchiectasis) came into hospital some years ago. It was almost impossible to go inside her screens—she was screened off because of the awful odour of breath and sputum. *Kreosotum* 200, not only banished the odour by the next day, but restored her to life, to the amazement of the then house physician. One has seen *Kreosotum* 200 also annihilative of the terrible odours that sometimes accompany cancer of cervix ; where, if it did nothing more, it made life more supportable for patient and her entourage.

* * *

BLACK LETTER SYMPTOMS

Anxious : full of fear : melancholic.
Very depressed, sad, suicidal thoughts.
Driven to despair by excessive itching.

Moist, suppurating, fetid, also dry eruptions on scalp.
Tinea capitis et faciei.

Discharge of fetid pus from ear.
Otorrhœa ; with headache ; thin, ichorus and horribly offensive, like rotten meat. Very offensive, purulent, with watery, stinking diarrhœa. Brown, offensive, from left ear, for almost four years.

Chronic cases following scarlet fever.

Humid soreness behind ears : scurfs on ears, and humid scurfs behind ear.

Swelled upper lip.

Tongue very dry.

Sensation of plug or lump in throat impeding hawking.

Great hunger.

Eructations tasting like rotten eggs.

Stool, dark-brown : very fluid, and foul-smelling.

Cough, with expectoration of green mucus, nearly like matter.

He perspires freely when walking :—profuse sweat with consequent debility.

Skin has a dirty, dingy look, as if patient never washed : in some places looks coarse, as if bathed in oil. Sebaceous glands secrete in excess.

Eczema behind ears, on scalp, in bends of elbows and armpits, accompanied by abscesses affecting bones.

Itch ; dry on arms and chest, most severe on finger joints ; followed by boils : inveterate cases with symptoms of tuberculosis, repeated outbreak of single pustules after main eruption gone. Suppressed eruptions.

Important, Characteristic Italic, or Peculiar Symptoms

Very irritable, easily angered ; always thinks of dying.

Great fear of death. Sad and joyless.

Greatest despondency, making his own life and those about him intolerable.

Religious melancholy. Despair of recovery.

Attacks of fear ; fear of fire, of being alone, of apoplexy, of becoming insane, etc.

Frontal headache, with sensation of weakness in forehead : not space enough in skull, as if everything were pushed out—on rising.

Better : for nose-bleed ; after washing and breakfast.

Fiery sparks before eyes : objects appear as if they were trembling, vibrating.

Discharge : from ears of reddish earwax, or fetid pus.

Herpes from temple, over ears to cheeks.

Right ear a mass of crusts and pus.

Looseness of teeth : so loose, feels they may fall out.

Thirst for beer : desire for acids ; loathing of pork.

Vomiting of sweet mucus every morning at ten and in evening.

Horribly offensive, nearly painless, almost involuntary, dark and watery stool : at night, and most towards morning.

Leucorrhœa, large lumps, unbearable in odour : violent pains in sacrum and right loin.

Suffocation and crawling in larynx : tickling ; throat seems narrowing, must cough.

Out for a walk, must return home in order to get breath, or to lie down, so that they can breathe more easily : < instead of > from open air.

Chest expands with difficulty : cannot get breath. Anxious dyspnœa. Worse when sitting up : better lying down. Worse the nearer arms are brought to body.

Asthma as if he would die.

Cough with salty-tasting, green and yellow expectoration.

Expectoration of blood, with hot sensation in chest ; yellowish-green.

Chronic blennorrhœa of lungs, threatening phthisis.

Suppuration of lungs.

Chest symptoms better lying down.

Pain in heart better lying down : thinks the stitches in heart will kill him if they continue.

Gurgling in region of heart, especially noticed when lying down.

Dyspnœa with palpitation.

Weakness in all joints as if they would not hold together.

Joints easily sprained : tends to overlift himself : troubles from tension or stretching of muscles.

Herpetic and itching eruptions, especially in bends of joints, in bends of elbows, in popliteal spaces.

Better bending forward.

Profuse sweat from slightest exercise.

Malaise : tired out.

Constantly increasing debility, with abdominal affections.

Child at night would twist and turn and fret from bedtime till morning, and next day be as lively as ever.

Children : emaciated. Children good all day, restless, troublesome, screaming all night. Or will not sleep, but worry, fret and cry day and night.

Very sensitive to cold air, or change of weather. Wears a fur cap, overcoat, or shawl even in hottest summer weather.

Restlessness before and during thunderstorm.

Averse to having head uncovered.

While in bed, body itches.

Profuse night-sweats of phthisis : or want of perspiration : dry skin.

All excretions, diarrhœa, leucorrhœa, menses and sweat have a carrion-like odour.

Body has a filthy smell, even after a bath.

Abnormal tendency to skin diseases.

Itching when body becomes warm. When rubbed small papules and vesicles arise, between fingers, in bends of knees, terrible, of whole body at night, preventing sleep.

Eruptions bleed easily and tend to suppurate.

PTELIA TRIFOLIATA

SOMEWHAT restricted as to space, in these war days, we will try to give some of the minor, but very useful remedies : less extensively proved, probably not known as to their utmost possibilities, yet recognizable and even more easily prescribed, than some of the polycrests.

Ptelia is a great stomach and liver medicine ; and, as seen in the provings, it causes *hurry,* and a sensation of burning heat of skin, face ; even breath that burns the nostrils.

Ptelia's MOST EMPHASIZED SYMPTOMS

General depression of spirits.

Bilious headaches.

Repugnance to animal food and rich puddings of which he is ordinarily fond ; to butter and fatty foods, even a small quantity aggravated epigastric pain.

Appetite poor, with muddled feeling, or pains in liver.

Hepatic and gastric symptoms : worse after meals.

Sense of weight and fullness, even after a moderate meal.

Burning distress ; oppression, vomiting ; chronic gastric catarrh.

Gastralgia.

Obstinate chronic dyspepsia.

Chronic gastritis : a constant sensation of corrosion, heat, and burning in stomach, with vomiting of ingesta, constipation, and afternoon fever.

Weight and aching distress in hepatic region ; dull pain, heaviness ; better lying on right side. Turning to left causes a dragging sensation.

Liver swollen, sore on pressure, causing dull and aching pains or stitches ; griping in bowels ; clothes feel too tight (Lyc.).

Congestion of liver ; chronic hepatitis.

Diarrhœa bilious, thin, faecal, dark, offensive ; even cadaverous in smell, or sulphuric : with tenesmus, preceded by griping pains and rumbling. Smarting in anus.

Constipation and diarrhœa alternately.

SOME OTHER NOTEWORTHY SYMPTOMS OR QUEER SYMPTOMS.

When walking, reeling as if intoxicated.

Dull aching in forehead, with depression and sour stomach ; racking pain, with hurried manner and red face . . . a great desire to hurry his business.

Sensation of a nail driven into brain (*Thuja*).

Sensitive to sounds ; impression of sounds last heard continue for a long time.

Headache in bones of skull (*Ipec.*).

Breath seems so hot that it burns nostrils.

Burning heat of cheeks and face.

Yellowish face, with dry, hot skin.

Teeth feel as if elongated.

Fine pricking sensation over whole surface of tongue.

Worse from cheese, meat, puddings.

Persistent nausea and vomiting, with giddiness and unsteadiness of legs. Better by walking.

Stomach feels empty after eating ; sensation of goneness (*Lyc.*, *Sep.*).

Griping in stomach, with dry mouth, yellow-coated tongue ; bitter taste.

Constant weight in both hypochondria when walking ; dragging pain.

Jaundice with hyperæmia of liver.

Pulsation and severe abdominal pain near umbilicus (comp. *Dulc.*).

Pressing suffocation when lying on back.

Walls of chest feel as if they would sink in ; asthma.

Hectic fever with purulent expectoration, and sweetish taste.

Tickling, prickling in fingers and hands, like that produced by electricity.

Wakes in a profuse perspiration. Chilly : wants to be near fire.

Has cured ague, with profuse vomiting of bilious matter.

Of *Ptelia* NASH says : " Another liver remedy, for it has one very characteristic symptom, viz. Aching and heaviness in the region of the liver, *greatly aggravated* by lying on the *left side* ; turning to the left causes a dragging sensation. (See *Bryonia*, which is also worse lying on left side and has the dragging sensation. Remember, *Bryonia* is generally better lying on the painful side.) *Magnesia mur.* has all these symptoms, termed ' bilious ', but, like *Mercurius*, it is worse when lying on the *right* side . . . *Ptelia* may have either constipation or diarrhœa, or like *Nux vomica*, constipation and diarrhœa alternately.

" I cured one bad case of liver trouble with *Ptelia* after œdema of feet and legs had set in ; she had the symptoms, could not lie comfortably on the left side, her breathing was becoming oppressed, and I thought the case looked as if it would not be very likely to be much better. I used the 30th in this case. The trouble rapidly disappeared and never returned. I considered it a brilliant cure."

PULSATILLA

THIS is not only one of the easiest of drugs to realize and learn, but it is also one of Hahnemann's Polycrests, or "drugs of many uses". In its provings it establishes symptoms on every part of the body and may be prescribed on its striking mental and peculiar symptoms.

Hahnemann says, "This very powerful plant produces many symptoms on the healthy, which often correspond to the morbid symptoms commonly met with." Hence the smallest homœopathic medicine chest, even one of a dozen remedies only, invariably contains *Pulsatilla*.

He says that "this, like all other medicines, is most suitably employed when not only the corporeal affections correspond but also when the mental and emotional alterations peculiar to the drug encounter similar states in the disease to be cured, or at least in the temperament of the subject of treatment".

Therefore "*Pulsatilla* will be the more efficacious when the patient exhibits a timid, lachrymose disposition, with a tendency to inward grief and silent peevishness, or at all events a mild and yielding disposition, especially when the patient in normal health was good-tempered and mild (or even frivolous and waggish)." "*Pulsatilla* is especially adapted," he says, "for slow phlegmatic temperaments ; and little suited for persons who form their resolutions with rapidity, and are quick in their movements, even though they may appear to be good tempered."

He tells us : "It acts best when there is a disposition to chilliness and adipsia. It is particularly suitable for females when their menses come on some days after their proper time ; especially also when the patient must lie long in bed at night before he can get to sleep, and when the patient is worse in the evening." "Useful for ill-effects from eating pork." He suggests the 30th potency.

Chilliness ! . . . One looks upon *Pulsatilla* as one of the " warm remedies ". But it has produced and cured chilliness, as we shall see when we go through its black letter symptoms. Among other things, it has *chilliness in a warm room*.

Pulsatilla hates and abominates warm rooms and stuffy rooms. Of all remedies it is *the* one that craves the open air.

Two of *Pulsatilla's* great characteristics are, " better from slow movement " (like *Ferr.*) and " *better in the open air* ".

One remembers that *Pulsatilla* cured distressing headaches in a man, who only found relief from " walking about on the Common at night " ; they were only tolerable *during motion, in the cool air.* *Pulsatilla* is not one of the drugs " better lying " !

With *Pulsatilla, walking* relieves vertigo, toothache, sticking pains in stomach and liver, bruised pain in back and knees. While *open air* relieves vertigo, pains in head, eye symptoms, fluent coryza, toothache, cough, etc., etc. But *Pulsatilla* cannot afford to get *wet.* This may mean colic, attacks of mucous diarrhoea, suppression of urine, ovaritis, metritis, suppressed menses, rheumatism. Cold air, yes : cold dry air : but not wet cold ! Thus we see that drugs have all the peculiarities and idiosyncrasies of mortals—and therefore are able to cure them, where these agree. *Pulsatilla* has a very wide range of action : but the mental symptoms, and the " modalities ", these peculiar distinguishing symptoms, must agree.

For instance, a case of severe erysipelas in a woman who had had frequent attacks, was cured in a couple of days by *Pulsatilla,* because her symptoms would not allow of any other drug being prescribed. And a recent case of terrible skin disease, that had resisted all treatments elsewhere, and came to our hospital as a last hope, is curing rapidly—is practically cured—after a few doses of *Pulsatilla.* Others of our doctors will tell of cases of psoriasis wiped out by *Pulsatilla,* . . . and so on. It is a great skin medicine—symptoms agreeing.

An interesting case was one of severe asthma of eight years' duration, attacks every fourteen days, confining her to bed, with absolutely and entirely *Pulsatilla* symptoms, " Irritable ; changeable ; laughs and cries easily ; fear of the dark : of death. Suspicious ; loathes fat, and dreams of cats." *Pulsatilla* has all these symptoms in the highest type, and has caused dreams of cats ! *Pulsatilla* in high potency was given in *September,* 1929, and again in *January,* 1930, for " a threat ". She was seen a few days ago : she has remained well ever since. If one could always get such clear-cut indications, prescribing would be indeed easy. This woman, after eight years of asthma, had actually only two attacks soon after her first dose of *Pulsatilla.*

A severe case of rheumatoid arthritis, one remembers, in hospital some years ago, utterly helpless and crippled, could hardly move arms, and they were useless ; but among her symptoms, she craved cold, open air, and liked a cold wind to blow upon her. *Pulsatilla* enabled her to put hands up ; behind her ; and in time she got onto her feet : and went out a different woman and with a very different manner of life before her.

Remember, it is not the disease but the drug that matters, and it must match, in its mentality, and its strange, rare, and peculiar symptoms, those of *the individual with that disease*.

Hahnemann says, " The occurrence of symptoms on only one-half of the body is a frequent peculiarity of *Pulsatilla*." And he draws attention to many such.

One curious symptom of *Pulsatilla*, which would take some explaining, is that it has one-sided sweat—profuse sweat on one side of the face !

Some years ago one of the Residents at hospital was in an acute state of worry, because he was perspiring profusely one side of the face and not the other. " What had he been taking ? "— " *Pulsatilla* "—and the symptom was looked up ; when it was realised that he was merely proving that drug.

Pulsatilla produces : " Sweat only on the right side of the body."—" Sweat only on the left side of the body." " Heat of one hand, and coldness of the other." " Hand and foot cold and red on one side, hot on the other." " Shuddering on one side of the face."

Nux also stands in black type for sweat on one side of face. And quite a number of remedies have one-sided perspiration, notably among them *Bar.c.*, *Chin.*, Nux, *Phos.*, Petrol, Puls., *Sulph.*, Thuja.

Lycopodium, like *Puls.*, has one foot hot and the other cold.

Thuja has a most peculiar symptom, which has led to striking cures, viz. profuse sweat on uncovered parts. Sir John Weir in his lectures quotes two such cases.

Hahnemann gives 1,156 symptoms, in all parts of the body, as produced by *Pulsatilla*. Allen, from further provings, adds to these, and gives 1,323 symptoms. The following are Hahnemann's black-letter symptoms, which he considers most characteristic of the remedy. Allen gives many more of these black-letter symptoms, caused and cured by *Pulsatilla*, but they are almost too numerous to quote in what must be a short article this time. As said, the drug attacks every organ and tissue in the body ; and to apply it successfully one only needs to see in the patient, Pulsatilla.

Vertigo, as from intoxication.
Vertigo especially when sitting.
Heaviness of head.
Transient obscuration of sight.
Itching burning in eyes, compels scratching and rubbing.
Smarting itching on hairy scalp.

A tension of face, as if parts would swell.
Alae nasi ulcerated externally and exude watery fluid.
Epistaxis. Flow of blood from nose with stuffed coryza.
Gums painful as if excoriated.
Tongue covered with viscid mucus, as with a skin.
Middle of tongue, even when moistened, a sensation as if it were burnt and insensible, at night and in the morning.
Throat painful as if raw. Sore throat :—scratchy : dry.
Dryness of throat in the morning.

Taste as of putrid flesh, with inclination to vomit.
A burnt taste in the mouth.
Bitter beer has to him a disgustingly sweetish taste.
After drinking beer, a bitter taste remains in mouth.
Dislike to butter.
Bilious eructations in the evening.
Diminished taste of all food.
Adipsia.
Frequent eructations with the taste of what has been eaten.
Sensation of sickness in epigastric region, especially after eating and drinking.
Inclination to vomit, with grumbling and rumbling in subcostal region.
Hiccough when smoking tobacco.
In the morning in the scorbiculus cordis, aching and drawing pain.
Immediately after supper flatulent colic : flatulence rumbles about painfully, especially in upper part of abdomen.
The flatus is discharged with cutting pain in the abdomen in the morning.
Bellyache as if diarrhoea must ensue, and yet there only occurs a good natural stool.
Bellyache after the stool.
Frequent urging to go to stool.
Frequent soft stool mingled with mucus.
Stools consisting of nothing but yellowish-white mucus, mingled with a little blood.
Quite white stool.

Frequent call to urinate.
The urine dribbles away when sitting and walking.
Itching, smarting inner and upper part of prepuce.
In the morning on awaking excitement of the genitals and desire for coitus.
Sneezing. Coryza.

Nocturnal dry cough, which goes off by sitting up in bed, but returns on lying down (Hyos.). Expectoration of blood.
Shooting pain in nape.
Heaviness of legs by day.

He moves about in his sleep. Sleeplessness from ebullition of blood.
He starts up in affright in his sleep.
At night he wakes up frightened and confused, not knowing where he is, and cannot rightly collect himself. Chattering in his sleep.
Yawning.

Chilly feeling with trembling, which recurs after some minutes, with little heat thereafter and no sweat.
External warmth is intolerable to him, the veins are distended.
Anxious heat as if hot water were thrown over him, with cold forehead.
Palpitation of the heart with great anxiety so that he must throw off the clothes.

Hypochondriacal moroseness : takes everything in bad part.
Everything disgusts, is repugnant to him. Breaks out into weeping.
Fretful : irresolute : trembling anxiety, relieved by motion.
Morose : ill-humoured : discontented : fretful.

Mothers come to hospital, " cannot think what is the matter with the child: it is so grizzly lately ". *Pulsatilla* generally cures.

Among other peculiar and characteristic symptoms of *Pulsatilla* that must be noticed, are the following. We will run through Kent's great lecture, quoting . . .

" The *Pulsatilla* patient is an interesting one, found in any household where there are plenty of young girls. She is tearful, plethoric, and generally has little credit for being sick from her appearance : yet she is most nervous, fidgety, changeable, easily led and easily persuaded. While mild, gentle and tearful, yet she is remarkably irritable—extremely touchy—feels slighted ; sensible to every social influence. Melancholia, sadness, weeping, despair, religious despair, fanatical ; full of notions and whims ; imaginative : extremely excitable. She imagines the company of the opposite sex a dangerous thing to cultivate. . . . These imaginations belong to eating as well as to thinking. They imagine that milk is not good to drink, so will not take it. That certain articles of diet are not good for the human race. Aversion to marriage is a strong symptom. . . . Religious freaks . . . misuses and misapplies the Scriptures to his own detriment,

. . . thinks he is in a wonderfully sanctimonious state of mind, or that he has sinned away his day of grace. . . . Tearful, sad and despondent, ameliorated walking in the open air, especially when it is crisp, cool, fresh and bright. . . .

" *Aggravations from fats and from rich foods*—worse for fat, pork, greasy things, cakes, pastry and rich things. The *Pulsatilla* stomach is slow to digest. . . .

" Can't breathe in a warm room ; wants the windows open ; chokes and suffocates in a warm bed at night. . . ."

Kent contrasts the *Chamomilla* and the *Pulsatilla* child (with pains in ears). " In *Chamomilla* you have a snapping and snarling child, never pleased, scolds the nurse and mother, ameliorated by walking about. The irritability decides for *Chamomilla*. You can detect a pitiful cry from a snarling cry. Both are ameliorated by motion, by being carried. Both want this and that and are never satisfied ; they want amusement. But the *Pulsatilla* child when not amused has a pitiful cry, and the *Chamomilla* child a snarling cry. You will want to caress the one and spank the other. . . ."

" *Pulsatilla* is one of our sheet anchors in old catarrhs with loss of smell, thick yellow discharge, and amelioration, in the open air ; in the nervous, timid, yielding, with stuffing up of the nose at night and copious flow in the morning. . . .

" *Pulsatilla* has *wandering pains*, rheumatism goes from joint to joint, jumps around here and there ; neuralgic pains fly from place to place ; inflammations go from gland to gland."

Here is the characteristic *changeableness* of *Pulsatilla*, carried from the mental to the physical sphere. But Kent says that *Pulsatilla*, " though it jumps around, does not (like some drugs) change to a new class of disease, so that the allopathic physician can say, as of the *Abrotanum* patient, ' This is a new disease to-day.' "

With *Pulsatilla*, as said, digestion is slow. And Kent says : " A striking feature here is, he never wants water. Dry mouth, but seldom thirsty. Craves ice cream, pastries, things which make him sick."

A picture of *Pulsatilla* that one has gradually evolved is :

Not hungry.

Not thirsty.

Not constipated.

Weepy : can't tell symptoms for tears.

Changeable ; and will laugh the next moment.

Very responsive to sympathy.

Like " *Phosphorus* ", fears :—alone—in the dark—in the twilight—in the evening. (*Pulsatilla* is worse in the evening.)

Great fear of insanity.

Imaginative : jealous ; suspicious.

Chilly, yet worse for heat.

Craves open air.

Craves movement, if in pain, mental or physical.

Pulsatilla is a great medicine for measles : for chilblains where they are unbearable *when hot* (*Agaricus, when cold*).

The classical description of *Pulsatilla* is, " sandy hair, blue eyes, pale face, easily moved to laughter or to tears ; affectionate, mild, timid, gentle, yielding disposition, inclined to be fleshy ". But cases wholly atypical may, by their symptoms, demand, and be cured by *Pulsatilla*.

PYROGEN

ANOTHER great FEVER remedy !—but not the remedy of simple acute fevers, like *Aconite*, but the remedy of septic conditions—typhoid conditions—typhoid.

Pyrogen is a weird medicine—weird in origin—weird in symptoms ; and it belongs to Homœopathy alone.

We owe this remedy to Dr. Drysdale, who published his pamphlet " *On Pyrexin or Pyrogen, as a Therapeutic Agent* ", in 1880.

Dr. Drysdale had been greatly struck by a remark made by Dr. Burdon Saunderson in a *British Medical Journal* in 1875. It runs thus : " *Let me draw your attention to the fact that no therapeutical agent, no synthetical product of the laboratory, no poison, no drug is known which possesses the property of producing fever. The only liquids which have this endowment are liquids which either contain Bacteria, or have marked proneness to their production.*" Drysdale says that : " *this last clause is qualified by statements elsewhere, and from other sources, that the fever-producing agent is a chemical non-living substance formed by living bacteria, but acting independently of any further influence from them ; and formed not only by the bacteria but also by living pus-corpuscles, or the living blood- or tissue-protoplasm from which these corpuscles spring. This substance when produced by Bacteria is the sepsin of Panum and others, but in view of its origin also from pus, and of its fever-producing power, Dr. B. Saunderson names it Pyrogen.*"

The above may not be the last word in bacteriology—or in Homœopathy—but one records it *in toto*, because to its inspiration we owe a unique and very useful remedy, as will be seen.

But Dr. Drysdale, of course, cannot admit that no other drug or poison can produce fever, because " *Aconite, Belladonna, Arsenic, Quinine, Baptisia, Gelsemium* and a host of other drugs do produce more or less of the febrile state, among other effects. But they produce it only after repeated doses and contingently on the predisposition of the subject of the experiment—or they produce it as a part of a variety of complex local and general morbid states. Therefore," he says, " it is practically true that no other known substance induces idiopathic pyrexia, certainly, directly, and after a given dose. *This directness of action ought to make it a remedy of the highest value, if it can ever be used therapeutically,* and if the Law of Similars is applicable here also, we ought to find it curative in certain states of pyrexia and certain blood disorders to which its action corresponds pathologically."

Drysdale gives Burdon Saunderson's experiments on animals which show that *Sepsin* or *Pyrogen*, given in lethal doses, kills—having produced changes in blood and tissues analogous to those of septicaemia after wounds : while in non-lethal doses, after severe symptoms," the animal, in a few hours, recovered its normal appetite and liveliness with wonderful rapidity . . . showing that this septic poison has not the slightest tendency to multiply in the organism."

So, pondering these things, Drysdale set out to prepare his remedy for fevers of the worst type—from *sterilized putridity*.

He chopped up half-a-pound of lean beef into a pint of tap-water, and set it in a sunny place for three weeks.

The maceration fluid was reddish, thick and fetid ; and the stench can be imagined when he set to work to render his material absolutely sterile and safe.

It was strained ; filtered ; evaporated to dryness at boiling heat ; rubbed up in a mortar with spirits of wine ; boiled ; again filtered ; again dried to form a brownish mass ; rubbed up now with distilled water, and again filtered. The clear amber-coloured resulting fluid was a watery extract, or solution of *Sepsin*. This, mixed with an equal volume of glycerine, was labelled *Pyrexin ø*.

(But Burnett, when it was prepared for him some eight years later, had it run up with spirits of wine to the sixth potency, which he used curatively in cases of typhoid fevers ; and some of Burnett's preparation went on to Dr. Swan, of high-potency fame, who prepared from this the very highest potencies of *Pyrogen* ; much used in U.S.A.)

To be absolutely sure that his " *Pyrexin* " or *Pyrogen* was pure poison—sterile—and incapable of carrying or breeding disease, it was tested, by injection, on white mice. And Drysdale was able to state that " *Sepsin* or *Pyrogen is only a chemical poison, whose action is definite and limited by the dose :* it is incapable of inducing an indefinitely reproducible disease in minimal dose, after the manner of the special poisons of the specific fevers."

He says : " The most summary indication for *Pyrogen*, would be to term it *the Aconite of the typhous, or typhoid quality of pyrexia.*"

Burnett, always on the look-out for curative agents, wrote a small monograph on *Pyrogen* in Typhoid, giving cases ; because Drysdale's work had been more or less passed over, and he realized and had experienced the importance of the remedy.

Then Dr. H. C. Allen (the Allen not of the *Encyclopedia of Pure Materia Medica*, but of Allen's *Keynotes*, and Allen's *Materia*

23

Medica of the Nosodes), by including *Pyrogen* among his remedies brought it into practical use.

But by far the most illuminating article on *Pyrogen* comes from Dr. Sherbino, of Texas, published in the *Homœopathic Physician*, in April, 1893 ; and in the same volume is to be found an article by Dr. Yingling, who " collates the reliable indications of *Pyrogen*". Yingling says : " As the larger part of this record is clinical, and as the *symptoms cured with a single remedy* are reliable data, I do not indicate the difference. . . ." (one supposes between the symptoms of the provings, and the symptoms cured.)

I have not been able to find, so far, a proper and complete proving of *Pyrogen* on humans. But Clarke used to insist that it was not only a case of " *what a remedy can cause it can cure*", but the other way about : *what it can cure, it can also cause.* In the latter case the remedy, according to him, was born by breach presentation : and he was jubilant when, later, his cured symptoms were found to have been also caused by his remedy.

Dr. Sherbino not only gives arresting indications for *Pyrogen*, but a set of telling cases which show its great power and utility, and also the rapidity of its action ; and he stresses the very striking and peculiar symptoms that should suggest its use.

We will give some of his pointers, and then, briefly, some of his cases.

The hard bed—hard pillow sensations—the intolerable aching, compared to lying on a pile of rocks, show the extreme *soreness* of *Pyrogen*. (*Arnica, Baptisia*.) The patient may " feel as if a train of cars has run over him ".

Extreme restlessness, *better when first beginning to move.* This is the great difference between *Rhus* and *Pyrogen*. *Rhus* is worse when beginning to move, but better for continued motion. As the relief from movement in *Pyrogen* only lasts a few moments, the patient *has to keep on moving*. Hence its frightful restlessness. Restlessness better sitting up in a chair and rocking hard. *Pyrogen* has only momentary relief from moving, but must move for that relief. (One thinks of *Pyrogen* as the dream of scientists— *perpetual motion*.)

Fan-like motion of the alae nasi (*Ant. t., Bapt., Bell., Brom., Hell., Lyc., Phos., Rhus tox.*).

Vomits water when it becomes warm in stomach (*Phos.*). Sick stomach, better by drinking very hot water (not *Phos.*). Coughs rusty mucus : pain in rt. lung and shoulder, agg. from coughing or talking.

Throbbing of vessels of neck (*Bell., Spig.*). Violent heart's action. Heart beats hard : sensation as if too full of blood : beats very loud, can be heard a foot away from thorax. Can't sleep for heart whizzing and purring so.

Delirium on closing eyes : sees a man at foot of bed, or in far part of room. Inclined to talk all the time at night during the fever. Talks to herself. Whispers to herself. If asked what she said, does not answer. Cries out in sleep that some one, or a weight is lying on her. Sensation of a cap on head. When she awakens and feels the cap, knows that she is not delirious ! Sensation as if she covered the whole bed : or she knew that her head was on the pillow, but could not tell where the rest of her body was. (Comp. *Bapt.*, *Petrol.*) Feels when lying on one side that she is one person, and that when she turns to the other side, she is another person. Felt as if existing in a second person, or as if there were two of her. The fever would not run in each alike. (*Bapt.* the fever wants to run separate.)

Feels crowded with arms and legs.

Can tell when fever is coming on, because he must urinate. Urine clear as spring water. Intolerable tenesmus of bladder.

Coldness and chilliness that no fire would warm. Sits by fire and breathes the heat from the fire. Then later, sensation of lungs on fire, and that he must have fresh air, which relieved.

Knife-like pains in side, go through to back ; worse from motion, coughing, and deep breathing ; better lying on affected side (*Bry.*). Groaning with every breath.

Face and ears red, as if the blood would burst through.

After the fever, the hallucination still persists that he is very wealthy, and has a large sum of money in the bank ; this is the last to leave him—this idea that he has the money.

Numbness hands and feet : extends over whole body. Hands cold and clammy.

Bowels so sore he can hardly breathe. So sore, can bear no pressure over right side abdomen.

Tongue coated white : yellow-brown streak down centre (*Bapt.*). Tongue dry : dry down the centre : not a particle of moisture on it. Bitter taste.

(Allen gives also, tongue clean, smooth and dry ; first fiery red, then dark and intensely dry ; smooth and dry ; glossy, shiny as if varnished ; dry, cracked, articulation difficult.)

Rolling of head from side to side.

And a most curious symptom. Bearing-down pain and prolapsus uteri, only relieved by holding the breath and bearing down. Pain starting at umbilicus, or just above, passing down towards uterus, but intercepted by just the same kind of pain starting from the uterus and passing up till they met midway and died away till another came. . . .

Dr. Sherbino calls *Pyrogen* a " *grand nosode—one of the greatest monuments to Hahnemann and to Homœopathy, as it covers a very wide range of action, and fills a place of its own that no other can fill* ".

The above is greatly condensed, as are the cases that follow. Dr. Sherbino uses Swan's very high potencies of *Pyrogen* in these cases. As we said, Burnett's work was done with the sixth potency, which is a very useful one.

PNEUMONIA. Girl of 14. Had been ill for a week. Temp. 105½ ; resp. 52 ; pulse 120 ; rusty sputum. Pain rt. lung and shoulder, worse talking and coughing. Fan-like motion alae nasi. Restlessness. Temp., on succeeding days, 102½ (improving fast) ; 100 ; 97½—subnormal in three days. She took four doses of *Pyrogen* cmm. " Cured " on the third day. (But pneumonias have a way of resolving rapidly by crisis or lysis. So, much cannot be claimed for this case.)

MRS. X. Aching all over : so very restless all last night ; couldn't keep still. *Pyrogen* dmm. Cured by next morning.

LITTLE GIRL with paralytic symptoms. Couldn't stand on her feet, and when they set her up in bed she would wave back and forward as if she had no control of herself. Her pulse was 120. Taking the increased heart-action as a leading symptom, I gave her *Pyrogen* cmm. which cured her quickly.

MRS. A. Fever began yesterday. Had a miserable night. Temp. 103, pulse 130. Very restless, especially after midnight ; constantly changing her position in bed. *Rhus* did not help. Next morning no better. Had had a bad night : no sleep : says it keeps her busy trying to get into an easy position, and she noticed that she was better while she kept up this motion all the time. *Pyrogen* cmm. Began to improve at once, rested better at night, and next day aching gone, pulse 108, temp. normal. She had a great deal of throbbing in vessels of thorax and neck, so violent it would shake the bed.

CHILD WITH LA GRIPPE. Her father called to ask for medicine. Said she was very restless, worse lying down, better sitting up. Vomited after drinking as soon as it gets warm in stomach. Better by vomiting. Cured with one dose of *Pyrogen* cmm.

LA GRIPPE. Mr. —. Coldness and chilliness no fire can warm. Grew more restless towards night. Had been breathing hot air from fire, now had a desire for fresh air, or his lungs would burn up. Groaned all night, and rolled and tumbled from one side of the bed to the other, not lying on one spot but a moment at a time. The bed was as hard as a board, the pillow was hard, and he was as sore as if a train had run over him. He tried to lie on his face, but found that that side of his body was sore too.

Before daylight he awoke and told his wife he was so glad that he had got rid of those arms and legs that had crowded him all night ; if he turned over they were there, and he was trying all night to get them out of the bed. . . . He took two or three doses of *Pyrogen* cmm.

DYSMENORRHOEA. Mrs. W. F. F. has had painful menstruation for several years, always preceded by aching in bones, causing her to complain of the bed being hard, and accompanied by intolerable restlessness. Better when first beginning to move—and she has to keep this up, as it affords some relief to the restlessness. I saw her have one of these spells, and she was on the floor, and she would curl up and then straighten out, and then turn and twist in every possible position. The cmm. of *Pyrogen* would always relieve her, till now she does not have the aching. This remedy has cured this condition, but other remedies had to be used . . .

I was called to see A COLOURED GIRL about twelve years old, who seemed to be partially paralysed. She could not sit up or stand, nor walk a step without help. She was very restless and kept rocking back and forth while sitting on the edge of the bed. She said that this rocking motion relieved her and so she kept it up. I gave her a dose of *Pyrogen* cmm. and she was all right in a day or two.

CHILD had a fever for several days and was getting worse. (*Bell.* and *Rhus* had failed.) I sat up all night with the case and it had all the restlessness of approaching death. There was more motion of the right leg and arm, and she would make a semi-circle from left to right, and her feet would get up upon the pillow, and she was not still for one moment all night long. She would make this peculiar circle and would have to be put on the pillow, and in a very short time she would be kicking the headboard with her feet. All of these symptoms passed away under the action of *Pyrogen* dmm.

MRS. M. has been troubled for some time with bearing down feelings in the uterine region, relieved by holding her breath and pressing down as if in labour. She was very restless at night and had to keep in motion, as only then could she get any relief. (Better when first beginning to move.) Cured by *Pyrogen* dmm.

Other cases, *Pneumonia—typhoid pneumonia—relapse after typhoid fever*, cured by *Pyrogen*, in very high potencies, are too lengthy to quote here. They are all on the same lines, as regards symptoms.

Dr. Yingling collates the reliable indications of *Pyrogen*, giving them in schema form. He " omits any symptoms where the action of other remedies used in connection with *Pyrogen* might have influenced its curative range."

Among his additional symptoms, one may quote :

Very loquacious. " I never talked so much in one day in all my life. I could think faster than ever I could."

Frightful throbbing headache, better for a tight band. Every pulsation felt in head and ears. Excruciating, bursting, throbbing headache *with intense restlessness* : with bleeding of nose, nausea and vomiting.

Sneezing every time he put his hand out from under the cover.

Terrible fetid taste, as if mouth and throat were full of pus, as if a broken abscess in mouth. (Proving.)

Tired feeling about the heart, " feels like taking it out to let it rest ; it would be such a relief to stop it, let it lie down, and stop throbbing ".

Perspiration horribly offensive, carrion-like : disgust, up to nausea, about any effluvia arising from her own body.

Great restlessness. " Thought she would break if she laid too long in one position."

Septic states. Typhoid conditions.

Yingling also gives a few cases—*Neglected pneumonia :* cough, night-sweats, frequent pulse, and to all appearance as if in the last stage of pneumonic consumption. An abscess had burst that day and was discharging a great amount of pus ; tasted like matter. Made a rapid recovery on *Pyrogen* cm., a few doses.

" Knew he was going to have typho-malarial fever, which he had had two years previously, after a malarious exposure on a foreign mission field." Had every other day what he called " dumb ague ". *Pyrogen* cured.

Yingling says, *Pyrogen* has cured cases of *blood poisoning*. It should be thought of in dissecting wounds ; and he quotes : " *In all fevers when other remedies do not act, think of Pyrogen* " (Swan).

" *In septic poisoning from wounds—after abortion—accouchment, etc., etc., think of Pyrogen* " (H. C. Allen).

" *Pyrogen* resembles *Ipecac.* very closely in uterine haemorrhage. If you have an *Ipecac.* case, and that remedy fails you, think on *Pyrogen*."

Kent says : " Septic conditions, where there is a continuous intermingling of little chillinesses and little quiverings throughout the body and the pulse has lost its proper relationship to the temperature, *Pyrogen* must be administered."

Allen's *Nosodes* has a chapter on *Pyrogen* : and here is a little quotation from " Notes from Lectures by H. C. Allen ", which sums up well the " inwardness " of this powerful and rapidly-acting remedy.

PYROGEN.

I have found this remedy invaluable in fevers of septic origin, all forms ; when *Bapt., Ech., Rhus* or the best selected remedy fails to relieve or permanently improve, study *Pyrogen.*

The bed feels hard (*Arn.*) ; parts lain on feel sore and bruised (*Bapt.*) ; rapid decubitis (*Carb. ac.*) ; of septic origin.

Chill :—Begins in the back between scapula, severe general coldness of bones and extremities.

Heat :—Sudden, skin dry and burning ; pulse rapid, small, wiry, 140-170 ; temp. 103-106°.

Sweat :—Cold, clammy, profuse, often offensive, generally exhausting. Pulse abnormally rapid, out of all proportion to temperature (*Lil.*).

In septic fevers, especially puerperal, where fœtus or secundines have been retained, decomposed ; fœtus dead for days, black, horribly offensive discharge.

When patient says : " Never been well " since septic fever, or abortion, or a bad confinement.

To arouse vital activity of uterus and enable it to expel its contents.

Much of this—and much more—will be found in Clarke's *Dictionary.* And, by the way, one of the indications for *Pyrogen* that we have forgotten to mention is : *Pulse very high, out of proportion to temperature.* One wonders whether it might not even save life in those desperate conditions when, with a soaring pulse, the high temperature suddenly drops.

One's experiences of *Pyrogen* seem hardly worth mentioning after the foregoing, and yet they are corroborative.

INFLUENZA. One recalls the early days of severe Influenza, which came, like a bolt from the blue, after many years' absence — so one was told. It was called the Russian Influenza, because it was supposed to have spread from the Foreign Office, having come in Despatches from Russia. One remembers the agonies of restlessness, with the utter impossibility of remaining for more than one moment in any position, till, from a chair, one wriggled and twisted, in search of relief, till down on the floor, when one had to start again. This was a cry for *Pyrogen*—had one then known it !

The year when the Duke of Clarence died, the doctors were writing to the papers, almost in panic (because so many people died), that it was imperative, since the disease was so severe and brief, to give the patients quantities of alcohol. With Burnett's

Pyrogen 6 we had a wonderful experience. At that time we had a number of adults and children living on the place—the family, indoor servants, out-door servants and their families (not the restricted families of 1932 !)—and as they went down with influenza one by one, or in batches, *Pyrogen* 6, given six-hourly for a few doses, cured every single case in from twenty-four to forty-eight hours ; and there was no alcohol, and there were no complications. And after that it was *Pyrogen*, a dose or two at the sudden onset of the violent pulsations, that used to announce a fresh attack of Influenza, that, for me, finished its bi-annual recurrences.

Of course, epidemics of what we call influenza vary greatly in their symptoms, and in the remedy of the "genus epidemicus", needed to combat them. One year it may be *Mercurius*—one *Gelsemium*; one year most of the cases will be of the *Baptisia* type, and so on. But the fever of violent pulsations and intense restlessness, because it is only constant movement that makes existence possible, needs *Pyrogen*.

A doctor was telling me the other day about a recent *Pyrogen* case. It was not yielding to likely remedies, when the symptom, " Felt as if he covered the bed ", led him to prescribe *Pyrogen*, which promptly cured.

American doctors find one of their most dramatic uses for *Pyrogen* in sepsis after delivery, with offensive discharges, and where part of the placenta has been retained. They say that they give *Pyrogen* and it " pops out ". Here is such a case :

A couple of years ago one of our cows calved away in the fields. Calf was found dead, and no placenta. Vet. removed some of it, but failed to get it all away. She had fever and was very ill, and he was thinking of exploring further ; but she was given *Pyrogen*, and the next day the fever was gone and she was well. I don't know if it was a case of " popping out", but there was no further trouble.

One has seen very great relief from *Pyrogen* in abscess and whitlow. But here Homœopathy has such a wealth of helpful remedies—*Crotalus, Lachesis, Anthracinum, Silica, Arsenicum, Hepar, Pyrogen*, etc.

One remembers a case of diarrhoea persisting for years after typhoid fever, and other cases of diarrhoea, cured by *Pyrogen* ; also a case of diabetes (indications forgotten) where *Pyrogen* removed the sugar.

Allen's *Nosodes* gives a number of cases showing rapid curative action of *Pyrogen* : cases of sepsis after parturition with offensive discharges : cases of varicose ulcer with offensive discharges ; of diarrhoea with frightfully offensive stools, after poisoning by sewer gas, etc. He quotes a case of Bogers : " An old woman dying of gangrene inoculated one of her nurses ; the nurse had chills, high fever and red streaks running up the arm following the course of the lymphatics. *Pyrogen* rapidly removed the whole process."

Allen says : " I can hardly mention *Pyrogen* without becoming enthusiastic, on account of the wonderful results I have had from it in blood poisoning. In any kind of septic infection, either puerperal or traumatic, *Pyrogen* will do wonders, when the symptoms correspond. It is similar to *Anthracinum* in some respects."

Pyrogen, as we saw, is made from *putrifying animal matter*. Allen, in his *Nosodes*, compares it with another powerful fever-producing and curing remedy, made from *decaying vegetable matter*, i.e. the decaying vegetable matter of a very malarial region on the Wabash river. He calls it " *Malaria officinalis*, the vegetable *Pyrogen* ", and describes its preparation, and the symptoms produced in its provers. He also says : " I know several localities in South America, Africa and Spain, where the marsh miasma has unquestionably arrested phthisis pulmonalis, without any other treatment or restriction in food or drink."

Provers of Malaria had fearful headache, nausea, vomiting in some cases, distress in stomach, hypochondria—" first in the spleen, then the liver and stomach, and on the third day pronounced chills, which were so severe that they had to be antidoted."

With one of the preparations, the stomach, spleen, liver and kidneys became involved, with quartan and tertian intermittent fevers. In one case a genuine typhoid condition was set up, which compelled the provers to take to bed.

It would be most interesting to try the effect of *Malaria officinalis* in G.P.I. It would be simpler and less risky than by imported mosquitoes.—P.S.

SEPTICÆMIN

A like remedy to *Pyrogen* is *Septicæmin* (another of Swan's *Nosodes*) : potencies made " from the contents of a septic abscess ".

Clarke (*Dictionary of Mat. Med.*) says that Skinner gave a supply to a volunteer going out to the Boer War, with instructions to take a globule every four hours if attacked by anything like typhoid fever. He wrote home, " *Septicæmin* is like magic in diarrhœa and dysentery in Camp life ", and asked for more, as his supply was largely drawn on by his friends.—ED.

RANUNCULUS BULBOSUS
(Buttercup)

WHO, coming on a field, golden in the springtime with buttercups, would dream of their poisonous properties and therefore their power of curing painful and intractable conditions, such as shingles can be?

It is because of one's happy experiences in the cure of shingles with *Ranunculus bulb.* that one is impelled, now in the springtime, to honour them, and to spread the knowledge of their devastating, and, therefore, healing power. In the course of years one has had many cases of herpes zoster to treat, and fails to remember a *Ranunc.* case where a few doses of a high potency did not wipe the trouble out in a couple of days—pain and all. In some cases, where the pain is burning and relieved by heat, with great restlessness and anxiety, *Ars.* would be the remedy; and many doctors swear by *Mezereum.* But even in the aged, and with extreme pain, one has seen the trouble simply wiped out and the pain which doctors have told patients would go on for the rest of their lives, has promptly ceased: we gave such a case recently in this Journal. But, one must not forget *Variolinum*, which, for Burnett, " wiped the trouble out, pain and all " and which is the more interesting because in these days, herpes zoster is associated with chicken pox. One remembers one terrible case, which had been under old school treatment, with extreme pain and great deformity, including the destruction of an eye, where the patient improved so far as pain was concerned, but ceased to come, because her eye, with its scarring and bulging hernia, was not restored.

In regard to its chest symptoms, one needs to diagnose between *Ranunc. bulb.* and *Bryonia.* Both have the stitching pains, worse from movement: but *Bry.* wants pressure on the suffering chest, to keep it still, while *Ranunc.* cannot bear touch or pressure. Again *Bry.* is worse in the dry, cold weather; *Ranunc.* in wet weather. The aetiology of *Acon.* is also " dry cold "—sudden attacks from exposure to dry, cold winds. While *Arnica*, that great remedy of pleurodynia, with its stitching pains that will not allow a deep breath to be drawn; with its sore, lame, bruised beaten sensations, is not particularly affected by cold or heat, damp or dry, but is physically over-sensitive, and finds the bed intolerably hard.

BLACK LETTER SYMPTOMS

*Headache over right eye: worse lying, **walking and standing.** Pressure and smarting in eyeballs.*

Pain in both hypochondria, with painfulness to touch.

In the evening, both hypochondria and lowest ribs in chest, feel painful, as if bruised.

Stitching with pressure, right abdomen, in region of last true rib (liver) arresting breathing, with stitches and pressure on the top of right shoulder.

Chest : stitches, neuralgic, myalgic, or rheumatic pains in chest. Pleurodynia, rheumatic, myalgic or neuralgic.

Pressure and tightness across lower part of chest, with fine stitches, felt first in outer parts of chest, then extend deep into the chest, now in the right, now in the left chest : increased by moving, stooping, or taking an inspiration.

The breathing is painful, even contact is painful.

Stitches left side above the nipple, in a space the size of a hand, worse during contact and motion.

Violent fine stitches in the middle of left chest, in front, during inspiration, in the forenoon.

Burning and fine stitches left chest.

Pain, as if bruised, in region of short rib, with pain in back, lassitude, ill-humour.

Violent sticking in right side chest, region of 5th and 7th ribs, arresting breathing, with stitches and pressure on the top of right shoulder.

Sticking pain in right side chest, region of 5th and 6th ribs, with great sensitiveness of the spot to touch and great debility.

Stitches about chest in every change of weather.

Chest feels sore, bruised ; worse touch, motion, turning body.

Intercostal or spinal neuralgia, pleurodynia.

Rheumatism of muscles, especially muscles about trunk : intercostal rheumatism : muscles sore to touch : as if they had been pounded.

Shingles and intercostal neuralgia.

Small, deep, transparent, dark-blue, little elevated blisters, blue, transparent vesicles. (Crowded together in oval shaped groups, with intolerable burning itching.)

In Italics; Important, or Curious and Suggestive Symptoms

Herpes zoster supra-orbitalis, with bluish black vesicles and the usual pains.

Hay fever, eyes smart, lids burn and are sore ; nose stuffed, with tingling and crawling inside ; or in posterior nares, patient hawks and swallows, and tries in every way to scratch the affected part ; ? neck of bladder also affected, with burning during micturition.

Pain about lungs from adhesions after pleurisy. (*Bry.*)

Pain in whole chest, as of a subcutaneous ulceration, on slight motion of trunk.

Violent sticking pain above left nipple, near axilla, when rising in a.m. Dares not move arm, or raise it, dares not even raise trunk lest he should scream with pain ; has to sit or stand stooping, with head and chest forward to the left.

Herpes or blister-like eruption palms ; blue blisters on fingers.

The well-covered chest is chilly out of doors.

As if cold, wet cloths were applied to different parts of thorax ; a knife thrust into side and through back.

Crawling and creeping in scalp, nose, skin of fingers.

Worse wet weather, change of weather, change of temperature.

Herpes zoster ; zona ; vesicles filled with serum which burn, may have a bluish-black appearance, especially when following course of supra-orbital or intercostal nerves, and followed by sharp, stitching pains.

Pain like that of shingles without eruption.

Pemphigus, eczema.

*   *   *

What have the Masters to say in regard to their personal experience with *Ranunculus ?*

NASH only says : " Blister-like eruptions on palms of hands."

*   *   *

GUERNSEY gives :

Biting or pungent pain ; pain as if parts would burst, were pressed or pushed asunder.

Pustulous exanthema, blue-coloured.

Waking too early in the morning.

Affections of any kind of the external angles of the eyes ; hypochondrium, particularly about the spleen ; lower region of abdomen ; palms of the hands.

Worse: entering a cold place ; from spirituous liquors ; with drunkards ; when stretching the limbs ; at changes of temperature, whether from hot to cold, or *vice versa*.

*   *   *

CLARKE (*Dictionary*) says : " Small, deep, transparent, dark blue little elevated blisters of the size of an ordinary pin's head, crowded together in oval shaped groups the size of a shilling, with intolerable burning, itching, emitting when opened a dark yellow lymph, afterwards becoming covered with a herpetic *horny* scurf : a complete picture of herpes. The pains, as well as the appearance of herpes are met with in the pathogenesis of

Ranunc. bulb. . . . pains lancinating ; pressing and out-pressing ; jerking and sticking ; as if bruised ; with external sensitiveness." He says its hay fever symptoms have led to many cures of hay fever with *Ranunc. bulb.*

" The general sensitiveness of *Ranunc. bulb.* to air—cold air—change, the grand keynote of the remedy ; another keynote is sensitiveness to touch—bruised soreness of the parts affected.

" *Ranunc. bulb.* has proved one of the most effective agents for removing the bad effects of alcoholic drinks ; hiccough ; epileptiform attacks ; delirium tremens. Quarrelsome, angry mood ; and fear of ghosts."

He gives a case of Burnett's in regard to the cold water feeling of *Ranunc. bulb.* A woman, after a fall two years before, had the peculiar sensation, whenever she goes out of doors feels as if wet cloths were applied to three different parts of anterior walls of thorax—both intraclavicular fossae, and under left breast. *Ranunc. bulb.* quickly cured. . . .

*   *   *

FARRINGTON has a good deal to say about *Ranunc. bulb.* and he gives valuable tips, which we have not found elsewhere except in the provings.

We will quote, condensing.

He says : " Compare with *Acon., Arn., Cact., Bry., Rhus, Ars., Mez.*"

" Both these plants " (*bulbosus* and *sceleratus*) " possess a juice or sap which is exceedingly irritating to the skin. Applied locally it produces erythema, followed by an eruption at first vesicular, and attended by burning, smarting and itching. If by reason of the intensity of the action of the drug, the symptoms continue, ulceration and even gangrene follow, the gangrene with fever and delirium.

" Think of *Ranunc. bulb.* in its action on serous membranes, especially pleura and peritoneum, with stabbing pains in chest, and effusion of serum into one or other cavity, according as one or other membrane is inflamed. Accompanying this effusion we find great anxiety, dyspnœa and distress, caused partly by the accumulation of fluid, and partly by the anxiety from the pains themselves. Now, these symptoms are not commonly known among physicians, yet you will find that here *Ranunculus* will serve you as well as *Apis, Bryonia* or *Sulphur*, or even better than these, if the character of the pains just described is present. . . ."

" Muscles." We find *Ranunculus* acting here as a curative agent. Particularly in muscles about the trunk. " Intercostal rheumatism yields far more quickly to this drug than to any other.

There is usually a great deal of soreness to touch, the muscles feel bruised as if they had been pounded. I know that *Aconite*, *Arnica* or *Bryonia* is often given when *Ranunculus* is indicated."

Ranunculus for persons who are subject to stitches about the chest in every change of weather.

May be used for sore spots remaining in and about the chest after pneumonia. A feeling of subcutaneous ulceration. (*Puls.*)

For pains from adhesions after pleurisy. For diaphragmitis with sharp shooting pains from hypochondria and epigastrium through to back. (*Cactus.*)

Again for the bad effects of drink . . . Then, the skin. (We have given this fully in regard to herpes zoster.) But also pemphigus, with large blisters which burst and leave raw surfaces. In eczema, with thickening of the skin, and the formation of hard, horny scales. (*Ant. crud.*) Hay fever. (We have given.)

Farrington warns us that *Sulphur* does not follow *Ranunculus* well.

He says that *Ranunc. sceleratus* develops more markedly large isolated blisters. When these burst, an ulcer is formed, with very acrid discharge, making the surrounding parts sore.

He says, even in diphtheria or typhoid it is indicated by denuded patches on the tongue, the remainder of the organ being coated. *Nat. mur.*, *Ars.*, *Rhus* and *Tarax.* have these patches (" Mapped tongue ") but none of these remedies have the same amount of burning and rawness that *Ranunc. sceleratus* has.

May be indicated in ordinary catarrhs with sneezing, fluent coryza, pains in joints, and burning on urination.

*   *   *

H. C. ALLEN (*Keynotes*) starts off with, " one of our most effective remedies for the *bad effects of alcoholic beverages ;* spasmodic hiccough, delirium tremens. . . ."

After the stitches, etc., he gives :

Pleurisy or pneumonia from sudden exposure to cold, while overheated (*Acon.*, *Arn.*).

Corns sensitive to touch ; smart, burn (*Salicyl. a.*)

And so on, as already recorded.

*   *   *

One recalls, very long ago, and before X-ray would inevitably have revealed the condition, a case of most extreme suffering, the pains being in the chest. The case was carefully gone into from the symptomatic point of view, and after a few doses of *Ranunc. bulb.* the pain disappeared. The man, an in-patient, had been almost heart-broken because one of the surgeons who examined him had suggested malingering. His symptoms, had suggested the successful "like" prescription, and he went out happy and (apparently) well. A couple of years later he was readmitted for some acute illness—a septic pneumonia, as a matter of fact, and died. A post mortem was done, and revealed what occasioned a gasp of surprise:—a large aneurism which had caused the text-book wasting of several intervertebral discs. This fully accounted for the old pain, but not for its cessation. *Ranunc.* had done for that man what nothing else could have done : it had made life endurable, even where it could not cure.

For Homœopathy, " incurable " does not mean that no relief of suffering can be given. Far from it.

*   *   *

BURNETT used to make play with *Ranunc. sceleratus* (the wicked buttercup). His indication was excessive external tenderness of chest. This, CLARKE says has led to the cure of many chest affections, including aneurism.

But, the best-known characteristic of *Ranunc. sc.* (which is a well-proved drug) is the mapped or peeled tongue, and when this is associated with smarting, burning and rawness, *Ranunc. sc.* will be the remedy. (CLARKE.)

RHODODENDRON

Rhododendron and *Rhus tox.* are linked in one's memory as rheumatic remedies of like modalities. Both are worse for cold, worse in wet weather, and relieved by motion. But *Rhododendron* is far more affected by electrical conditions : all its sufferings and pains are worse before thunder.

CLARKE says of *Rhododendron*. " Growing among the fogs and storms of the Siberian mountains, its provings show that it produces sensitiveness to storm and weather changes, and this gives the grand key-note of its use in medicine."

GUERNSEY tells us to think of this remedy for the sufferings made worse in windy weather. " The patient may be in bed, or in a warm comfortable room, but the blowing of wind aggravates his symptoms."

Rhododendron is a remedy of general rheumatic pains, brought on by damp, cold weather, and worse during wet weather.

HUGHES says it has a high native reputation for gout and rheumatism.

It is one of the remedies of wandering rheumatism (*Lac. can.*). The acute inflammatory swellings wander from joint to joint (unlike those of *Rhus*) and may even reappear in the first joint affected. Note ! that in this wandering of inflammatory conditions it parts company with *Rhus* : though, with *Rhus*, " the pains do not admit of the limbs being at rest "

It is also a remedy of chronic rheumatism, affecting the smaller joints and their ligaments.

Among the special localities affected, it has, sensation as if wrists (*Ruta*) were sprained : sprained pain in wrist joint, impeding motion : worse at rest in rough weather.

It is also a remedy of arthritic nodes.

It affects especially fibrous tissues (*Rhus, Ruta*).

It has cured pleurisy, where breath and speech failed from violence of pleuritic stitches, running downwards, after standing on cold ground and getting chilled. Also rheumatic pains, left side, below the short ribs, after taking cold by getting wet.

The head pains of *Rhododendron* are worse when lying in bed in the morning, worse from wine and in wet cold weather. It is very sensitive to alcohol : " intoxicated from a little wine ". The painful head is better when wrapped up warmly ; from dry heat ; from exercise.

There may be *ciliary neuralgia* before a storm.

Diarrhœa or dysentery in cold wet weather, and renewed before a thunderstorm.

One remembers curing a small boy of hydrocele with *Rhododendron*. It has a great reputation for hydrocele, especially in children—even from birth. It is also a remedy of orchitis ; testicle indurated ; it feels as if being crushed.

There are profuse debilitating sweats especially when walking in the open air, and perspiration has the odour of spice.

BLACK LETTER SYMPTOMS

The approach of a thunderstorm, or of cloudy windy weather, is always preceded by pain, drawing-aching (and cutting).

The testes, especially the epididymis, are intensely painful to touch, for many days. Contusive pain in testes, with alternate drawing. Worse now in the one, now in the other.

Very painful drawing in the hard, somewhat swollen testes, extending as far as the abdomen and thighs, especially on the right side.

CLARKE says *Rhododendron* disturbs all parts of the economy producing delirium, fever, headache, neuralgias (earache, toothache), and inflammations ; but its chief determining characteristic is that the symptoms come on or are worse on the approach of a storm, during a storm, or in wet weather. Sensitiveness to electric changes.

Suited to nervous persons, who dread a storm and are particularly afraid of thunder. . . .

But *Rhododendron* has other characteristics, among these is loss of memory. Words are omitted while writing ; sudden disappearance of thought ; forgets what he is talking about. . . . Vertigo when lying in bed, better while moving about. Intense degree of tinnitus aurium gives *Rhododendron* a place in Ménière's disease. (We have seen *Salicylic acid* curative here.) Clarke says chorea of left leg, arm, face, worse at approach of a storm, has been cured by it.

He tells of a flock of sheep poisoned by eating the leaves ; a number died immediately—" from paralysis of the swallowing muscles ".

He gives interesting cases of cure—neuralgias, where other remedies had failed ; but worse in bad weather. In one case there was instant relief when the sun came out. A curious symptom, one pupil dilated, the other contracted.

Rhododendron is a powerful drug, and a fascinating study, because of its very marked characteristics. But remember, the *Rhododendron* joint pains wander from joint to joint : even return to the same (*Lac. can.*).

Rhus, Rhododendron and *Ruta* affect especially fibrous tissues— *Bryonia* especially serous tissue.

RHUS

(" *Rhus radicans,* also called *toxicodendron."* HAHNEMANN.)

Rhus is a native of North America, and is one of those most valuable medicines which we owe to the domestic practice of the North American Indians :—*Baptisia, Gelsemium, Caulophylum,* etc. It was proved and included in his *Materia Medica Pura* by Hahnemann, as " a remarkable and valuable medicinal substance ". He notes " *a great number of characteristic peculiarities in its action* ", and says :

" To mention one only : we observe this curious action (which is found in very few other remedies, and in these never to such a great degree), viz. *the severest symptoms and sufferings are excited when the body or the limb is at rest and kept as much as possible without movement."* And adds, " the opposite, an increase of the symptoms by movement, is much more rarely observed ".

Then he contrasts the action of *Rhus* with that of *Bryonia.* Here, " with almost identical symptoms ", there is " *the striking amelioration by avoiding all movement* " of *Bryonia,* " exactly the opposite of what *Rhus* does ".

Hahnemann calls them " these two antagonistic sister remedies " and tells of their inestimable value in the disastrous war pestilence of 1813, when these patients were " dying in thousands while the doctors carried on vain disputations as to the *presumed internal nature* of the disease ".* Hahnemann treated it symptomatically with *Rhus* alternated with *Bryonia, as the symptoms changed and demanded the one or the other remedy.* And he says that, of the 183 cases he treated in Leipsic, not one died, " which created a great sensation among the Russians then ruling in Dresden, but was consigned to oblivion by the medical authorities." He says, " If ever there was a triumph for the only true, the homœopathic treatment, this was one."

Farrington says : " You must remember *Rhus* as complementary to *Bryonia,* a fact discovered by Hahnemann in his experience with an epidemic of war-typhus. . . . The success he gained was acknowledged on all sides. Many lives have since been saved by the exhibition of these two remedies in alternation ; i.e. an alternation which consists in giving *Bryonia* when *Bryonia* symptoms are present, and *Rhus tox.* when the patient manifests

---

* *See Hahnemann's account of this epidemic,* HOMŒOPATHY, *Vol. IV., p.* 202.

symptoms calling for that remedy. This is a legitimate alternation."

Farrington tells us that Boenninghausen's* son had typhoid, and was attended by his father. Among his symptoms was the *Rhus* restlessness, yet *Rhus* gave no relief. Looking up the *Materia Medica* Boenninghausen found that *Taraxacum* had this same restlessness of limbs with tearing pain, and in addition a symptom present in his son's case, mapped tongue. He gave *Taraxacum* with prompt relief.

Farrington describes the use of *Rhus* in FEVERS. . . .

"*Rhus*, when acute diseases take on a typhoid form—dysentery—scarlet fever—diphtheria—pneumonia. . . .

He says, " *Rhus* is indicated in DYSENTERY, when there are tearing pains down the thighs during defæcation. I once cured a case of small-pox which had degenerated into a hæmorrhagic type, the pustules containing bloody pus, with *Rhus* ; the indications for the remedy were, *Stools of dark blood, with pains tearing down the thighs during stool.*"

He describes *Rhus*, in TYPHOID . . . " mild temperament, delirium mild : though may try to jump out of bed to escape. Restlessness : cannot lie still. Sometimes the hallucination, fear he will be poisoned. Will not take the medicines, or food, as fears people desire to poison him (*Hyos., Lach.*). Tongue dark-brown, dry, cracked : cracks may gape and bleed. Triangular red tip. Typhoid pneumonia, rusty sputum. Almost intolerable backache ".

Dunham says, " These remarks " (i.e. to above effect) " will suffice to give an idea of the application of *Rhus* in FEVERS. They have included no name except that of typhoid fever—but surely I need not at this hour remind you that, *no matter how different may be the names that are applied to morbid conditions, if the conditions be similar the remedy may be the same.* It often happens that in the course of the exanthematous fevers, measles and scarlatina, a similar train of symptoms to those already described makes its appearance and calls for *Rhus*. Especially is this the case with scarlatina, a disease in which the value of *Rhus* is not well understood by the profession."

Farrington says, " In INTERMITTENT FEVER it is very important to note the point at which the chill starts.

" *Rhus* starts in one leg, usually in the thigh, or between the shoulders, or over one scapula.

" *Eupatorium*, sometimes *Nat. mur.*, begins in small of back.

" In *Gels.* it runs up the spine."

* Hahnemann's friend and great disciple.

In regard to the extraordinary action of *Rhus* on the Skin—even the exhalations of the plant will effect this in sensitives, Carroll Dunham says :

" *Rhus* produces a most remarkable imitation of vesicula erysipelas and is our most valued remedy here. . . . But its grand rôle is in the treatment of the pustular form."

And he quotes Trousseau, " no advocate or friend of Homœopathy ", who " relates an interesting proving of *Rhus* " (which accords with its other provings). . . .

" ' Dr. Savini applied two drops of the juice of *Rhus rad.* to the first phalanx of his forefinger ; he left it there only two minutes, and yet, at the end of an hour, it had produced two black spots. Twenty-five days afterwards the following symptoms suddenly manifested themselves : great heat, mouth and gullet ; rapid swelling of left cheek, upper lips, and eyelids. The following night, swelling of forearm, which had acquired double its normal volume ; the skin was rough, the itching intolerable, the heat very great, etc. ' This singular action of *Rhus* ', says Trousseau, ' induced the homœopaths to use it in skin diseases ; but already, before them, Dufresnoy, of Valenciennes, had published a pamphlet extolling the virtues of this plant against cutaneous diseases, and subsequently against paralysis . . . ' and Trousseau says that he had often used *Rhus radicans* for paralysis of the lower extremities ' succeeding on a concussion of the spinal marrow, or a lesion of that organ, which did not destroy its tissue. On this point we have collected facts enough to place beyond a doubt the therapeutic efficacy of *Rhus radicans.* ' "

Skins, then, and Traumatic Paralysis without destruction of nervous tissue ! We shall amplify, and detail some of its other uses.

Dunham points out that " in fevers, the special senses are dulled, but not perverted ".

Dunham also explains the apparently contradictory symptoms of *Rhus*, as hinted by Hahnemann.

" The great and characteristic peculiarity of *Rhus* is that, with few exceptions, they occur and are aggravated during repose, and are ameliorated by motion . . .

" *Rhus* has *symptoms which resemble paralysis*, also *groups of symptoms resembling muscular and articular rheumatism.* These latter come on with severity during repose and increase as long as the patient keeps quiet, till they compel him to move. Here the first movement is exceedingly painful : but by continuing to move the stiffness is relieved and pains decrease, and he feels much better. But, after a period of continuously moving and finding comfort therein, the paralytic symptoms interpose their exhausting protest, and he is compelled by lassitude and power-lessness to suspend his movements and come to repose. This repose is at first grateful and relieves, not the aching pains, but the sense of prostration. Before long the pains come on again and the patient is forced to move again, as before. . . . This will explain the seeming contradictions in the symptoms of *Rhus*."

Kent says of *Rhus*, " *He is never perfectly at ease, and never finds rest.*"

In regard to the *Rhus* characteristic, worse first morning, then better, Guernsey says, " We are led to think of this remedy where we find an irresistible desire to move, or change *the position every little while, followed by great relief for a short time,* when they must again move, and again experience the same relief for a short time. *After resting, when first moving a painful stiffness is felt which wears off from continued motion.*"

He says " a nursing mother may have sore nipples, and when the child begins to nurse, the nipple hurts exceedingly, but on continued nursing it becomes much easier ".

And Kent has it, " Hoarseness on first beginning to sing which wears off on singing a few notes, or wears off after talking a little while."

DILATATION OF HEART with distress; from over-exertion (*Arn.*). Uncomplicated hypertrophy of heart, i.e. not associated with valvular lesions . . . from the effects of over-exertion— athletes and men who handle heavy tools. (*Arn.*) Palpitation of heart following over-exertion, with usually numbness of left arm and shoulder.

Farrington tells us that *Rhus* is the great remedy of over-exertion.

" *Over-exertion.* A player of wind instruments gets pulmonary hæmorrhage : *Rhus* will be his remedy. If from violent exertion a patient is seized with paralysis, his trouble may yield to *Rhus tox.*" (*Arn.,*—but *Arn.* has not the *strained feeling of Rhus*. Hill-climbing, *Ars. Rhus* is almost the specific of STRAINS and SPRAINS.)

But of *Lumbago* he says, " Here *Rhus* is the remedy whether the patient is better from motion or not. *Rhus* has ' great pains in attempting to rise : stiff neck from sitting in a draught ; interscapular pains, better from warmth and worse from cold.' "

And he says, " *Rhus* is especially indicated in what has been termed rheumatic gout. Especially indicated in a rheumatic hard swelling of the big-toe joint, often mistaken for bunion."

Rhus has " Colic, better by bending double *and moving about.* (*Coloc.* better bending, but not from motion.)"

" In orbital cellulitis, *Rhus* is almost a specific."

Rheumatism of maxillary joints, as if jaw would break. Easy dislocation of jaw.

"RHUS is very freaky. For instance, hunger without appetite : hungry sensation, or sensation of emptiness in the stomach without desire for food. Dryness of the mouth and throat with great thirst; unquenchable thirst for cold drinks, especially at night, with great dryness of the mouth. Yet many times the cold drinks bring on chilliness, and bring on the cough." KENT.

The relentless periodicity of *Rhus* poisoning, on sensitives, is instanced by one case where the symptoms returned on the same day—even hour, for sixteen years, till *Tuberculinum* stopped the trouble (Clarke) ; and another case (Hering) where the burning itching of skin, lasting twenty-four hours, recurred on May 13th each year.

In a previous number of HOMŒOPATHY we quoted a letter to Dr. Kent, alluding to his statement that " when a person was poisoned by *Rhus* it was because he was in need of that poison, and had it been given in a high potency, he would not have been poisoned by contact with the plant " ; and saying, that in travels in northern and western parts of New York, the writer, a Dr. Peters, " learned from the farmers that as soon as the leaves come out, they pick off two or three and chew them, after which they can handle the plant with bare hands with impunity". Personally, one would not care to risk either !

Farrington speaks of *Rhus* as useful in various forms of PARALYSIS, especially in rheumatic patients from over-exertion, or exposure to wet (as lying on damp ground (*Dulc.*). He thinks it originates in a rheumatic inflammation of the meninges of the cord. The three drugs he contrasts for paralysis from *cold* are *Rhus*, *Sulph.* and *Caust.* *Rhus* especially affects fibrous tissues, tendons, fasciæ, sheaths of nerves, ligaments and tissues external to joints, rather than the joints themselves (*Bry.*). It has a great record in the treatment of lumbago and sciatica, where not from mechanical cause ; and, as Hahnemann insists, *Sprains.* We seem to remember that it was the prompt relief from a very bad sprained ankle that caused one of our doctors to look into Homœopathy.

BLACK LETTER SYMPTOMS

(*Allen, Hering and Hahnemann*).

Worse in the house, relieved by walking in open air (Puls.).
Sad, begins to weep without knowing why.
Very restless mood.

Great apprehension at night ; cannot remain in bed.

On rising such dizziness, it seemed she was going to fall forward and backward.

Inflammation of the EYES.
Very sore around the right eye.
The eyes are closed, or greatly swollen and inflamed.
Great swelling of the lids.
Left eye closed from swollen lids.
Inflammation of the lids.
Eyes red and agglutinated with matter in a.m.
Eyes agglutinated with purulent mucus in a.m.
Heaviness and stiffness of lids, like a paralysis : difficult to move the lids.

Nasal mucus runs in profusion out of nose, as in the most severe coryza in a.m., after rising from bed (Nux). Frequent, violent, spasmodic sneezing.

Great swelling of the FACE.

Yawning so violent and spasmodic : causes pain in maxillary joint which is in danger of being dislocated.

Sore sensation with redness at apex of TONGUE.
Tongue dry.   Salivation.

THROAT *much swollen externally, maxillary and parotid glands greatly enlarged.*
Parotid and submaxillary glands hard and swollen.

Great thirst.
Thirst and dryness of throat.

Acute diseases take on a TYPHOID *form—dysentery.   Peritonitis, Pneumonia, Scarlatina, Diphtheria.*
Typhoid fever : mild temperament ; mild delirium ; at times may try to jump out of bed or try to escape. . . .   Mental and physical restlessness.   Constantly tosses about bed, lies first on one side then the other, one moment sitting up, the next lying down.   At beginning of disease wants to lie perfectly quiet on account of great weakness—prostrate—indifferent.   Hallucinations : fears he will be poisoned ; refuses medicine and food.

Short COUGH, *from severe tickling and irritation behind the upper part of sternum, followed the feeling of discouragement and apprehension.*
Pneumonic cough, rust-coloured sputum.

Stiffness in small of BACK, *painful on motion.*

Small of back feels bruised.

While sitting the small of back aches, as after long stooping and bending the back.

Pain as if bruised in small of back, whenever he lies quietly upon it or sits still : on moving about he feels nothing.

Heaviness and pressure in small of back, as if one had received a blow, while sitting.

The LIMBS *tremble after exerting them.*

All the limbs feel stiff and paralysed, during and after walking ; with a sensation of a hundred-weight on nape of neck.

Sensation of stiffness on first moving the limb after rest.

The limbs upon which he lies, especially the arm, fall asleep.

A sensation as of trembling in arms and lower extremities, even while at rest.

Drawing in all the limbs, while lying down.

Trembling of arms after moderate exertion of them.

Violent tearing pain in arm, most violent while lying still.

Drawing and paralysed sensation left arm, at night.

Sticking and drawing in left arm extending from above downward and out at tips of fingers.

Pain in left upper arm as if muscles or tendons were unduly strained, when the limb is carried by them far upwards and backwards, at 2 and 3 p.m.

Jerking tearing in elbow and wrist joints, during rest, better during motion.

Loss of power and stiffness in forearms and fingers on moving them.

A powerless sensation in upper right forearm, on motion, and pain as if sprained in wrist, when grasping anything.

Sensation on upper surface left wrist on bending it, as if it had been sprained.

When grasping, feeling as if pins were pricking tips and palmar surface of first phalanges of fingers .

Great weakness of legs while walking in open air (afternoon), hardly able to proceed, because they are so heavy and weary (Gels.): after sitting an hour, weariness disappears.

Great heaviness in legs while sitting, disappeared on walking.

Aching pains in legs, inability to rest in any position but for a moment.

Pressive pain in both hip-joints on every step, and paralysed sensation in anterior muscles of thighs.

Tension, left hip-joint, while sitting.

When lying on the side the hips hurt, and when lying on the back, the small of the back hurts.

Stiffness, especially knees and feet.

Tension left knee joint, when rising from seat.

Tension knee, as if it were too short.

Uneasiness in foot (from pulling and tension in tendons.)

Tearing in knee and ankle, worse during rest.

Legs heavy and weary, as if he had walked a long distance.

Pain like a tingling in tibiæ at night, when feet are crossed.

Constantly obliged to move legs back and forth, and so unable to sleep.

Heaviness and tension in feet while sitting, but only weariness when walking.

Feet painful, as if sprained or wrenched on rising in a.m.

A drawing, like paralysis, in whole foot, while sitting.

Unusual weakness of limbs, mostly during rest.

Very great weakness, especially walking in open air.

Weariness, worse sitting, relieved while walking : decided stiffness on rising from seat.

Unusual RESTLESSNESS *at night. Great restlessness.*

Could not sit still on account of internal uneasiness, but was obliged to turn in every direction on the chair, and move all her limbs (Pyrogen).

Great uneasiness at night.

Stiff on rising from a seat.

Soreness in every muscle, passes off during exercise.

SKIN: *erysipelas, with numerous vesicles that burst, and secreted for eight days a slimy liquid.*

After 24 hours itching and burning commenced, lasting from half-an-hour to two hours.

After 36 hours, swelling of the parts, with violent itching and burning, increased on touching or moving; the parts affected as if pierced by hot needles (Ars.) White transparent vesicles appeared on the highly red and inflamed skin (Ran. bulb.).

Covered from head to foot with a fine red vesicular rash, itching and burning terribly, especially in the joints ; worse at night causing constant scratching, with little or no relief, and which felt very hard when pressed with the finger : skin burning hot.

The face became red, enormously swollen and œdematous, then also the hands and the skin of the whole body became covered with a scarlet-like exanthema, with intolerable itching biting ; on the fourth day, the backs of the hands and legs became covered with blisters, which burst and slowly desquamated. Violent vesicular erysipelas of the face and hands, attended with a high state of fever.

Burning, itching eruptions.

Urticaria from getting wet : during rheumatism : with chills and fever. Worse in cold air.

Eczema : raw, excoriated : thick crusts, oozing and offensive.

Burning, itching, tingling pains. Incessant itching and scratching. The more they scratch, the greater the urgency to scratch.

Acts on fibrous and muscular TISSUES.

Flesh of affected parts sore to touch.

Pain as if flesh torn loose from bones : or bones being scraped.

Pains as if sprained : disposition to sprain a part by lifting heavy weights, or stretching up to reach things.

Inflammation of tendons and muscles from over-exertion, or sudden wrenching as in a sprain.

Bad effects of getting wet, especially after being heated.

Smooth red and shining swellings, the inflamed skin being covered with small painful, white vesicles.

Glands swollen, hot, painful ; indurated : suppurating.

PARALYSIS : *after unwonted exertion : parturition : rheumatic, from getting wet or lying on damp ground : after ague or typhoid.*

Parts painless, or painfully stiff and lame, with tearing, tingling numbness.

Twitchings of limbs and muscles.

Restless at night, has to change position frequently.

Bad consequences from getting wet, especially after being heated.

FEVER. *Cough during chill : dry, teasing, fatiguing.*

Slow fevers : tongue dry and brown, or red as if skinned ; sordes on teeth ; bowels loose ; great weakness ; powerlessness of lower limbs, can hardly draw them up. Great restlessness after midnight ; must move often to get relief.

*　　*　　*

As we have seen, *Rhus* has *very definite spheres of action.* SKIN, to vesication and erysipelas ; glands throughout the body, enlarging and inflaming them, including the parotids and Peyer's patches (*Dros.*), which suggests its deep utility in typhoid. It " depresses nutritional activity ; depresses the sensorium, and the capability of the mind for continuous thought ; thus a patient meaning to write the number 12 will write the figure 1, but cannot recollect the figure which should follow " (DUNHAM). The *Rhus* powerlessness, approaching paralysis, is more pronounced in the lower extremities (DUNHAM). And Dunham sums up the action of *Rhus*, as follows : " It produces a kind of rheumatic affection of muscles and ligaments, alleviated by motion ; a paralysis aggravated by motion ; an apparent passive congestion of head, relieved by repose ; a debility of the organs of nutrition marked by deficient and depraved appetite and by tympanitis ; a serous infiltration of the cellular tissue in various parts, as face, fauces, genital organs, feet ; a vesicular eruption generally ; an acrid state of the secretions generally, tears, nasal mucus, urine, menstrual flow, contents of cutaneous vesicles ; general depression of sensorium."

But *Rhus* is practically only prescribed on its peculiar modalities and that in *any* disease : its restlessness : its temporary relief from motion ; its intolerance of damp and cold : and the etiology of most of the conditions it causes and cures—A COLD WETTING : A CHILL FROM DAMP, especially when warm (*Dulc.*).

*　　*　　*

There are other species of *Rhus* used in homœopathic medicine. *Rhus radicans* (Poison Ivy), which Jahr makes much of, and which has seemed to us a more potent remedy in lumbago, sciatica, and even headache, than *Rhus tox.* (Poison Oak), but which Hahnemann, as seen from our heading, has included in his provings with *Rhus tox.* Then there is *Rhus aromatica* (Fragrant Sumach), a non-poisonous shrub, which has a reputation, in the tincture, for diabetes. *Rhus venenata* (Poison Sumach), said to be more poisonous than *Rhus tox.* and which has to be handled with extreme caution, and it is said to be more actively curative in skins. It seems to affect bones more than *Rhus tox.* especially where bones are near the surface, " directly covered with skin ". *Rhus diversiloba*, again, a remedy of eczema and erysipelas, and *Rhus glabra*—all to be found in *Clarke's Dictionary*.

RUTA GRAVEOLENS

"THERE'S Rue for you!" . . . An ancient herb of great virtue: "Herb of Grace";—"Herb of repentance":—supposed to be a valuable defence against witches;—and "an antidote to all dangerous medicines and deadly poisons", so Culpepper tells us; a "Mithridate", i.e. one of the poisons on which the King of Pontus fed daily, to the intent that "*they should have no power, but be a kind of nutriment*". He is said to have eaten, among the rest, by which he sought to render himself acclimatized, as it were, and so immune from poisonings, two of the tiny leaves of Rue daily. And Rue is a poison, and therefore a medicine.

Used for purposes of abortion, it has encompassed its end in the most protracted and suffering way—at times ending with death : like other methods to the same intent.

Rue is a dear friend among medicines ; One met with it first as a plant which our gardeners always kept in an odd corner of the kitchen garden, from which to make an ointment for the cows' udders, should they get sore. As an ointment, it is also a fine application for chilblains : one used to get appeals for some more Rue ointment for a young nephew's chilblains, which otherwise were bad enough to keep the poor schoolboy in bed. One discovered its virtues also in housemaid's knee, and generally in inflammations of synovial membranes. But here it seems to do equally well internally in the 200th potency.

It was proven by Hahnemann and some of his band, and has very definite spheres of action—as we shall see : viz. *eyes*—*anus*—*ganglia* and such-like—*injuries to periosteum*—*sprains*, especially of *wrist and ankle*. It is one of the great vulneraries (with *Arnica*), helping in injuries not only of soft parts, but of bones and periosteum—and as said—sprains (with *Rhus*)—and skins, even to erysipelas. Like *Rhus* it has caused, in some persons who have handled it, severe skin troubles. *Some* persons !—not all, for one has handled it, from time to time, for years, and taken no hurt.

In regard to *Rue*, hear Hahnemann (*Materia Medica Pura*). "This powerful plant, hitherto almost only employed in haphazard fashion by common folk as a domestic remedy in indeterminate cases, acquires considerable importance from the following (all too meagre !) symptoms observed from its administration. The homœopathic practitioner sees what peculiar serious cases of disease he is able to cure by its means.

"If Rosenstein cannot sufficiently commend the virtues of *Rue* in affections of the eye and dimness of vision from *too much*

reading, in which Swedjaur and Chomel agree with him, he must
be very blind who fails to see that these are solely owing to the
homœopathic power of Rue to cause a similar condition in healthy
persons." He refers to the symptoms, 44, 45 :

" His eyes feel as if he had strained the sight too much by
reading.

" Weak, pressive-like pain in right eye, with dimness of
surrounding objects, as if from having looked too long at an object
that was fatiguing to the eyes.

" A feeling of heat and burning in eyes and pain in them when
he reads."

He goes on : " By this so similarly acting medicine the malady
is certainly not increased and aggravated as our opponents, who
think themselves so wise in their ignorance, would conclude, with
ridiculous expressions of alarm, and *without interrogating experience*.
On the contrary, it will be cured (if not dependent on a miasmatic
dyscrasia) to the bitter disappointment and confusion of learned
routinists who reject the most beneficent of all truths."

Hahnemann is delightful in his happy expressions. " *A
domestic remedy in indeterminate cases* " ; opponents " who without
interrogating experience *think themselves wise in their ignorance* ".
But, I suppose we all do that, more or less : like madness, " it is
only a case of degrees ". " Ridiculous expressions of alarm
without interrogating experience."

The black letter symptoms give one a great idea as to the
range of action of a drug, and the special localities it attacks.
Glancing down these, there is no doubt as to the effect of *Ruta*
on the *eye* ; but it is chiefly on the eye muscles, tiring, and failing
to accommodate, that *Ruta* acts. It does not appear to violently
inflame the eye, like *Arg. nit.* for instance : but Milton hits it very
cleverly when he says, " *Euphrasie* and *Rue to clear his visual ray.*"
One remembers a case of a woman, away in the country, with
lengthening sight and imperfect vision therefrom, needing glasses :
but a dose of *Ruta* (ϕ so far as one remembers) so improved the
eye strain, that the necessity for glasses was deferred.

Again reading down the black letter symptoms, one is struck
with the *Ruta* sensations " *weariness* "—" *as from a strain* "—
" *as from a blow* "—" *as from a fall* "—and again and again,
" *as if bruised* ",—even, " *as if broken through the middle* " (the
thigh). Then, *loss of power*, especially in the thighs and lower
extremities.

Its kindly effects on painful and sprained wrists one has seen
often : it seems to have a specific action on wrists and ankles.
It has been permitted to torture the wrists of a few provers, in

order that it should prove curative to the sprained wrists of the multitude—*in der evigkeit*. In Homœopathy it is good indeed that the few have suffered for the many.

In regard to *Rue*, GUERNSEY (" *Keynotes* ") says : " Injuries to periosteum, as when one has had a fall or an accident which injures the periosteum, making it very sore and causing a bruised sensation.

" When the rectum protrudes from anus after confinement ; prolapsus ani, which may come down every time the bowels are moved.

" Pain, as if bruised in the outer parts and in the bones ; painfulness of bones in general : wounds where the bones are injured. . . .

" Affections in general of left side head ; of bladder ; wrist joints ; lumbar region ; bones of lower extremity.

" Worse lying on painful side : looking fixedly at an object, as those who have looked closely at watch-making, fine sewing, etc. ; from taking uncooked food."

Ruta is worse from cold : worse from wet : relieved by motion. (All *Rhus* !)

Nausea may be felt in various parts of the body, in throat, as CYCL., PHOS. A., STANN ; in stomach, nearly a half-page of drugs, including, *par excellence*, IPEC. ; in abdomen, a few drugs, including *Puls*. Clarke gives a curious " clinical symptom of *Ruta* : *A sensation of nausea located in the rectum.*"

NASH says, " *Ruta* is also one of our best remedies for *prolapsus of rectum.*" (*Ign.*, *Mur. a.*, *Pod.* and *Aloe.*) And for eye-strain he says, " *Nat. mur.* and *Senega* must be remembered."

By the way, in regard to *Ruta* for " backs ", synovial membranes and sciatica : After manipulating sub-luxations of pelvis, it seems to be good practice to give a dose or two of *Ruta*. So far as one has observed, the pain, sometimes felt for a day or two after such manipulations, may be thus lessened or obviated.

In conclusion, KENT tells us that the symptoms of *Ruta* are difficult to classify in the Repertory ; its *nature* must be obtained. It resembles RHUS, as sensitive to cold, and cold damp ; as suffering from strains and over-exertion :—with him *Ruta* is *Rhus*, but more so. *Ruta* has more than any drug, periosteal troubles from injury : as when lumps persist in the periosteum, sore : slow repair : bruises leave indurations : hardened masses in tendons, after gripping and clasping, as in hands : with gradual contraction of flexors, till hands are permanently flexed. Feet become also contracted, and so flexed that the sole becomes concave, and toes drawn under. (Comp. *Caust.*)

In eye troubles he contrasts *Ruta* with *Arg. nit.* But *Ruta* is worse from cold : *Arg. nit.* from heat, and wants a cool place.

He says both *Ruta* and *Phos.* have violent unquenchable thirst for ice-cold water, and can never get enough of it.

Neuralgias, etc. He says, *Ruta* " has all the pains in the books, described by all the adjectives that apply to pain, but it is worse lying down, and worse from cold. Neuralgias of all sorts— severe." The severest forms of sciatica—worse as soon as he lies down at night. Restlessness like *Rhus* : bruised sensations like *Arnica*. . . .

One of our greatest vulneraries, unquestionably.

Black Letter Symptoms

HEAD. *Shooting pain from frontal to temporal bone : from temporal bone to occiput : in the periosteum : pain as if from a fall.*
Stitches in left frontal bone, only from reading.
Rhythmical pressive pain in head.

— *Sensation of heat and fire in* EYES *: aching while reading, in the evening, by the light.*
— *Eyes feel fatigued, as after reading too long.*
— *Weary pain in the eyes while reading.*
— *Aching in and over eyes, vision blurred, after using eyes and straining them over fine work.*
Vision very weak, as if eyes were excessively strained.
Asthenopia : irritability of every tissue of eye, from overwork, or using eyes on too fine work ; heat and aching in and over eyes ; eyes feel like balls of fire at night ; blurring of vision ; letters seem to run together ; lachrymation.
— *A burning under left eye.*
Itching inner canthi and on lower lids, which smart after rubbing them, when eyes become filled with water.
Spasm in lower eyelid ; the tarsus is drawn hither and thither, and when it ceases, water runs from both eyes.

Sensation in EAR *as if a blunt piece of wood were pushed about in it : a scratching pressure.*
Cartilages of ears pain, as from a blow or fall.
Under the mastoid process pain as from a blow or fall.

Tension in STOMACH *> by drinking milk.*

< *In the* HEPATIC REGION *an aching, gnawing pain.*

When sitting, tearing stitches in the rectum.

Tearing in rectum and urethra, when not urinating.

Prolapsus of rectum. Fæces pass involuntarily while bending over. Prolapse always with and sometimes without stool.

Protrusion of rectum after confinement. After dysentery half a year previously.

A gnawing in left side of chest.

In right CHEST *a gnawing sensation, combined with something corrosive and burning.*

Pain, as if beaten in the SPINE.

Itching in left upper ARM : *excites scratching.*

In left elbow-joint pain, as from a blow, with weakness in the arm.

The bones of wrist and back of hand are painful, as if bruised, when at rest and when moving them.

In the bones about the hips pain as from a blow or fall.

He cannot bend his body, all the joints and the hip bones are painful as if bruised.

On touching the painful parts, especially hips and thigh bones, they are painful as if bruised.

The whole anterior surface of the thighs is as if bruised and painful to touch.

If he stretches out lower extremities, even a little, the thighs are painful, as if broken through the middle.

Posterior part of thigh and above the knee, feels bruised.

After sitting, he cannot walk immediately : falls back again.

When walking, falls from one side to the other ; his legs cannot support him ; no power and no stability in thighs.

Difficulty in going up and down stairs, legs bend under him.

Dare not tread strongly on feet : bones of feet painful, with feeling of heat.

On the front of left ankle joint a pain, throbbing and hacking, as if an ulcer were there.

Burning and corrosive pain in bones of feet when at rest.

Knows not where to put legs because of restlessness and heaviness, puts them first in one place then another, and turns body from side to side.

Lameness after sprains, especially of wrists and ankles.

Yawning, stretching and extending the hands.

24

All parts of body on which he lies, even in bed, are painful as if bruised.

Bruises and mechanical injuries of bones and periosteum : sprains ; periostitis ; erysipelas.
Bone lesions and fractures : scrofulous exostoses.

Coldness from the spine downwards.
Frequent waking at night : vivid confused dreams.

One of the peculiar sensations of Ruta *is cramp in the tongue.*
" Spasm of tongue with difficulty of speech."
Another, nausea felt in rectum.

SALICYLATES : SALICYLIC ACID

ONE of the drugs greatly used and sometimes greatly abused by
Old School, and therefore worthy of careful study from our point
of view.   Because, in order to know beforehand and with assurance what a drug can cure, it is necessary to discover just what
it can cause of damage to mind and body.   So we will endeavour
to consider its uses and abuses, in order to gather how best it may
be employed.

We are told that " it is chiefly used for its effect in articular
rheumatism, in which it is highly efficacious, but that it is of no
value in gonorrhœal arthritis or in arthritis deformans, and is
of little use in gout ".

" In acute rheumatism it promptly relieves all the local joint
symptoms, but it does not affect the endocarditis, and is in no
sense a specific remedy."   One can now see why homœopaths
with their host of remedies for rheumatism (*or for the patient with
rheumatism*), are not too ready to bow the knee to any remedy,
however popular, which, brilliantly relieving the local condition
and the fever, leaves the real menace—to heart—untouched.
One must remember that in children, acute rheumatism is a heart
disease, and that anything that suppresses external manifestations
with their pains and inconveniences, must be a very dangerous
remedy.   Acute rheumatism may be easily recovered from,
whereas a damaged heart is apt to be a life-sentence and a terrible
handicap.

By the way, though we are told of its uselessness in gonorrhœal
arthritis, arthritis deformans and gout, yet, given on homœopathic
indications, and in homœopathic preparations, salicylic acid, like
any other drug, has proved its curative powers.

The following are its subversive properties, from which we may
glean its homœopathic virtues.   Though " analgesic, antipyretic
and a feeble antiseptic", it has been used with success, homœopathically, in puerpural fever.

" It irritates mucous membranes and may cause vomiting
when given in large doses on an empty stomach.   In old school
text books, again, we are told that ' large therapeutic doses '
produce ringing in the ears, nausea, sometimes vomiting, and an
increase in the amount of urine ; they may also cause albuminuria
and renal irritation, which generally disappear after the drug is
excreted. . . .   In very large doses it may produce depression
of the central nervous system, rarely convulsions . . . is
useful in some forms of eye disease. . The dose, 15 grains, may be

repeated every hour till salicylism occurs, and then three times a day.   After death from poisoning by *Salicylic acid*, echymoses and ulceration of the mucous membrane of stomach have been found."

Our main experience with *Salicylic acid* has been in a few cases of Meniere's disease, where its action, in the usual small doses of Homœopathy, has been prompt and satisfactory.   And it has been interesting to see that in some old school text books the drug is recommended for that disease,—because of its power to produce the symptoms !

Black Letter, Italic and Suggestive Symptoms

Ulceration of mucous membranes.
Acute articular rheumatism.
Delirium ; stupid ; can hardly collect thoughts ; laughed without cause ; talked incessantly and disconnectedly ; frequently looked about him with apparent hallucinations.

Vertigo, inclined to fall to left ; while surrounding objects seen to fall to right.
Ménière's disease ; *vertigo comes and goes from no cause ; headaches frequent, not always present ; noises in ear ; defective or perosseous hearing ; no gastric symptoms, or too slight to account for the rest ; indeterminate giddiness in horizontal position, considerable when raising head, or sitting up.*
Deafness, with noises in ears.
Auditory nerve vertigo ; troublesome nausea accompanies head symptoms.

Incipient catarrh ; sneezes all day.

Mouth and throat dry; burning and dryness of mouth and fauces.
Stomatitis ; mouth dry and hot ; tongue covered with burning vesicles.
Canker sores ; with burning soreness and fetid breath.
Canker of mouth, stomach and bowels.

Burning in throat.
Tonsils red, swollen, studded white.
Difficulty in swallowing ; violent efforts to swallow.   Worse right side.   Throat and fauces red, swollen, ulcerated.

Ecchymoses and ulceration in mucous membrane of stomach and bowels (found P.M. in poisonings).

Burning in epigastric region.

Dyspepsia ; putrid eructations and much gas in stomach.

Diarrhœa ; cholera infantum, when eructations have a peculiarly putrid and offensive odour.

Urine very offensive ; with mucus, pus, blood.

Urine, 3 hours after passage has a green tinge and deposits a feathery precipitate—salicyluric acid ; if these are removed it becomes at once putrid ; if not, it remains fresh for above a week.

Rheumatism : heat, redness, soreness, swelling about joints, worse knees, with acute piercing pains. Worse motion. Worse touch of anything cold.

Worse at night. Better dry heat : hot applications.

Copious foul-smelling foot sweats. Sensation as if foot wanted to perspire.

The pains are burning ; also shooting and stitching.

Purpua hæmorrhagica, with hæmorrhages from all mucous membranes ; with constant dull aching distress in stomach, and occasional vomiting of blood and mucus.

Has a very specific action on serous membranes.

*   *   *

DR. HUGHES, *Pharmacodynamics :* " The physiological effects of the acid and of its compounds with soda, we know mainly from observations of over-dosing. . . . Resembles quinine in pathogenetic as well as curative action. . . . Its most striking effects were manifested in a non-contagious fever, which had hitherto been classed separately from the zymoses, I speak of acute rheumatism. As a remedy for this malady it has received the warmest commendation from all quarters. It seems to find its opportunity when the temperature is high, and joint after joint is being involved, with severe pain. Its administration at this time rarely fails to bring down the fever and relieve the pains in the space of 36 to 48 hours. . . . In the face of these facts, we disciples of Hahnemann had to consider what we ought to do. Our results in acute rheumatism, though satisfactory enough, were certainly not so good as those·claimed for this remedy. . ." He gives cases in which Salicin in provings and one in enormous dosage in a case of acute rheumatism, provoked fever : in the latter, the temperature rose steadily till death occurred, when the thermometer registered 110 degrees. Also,

in experiments on animals, that Salicylic acid, both free and in
the state of Salicylate, lowers the temperature, but within
restricted limits. In a somewhat larger dose, it not only does
not lower the temperature, but sometimes considerably increases
it. . . .

He says further, that there are three ways in which acute
rheumatism has been and can be treated, and the medicines
which have been in repute for it fall into three classes accordingly.
You may endeavour to neutralize chemically the presumedly
acid *materies morbi*, as by alkalies, neutral salts or lemon juice.
You may seek to check the formation of this peccant matter.
Or you may forcibly (as it were) repress fever and deaden pain,
while leaving untouched the specific morbid process present.
. . . The great defect of such remedies is that, leaving the
essential malady untouched, and only hushing up its expressions
they favour the tendency to relapse, and so unduly protract the
illness.

He then discusses the symptoms now known as salicylism—
deafness, noises in the ears, vertigo—the essential features of
Ménière's disease : " auditory nerve vertigo " for which even
old school authorities have found it useful.

* * *

BOERICKE, *Materia Medica,* says : " The symptoms point to
its use in rheumatism, dyspepsia, and Meniere's disease. Prostration after influenza : also tinnitus aurium and deafness.
Hæmaturia."

* * *

The *Cyclopædia of Drug Pathogenesy* gives interesting cases,
especially where it details over-dosage, and poisonings. Their
salient features are practically contained in our extracts from
Symptomatology, above. Its effects on mucous membranes :
its pains, especially burning pains, with inflammation leading to
ulceration, foulness and putridity ; its specific effects on ears
and hearing, with all the symptoms of Ménière's disease : its
hæmorrhagic tendencies, very pronounced in regard to nose,
gums, and stomach, make it an important remedy. In one case
a young married woman of 27 was dosed with Salicylic acid for
acute rheumatism and developed first the usual deafness, singing
in ears and hallucinations of hearing. A few days later, nose and
gums began to bleed, and the bleeding from gums became so severe
that she grew pale and weak with a small rapid pulse. Large
clots collected in mouth, and stools were blackened, it was supposed
from swallowed blood. The Salicylic acid was stopped; though the

idea was that it might be a purpuric or scorbutic affection:—whereupon the hæmorrhage also ceased. But when in a few days, for a slight relapse of the articular rheumatism, the salicylate was again given, the very next day, the gums began to bleed again—which finished the treatment by Salicylic acid. It was ascertained that she had never before suffered with bleeding from gums ; nor were they spongy or inclined to bleed between these attacks of hæmorrhage.

In another case, a patient suffering from a very severe and painful attack of acute rheumatic fever, was given large doses of Salicylic acid ; after the fifth dose, the pains disappeared by magic ; but on the third day he felt all at once a violent pain in epigastric region, and suddenly expired. Quite a number of sudden deaths have been recorded.

Besides epistaxis, other hæmorrhages had been frequently observed from the administration of large doses of Salicylic acid for acute rheumatism ; among them hæmaturia, and even retinal hæmorrhage.

One has an idea that Salicylic acid is used to preserve jams from deterioration. It should,—in small doses—since in "heroic" doses it produces, everywhere, putridity. In susceptibles one should look out for even such small salicylic poisonings. One is beginning to think that in our day the devil has special methods of torture and damage for civilized humanity, in the Knowledge of Good and Evil that comes through such sciences as chemistry. The simpler our foods and lives and the more natural, the safer—as regards vigour and well-being. But always the question of *individuality* and *idiosyncrasy* creeps in ; and the many seem to tolerate without notable damage what is destruction—perhaps death, to the few. And yet, the many must also suffer, to a less appreciable extent.

Moral : the more one learns, the more convinced one is, that the rapid, safe and successful methods of Homœopathy are preferable, every time, in the treatment—of even such painful conditions as acute rheumatism. Where an indifferent prescriber may not get quick and full results, he, at least, does not endanger life.

SANGUINARIA CANADENSIS
(*Bloodroot*)

WHEN one thinks of recurrent sick headaches, one's thoughts are apt to fly beyond the polycrests to, especially, *Iris* and *Sanguinaria*; and it may be well to take them one after the other, in order to realize their great differences, as well as their correspondences: because there is no such splendid way of learning anything, as teaching it. The person you teach may absorb little or much— depends perhaps a bit upon the way the thing is presented and the extent to which it interests him and gets his attention : but the person who teaches is obliged to really study and get the subject up, and it probably goes in a little deeper, and more ought to stick.

Sanguinaria, like *Iris*, has won a great reputation in *sick headaches* ; but *Sanguinaria* is of the " sun headache " variety : starts with sunrise, grows more intense as the day wears on, and declines towards evening. There is nothing like this in *Iris*. Other drugs that come in here are GLON., *Nat. m.*, *Phos.*, *Spig.*, *Stann.*

Sanguinaria also lacks the burning acridity of *Iris*, while it affects lungs more than, like *Iris*, the length of the digestive tract. *Sanguinaria* is a great chest medicine : useful even in phthisis. Hahnemann, in his arrangement of provings (and all his followers in their arrangement of materia medica and Repertories, following his useful lead), starts with mouth, runs through the whole of the digestive tract, œsophagus, stomach, intestines, rectum, anus and stool, adding the organs of digestive secretions, liver, pancreas;—in all these *Iris* meddles fearfully, and therefore heals. Then he starts again at mouth, and runs through the respiratory system, and here *Sanguinaria* especially interferes, for evil and for good. So, after all, one can place these two remedies, and realize their possibilities and peculiarities very easily, if one "figures it out" thus.

We are trying to stress the spheres of these two sick headache remedies : but they are only two among the many.

* * *

Sanguinaria's BLACK LETTER SYMPTOMS (most often confirmed by caused and cured symptoms) are of course emphasized by every teacher and every text book that treats of " Bloodroot ".

Determination of blood to the head, with whizzing in the ears and transitory feeling of heat, then a sensation as if vomiting was about to take place.

HEADACHE *begins in occiput, spreads upwards, and settles over right eye.*

Periodical sick headache ; begins in the morning, increases during the day, lasts until evening. Head feels as if it must burst, or as if eyes would be pressed out. Throbbing, lancinating pains through brain, worse on right side, especially in forehead and vertex ; followed by chills, nausea, vomiting of food or bile ; must lie down and remain quiet ; relieved by sleep.

Paroxysmal headache. Headache, with nausea and chilliness, followed by flushes of heat, extending from the head to the stomach.

Neuralgia in and over right EYE.

NASAL *polypi.*

Red CHEEKS *with burning in ears, with cough.*

Burning in PHARYNX *and* ŒSOPHAGUS.

VOMITING *of bitter water ; of sour acrid fluids ; of ingesta ; or worms ; preceded by anxiety ; with headache and burning in stomach ; head better afterwards ; with prostration.*

Dry COUGH, *with considerable tickling in throat-pit, and a crawling sensation, extending down beneath the sternum. Teasing, dry, hacking cough, with dryness in the throat. Hacking cough, caused by tickling in the throat, several evenings after lying down. Tickling cough with very dry throat.*

Severe cough occurring after whooping-cough, when patient takes cold, which partakes of the spasmodic nature of whooping-cough.

Catarrhal irritation in chest ; night sweats ; after a cold, several months previously.

RHEUMATIC PAIN *in right arm and shoulder ; worse at night ; on turning in bed ; cannot raise arm.*

Lassitude, torpor, languor, not disposed to move or make any mental exertion. Worse in damp weather.

Lameness of right arm.

ITALIC OR CURIOUS SYMPTOMS

Flushes of heat, *extending from head to stomach.*

Some hard substance in stomach.

Head drawn forward : will burst : as if eyes would be pressed out.

Temples and scalp alive with irrepressible pulsations.

As if in a vehicle, moving and jarring her : as if all about her moved rapidly.

Tongue as if scalded : as if in contact with something hot.

Throat so dry, as if it would crack.

As if something alive in stomach (*Croc. Thuja*).

As if hot water were pouring from breast into abdomen.

Cough as if head in a blanket.

Upper part chest as if too full of blood.

Severe pain : head : root of nose : frontal sinuses ; right breast, extends to shoulder.   Right side chest.

The pains are burning : stitching : constricting.

Rheumatic pain, in places least covered with flesh.

*　　*　　*

Guernsey briefly epitomizes *Sanguinaria* : hitting, as usual, the principal points helpful in prescribing.

Useful where there is a pain rising from the back of the neck over the top of the head, running down the forehead : this symptom may occur alone, or in connection with some other trouble.

Headache begins in the morning, gets worse during the day, and lasts until evening.   Comes every seventh day (*Sabad.*, *Sil.*, *Sulph.*).

He says it is useful often for menopausic troubles, flashes of heat, etc.   *Rheumatism of right shoulder.*

*　　*　　*

Nash emphasizes the service *Sanguinaria* has rendered him. The headache coming up from the back of head, and settles down over the right eye (left eye, *Spigelia*), with nausea and vomiting : better quiet in a dark room.   " It will probably cure, or greatly relieve the ordinary American sick headache as often as any other remedy.   I use the 200th."

He italicizes, " *Loose cough, with badly smelling sputa ; the breath and sputa smell badly to the patient himself.*"   Sometimes pain behind sternum.   This kind of cough usually comes on after severe bronchitis or pneumonia, and it looks as if patient were fast running into consumption.   There may be flushes of fever, with circumscribed redness of cheeks, like hectic fever.   Many a case of this kind has been helped by this remedy.   He says Dr. T. L. Brown used the first trituration of the alkaloid with fine effect. The 200th has made just as good cures.   *Sanguinaria* in my hands has done good service in typhoid pneumonia with great dyspnœa and circumscribed redness of the cheeks.   The right lung seems to come under its influence, in either acute or chronic troubles.

He says that in the right shoulder and arm pain, *Sang.* has won him much credit. He has seen one dose of the first trituration cure such cases of long standing : also the C.M. do the same thing.

Acts intensely on right lung and chest.

* * *

ALLEN (*Keynotes*) emphasizes a curious symptom, which when it occurs should be very helpful in fixing the remedy. " Neuralgia of face, relieved by kneeling down and pressing head firmly against floor: pain extends in all directions from the upper jaw." "Again, *re* cough, this peculiarity ; cough dry ; wakes him at night, does not cease till he sits up and passes flatus."

* * *

KENT says, *Bloodroot* is an old domestic remedy. Eastern farmer's wives will not go into winter without bloodroot in the house. In cold winter days, for " cold " in head, throat and chest, then they make a bloodroot tea : their routine remedy . . . . and provings show its relation to " colds " that go to the chest.

Headaches, when headaches come once in seven days : begins on waking in the morning, or wakes the patient. Begins occiput, travels up to settle over right eye and in temple. Patient is driven into a dark room, and has to lie down. Then vomiting —bile, slime, and food taken the day before : then relief of pain, and sleep. If there are hot palms and soles, which he must put out of bed, this is an additional striking feature.

He says, it is not a long-acting remedy, and only of medium depth. Needs a deeper drug, an antipsoric, later, or headache may return—or worse, as *Sanguinaria* does not go deeply into the nature of the case. He says, Hahnemann warns against the use of *Phosphorus* in such cases of deficient vitality : here *Sanguinaria* is an excellent surface remedy : it does excellent palliation.

Sanguinaria has " rose colds " in June : is sensitive to flowers and odours :—hay fever . . . . palms and soles dry, wrinkled and hot to touch ; toes burn : corns burn : put hands and feet out of bed for relief. (An addition to *Sulph.*, *Puls.*, *Cham.* and *Meddorrh.* here.)

With the headache and many complaints *Sanguinaria* has a faintness : like a hunger, yet not for food. A sinking, faint, all-gone feeling. *Psorinum* leads all others in hunger headaches, but *Psor.* wants to eat and can't get enough. *Sang.* has a hunger, but not for food : aversion at the thought and smell of food . . . . it is a false hunger with the headache in *Sang.*

SANICULA AQUA

FROM water of a mineral spring of Ottawa, proved as to its deleterious effects by Dr. J. G. Gundlach, who, with his family drank it for more than a year, and who was still suffering from its effects five years later. The evaporated, triturated and potentized salt, was proved in the usual way under the auspices of the American doctor, Sherbino.

Clarke says, " In *Sanicula* we have one of the best proved remedies of the Materia Medica ; a polycrest and anti-psoric of wide range."

Personally one has used the remedy, in pretty high potency, from time to time with great satisfaction in the case of unflourishing children. It is very like *Silica* in the kind of children it benefits : many of their queer symptoms being almost identical : such as the sweating head at night, drenching the pillow : the " bashful stool ", very large, and slipping back when almost voided ; and the offensive foot-sweat. The appearance of the child it benefits, also suggests *Silica*.

ALLEN'S *Keynotes* has the most useful presentment of *Sanicula* : We will extract some of its salient features, re-arranging.

Child looks old, dirty, greasy, brownish. Skin about neck wrinkled and hangs in folds.

There is progressive emaciation.

Mentally: obstinate, headstrong. Cries and kicks. Does not want to be touched. (*Ant. crud., Cham.,* etc.)

"Constantly changing" is a feature that runs through *Sanicula*. Cross and irritable, then quickly laughs. Constantly changing occupation. Physical symptoms are also constantly changing. The diarrhœa is changeable in character and odour; like scrambled eggs ; or frothy and green—" like scum on a frog pond " (*Mag. carb.*).

The constipation is a great feature. Stools large, hard, impossible to evacuate. After great straining, the stool, partially expelled, recedes (*Op., Sil.,* LAC. D., NAT. MUR., THUJA, etc.), and must be mechanically removed.

Then, a *Sulphur* symptom, the odour of stool persists, despite bathing. Strong, offensive odour from ear ; of leucorrhœa ; of foot-sweat.

The uterine symptoms remind one of *Sepia* and *Lilium tigr.* Bearing down as if contents of pelvis would escape. Worse walking; jar. Must support parts by hand against the vulva.

The *Silica* foot-sweat, as said ; not only offensive, but causing soreness between toes. (*Graph.*, BAR. C., ZINC., *Sil.*, etc.)

Feet as if in cold water (comp. *Sepia*) or burning : must uncover them, or put them in a cool place (with SULPH., CHAM., MEDORRH., PULS., etc.).

And, again, like *Sulph.*, child kicks the clothes off.

Sanicula is a remedy of symptoms that appear to be picked out of a dozen other better known remedies, and here assembled bewilderingly.

But one sensation is probably peculiar to itself—*Bursting*:—in perineum—bowels—bladder—vertex—chest.

* * *

CLARKE (*Dictionary*) gives some of the rare and peculiar symptoms of *Sanicula*, and since the complete provings of the drug are not easily come by—not to be found in ALLEN's *Encyclopaedia* or HERING's *Guiding Symptoms*, we will give a number of them: remembering, always, that a rare symptom may really be common to several drugs, only perhaps not yet brought out in their provings. Yet, the queer experiences of provers may draw attention to a remedy that would not be otherwise considered, and which may be found, on examination, to cover the case. Again, almost more than any other remedy, this drug displays over and over again, exactly opposite conditions.

Restless desire to go from place to place (*Tub.*, etc.).

Great fear of darkness (*Stram.*, *Phos.*, CANN. IND., etc.).

Constant irresistible desire to look behind her (*Brom.*, *Lach.*, MED., etc.).

Sensation that head was open and wind went through it.

Sensation of a cold cloth round brain.

Awoke with dryness of whole eye, and sensation that eye is sticking to eyelid.

Soreness behind ears with discharge of white, gluey, sticky substance. (Comp. *Graph.*)

Large scabs on upper lip; picks them till they bleed. (Comp. *Arum triph.*)

On waking, dark brown streak down centre of tongue, which is furred and dry like leather.

Sides of tongue turn up. Tongue adheres to roof of mouth.

Teeth sensitive to cold air as if they were very thin.

Roof of mouth feels raw.

Child wants to nurse all the time, yet loses flesh. (Comp. *Nat. mur.*, *Abrot.*)

Child craves meat ; fat bacon, which aggravates. Craves salt.

Loss of desire for bread (*Nat. mur.*).

Child gets frantic when it sees a glass of water : drinks large quantities greedily. Or, thirst for small quantities very often, which are vomited almost as soon as they reach stomach.

Bloating of stomach on beginning to eat.

Feels terribly stuffed after a meal, must loosen clothing (*Lyc.*).

Shortly after nursing, food all comes up with a gush, and child drops into a stupid sleep. (Comp. *Aeth.*)

Sudden nausea while eating, vomits all the food taken.

(Falls asleep after vomiting is a feature of *Sanic.*) (*Aeth., Ip.*)

Vomits large tough curds like white of a hard-boiled egg (*Aeth.*).

Vomits after drinking cold water.

Food turns sour and rancid, with burning desire for water, which relieves for a short time, then aggravates.

(*Sanicula* is rich in stomach symptoms: in nausea and vomiting; in the vomiting of infants.) (Comp. *Aethusa*).

Sensation of a lump in stomach (*Bry.*).

Stomach sensitive to pressure and jar ; cannot laugh without holding stomach and bowels : worse when stomach is empty.

Morning sickness : sea sickness : nausea and sickness from riding in cars or close carriages, with desire for open air (*Cocc., Sep.*, etc.).

Rumbling and gurgling " like distant thunder " along course of large intestine : bowels bloated as if they would burst.

Pot-bellied children.

Rumbling relieved by eating (GRAPH., MOSCH., SUL., etc.).

After intense straining, stool which was partly evacuated, recedes. (*Sil.*, THUJA).

Even soft stool requires great effort to expel (*Alum.*), or—

Slim yellow stool at least ten inches long (Comp. *Phos.*), not requiring much effort.   .   .   .

Large evacuation of small, dry, grey balls ; must be removed by finger, lest it rupture the sphincter.

Great pain in perineum while at stool as though it would burst.

Perineum sore and burning for hours after stool. (Comp. *Nit. ac.*)

Stool feels full of jagged particles.

Stools as often as food is taken : must hurry from table after each meal. Must cross legs to prevent stool from escaping.

Stool square as if carved by a knife.

No control over sphincter : often soils himself, standing, running, even at night.

Frequent, profuse, sudden urination. Great effort to retain urine, yet if desire resisted, the urging ceases.

Urgent calls to pass urine, as if bladder would burst.

Feels as if a hard body like a lead pencil were forced up and back from bladder to kidney.

Child cries before urinating. Urine stains diaper red (Comp. *Lyc.*).

Odour like fish brine about genitalia. Child's parts smell like fish brine even after bathing.

Leucorrhœa or watery discharge from vagina with strong odour of fish brine.

During pregnancy, swelling and stiffness of hands and feet : sensation that os uteri is opening (Comp. *Lach.*), or dilating.

On swallowing, sensation of a hard substance in trachea.

Bursting feeling in vertex on coughing.

Asthmatic breathing : wheezing, rattling under sternum ; worse eating.

Tickling under sternum.

Sudden terrible sensation of a burden in chest : for a few moments it seems as if she would burst.

Neck so weak and emaciated that child cannot hold its head up ; (*Nat. mur., Abrot.*). Muscles back of neck seem too short.

Skin of neck wrinkles and hangs in folds.

Sharp pain from least turning : must hold himself stiff and turn whole body in order to look round.

Inclines head forward to ease pain in muscles of back of neck.

A dislocated sensation in last lumbar vertebra. Sensation in lower lumbar region that the vertebrae were gliding past each other.

Sensation that the back is in two pieces.

Region of coccyx sore (*Sil., Hyper.*).

Burning in spine (*Phos. Zinc.* etc.) : coldness in spine, worse cold.

A feature ; boils that do not mature, in various localities.

Deep, ragged, angry cracks of hands (*Petrol*), even exuding blood.

Hands as cold as though handling ice : or burning palms (*Phos.*, etc.).

On putting hands together they sweat until it drops from them.

Knuckles of fingers crack and leak.

Feet clammy cold : cramp in feet in bed, they are so cold.

Or, burning of feet, especially soles, wants to put them in cool place, in water, or to uncover them (Comp. *Sulph., Puls., Cham., Medorrh.*).

Sweat between toes, making them sore, with foul odour (*Baryta c.*, etc.).

Child kicks off clothing in coldest weather (*Sulph.*).

Wants to lie on something hard.

Child looks old, dirty, greasy, brownish. Progressive emaciation.

Wakes her companion to look for a tramp in her room ; gets up and looks under the bed for him (Comp. *Nat. mur.*).

On waking, child rubs eyes and nose with its fist (Comp. *Cina.*).

Cannot bear anyone to lie close to him or touch him.

Begins to sweat as soon as covered.   (Uncovered parts *Thuja*).

Sweat on first falling asleep (Comp. *Con.*), especially occiput and neck, wetting the clothes through.   Cold clammy sweat, those parts feel like a wet stone (*Verat. a.*).

Hungry during sweat.

Fevers with periodicity.

We have come across, in an old copy of *The Homœopathic Physician*, 1893, a few of Dr. Gundlach's cured cases, showing the range of the remedy, remedially.   The first is a case of polyuria with pale colourless urine, S.G. 1,000, day and night, but worse by day.   The man, an attorney, felt tired out and exhausted ; small of back weak and aching.   Bad taste, not much appetite : very thirsty for very large drinks : " wants to drink all the time. Feet cold and damp : sweat offensive."   He had seen two doctors— an allopath, and " our biochemic friend ", but was no better. Remembering his own case, and also its subsequent provings, Dr. Gundlach gave him *Sanicula*, and cured him.   A year later, the trouble had not returned.

A second case, " headache and mental ", in a printer, aged 40. Suffering from over-work, with dull pain in forehead over eyes : eyes felt as if being drawn back into head.   All worse in warm or close room : better in open air.   Mind wanders trying to apply it. Can't keep at anything in the office for any length of time.   Starts a thing ; drops it and picks up another.   Was his own master, with work that must be done, yet for the most trifling reason he will drop it and run out.   No appetite : tongue coated ; mouth dry.   In this case, no thirst.   The man was in great distress. Was sure he would lose his reason if not helped soon.   *Sanicula* 10*m* cured him at once : and three months later, he was still perfectly well.   *Puls.*, first given, " did not help any ".

His third case, a woman of 45, chilly with flushes of heat. Chills worse from moving round, or turning in bed : better from external warmth.   They come at irregular times.   Spread up from below.   During chill wants to be covered ; when heat comes, wants covers off (rev. of *Camphor*) ; feels sore and bruised all over, in flesh and bones.   Pains and aching in limbs.   Can't get hand up behind head, or on head, from pains in shoulder.   Warmth is good to pains in body, but not to head, which wants to be cold.

Can't stand heat of stove to head. Bad taste : nothing tastes good. Wants sour things. Some thirst with the fever. Urine dark and scanty. The trouble had been going on for some weeks, and the doctor did not seem to hit it, till he gave *Sanicula* 10*m*, which cured.

N.B.—The people who have themselves experienced the effects of a remedy can always best recognize and apply it. In Germany, recently, students of Homœopathy had to prove remedies, as part of their training.

*   *   *

NASH mentions *Sanicula* ten times in his LEADERS, comparing it with other drugs of like symptoms. He shows that it has the " no two stools alike " of *Pulsatilla*—the crying infant, after which sand appears on the diaper, of *Lycopodium*—the " bashful stool " of *Silica* and *Thuja*—the immense stool, long retained, painful and receding when partly expelled of *Silica*—the thin neck of *Natrum mur.* and *Lycopodium*—the emaciation while eating well of *Iodum*—the terror of downward motion, of *Gelsemium* and *Borax*.

*   *   *

DR. OSCAR HANSON (Copenhagen) in his text book of *The Materia Medica and Therapeutics of Rare Homœopathic Remedies*, notices especially in regard to *Sanicula* the profuse sweat on occiput and nape of neck during sleep ; its great photophobia, and lachrymation from cold air, or cold externally applied ; the thick tenacious, ropy mucus from throat, like *Kali bichrom.* ; the stools, large and painful enough to rupture the sphincter, *with pain in whole perineum*. And its therapeutics, for him, concern " Ophthalmia scrofulosa : Sea sickness (good remedy). Enuresis nocturna (many cases cured). Constipation ".

The water contains *chlorides of sodium, calcium, magnesium*, etc. etc., also *Silica*.

SEPIA

(*Cuttlefish*)

OF *Sepia* Hahnemann says, " This brown-black juice which, before me, had only been used for drawing, is contained in the abdomen of the sea-insect, *ink-fish* (*sepia octopoda*), and is sometimes jerked forth by the insect to darken the water around, either for the purpose of securing a prey or opposing an attack."

(For the manner of Hahnemann's spotting this great remedy, which he introduced, after provings, into his Materia Medica, see p. 652.)

It is imperative to get a true realization of SEPIA : one of our most important remedies in chronic diseases—related to *Nat. mur.* and *Phos.*, both of which enter into cuttlefish juice and determine some of its symptoms. Yet *Sepia* provides a special stimulus all its own, that neither of the others can supply.

I am told that Dr. Gibson Miller, that great prescriber, used to say that, if he might have only one drug, he would choose *Sepia*. And *Sepia* has made some very wonderful cures, when the unit dose has been left to act over several months,—goitre—insanity—rheumatoid arthritis, etc. *Sepia* is one of the drugs that does not bear repetition—anyway in chronic cases, and in the potencies.

Now, *how to spot Sepia* ? . . . And here, as it seems to give, pretty graphically, the *Sepia* mentality, we will reproduce our *Sepia drug picture* from a paper read to the British Homœopathic Society some years ago, and still to be found with a few other drugs in a small pamphlet.

Sepia has been called the Washerwoman's Remedy, and not without cause.

Picture her—the sallow, tired mother of a big family, on " washing day ".

She is perspiring profusely : pouring under the arms. She cannot be shut in, because of the heat and the stuffiness which make her feel faint—yet the cold wind that rushes in at the open door is almost unbearable.

Her back aches fearfully. She wants to press it—to support it (*Nat. mur.*). She feels she MUST sit down, or cross her legs, as her whole inside seems to be dragging down, and coming out of her. She simply must sit down to keep it in (*Lil. tig.*).

The worry of the children is more than she can bear. Her *Cham.* baby wants to be picked up and carried, and wails and screams. The quarrels of the penultimate babies engaged in scratching out each other's eyes, are more than she can bear. And when her six-year-old starts drumming with a spoon on a tin pot, she can stand no more. She snatches the tin pot and hurls it away, and smacks her small son ; which does not improve matters. He howls dismally, and she *does not care*.

Oh ! how she wants to run away and leave it all, and have a little peace !

Her head aches. The pain is left-sided to-day : last time it was on the right side, as she remembers dully.

She is so nervous and jumpy, she has to hold on to the edge of the wash-tub to prevent herself from screaming. If she could only go away from everybody and everything, and lie down, alone, in the dark, and close her eyes !

Her husband comes in : she has no smile to greet his. Nothing but dull indifference, and weariness, and suffering. He must leave her alone. She has her work to do.

Ptosis—ptosis everywhere. Her whole body dragged down, " inside " and out. Veins—piles—all stagnant and dragging her down. Even her eyelids are too heavy to hold up.

If she could only lie down and close them ! She knows even ten minutes sleep would make her a new woman !—but there are the soapsuds—the steam—the stuffiness—the terrors of her restless children, with their noise and fidgeting. Sleep is not for her.

Her little *Pulsatilla* maid creeps up. " Can't I help you, Mummie ? " but she pushes her off. And the little maid creeps away, weeping : and Mummie feels that she is indifferent to her tears.

The dinner is cooking—and the smell of the cooking makes her feel deadly sick. The children are hungry, and her husband waits for his dinner. She is indifferent. Let them wait. She is irritable—indifferent—apathetic.

He looks at her sadly. Her dull face has lost its contour—its bloom—its pleasing lines. Browny bands or blotches are on forehead, and saddlewise across nose and cheekbones.

She was a bright and bonny girl when he married her—now she is Sepia.

Give her her drug, and he will come and bless you for giving him back the wife he chose and loved. (This has actually happened : for out of ten, *one* sometimes returns to give thanks !)

Black Letter and Suggestive Symptoms

(from Hahnemann, Allen's *Encyclopedia*, Hering's
Guiding Symptoms.)

Very irritable.

Very indifferent towards everything, and apathetic.

Aversion to one's occupation and family.

Great indifference to one's family—to those they love best.

Indolent mood.

Uneasiness in the presence of strangers.

Propensity to suicide from despair about his miserable existence.

" One dose takes away my ambition, I simply do not want to do anything, either work or play : an exertion even to think."

" So nervous that I felt unless I held on to something, I should scream."

Headache, right side head and face, with surging sensation like waves of pain rolling up and beating against frontal bone.

Darting pains, from left eye over side of head towards occiput.

Tearing in left temple to upper part of left side of head.

Headache with aversion to all kinds of food, a feeling of emptiness and goneness in stomach, very distressing.

Headache every morning with nausea, vertigo, epistaxis.

Headaches in women of sallow complexion, or moth-patches on forehead : smell of food repulsive.

Headache better after meals.

Great falling out of the hair.

Smarting right eye, evening ; lids close against one's wish.

Grain of sand sensation, especially right eye.

Inflammatory affections of asthenic character ; conjunctivæ dull red, some photophobia and swelling of lids, worse in a.m.

Lachrymation morning and evening.

Drooping of eyelids, heavy or not enough sense to lift them.

Fiery sparks before eyes. Flickering looking at light. Black spots. Fiery zigzags: zigzag wreath of colours (*Nat. mur., Graph.*).

Pale face. Yellowness of face and whites of eyes.

Yellow spots on face and a yellow saddle across the upper part of the cheeks and the nose. Yellow saddle across bridge of nose.

Large offensive-smelling plugs from nose (ozæna).

Crack middle of lower lip (*Nat. mur., Dros., etc.*).

Dry coryza : nostrils sore, swollen, ulcerated and scabby ; discharging large, green plugs.

Very sensitive to noise, music and odours.
Smell of cooking nauseates (*Ars., Cocc., Colch., Dig., Ip., Thuja*).

Nausea, mornings only, passing off after eating something.
Gnawing and weakness in stomach, which ceased at supper.
Emptiness of stomach, with nausea as soon as she thinks of food
which she would like to take. *Peculiar faint, sinking emptiness.*
Nausea: after eating, also in the a.m. fasting: from smell of
food or cooking: when riding in a carriage: with anxiety when
exerting eyes: with weakness.
Morning sickness of pregnancy. Toothache, esp. of pregnancy.
Vomiting: of food and bile in a.m.: frequently strains her so that
blood comes up: of mucus, after taking the simplest food.
Burning in pit of stomach. Stitches in pit of stomach.
Canine hunger, or no appetite.
Desire for vinegar, for wine, for sweets.
Aversion to food, particularly to meat and fat, to bread during
pregnancy; to milk which causes diarrhœa. Loathing.
Worse for bread, milk, fat food or acids.
" *Sepia* creates an aversion to drinking beer."

Feeling of bearing down of all pelvic organs.
Pot belliedness of mothers.
Many brown spots on abdomen: chloasma.
Weight in abdomen: distension: rumbling and grunting.
Sensation of emptiness in abdomen.
Pain and weight in abdomen, on rising in a.m.
Pain, tenderness; heaviness, load during motion in abdomen.
Sensation of bearing down in pelvic organs, with slow dragging
pain from sacrum.
Pressure in abdomen as though the contents would issue through
the genital organs. Pressure in uterus, as if everything would issue
through vulva. Feeling of crowding and pressing downwards.
Rolling in abdomen, as if something alive were there (*Croc.,*
Thuja). Then rises up towards her throat. . . .
Constipation: during pregnancy: slow and difficult discharge
even of soft stool: excessive straining. . . .
Sensation of weight, or ball, in anus, not > by stool.

Pressure on bladder and frequent micturition with tension and
painful bearing down in pelvis.
Involuntary discharge of urine at night, especially during first
sleep. The bed is wet almost as soon as the child goes to sleep, or
passed within two hours after going to bed.

Urine clear like water : thick, slimy and very offensive, depositing a pasty sediment next morning. Sediment adheres like cement.

Turbid, clay-coloured urine, with reddish sediment in the chamber.

Uterus congested, and a yellowish leucorrhœa pouring from it ; beginning to prolapse. Slightly displaced.

Great dryness of vulva and vagina, causing a very disagreeable sensation when walking, after cessation of menses.

Pressure in uterus, as if everything would issue through vulva.

Sensation in rectum not > by an evacuation : sensation that limbs must be crossed to prevent everything being pressed out of vagina. (See *Lil. tigr.*)

Pain in uterus, bearing down, comes from back to abdomen : crosses limbs to prevent protrusion of parts.

Prolapsus of uterus, of vagina, with constipation.

Pressure in uterus, causing oppression of breathing ; the pressure downwards is as if everything would fall out, with pain in abdomen. She must cross her limbs in order to prevent the protrusion of the vagina, yet nothing protruded, but there was an increase of gelatinous leucorrhœa. Yellowish leucorrhœal discharge.

Leucorrhœa like milk, only by day, with burning and excoriation between thighs.

Before menses acrid leucorrhœa, with soreness of the pudendum.

Metrorrhagia, during climacteric or pregnancy, especially fifth and seventh months.

Menses : too late : too early : causing faintness, chilliness, shuddering. . . .

Amenorrhœa : at puberty : from a cold : in feeble women with delicate skin.

Sudden hot flushes at climacteric with momentary sweat, weakness and tendency to faint.

Short, hacking cough, in the evening, on lying down.

Spasmodic cough.

Cannot sleep at night on account of incessant cough.

Short, dry cough, seems to come out of stomach.

Oppression of the chest morning and evening.

(One remembers an asthma case, where nothing helped till *Sepia* was given, on his general symptoms.)

Hering gives, " Tuberculous and other chronic diseased conditions of the central third of right lung.—*Ars.* the upper third."

Pain in back across hips.

When stooping sudden pain in back as if struck by a hammer : > by pressing back against something hard.

Pain in small of back : pain and weakness : weakness when walking : pain as if sprained. Pain with stiffness, better by walking.

A short walk fatigues much.
Sudden prostration and sinking faintness.
Great faintness with heat, then coldness.
Faintness while kneeling in church : at trifles.
Great exhaustion in a.m. during menses.

Hands generally cold, but moist with perspiration.
Very cold feet with headache (feeling as if they stood in cold water up to the ankles).
Attacks of flushes of heat, as if hot water were poured over one with redness of face, sweat of whole body and anxiety, without thirst.
Profuse night sweats. Cold night sweats, chest, back and thighs.
Perspiration of head at night in sleep. (*Calc., Merc., Sil.*)
Sensation of icy-cold hand between the scapulæ.

Herpetic eruption on lips; about mouth. (*Nat. mur., Rhus.*, etc.)
Itching often changes to burning when scratching.
Itching on the bends of elbows.
Soreness of skin : humid places on bends of knees.
Brown or claret-coloured tetter-like spots : cloasma.
Herpes circinatus.
Brown spots on skin with leucorrhœa.
Tettery eruptions : humid : with itching and burning.

Queer sensations :
As if heart stood still.
As if suspended in air : brain crushed : head would burst.
As if eyes were gone and a cool wind blew out of sockets.
As if lids too heavy to open. As if lids paralysed.
Eyes as if balls of fire : lids too tight to cover eyeballs.
As if everything in abdomen were turning around : as if viscera were turning inside out.
As if ribs broken and sharp points sticking into flesh.
As if a strap, wide as her hand were drawn tightly round waist.
Liver as if bursting : as of something adherent in abdomen.
As if everything would issue through vulva.
As if something alive in abdomen. (*Crocus, Thuja.*)
A weight in anus. Bladder full, as if contents would fall out.
As if urinary organs would be pressed out.
As if everything would fall out of uterus : uterus as if clutched.
As if vulva were enlarged : something heavy would force itself from vagina.

Chest as if hollow : sore.

As if stomach being scraped.

As if knife thrust into top of left lung.

Back struck by hammer, as if going to break in back.

Shoulder dislocated, feet asleep.

A mouse running in lower limbs.

As if bones of legs were decaying.

Icy hand between scapulæ. (Burning, *Lyc.*, *Phos.*)

As if she would suffocate.

Something twisting in stomach and rising to throat.

Feet in cold water up to ankles. . . . (Compare *Calc.*)

Pains, ailments, disease, in any part of the body, and of every description—*in a Sepia patient.*

Ptosis suggests *Sepia.*

Intertrigo suggests *Sepia.*

" Bearing down " suggests *Sepia.*

Sepia is an important remedy in insanity, and in " borderline cases". We will reproduce a couple of little cases, quoted elsewhere, but especially pertinent here :—

" Lady is going to foal. Last year she bit and kicked her first foal, and would not let it suck, and it died. What can we give her ? " " Oh ! *indifference to offspring ? Sepia*, of course ! Give her a dose of *Sepia*." . . . And the foal arrived in due course, and Lady was the most devoted mother of all the mares that year ; couldn't bear the foal a moment out of her sight ; grazed round it where it lay in the grass. . . .

" Doctor, can you help a young man ? It is his first baby, and he hates it. He cannot bear his wife to touch it. Her people had him shut up, but his people got him out again. I stayed with her all last night, and he was raving in the next room, banging about and smashing things. They are afraid he will kill the baby." . . . " Oh ! *indifference to offspring* " . . . he got a dose of *Sepia*. In a week he came up himself, weepy, shaky, frightfully upset still, but better. The next report was, " Doctor, you know that young man who hated his baby ? Well, he is *devoted* to it now. He can hardly bear anyone to touch it when he is there. He is quite cured."

You see, *Sepia* is the drug that has caused and cured indifference to offspring. Mental symptoms, where they exist, are the most important in determining the required remedy.

Here is another striking and well-remembered *Sepia* mental case. . . . A handsome young woman, statuesque not only in features and in colour—stony white—but in immobility, was brought to " Out-patients " some years ago. It was impossible to get an answer out of her, except after a long wait, and then it was monosyllabic. The shock of her brother's going abroad was said to be the cause that had unhinged her. Her expression never changed : one could get no response : she just sat there immovable, while her mother gave what symptoms she could and then took her away. *Arsenicum* suggested itself, and *Sepia* : —one can see now, and at this distance of time, that *Ars.* might have been distrusted in a patient so devoid of restlessness—so entirely atypical. (And yet, recently, one has seen *Arsenicum* work the miracle in a girl with acute heart disease, with endocarditis and great effusion, who was absolutely atypical as regards anxious restlessness :—though her symptoms, otherwise, were *Ars.*)

Well, on further consideration (*Ars.* having failed to touch the handsome statue) *Sepia* was given, and a few weeks later a veritable tornado of a girl swept in on out-patient work, all expression and animation ; all eagerness to tell her story . . . what she had done and felt ; all the ways in which she had failed to commit suicide. She had tried to drag her mother in front of an omnibus : she had tried to hang herself from a skylight, only someone came in : she had even gone to the lavatory and tried to drown herself by pulling the plug. All this and more she poured out with intense and indescribable animation. That dose of *Sepia* had unfrozen her, and redeemed her life. For several years after that she used to present herself, and she remained normal and commonplace, and never relapsed even under circumstances, a little later, of trial and distress. . . . Homœopathy may be beneath contempt—" nonsense "—" sugar pills "— " imagination "—but *it works*, provided that you hit the remedy (as here, where the one drug did nothing, the other cured). Otherwise it is all the things they say against it—but that is *when it did not happen to be Homœopathy at all.* Get it out of your head that a drug is homœopathic, and that Homœopathy must stand or fall by it because it comes out of a homœopathic case, or has been prepared after the manner of Hahnemann by a homœopathic chemist, or has been potentized, or prescribed by a homœopathic doctor (or even by a lay homœopath !) or because it has been " worked out " and has, more or less, " come through ". Whereas, on the other hand, a remedy may be absolutely homœopathic when it comes from an ordinary chemist's shop, is prescribed by an old school doctor, and is supposed to be an ordinary " allopathic " drug :—As for instance, *Ipecac.* for incessant nausea and vomiting—which it causes : *Pot. iod.* for gummata (which it has produced, and cures) : *Salicylic acid* for Ménière's disease, whose symptoms it evokes, and so on, a large number of drugs : I think it was Dr. Dyce Brown who discovered enough of these to fill a pamphlet. So, when we have failed (as with *Ars.* in the above case), it was not because Homœopathy was incapable of curing, but because we were incapable of finding the homœopathic remedy. This applies to our failures everywhere ; in some cases of rheumatoid arthritis, for example, where the remedy is sometimes terribly difficult to spot, but when found can do astonishing work in relieving what is incurable in advanced cases, and in curing early cases.

Which reminds one !—that *Sepia* is one of the remedies that has cured rheumatoid arthritis—in *Sepia* patients. It has helped within our knowledge several times. Here is a case. But remember that Homœopathy does not treat diseases, but patients with diseases : and don't on any account write down in your memory that *Sepia* is " a cure " for that disease. That is the perfect way of demonstrating—to the satisfaction of your inexperience—that " Homœopathy is no use for rheumatoid arthritis any way ! "—you have "*proved* that it is not !"—with remedies that did not happen to be *en rapport* with the patient.

Woman of 42, sent up by a country doctor, who told her that she would never walk again. She had a fifteen-years' history of supposed hopeless rheumatoid arthritis. She was wheeled in in a bath chair :—could not feed herself or dress herself without help ; could not even pull the sheet up at night. There was rapid improvement after *Sepia* 30, a dose in December (1915). In February she was walking. In six months the hospital note is, " Hands look normal : walks with a very slight limp." Seen again, from time to time for " stomach ", for " slight return of rheumatism ", etc. Notes extend over fourteen years, and no return. Here, of course, the bony changes cannot have been great. But such cases show the wide range of *Sepia*—in *Sepia patients !* And here let us retell its chief characteristics, in the words, this time, of KENT.

" *Sepia* is suited to tall, slim women with narrow pelvis and lax fibres and muscles. . . . One of the strongest features of the *Sepia* patient is found in the mind, the state of the affections . . . the remedy seems to abolish the ability to feel natural love, to be affectionate. . . . ' I know I ought to love my children and my husband, I used to love them, but now I have no feeling on the subject.' . . . The love does not go forth into affection. . . . An absence of all joy, inability to

realize things are real : no affection for the delightful things of
life : no joy : life has nothing in it for her. . . . Sallowness
and jaundice . . . the yellow saddle across nose and down
sides of face . . . enormous freckles, great brown patches
. . . brown warts . . . Face sallow and doughy, as if
muscles were flabby. . . . *You will seldom see* Sepia *indicated
in the face that shows sharp lines of intellect* . . . and possesses
will. *Sepia* is rather stupid and dull, thinks slowly and is forgetful . . . or a quick patient :—but the dullness of intellect is
the most striking feature. . . . Face generally puffed, often
smooth and rounded and marked by an absence of intellectual
lines and angles. . . . Anæmic . . . skin becomes wrinkled.
. . . Constipation with sensation of lump in rectum. Gnawing
hunger, seldom satisfied : eats plentifully, yet feels a gnawing,
all-gone, empty, hungry feeling in stomach. . . . When these
symptoms are associated with prolapsus, *Sepia* will almost certainly cure, no matter how bad the prolapsus has been, or what
kind of displacement there is. . . . Inner parts as if let down,
wants a bandage to hold parts up, or to place a hand or napkin
on the parts : a funnelling sensation, better sitting down and
crossing the limbs. *When these symptoms group themselves, the
gnawing hunger, the constipation, the dragging down, and the mental
condition, it is* Sepia *and* Sepia *only.*"

Sepia comes in for menstrual troubles ; leucorrhœa ; eruptions, herpetic, and crusty, and weepy, especially on the bends of
joints : " induration like some forms of epithelioma." Kent
says " *Sepia* has cured epithelioma of lips, wings of nose, and
eyelids." He says Fear of ghosts, etc. " *Never happy unless
annoying someone.*" Fear : fear of insanity . . . very easily
offended. And then the *Sepia relief from sleep*—even a short
sleep : (Phos.) and *relief of most complaints from eating.*

* * *

And now a few gleanings from Farrington's masterly article
on *Sepia (Comparative Materia Medica).*

He tells us that *Sepia is* a remedy of inestimable value. Acts
on the vital forces as well as upon the organic substances of the
body. Soon impresses the circulation, which becomes more and
more disturbed. Even as early as the fourth hour there are
flushes of heat and ebulitions which end in sweat and weak feeling. . . . Hand in hand with this orgasm is an erethism of
nervous system, with restlessness, anxiety, etc.

Quickly following are relaxation of tissues and nervous
weakness. Joints feel weak, as though they would dislocate :

the viscera drag—the "goneness". The prolapsed uterus becomes more and more engorged : the portal stasis augments : liver is heavy and more sluggish : blood vessels full, and limbs feel sore, bruised, tired, heavy. . . . The sphincters, and all structures depending for power on non-striated muscle, are weak, i.e. rectum prolapses ; and evacuations of bowels and bladder are tardy and sluggish.

Organic changes are seen in complexion, yellow, earthy : in the secretions, sour, excoriating : in skin, with offensive exhalations, and disposed to eruptions, discoloration, desquamation, ulcers, etc.

Rather violent motion, by improving the circulation, relieves. . . . "The hands are hot and the feet are cold ; or as soon as the feet become hot, the hands become cold. This is an excellent indicating symptom for *Sepia*."

"A common attendant, clearly expressive of the *Sepia* case, is the excellent Keynote of Guernsey, 'with sense of weight in the anus like a heavy ball.'"

*　　　*　　　*

To show how deep-acting *Sepia* can be, we will retail rather an astonishing memory from early Dispensary days.

She was a gaunt, grey and grey-haired widow with multiple T.B. manifestations, whose husband had died of tuberculosis. One remembers especially the large, highly inflamed prepatellar bursa, for which she would not hear of operation : and three T.B. sinuses in particular, one on the palmar aspect of the right forearm, and one on each side of the middle finger of the right hand, going down to the first and second phalanges. *Tub. bov.* and *Silica*, to one's astonishment, left the condition I.S.Q. :—as did three weeks at our Eastbourne Convalescent Home, with good air, cleanliness and dressings.

Then, tardily, the idea came, to "find her remedy, and give her that, and afterwards try to deal with the tubercular manifestations." Her remedy turned out to be *Sepia*, which rapidly cured the sinuses, although, being "scrub-lady" in a public house, her hand was apt to be steeped, from morning to night, in dirty water, as she scrubbed floors and washed the pewter pots. The sinuses closed, the finger healed, with all the rest : and the "stuffing" of the prepatellar bursa could be felt breaking up into smaller india-rubber-like masses, before finally disappearing.

It is worth while to make friends with Sepia! Small wonder that Dr. Gibson Miller should have said, "If he were only allowed one remedy, he would choose SEPIA."

SEPIA IN MALARIA

In old cases of suppressed malaria, *Sepia* brings back the chill, but its most useful sphere is after a bad selection of the remedy and the case becomes confused. Where a remedy has been selected for only a part of the case and changed it a little but the patient gets no better. When the case gets into this kind of a fix, stop right off and give *Sepia*. It will be seen that the fever, chill and sweat are just as eratic as can be. *Natrum mur.* is one of the greatest malarial remedies, but it is full of order, like *China*. *Sepia* is full of disorder. In cases confused by remedies think of *Calc.*, *Ars.*, *Sulph.*, *Sep.* and *Ipecac.* Never give *China* or *Natrum mur.* for disorderly cases.   Kent.

Farrington tells the history of the introduction of this substance into our Materia Medica. " Hahnemann had a friend, an artist, who became so ill that he was scarcely able to attend to his duties. Despite Hahnemann's most careful attention he grew no better. One day when in his friend's studio, Hahnemann observed him using the pigment made from the Sepia, and he noticed also that the brush was frequently moistened in the artist's mouth. Immediately the possibility of this being the cause of the illness flashed across Hahnemann's mind. He suggested the idea to the artist, who declared positively that the Sepia paint was absolutely innocuous. At the physician's suggestion, however, the moistening of the brush in the mouth was abandoned, and the artist's obscure illness shortly passed away. Hahnemann then instituted provings with *Sepia succus*. All the symptoms observed by him have since been confirmed. In 1874, the American Institute of Homœopathy, acting under the notion that our old remedies should be re-proved, performed this task for *Sepia*. There were made some twenty-five provings of the drug in from the third to the two hundredth potencies. These were reported at the Meeting of the Association in 1875. They testify to the fact that the provings left us by Hahnemann cannot be improved on."

SILICA

TYPICAL *Silica* crawls nervously in, or is dragged in on his mother's hand, and you can hardly miss him.

He is the most homœopathic drug you can imagine ! Read the black type only in Allen's *Cyclopedia*, and see how extraordinarily suggestive the provings are in regard to tuberculosis, especially abdominal ; to pustules, boils and abscesses ; to effects of splinters, stings and abrasions ; to lack of reaction against injury and disease.

Silica, they say, lacks grit—needs sand. And doses of *Silica* stimulate mightily these weaklings who are going under, to put up a fight, mental and physical.

You look up, as poor little *Silica* is dragged reluctantly in. He is listless ; not interested ; not frightened.

You see a pale, sickly, suffering face ; and you realize at once that there is something deeply wrong here ; no mere ailment— DISEASE.

Now for the mother's story—in Allen's black type—for they are identical :

" He doesn't get on, he doesn't. He doesn't thrive. He doesn't learn ; he doesn't even play. He is irritable and grumpy. He is always at the bottom of everything, and his teacher can't make nothink of him ; she writes, see !—' he shrinks from effort, from the least responsibility, and is utterly lacking in self-confidence and self-assertion.' Doesn't seem to have no ' go ' in him. He doesn't seem to be able to think ! He can't fix his mind. He can't read or write. And yet he's always worried to death over little things he's done wrong. That's it : he's so odd, and so unlike the others.

" He gets violent attacks of headache, she says, and complains that the back of his head is cold. That's where the pain is, but it goes all over his head. He says his head will burst. He wants it tied up tight. He wants it warm. Warm and tight, that's what his head has got to be—when he gets one of his attacks.

" And a funny thing she has noticed, he's always ill with the new moon !

" And he's got a shocking cough, pore little mite. He spits up awful stuff with it—lumpy and yellow, or greeny, it is ; and it sinks to the bottom of any fluid, and smells horribly. It's more like ' corruption ' (matter).

" And he's all wrong somehow, all over, he is ! Look at his nails—rough and yellow; and feeling as if he had got a splinter in his finger. Or gets a red, swollen finger that throbs and feels like a felon. Or look at that finger, how it is swollen, and the bone feels big. He wakes crying, and says his hands have gone to sleep.

" And then his skin won't heal. He's an awful boy for knocking bits off of hisself, or falling and scratching his knees ; and every little scratch and hurt festers and ulcerates, and they won't never heal. And in every sore he gets sticking pains or burning pains. He is so thin ; and such a lot of sore places.

" Boils, too !—such a boy for boils as you never see. A boil on his chin; then boils on his neck ; pustules or boils anywhere on his body. To her mind he has never been right since vaccination.

" And the child is so cold ; never seems to be warm. Chilly with every movement. Why, he seems extra chilly in a warm room ! That ain't natural in a child ! Cold up to his knees, he is. Can't sleep for cold feet.

" And then with all his coldness, he's an awful one for sweating ! He's just drenched at night ; with no appetite ; and so tired always !

" So weak and tired. Always wants to lie down. Going into a decline, that's what she thinks he is, if you ask her. At night he's a terror one way or the other. Feels as if he was all sore on the side he lies on ; yet if he turns over, shifting the clothes and moving makes him more cold. And then his dreams— frightful!

" Sometimes it's only his head that perspires, and in sleep. But that's not all ; it's the awful smell of the perspiration of his feet. You see, the perspiration on his feet not only smells enough to turn you, but it makes his poor little feet that sore ! Sore between the toes, they are, till he can scarce shuffle along. In his armpits too, there's a very smelly sweat.

" If he runs, he goes deathly white.

" Oh! and she had forgotten that. He seems always wet about the back passage ; and he seems to have a lot of pain there, as if it was tight closed. And he always seems to be wanting to pass something, though as often as not it is only a little jelly stuff. But he has horribly offensive stools ; often hard and difficult. He has to strain that awful, it makes his whole stomach wall sore ; and sometimes when the motion is half out, why, it slips back again. (Were this mother an American doctor, she would describe it as a ' bashful stool '.)

" Oh, and she had forgotten that, too, his stomach is so hard, and swollen, and big. He seems to have an awful lot of wind, and it is awful smelling. And that don't seem right somehow.

"And—such a funny thing for a boy!—one nipple seems to be swollen and painful, it almost seems as if it was gathering ; and he says he has shooting pains in the other. All his pains are like splinters ; or stitching pains ; or pains like a gathering."

That is Allen's black type. What is your diagnosis, before you put a finger on the child ? Is it not all graphic ? You would expect a T.B. abdomen—a T.B. chest—T.B. dactylitis—a T.B. family history. Not the acute-phthisis type—he cannot even put up an acute tuberculosis—he is just—*Silica*. And *Silica* and *Tub. bov.* may make a man of him yet.

No wonder *Silica*, with such a proving should be a drug to think about in abscesses, whitlows, unhealthy skin, smelly feet, mammary abscess, mammary cancer, wounds that refuse to heal, tubercle of skin, bone, abdomen. But the old homœopaths say, " Use *Sil.* with caution in pulmonary phthisis." It has a well-known trick of ulcerating out foreign bodies and breaking down scar tissue. It may liberate tubercle. Do not use it high in tuberculosis.

Its great sphere is connective tissue. We know now, since Old School experiments with colloidal *Silica*, that it not only breaks down scar tissue, in potencies, but, in poisonous doses, has produced cirrhosis of liver and kidneys, etc.

Black Letter Symptoms

And a few very important italic symptoms given in brackets.

Sensitive to noise.
(*Most excessive scruples of conscience, about trifles frequently.*)
(*Great difficulty in fixing the attention. Thought difficult.*)

HEADACHE *rising from nape of neck to vertex.*
(*The most violent headache.*)
Tearing in the whole of the head, starting from the occipital protuberances and extending upward and forward over both sides of the head.
(*As if head would burst*) *relieved by binding the head tightly.*
Pressive pain in occiput, relieved by warm wrapping up of the head. . . . soon followed by stitches in the forehead, with chilliness nape of neck and back.
The head was sore to touch externally.
The itching spots on head are painful, as if sore, after scratching.

⌐ *Swelling in the region of the right lachrymal gland and sac.*
⌐ *Painful sensitiveness of the ear to loud sounds.*
⌐ *The gum is painfully sensitive on taking cold water into the mouth.*
   Sensation of a hair lying on forepart of tongue.
   Inflammation and suppuration of salivary glands.

ABDOMEN *hard, tense.*
Very offensive flatus.
Moisture in the ANUS.
Hæmorrhoids painfully sensitive.
STOOL *remains a long time in rectum.*
Cutting in rectum. Stinging in rectum.
Tension in the anus.

Pain in the anus as if constricted during stool.
Burning in anus after a hard, dry stool.
Frequent desire for stool, but discharge of only mucus, with chilliness of the body.
Constant but ineffectual desire for stool.
Horribly offensive stools.
Stool of hard lumps evacuated only with great effort.
Stool scanty, difficult : after great urging and straining until the abdominal walls are sore, the stool that has already protruded slips back again.
Very hard stool, followed by burning in anus.
Very hard, nodular stool, like clay-stones, evacuated only with great effort.
Very hard, unsatisfactory stools, with very great effort.
Fissura ani and fistula in ano.

EXPECTORATION *thick, yellow, lumpy.*
Purulent expectoration when coughing.

The right BREAST *is hard, painful, and swollen at the nipple— it feels as if it were " gathering ".*
Darting and burning pain in left nipple.
Aversion to mother's milk : if child nurses, it vomits.

⌐ *Stiffness nape of neck, with headache.*
⌐ *The* COCCYX *is painful, as after a long carriage ride.*
   Stinging in the os coccyx, which is also painful to pressure.

Weakness of all the LIMBS.
Falling asleep of the hands at night.
⌐ *Finger nails rough and yellow.*

25

Sensation as if the tips of the fingers were suppurating.

Pain in the left index finger as if a panaritium would form.

Whitlow extending to tendons and bone.

Weakness of lower extremities.

Pain in hips.

The knee is painful, as if too tightly bound.

Intolerably bad, carrion like odour of the feet, without perspiration, every evening.

Offensive perspiration on the soles and between the toes ; they become quite sore while walking.

Offensive perspiration on the feet.

Every morning perspiration which sometimes was very profuse.

Sense of great debility ; she wants always to be lying down.

Great weariness.   Great weakness.

Internal restlessness and excitement.

Sensitiveness to cold air.

He took cold very easily.

Takes cold easily and has a cough.

Bruised feeling over the whole body after coition.

The whole side of the body on which he is lying is painful, as if ulcerating, with constant chilliness on the slightest uncovering : with intolerable thirst, and frequent flushes of heat in the head.

The whole body is painful as if beaten.

Most of the symptoms of Silica occur at the new moon.

Pain aggravated by motion.

Small wounds in the SKIN *heal with difficulty and easily suppurate.*

Variola-like pustules on forehead, occiput, sternum and spine : they are extremely painful, and at last form suppurating ulcers.

Several boils come out on different parts of the body : with stinging pain when touched.

A boil on the nape of the neck.

Some boils on the posterior portions of the thighs.

Frequent ulcers about the nails.

A large corrosive ulcer, with violent itching, on the heel.

Sore, painful scabs below the septum of the nose, with sticking pain when touched.

Itching suppurating scabs upon the toes.

Pressive-stinging pain in the ulcerating part of the leg.

Sticking in an ulcer on the leg.

Restless sleep.
Frightful dreams.
Dreams of his youth.

Very CHILLY *all day.*
Chilliness on every movement.
Chilliness in the evening.
Distressing sensation of chilliness in the afternoon—in a warm room. He feels very chilly even in a warm room.
Cramp-like chill in the evening in bed, so that he shivered.
Icy-cold shivering frequently creeps over the whole body.
Coldness of the legs, as far as the knees, in a warm room.
Icy-cold feet in the evening, even in bed.
Icy-cold feet during the menses.
Cold feet in the evening in bed, preventing sleep.

FEVER *with violent heat in the head.*
Febrile heat all night, with violent thirst and catching respiration.
Heat of the head.

General sweat at night.
Profuse PERSPIRATION *every night, towards morning.*
Profuse general nightsweat.
Profuse perspiration every night, with loss of appetite and prostration, as if he would go into a decline.
Perspiration of a strong odour.
Sweat on the head.
Sweat only on the head, running down the face.
Offensive perspiration on the soles and between the toes; they become quite sore while walking.
Offensive perspiration on the feet.

We will now let NASH speak in regard to *Silica*.

Weak, puny children, not from want of nourishment taken, but from defective assimilation. . . . Sweaty-headed children, over-sensitive, imperfectly nourished. The *Silica* child is not larger than natural except in its " big belly ", which is due to diseased mesentery. Its limbs are shrunken and its face pinched and old-looking. It does not increase in size or strength, learns to walk late : . . . everything seems to have come to a standstill so far as growth and development are concerned . . . strains and strains, the stool partly protruding and then slipping back (*Sanicula, Thuja*). Or bowels very loose . . . in spite of abundant nourishment, goes on emaciating and growing weaker until it dies of inanition, unless *Silica* checks this process. Many such cases have I saved with this remedy, and made them healthy children. (I have always used the 30th and upwards.)

Inflammations tending to end in suppuration or refusing to heal : becoming chronic.

Coldness, lack of vital warmth, even when taking exercise ; must be wrapped up, especially the head.

Suppressed sweat, especially of feet, which is profuse and offensive.

Weak, nervous, easily irritated ; yielding, giving up disposition, " grit all gone ".

Worse from cold or draught, motion, open air, at new moon : better in warm room, wrapping up head. . . .

Diseases caused from suppressed foot-sweat ; exposure head or back to any slight draught of air : from vaccination (*Thuja*), dust complaints of stone-cutters, with total loss of strength. . . .

Unhealthy skin : every little injury suppurates.

Ulcers, a curious symptom : *Mercury* has " shivering in abscesses ", *Silica* has " a sensation of coldness in ulcers ".

Promotes expulsion of foreign bodies from the tissues : fish-bones, needles, bone splinters.

And among NASH'S TIPS we find :

" In the marasmus of children we may have to choose from among remedies such as *Silica, Abrotanum, Natrum mur., Sulphur, Calcarea* and *Iodine*.

" Under all these remedies we may find emaciation of the rest of the body, while the abdomen is greatly enlarged.

" Again, under every one of them the child may have a voracious appetite ; eat enough, but grow poor all the time. *It is a defective assimilation*."

" There are strong points of resemblance between *Baryta carb.* and *Silica*, namely : *Offensive sweat on the feet. The head is disproportionally large for the body*. Both suffer from damp *changes in the weather and both are sensitive to cold about the head*.

" But *Silica* has the important diagnostic difference—*profuse sweat on the head* (equal to that of *Calc.*), which *Baryta* has not. And there is not that weakness of mind in *Silica* that is found in *Baryta* : on the contrary the child is self-willed and contrary."

GUERNSEY says :—

" Feet perspire very much and smell very offensively ; feet become sore and blistered between the toes. Head perspires very

much in the evening on going to sleep. This looks like *Calc.*
but in *Silica* the perspiration extends lower down the neck and is
apt to have an offensive smell.

"Worse from getting the feet wet:—when single parts are cold :
—from uncovering the head."

HUGHES, writing of rickets, says, " I am accustomed to
prescribe it (*Silica*) in the earliest manifestations of the diathesis,
which are generally *unhealthy evacuations, sweats of the head*, and
tenderness of the surface ; with the best results."

He gives the classical uses of *Silica* :—its power over
suppurations, once established or long-enduring : for external or
internal ulcers. Of its effect on brain and cord, " affecting the
centres of nutrition " : in children not able to stand or walk.
Of its importance in the treatment of lachrymal fistula—housemaid's knee—suppressed *foot-sweat*, and ailments therefrom.
To abate the pains of cancer, etc. etc.

And Hughes quotes Dunham, *re* the *Silica* mentality : " *Silica*
' cannot possibly do a thing ! ' but when urged to the doing, goes
off in a paroxysm of overdoing."

Clarke says :—

" A curious symptom, and one of great value, is this : ' Fixed
ideas : the patient thinks only of pins, fears them, searches for
them, and counts them carefully.' This symptom helped me to
make a rapid cure of post-influenzal insanity in the case of a man
of bad family history, one of whose sisters had become insane
and drowned herself, another sister being affected with lupus.
The patient's wife told me one morning that he had *been looking
everywhere for pins*. *Sil.* 30 rapidly put an end to the search for
pins and restored the patient to his senses.

" *Silica* has another link with insanity in its aggravation at
the moon's phases : epilepsy and sleep-walking are worse at the
new and full moon."

Silica is one of the great medicines to be thought of in epilepsy
—and in petit mal—*in the Silica patient*. One has lately had
news of a girl—a pale and feeble young epileptic of many years
ago—who used to come to Hospital, and improved so much with
Silica that (as one hears now) she " has never had another fit."
It is " curses and chickens "—and bad prescriptions—" that
come home to roost " !—often one hears of one's very best work
only accidentally, years afterwards,—or never.

And now a few more gleanings from Kent. . . .

"The action of *Silica* is slow. In the proving it takes a long time to develop the symptoms. It is suited, therefore, to complaints that develop slowly. . . . The long-acting, deep-acting remedies are capable of going so thoroughly into the vital disorders that hereditary disturbances are routed out. . . .

"The mental state is peculiar. The patient lacks stamina. What *Silica* is to the stalk of grain in the field, it is to the human mind (Farrar's ' shining siliceous sheath.'). . . . When the mind needs *Silica* it is in a state of weakness, embarrassment, dread, a state of yielding. . . . A prominent clergyman or lawyer will tell you that he had come to a state where he dreads to appear in public, he feels his own self-hood, so that he cannot enter into his subject, his mind will not work . . . but he will say that when he rouses and forces himself into harness he can go on with ease, his usual self-command returns to him and he does well—with promptness, fullness and accuracy. The peculiar *Silica* state is found in the *dread of failure*. . . .

"It is the natural complement and chronic of *Puls.* because of its great similarity ; it is *Puls.* only more so, a deeper, more profound remedy. . . .

"A lawyer says, ' I have never been myself since that John Doe case.' He went through a prolonged effort and sleepless nights followed. *Silica* restores the brain to its tone. . . .

"It produces inflammation about any fibrinous nidus and suppurates it out ; acts on constitutions that are sluggish, and inflames fibrous deposits about bullets, etc. It will throw out abscesses in old cicatrices and open them out.* . . . (He warns against the use of *Silica* therefore where the whole lung is tubercular since *Silica* establishes an inflammation about tubercles—as other foreign bodies, and throws them out ; and in such cases it may lead to a general septic pneumonia. . . .)

"Complaints from the suppression of discharges—suppressed sweat—foot-sweat. *Silica* cures long-lasting foot-sweat when the symptoms agree, or complaints that have lasted since the suppression of a foot-sweat.

"There is no deeper remedy than *Silica* in eradicating the tubercular tendency, when the symptoms agree ; most tubercular

---

* *Cyclopedia. of Drug Pathogenesy*, one reads, among the re-provings of *Silica* : Girl of 17. Has several enlarged cervical glands, one of which had suppurated and discharged some years previously. After taking two doses of the 21st dilution, the gland recommenced to discharge yellow matter. This continued while trying other dilutions, viz. the 12th, 4th and 1st. While taking the 4th she got a cough with scraping in throat and mucous expectoration. The cough lasted about a fortnight, the discharge for over a month.·

cases are worse from cold, wet weather ; better in cold dry weather.

" *Silica* has an aggravation from milk.   Many times the infant is unable to take any kind of milk and, hence, the physician is driven to prescribe all the foods in the market as he does not know the right remedy.   *Natrum carb*. and *Silica* are both useful when the mother's milk causes diarrhœa and vomiting.   The routinist is likely to give such medicines as *Aethusa*, entirely forgetting *Silica*.   The latter, as well as *Nat. carb*. has sour vomiting and sour curds in the stool.   ' Aversion to mother's milk and vomiting.'   ' Diarrhœa from milk.' "

In skin troubles Kent says, " There is a tendency to make the soft tissues harder and the hard tissues harder.   Indurations, cracks and fissures.   Crusty formations."

Abscesses—fistulæ.   One remembers a doctor with whom one was working suddenly exclaiming, " If you wore a cap, I'd put a feather in it."   He said that for months he had been trying to cure a case of fistula ani with *Silica* low, and a dose of the *cm* had finished it.

But of course *Silica* is one of the polychrests, one of the drugs of many uses ; affecting especially mucous membranes, skin, with nails, connective tissues, glands, in a *Silica* patient—i.e. chilly, easily-perspiring, with want of self-confidence, of grit ;—*to build up and give backbone to the weaklings*.

* * *

By the way :

Silica is one of the remedies of ANTICIPATION.   These are not all collected into one rubric in Kent's *Repertory*, but we will give them, so far as discovered ; there may be more.

They are :—
ARG. N., *Ars.*, *Carb. v.*, GELS., Lyc., Med., Pb., *Phos. a.*, SIL.,
(? *Thuja*), viz.
Complaints from anticipation (p. 4)—*Arg. n.*, Ars., *Gels.*, Lyc.,
Med., Phos. a.
Anxiety, anticipating an engagement (p. 5)—ARG. N., Gels., Med.
Anxiety when anything is expected of him (p. 6)—*Ars.*
Timidity appearing in public (p. 89)—*Carbo veg.*, GELS., Pb., SIL.
Diarrhœa after anticipation (p. 611)—*Arg. n.*, Gels., Phos. a.
Diarrhœa from excitement, as before a theatre (p. 612)—ARG. N.
Diarrhœa from excitement—ARG. N., Gels., Phos. a., Thuja, and a
few in small type.

STAPHISAGRIA

HAHNEMANN, Materia Medica Pura, in his introduction to the provings of *Staphisagria*, says :

"*It is just to the most powerful medicines in the smallest doses that we may look for the greatest curative virtue in the most serious diseases of peculiar character for which this and no other medicine is suitable.*

"·For these reasons I anticipated a great treasure of curative action in the most peculiar diseases from *Staphisagria ;* and these reasons led me to make careful trial of it on healthy subjects. Thus, curative.virtues have been elicited from this medicinal substance which are of infinitely greater value than its power to kill lice ! (the only medicinal property the ordinary quackish medical art knew it to possess)—curative virtues which the homœopathic practitioner may make use of with marvellous effect in rare morbid states, for which there is no other remedy but this."

He says this seed got its name as an exterminator of head vermin. That a certain physician, when suffering from toothache, took some of it in his mouth, but it gave him such a violent exacerbation that he thought he should go mad. " What enormous power must not this drug possess ! "

It is in this little preface he writes, " Now, as our new and only true healing art shows by experience that every drug is medicinal in proportion to the energy of its action on the health, and that it only overcomes the natural disease by virtue of its pathogenic power provided it is analogous to the latter ; it follows that a medicine can subdue the most serious diseases the more injuriously it acts on healthy human beings, and that we have only to ascertain exactly its peculiar injurious effects in order to know to what curative purposes it may be applied in the art of restoring human health. Its power, be it ever so energetic, does not by any means call for its rejection ; nay, it makes it all the more valuable ; for, on the one hand its power of altering human health reveals to us all the more distinctly and clearly the peculiar morbid states which it can produce on healthy human beings, so that we may all the more surely and indubitably discover the cases of disease in which it is to be employed similarly (homœopathically), and therefore curatively. Whilst, on the other hand, its energy, be that ever so great, may be easily moderated by appropriate dilution·and reduction of dose, so that it shall become only useful and not hurtful, if it is found to correspond in the greatest possible similarity to the symptoms of the disease we wish to cure."

The keynote to *Staphisagria* is its peculiar *mentality*, " Complaints that come from pent-up wrath : suppressed anger : suppressed feelings. Speechless from suppressed indignation . . . he controls it, and then suffers from it . . . a *Staphisagria* patient when he has to control himself, goes all to pieces, trembles from head to foot, loses his voice, his ability to work, cannot sleep, and a headache follows." Thus, graphically, KENT.

As one has seen : when an officer, after the strain of the Great War, comes out of it with a feeling that he has not been fairly treated, that he has not received due recognition ; and his health suffers, and month after month he cannot get himself together, till a dose of *Staphisagria*, with its hidden magic effect ;—and health improves, to his great astonishment. He wonders what that marvellous medicine could have been.

Staphisagria also affects the *eyes*, and especially the lids. It has a great reputation for recurrent styes, and for styes that leave induration, and for scurfy margins to the lids. Also for injuries to the eyes:—for clean cuts, as in operations: for stretched sphincters, with the agonizing pain that ensues,—as when a hospital patient, after operation on the anus, was in such pain and distress that a male nurse had to be arranged for to keep him in bed. Luckily the R.M.O. knew his work, and fetched a dose of *Staphisagria :* and came back an hour later, to find patient and watcher both asleep. These things, once realized, are never forgotten. They are more rapid, and more satisfactory than morphia, since they are *curative*. Not merely a drugging, till, as is hoped, the worst of the suffering will be over.

Staphisagria is one of the drugs that greatly affects the *teeth*. Useful where teeth turn black as soon as erupted : and the first teeth quickly decay (comp. *Kreos.*) : or in toothache with such exquisite tenderness that no liquid even, to say nothing of the tongue, must touch the teeth.

It is also a *skin* medicine : " Eczema : yellow acrid moisture oozes from under the crusts; new vesicles form from contact of exudation. Humid, itching, fetid eruption on head and behind ears :—scratching changes the place of itching, but increases oozing."

BLACK LETTER SYMPTOMS

(Hahnemann and Hering, chiefly :)

Weakness of memory ; when he has read something, after a few minutes he remembers it only dimly, and when he thought about anything for himself, it soon after escaped him, and after long reflection he could hardly recall it.

Indifference, low-spirited, dullness of mind.

Children are ill-humoured and cry for things, which after getting they petulantly push or throw away (com. *Cham.*): *worse early morning.*

Great indignation about things done by others, or by himself; grieves about consequences.

Ailments from indignation and vexation, or reserved displeasure; sleeplessness.

Aching, stupifying pain, in HEAD, *especially in forehead.*

As if brain compressed, especially forehead, with roaring in ears which goes off sooner than headache.

Feels as if occiput were compressed inwardly and outwardly.

Heaviness of head; hard pressure in head, right temporal bone and vertex.

Pressive pain in left temple outwardly and inwardly, as if the finger were strongly pressed on it.

Pressive boring stitch, left forehead, from within outwards, its violence wakes him from sleep in the morning.

Sharp, burning needle-pricks in left temple.

Obtuse shooting in right temple, outwardly and inwardly, as if the bone would be pressed out: more violent when touched.

Painful drawing externally on several parts of head, more violent when touched.

Itching papules on nape.

EYES. *Very dilated pupils for many hours.*

Blepharitis, margins of lids dry, with hardened styes or tarsal tumours.

Styes, nodosities, chalazæ on eyelids, one after another, sometimes ulcerating.

Pressure on upper lid: smarting sore pain in the inner canthi. (Hahnemann adds footnote " in a man who had never had anything the matter with his eyes in his life ").

Inflammation of white of eye, with pains.

The eyes are excessively deeply sunk, with blue raised borders— as after great excesses.

Tensive stitch in left ear.

Tearing and tugging from head down through cheeks into TEETH. *Burning, sharp shooting in left cheek: must scratch.*

Teeth turn black, or show dark streaks. Gums ache.

Gums bleed when pressed, or when brushing teeth.

While eating, tearing in gums and in the roots of lower molars.

Much toothache:—in decayed teeth: in a whole row of teeth; during menses, shooting into ear. Worse cold drinks and touch, not from biting; from drawing in cold air; after eating.

Toothache when eating : teeth are not firm, but when touched waggle ; when eating, feels as if teeth were pressed deeper into gums, and the same when the two rows of teeth only touch one another ; but the gums are white.*

Tickling pricking in right lower molars.

Rough throat.
Constant accumulation of mucus in mouth, without bad taste.
Frequent hiccough.
Adipsia : drinks less than usual.
After indignation, cardialgia.†

Colic, after indignation : after lithotomy ; with urging to stool : or urging to urinate and squeamishness.   < food and drink.
Flatulence becomes displaced in hypogastrium.
Hard painful pressure in right ABDOMEN *below navel.*
Pinching stitch in abdominal viscera.
Violent, twisting about, pinching pain in whole abdomen, now in one part, now in another.   Hot flatus ;   much flatus is developed.
Itching needle-pricks in renal region.
Costiveness.
With the feeling as if flatus would be discharged, a thin, unnoticed stool occurs.
Itching in anus while sitting, independent of stool.

Frequent call to URINATE, *when very little dark urine is discharged.*
Call to urinate ;   scarcely a spoonful passes, mostly reddish or dark-yellow in a thin stream, or by drops, and after he has passed it always feels as if the bladder were not empty, for some urine continues to dribble away.
On awaking from sleep, pressure on the bladder.
Every time water is passed, burning in the whole urethra.

Violent drawing burning stitches out of right inguinal ring, as if in the spermatic cord as far as right testicle.
Aching pain in left testicle, when walking, and whenever rubbed ; the pain is more violent on touching it.
Effects of onanism or sexual excesses.   Seminal emissions followed by great chagrin and mortification :   prostration :   dyspnœa.

---

* Hering gives a cured case, " Prosopalgia in an old lady, made life unendurable ; on touching spoon or fork to lips inexpressible pains shot from lips over face ; fluid food had to be eaten with fingers (sic.), could take no solid food, mastication impossible."

† [" After indignation, after becoming angry, *all sorts of complaints*." *Comp*. Chamomilla, Colocynth.]

Frequent sneezing without coryza—or with.

Coryza : at first blows only thick mucus from nose, afterwards thin discharge.

Adhesive mucus lies in his CHEST.

At top of sternum, immediately below pit of throat, itching, fine, sharp pricks : must scratch.

Tightness in chest at end of coitus.

Pricking itching between the cartilages of the ribs. .

Sharp stitches in region of fourth costal cartilages of right and left sides, intermitting . . . they penetrate slowly from within outwards, without relation to respiration.

Itching pricks in both axillae.

Pains like dislocation in right shoulder joint, only on moving.

Obtuse shooting pains, shoulder-joint, < moving and touched.

Violent aching pain in left shoulder joint, not > motion.

Paralytic aching pain left upper arm, < touch and motion= arm weakened. Paralytic pressure on both upper and forearms, < by motion and touch.

Paralytic drawing pain in proximal joints of fingers : < by movement.

Fine twitching tearing in muscles of thumb, and several fingers ; especially in their tips.

Deep, itching, burning, sharp needle-pricks in thumb, must scratch.

Feeling of a hard skin drawn over finger-tips left hand : little feeling in them, and loss of sense of touch.

Prickling itching muscles of buttocks : on inner sides of thighs.

When walking, pain in thighs.

Drawing shooting, or obtuse stitches in knee joint < movement. On touching, stitches change into an aching pain.

Burning shooting under left knee, outer side : (?) in paroxysms.

Boring stitch in right tibia, when at rest.

Tearing in muscles of one or other leg : shooting under and in right calf and above left heel.

Pricking itching just above right outer ankle. Must scratch.

Drawing pains here and there in the muscles of the whole body.

Itching, sharp pricks on various parts of the body.

Pain in all the bones.

Weak in body, especially knees when walking.

Violent yawning, so that tears come into eyes.

Drowsiness in afternoon, so that eyes close.

Amorous dreams and seminal emissions.

Styes, nodosities, chalazæ on eyelids, one after another, some-times ulcerating.

Burning in urethra when *not* urinating.

Very sensitive to slightest mental impressions ; least action or harmless word offends.

Bad effects of sexual abuse ; mind dwelling continually on sexual subjects.

Teeth decay early in children ; cannot be kept clean.

Sensation as if stomach and abdomen were hanging down, relaxed. Craving for tobacco.

NASH says, in regard to its usefulness in the cure of condylo-mata, fig-warts or cauliflower-like excrescences. " In one case, with the 200th of this remedy, I removed an excrescence on the perineum of a lady in which the growth was an inch long and the appearance was exactly in appearance like a cauliflower. It rapidly disappeared under the action of the remedy and never returned."

" *Incised wounds.* It is the best remedy here, where there is a clean cut as after surgical operations. It is to such wounds what *Calendula* is to lacerations, *Arnica, Hamamelis, Ledum* and *Sulph. acid* for bruises, *Rhus tox., Calcarea* and *Nux* for strains ; *Calc. phos.* and *Symphytum* for fracture."

GUERNSEY, *Guiding Symptoms*, sums up *Staphisagria*, and one sees how greatly, mentally and physically, it resembles that most sensitive of sensitive remedies—*Hepar.*

" Patients are so sensitive that the least action or word troubles or annoys his feelings : anger and indignation. . . .

" Worse from mental affections, from anger with indignation.

" From grief : from mortification, especially if caused by offences.

" From loss of fluids : tobacco : mercury : sexual excesses.

" From sleeping in the afternoon.

" From touching the part, as in toothache : can't bear the tongue, drink, or anything to touch the teeth.

" From least touch on affected parts."

*   *   *

Among Hahnemann's symptoms, the last one reads. " *Good humour ; he was cheerful and talkative in society, and enjoyed existence.*" And in a footnote, he adds, " *Curative secondary action of the organism, in a man of an opposite character of dis-position.*" *Staphisagria* is indeed one of the mighty remedies of *warped mentality.*

STRAMONIUM—DATURA STRAMONIUM

(Thorn-Apple)

HAHNEMANN says : This narcotic plant shows in its primary action (with the exception of disagreeable sensations, which the prover cannot call " pain "), no actual pains.

Sensations which can strictly be called *pain* occur only in the secondary action, i.e. the subsequent reaction of the organism. This restores not only normal sensation as opposed to the sensation-destroying action of the drug, but when given in large doses, causes morbidly exalted sensation, or *pain*.

Again : in its primary action it produces great mobility of voluntary muscles and suppression of all secretions and excretions ; the reverse of which occurs in the secondary action—to wit, paralysis of muscles, and excessive secretions and excretions.

Therefore, in suitable doses it curatively allays spasmodic muscular movements and restores suppressed excretions in several cases in which absence of pain is a prominent symptom.

It can only cure homœopathically the morbid states produced by its primary characteristic action.

The symptoms of the secondary action (which, as with all narcotic drugs, are much more numerous, better expressed, and more distinct than with non-narcotic drugs), teach the observant physician to refrain from its employment in cases where the patient is already suffering from ailments resembling those of its secondary action. He would never administer *Stram.* in complete paralysis, or inveterate diarrhœas, or where violent pains constitute the chief feature of the disease.

He speaks " from experience " of the incomparable curative action of *Stram.* " in similar natural *mental maladies*", and of its usefulness in *convulsive ailments similar to those it causes*. . . . Its efficacy also in some epidemic fevers, with the symptoms it can excite in mind and body :—in varieties of hydrophobia, from the bite of rabid animals, which cannot all be cured with one remedy, but some of which require *Belladonna*, some *Hyoscyamus*, and yet others *Stramonium*, according as their morbid symptoms are more similar to one or other of these three plants. . . .

* * *

HUGHES (*Pharmacodynamics*) : " *Stramonium* is, as Hahnemann points out, exquisitely homœopathic to hydrophobia, even more so than *Belladonna*. He says that in China, the different species of *Datura*, among them the *D. Stramonium*, are in popular use as prophylactics against hydrophobia. It is said that enough of the plant should be taken to provoke an attack of ' rage ', the patient is then safe."

He says there are few neuroses in which *Stram.* is not more or less useful. It is our chief remedy in acute mania, to which it is more homœopathic than the more inflammatory *Belladonna.* It is hardly less valuable in delirium tremens, in the active form—the *mania-a-potu* of the older writers. The constant association of hallucinations with its delirium, make it very appropriate here. . . . In nymphomania and puerperal mania it stands highest among remedies, owing to its special action on the sexual functions. . . . Epilepsy, brought on by a fright . . . In chorea, one of the best vegetable medicines. . . .

He quotes *Guernsey,* in regard to the following indication : " Parturient women show such signs of fear as to cause them to look frightened and to shrink back from the first objects they see after opening their eyes. If they have had no spasms, they soon will have, after betraying such symptoms, unless *Stramonium* be immediately administered. . . . His other indications are : Great loquacity, expressing wild and absurd fancies ; desire for light and society ; an imploring, beseeching mood."

* * *

ALLEN's *Encyclopedia* gives six and a quarter pages of references for the 243 different poisonings and provings, whose symptoms are more or less set forth in the 1,680 given. The majority are poisonings by the drug, but there are provings, even in high potency.

Glancing down the black letter symptoms only, apart from the important symptoms in italics, one sees hydrophobia, mania, violent delirium and delirium tremens, epilepsy, chorea, with a high degree of hallucination, and FEAR. It is not the vague fear of *Aconite,* but something more concrete—fear of objects seen in imagination : seen more at the side than in front, curiously.

Stramonium has much that is in common with its cousins, *Belladonna,* and *Hyoscyamus* : and comes up for consideration for many of the maladies that both mirror forth. But *Stramonium* seems to lack the inflammatory intensity of *Belladonna.*

* * *

HALE WHITE, who supplies the teaching in Materia Medica for medical students, describes in twenty-one short lines the ACTION and THERAPEUTICS of *Stramonium.*

He says its action is almost the same as *Belladonna,* and that there is no reason why *Stramonium* should not be applied for the same purposes as *Belladonna.* And the only use he has for this powerful and valuable drug, is that of a palliative to relax the muscular coat of the bronchial tubes—more powerfully than *Belladonna*. He describes a powder, which, burnt, gives off dense fumes, and affords great relief in asthma ; and he adds that " Himrod's, Bliss's and other ' cures ' for asthma, are of similar composition ". He wisely puts *cures* in inverted commas, because palliatives do not cure : they relieve *pro tem.* ; and as we know, such powders may have to be burnt again and again in one night. And yet *Stramonium* should cure some cases of asthma, because it has caused difficult breathing : especially in connection with spasm of diaphragm.

* * *

CULPEPPER (*Herbal*, 1653) mentions *Stramonium* for epileptic disorders, convulsions and madness:—its ancient reputation, as we see, amply confirmed from the homœopathic standpoint by poisonings, provings and practice.

* * *

To get an all-round knowledge of the uses of any drug, one has to get the impressions of many prescribers and their experience in regard to its usefulness.

BOGER (*Synoptic Key*) stresses : " A REMEDY OF TERRORS, BUT LACKING IN PAIN. . . . *Disorderly, graceful*, or rhythmic movements. . . . DREADS DARKNESS, and has a horror of glistening objects. . . . Great thirst, but *dreads water*. . . . Putrid, dark, painless, involuntary diarrhœa. . . . *Awakes in fear*, or screaming."

* * *

GUERNSEY (*Keynotes*), who has a talent for going straight at the main features of a drug, says, of *Stramonium* :
" The principal range of this remedy is found in the mental affections. In young people, sometimes hysterical, praying, singing devoutly, beseeching, entreating, etc. (Young women with suppressed menses may be thus affected.) In fevers where the patient *cannot bear* solitude or darkness ; if they are left alone in a dark room, the mental affections are very much aggravated. Also in unconscious delirium when the patient will now and then jerk the head up from the pillow, and then let it fall—this being kept up without intermission for a long time. Women in puerperal fever may have absurd notions—that they are double, that some-one is in bed with them, and other strange unmeaning fancies. Affections of the intellect ; madness. . . .
" Face red and bloated. Cannot walk, or keep on the feet in a darkened room, falls. . . ."

* * *

NASH sums up *Stramonium* thus :

" Wildly delirious with red face and great LOQUACITY.

" Pupils widely dilated ; wants light and company ; fears to be alone.   Wants hand held.   (*Zinc.*)

" One side paralysed, the other convulsed.

" Wakes with a shrinking look : frightened   afraid of the first object seen.

" Painlessness with most complaints (*Opium*).   Jerks the head suddenly from pillow in spasms."

He calls it one of the trio of pre-eminently high-grade delirium remedies, differing from the other two chiefly in the degree of intensity.   He says :

" The raving is something awful.   Singing, laughing, grinning, whistling, screaming, praying piteously or swearing hideously, and above all remedies *loquacious*."

Again the patient throws himself into all shapes corresponding to his changeable delirium, crosswise, lengthwise, rolled up like a ball, or stiffened out by turns. . . . Things look crooked or oblique to him.

Mouth as if raw : tongue stiff as if paralysed.   Stools loose, blackish, smelling like carrion, or *no stool or urine*.   Later, loss of sight, .hearing, speech with dilated, immovable pupils and drenching sweat that brings no relief.   Death must soon close the scene, unless *Stram.* helps them out.

He contrasts the three :

Stram. is the most *loquacious*.

Hyos. is the most insensibly *stupid*.

Bell. stands half-way between.

Stram. throws himself about, jerks head.

Hyos. twitches, picks and reaches, otherwise lies pretty still.

Bell. starts or jumps, falling or awaking from sleep.

All have times of wanting to escape. . . .

*　　*　　*

Now for some of KENT's special points :—When considering *Stramonium*, the idea of violence comes into mind, . . . one wonders seeing a patient poisoned by, or needing *Stramonium*, at the tremendous turmoil, the great upheaval taking place.   Excitement, rage, everything tumultous, violent : face wild, anxious, fearful ; eyes fixed on a certain object : face flushed : hot, raging fever with hot head and cold extremities.   Turns from the light : wants it dark : aggravated especially by bright light.   High fever with violent delirium : heat so intense it may be mistaken for *Belladonna* : but usually a continuous fever, while the intense fever of *Bell.* is remittent always.

Like an earthquake in violence.   Mind in an uproar, cursing, tearing the clothes, violent speech, frenzy, erotomania, exposing the person.   (Useful in violent typhoids.)

Mania that has existed for some time.   A single attack would look like *Bell.*   But *Bell.* might be a palliative in the first attack, and in the second would do nothing.

When the delirium is not on, patient has the appearance of great suffering : forehead wrinkled : face pallid, sickly, haggard. Anxious look, indicative of intense suffering from meningeal involvement.

Delirium, bland, murmuring, incoherent chattering with open eyes ; vivid ; merry, with spasmodic laughter : furious, raving, wild : attempts to stab and bite ; with queerest notions . . . fear as if a dog were attacking him.   Strange ideas about the body, that it is ill-shapen, elongated, deformed . . .

Sees animals, ghosts, angels, departed spirits, devils : knows they are not real, but later is confident they are. . . .

Sings amorous songs and utters obscene speech. . . . Screams till hoarse and loses voice.   Screeches and screams day and night with fever, or mania.

Hyos. has wild maniacal delirium, but very little fever.   In *Stram.* there is considerable fever.   In *Bell.* the fever is afternoon and evening (3 p.m. to 3 a.m.), and then a remission.

Puerperal convulsions and insanity.   It has the septic nature. " Has sinned away her day of grace," yet has lived an upright life. . . .

Cerebral congestions ; profound intoxication : stupor : stertorous breathing : lower jaw dropped. . . . Typhoid, with oozing blood from mouth, tongue dry, swollen, fills mouth, pointed, red, like a piece of meat. . . .

Basilar meningitis from suppressed ear discharge.   Forehead wrinkled, eyes glassy . . . awful pain through base of skull with a history of necrosis about the ear.

Violent headache from walking in the sun : worse lying down. Worse motion and jar. . . . Pain in occiput.

High grade inflammation—pus forms, abscesses with excruciating pain, . . . vicious septic states.   Chronic abscesses :— the left hip-joint is a special locality.

Stram. stands alone among the deep-acting remedies, in its violence of mental sufferings. . . .

Suppuration of lungs where cough is worse from looking into the light.

Delusions in regard to personal identity. . . . Great anxiety when a train is going through a tunnel.

*   *   *

Black Letter Symptoms

Maniacal delirium : symptoms resembling HYDROPHOBIA.

Delirium of fear, as though a dog were attacking him.

Impression of danger : clings to person who had him in her lap.

Noisy DELIRIUM *with* HALLUCINATIONS.

Appearance of patient suggested mania.

" There are those bugs, help me catch them."

" There, a long trail of bedbugs, and after them a procession of beetles, and here come crawling over me a host of cockroaches." He shrank back in alarm : then suddenly, " I believe I know they are not really bugs : but except once in a while, they seem real to me."

(Biting a man's hand), sometimes crying out that she saw cats, dogs and rabbits, at the top, sides and middle of the room.

(Speaking) the sound resembled a squeak more than the natural tone of the voice.

Manifested great aversion to fluids of every kind. When a cup of water was put to her lips, she would start from it, and sometimes relapse into her paroxysm : such great aversion to it, that it was with the utmost difficulty that any liquid could be forced down her throat.

Hydrophobia : Aversion—even rage, when it was attempted to administer any liquid. Had even spasmodic irritation of pharyngeal muscles, and anything taken choked him and, was regurgitated.

Asked her mother not to leave her, "something was going to hurt her".

Constant staring about, then a fixed gaze, with sudden startings of arms and lower limbs, with low mutterings, then sudden and furious screaming, scratching, tearing with the hands, and kicking.

He makes all motions hastily.

From the expression of face and movements, he seems at times to be chasing, or fleeing from imaginary objects.

Terrified by fanciful delusions : they appear to grow out of the ground at his side—large dogs, cats and horrible beasts, from which he springs away with signs of terror, but cannot get away from them.

Continually strange objects intrude on his fancy, frightening him. He sees more horrifying images at his side than in front of him.

The boy seemed to see black objects.

(An executioner standing before him) seemed to him a reality.

All ideas seemed to consist of mere reproductions : there was nothing original, no new combinations.

Occupied with hallucinations : gaze fixed ; seemed trying to reach towards something she saw. Solely occupied with objects of his fancy.

The sight of a light, a mirror, or water, excited horrible convulsions.

Quite irrational : picked the bedclothes, saw bugs, etc.

Shuddering and seeming much frightened. Starts up in affright.

FEAR *of being in the dark, and (less) of being alone in the evening after sunset.*

Conduct and countenance like that of a child severely frightened, and apprehending some terrible calamity.

DELIRIUM : *bland : murmuring : violent : foolish : joyful : loquacious : incoherent : chattering : with open eyes : vivid : merry : with spasmodic laughter : furious : raving : wild attempts to stab and bite : with queerest notions ; with sexual excitement : fear as if a dog were attacking him : conscious of her condition : calls for papa and mamma, who are present and trying to console child : with open eyes : noisy, with hallucinations ; shy, hides himself : tries to escape : full of fear : talks incessantly, absurdly, laughs, claps hands over head, wide-open eyes.*

Mania for light and company : cannot bear to be alone.

DELIRIUM TREMENS. *Hallucinations which, especially at night, put patient into wildest restlessness. . . .*

Laughing. Intoxication.

Rush of blood to head. Violent congestion of head.

EYES *wide open, prominent : pupils exceedingly dilated, insensible, with injected conjunctivæ, as if vessels filled with dirty liquid. Complained that it was dark and called for light.*

Hallucinations DARK. *(Bell., fiery, shining.)*

Hot cheeks. Blood rushing to FACE.

White circle round mouth.

Wild staring look : expression of great fear and terror. (Acon.)

Glairy saliva dribbling from MOUTH.

Speech stammering, difficult and unintelligible.

Has to exert himself a long time before he can utter a word.

(Distorts face, makes great efforts to speak.)

Dryness of THROAT. *Constriction.*

Spasmodic constriction of throat, a kind of paralysis, so that swallowing was very difficult—almost impossible.

Fauces dry : very red : with difficult swallowing   Terrible spasm of throat on each attempt to swallow, like hydrophobia.

Dryness of throat not removed by frequent draughts of water.

The child had not only lost power of utterance, but that of voice. Could only utter a hoarse croaking sound, alternating with sonorous croupy barking cough : unable to swallow for the violent spasms.

Thirst violent, for sour drinks. Fear of water : and aversion to all fluids.

ABDOMEN *distended, not hard.*
Stool and urine suppressed.

VOICE *hoarse and croaking. High, squeaking, out of tune.*
Usual modulation quite lost : higher and finer than usual.

Twitching of hands and feet ; of tendons ; of extremities : during chill ; through body like CHOREA.

Trembling of limbs.
Trembling of whole body, seemed as if in a great fright.
CONVULSIONS.
Frightful convulsions at sight of a lighted candle, a mirror, or of water.
Now rejected every liquid, and seemed to labour under hydrophobia, for the moment a cupful of drink touched lips, the spasms returned with great violence.
Child became restless : tossed about : called for water : could swallow with great difficulty.
Constant restless movements of all limbs and the whole body.
Convulsions, alternating with rage : opisthotonic, from bright, dazzling objects, a lighted candle, a mirror, or touch. Child rigid as a board, when loudly spoken to or when touched. Shrieks in hoarse voice.

Scarlatinous redness of SKIN.
Intensely red rash in skin, resembling scarlet fever, but having a more shiny appearance.
Scarlet efflorescence over the whole body.

HEAD *very hot. Skin hot, dry, burning : scarlet.*

Child will not go to SLEEP *in the dark, but soon falls asleep in a lighted room.*

" STRANGE, RARE AND PECULIAR " SYMPTOMS

Hands and arms in motion, as if spinning or weaving.
Grasps about in air, catching at imaginary objects.
Motionless, pulseless : then tossed about in great rage : made signs to those about him, not understood.
Condition resembles highest state of intoxication from alcohol.
· · Calls things by wrong names, his boots, logs of wood ; his bedroom, the stable.
No correct estimate of distance or size : reaches for things across the room : bumps into persons and things which appear to be distant.

Uses wrong words, cannot find right words.

Talks in different languages.

Sits silent, eyes on ground, picking at her clothes.

Mind wanders, with quick motions of eyes and hands.

Excessive dilatation of pupils, with slow pulse.

Aberrations of mind.   One carries home wood to manufacture brandy : another places two axes across each other to split wood : a third burrows in ground like a pig with his mouth : a fourth was " a wheelwright ", and began to bore holes : a fifth ran into forge, to catch fish which he saw swimming there   . . .   a girl ran about the room and cried that all evil spirits were pursuing her.

Face expresses perturbation—stupidity—FEAR.

Converses with spirits : is under influence of spirits ; has communications from God ; delivers sermons : prophecies.

Animals jump out of the ground sideways : he moves quickly to other side, where others start up and pursue him.

Thinks he is tall : double : lying crosswise : that he was killed, roasted, and being eaten.

Sees more horrifying images at his side, than in front of him : they all occasion terror.

Seemed to see black objects : spoke of black people and black clouds : grasped at air.

Rush of blood to head with furious loquacious delirium.

" A dog is biting him and tearing flesh off his chest " ; complains of violent headache : confessing and praying : wants to be killed : to be kissed : accuses his wife of unfaithfulness : will not be touched ; takes people for dogs and barks at them.

Is a distinguished person.   Threatens to use knife on those about him: to break furniture: to throw himself out of the window.

Thinks he has snakes in him : lizards : worms in his clothes.

Religious mania : pious looks : praying : inspired talking : despair of her salvation.

Water, or a mirror, or anything bright excites convulsions.

Screams and howls.   Wants to kill people, or himself.

Changeable : anticipation of death, and rage ; then laughable gestures : then haughtiness and inconsolableness.

Obscene thoughts and actions.   Sought to bite, or to catch flies.   Sings and utters obscene things.

Laughing.   Makes faces : imitates motions, gestures and voices of different animals.

Suicidal : wants a razor to cut his throat.

Pangs of conscience : thinks he is not honest.

On being reprimanded, pupils dilate immediately.

Child very cross ; strikes or bites.

Going down stairs takes two steps for one, and falls.

Alae nasi white, face red.

Taste bitter : all food bitter ; all taste lost.

Tongue whitish with fine red dots ! In constant motion : swollen ; hangs out of mouth.

Averse to fluids : to water, even the sight of it causes spasms.

Violent desire to bite and tear things with his teeth.

Sight of a light, mirror, or water excites horrible convulsions.

Froths at mouth and constant spitting.

Violent thirst with desire for sour drinks.

Great desire for acids. Better for vinegar.

Very violent hiccough. Flow of very salt saliva.

Vomits water, bile, dark-green substance : green bile.

As if navel were to be torn out.

Wind in abdomen wakens her : screams, thinking herself full of creeping things.

As if urine could not be passed, for narrowness of urethra.

As if cylindrical body were being pushed through urethra : better after drinking vinegar.

Sexual irritation : hands constantly on genitals.

Nymphomania.

Metrorrhagia with excessive loquacity, singing, prayers, praise.

Shrinking look, when awaking.

Aphonia : aphasia : stammering.

Excessive sense of suffocation.

Hard pressure on cartilages of third and fourth ribs with difficult breathing : unable to inhale enough to breathe without anxiety.

When coughing while sitting, lower extremities are jerked up.

Something turns round in chest.

Diaphragmitis.

As soon as she falls into a doze, profuse sweat breaks out (*Con.*).

Arms thrown about : thrown upwards.

Beating with one arm, grasping with the other.

Falls over his own feet. Fingers and heels numb.

Falls with full consciousness, bent backward so that heels touch occiput ; suddenly snaps forward again.

Falls in the dark : can walk well in light.

Voluntary muscles do not obey will.

Continual cramp in hands and feet.

Great movability of limbs.

Strange involuntary motions : great agility.

Sensation in joints as if all parts of limbs were completely separated from each other. Arms and legs separated from body : hands and feet loosened in joints. . . .

(And so on : convulsions : chorea : hysteria : epilepsy : etc.)

Awakes : does not know where he is : with a solemn air of importance ; screaming, frightened, knows no one, shrinks away or jumps out of bed ; with staring eyes at one point : assumes a comically majestic appearance. . . .

As if cold water poured down back.

As if sparks of fire rushing from stomach to eyes.

*   *   *

It is important to recognize the exactly opposite conditions produced (and curable) by *Stramonium*. *Cursing*, and *praying* (as the boy who gets hauled to his feet in passages and odd corners, where he has fallen to his knees in prayer—one remembers such a case). *Desire for light*, unable to walk, or to sleep in the dark (like the young man who has to have a night light, because he " screams the house down" if it goes out), and yet convulsions *renewed by the sight of bright objects*. Again, *the violent convulsions*, with *horrible distortions of the face ;* or only the (characteristic) " *disorderly*, *graceful, rhythmical movements in delirium or chorea*, utterly unlike the angular jerkings of *Hyos*." (All remembered cases.)

One recalls several striking instances of the rapid curative action of *Stramonium*. Two cases, scribbled into the margin of Allen's *Encyclopedia*, at the time, come up opportunely. (1) A big, strong Scotchman, years ago, when influenza, after many years absence, came back to mightily stampede the doctors, and to claim a large number of victims including one of the princes, went down with a bad attack of the prevailing epidemic. He had a very high temperature, frightful pain, " right in the hairt of my heed ", as he afterward expressed it ; with delirium, and vomiting of green matter. But the " strange, rare and peculiar " symptom here was, that he said that the glass of water his wife brought him was *black*, and that her face was *black*. This black vision suggested *Stram*. and he was cured in a few hours by *Stram*. 30. (No. 2), long forgotten but scribbled in below, at the same time, reads : " Alice " (a housemaid). " Bad pain all day across head, but right *inside it*, cured by one dose of *Stram*. 30."

A third, a more recent Hospital case, already given, must be retold here, where it belongs. It was an amazing case. . . .

A woman of 33 was brought into L.H.H. on January 17th, 1930. The old school doctor who sent her in had been treating her for the last 14 days for pyelitis and frequent heart attacks, *with a temperature of* 104 :—and the previous year for " mitral incompetence and albuminuria ".

On admission there was much pus and blood in urine ; some lumbar pain, and difficulty in urination. She appeared to be very ill ; but on admission there was nothing abnormal found in the lungs.

Next day, she was restless and delirious towards evening, with morbid fears, and a temperature of 104·8, respiration 24.

On the third day temperature 104-104·8, respiration now 44. She had developed *a very rapid double pneumonia*. Skin flushed, hot, dry. Delirium. Thirst. And at night restlessness with twitchings of face and hands. Temperature 104. Respiration 34-48 (in spite of *Phos.* 30, which she had been having at six-hourly intervals). And she had only passed 11 oz. of urine in twenty-four hours.

On the fourth day, pretty twitchings of face : hands twitched:— a peculiar " angelic " smile in delirium. She was conscious when roused. It was observed that the temperature was always at its highest at NOON (" as now 104·6 ").

The case was reconsidered, having regard to its unusual and characteristic symptoms.

For *fever at noon*, there is only one drug in italics—*Stram.*

The graceful spasms and twitchings of face—" *facial muscles constantly play in delirium* "—again *Stram.*

Then, the character of the delirium, lacking the violence of *Bell.*, together with the fever, the dry hot skin, and the suppressed urine, again suggested *Stram.* So at noon on the fourth day of admission—the second day of the pneumonia, she was given *Stram.* 1m., *three doses, four-hourly.*

The result was dramatic ! viz. a quieter night ; no twitching ; no delirium. Quite sensible. *Temperature coming down.*

Next day it rose once more, *but at* 8 *p.m., not noon,* and only to 103·8—a degree lower ; when she got three more doses of *Stram.* 10m. After which, with one more small rise, it dropped—to remain sub-normal for some days.

A day later, as she was weak and drowsy, and " looked toxic ", she was given three doses of *Arnica* 200 ; *after which she needed no more medicine.*

Stram. was given on the second day of the double pneumonia, and she was sub-normal three days later.

By February 18th she was walking about the ward ; and was discharged a fortnight later, " *lungs normal, heart normal, urine normal. Quite well.*"

The interest in this case was its *great severity* (the doctor who sent her in believed her to be dying of pyelitis and heart trouble before the double pneumonia supervened), and *the unusual drug for pyelitis and double pneumonia.* This case shows how the curative remedy was found on a very few, but *characteristic* symptoms, not of pneumonia, or pyelitis, but of that individual patient exhibiting those disease-conditions.

Here, Hahnemann's " *totality of Characteristic Symptoms* ", suggested a remedy to which the patient undoubtedly owed her life.

And with this we may quit *Stramonium*. A marvellous drug, rightly applied—they all are !—yet only worthy of twenty-one short lines in *Hale White's Materia Medica*, the text book for students of medicine.

Things are moving at last : and one wonders how long it will be before medical students are allowed to take their course of Materia Medica with us ! We have no desire to run a medical school : all the rest can be better taught elsewhere, with appliances and first-class teachers : but—*Materia Medica ! Good Lord !* No wonder so many doctors have " lost their faith in medicine ".

*　　*　　*

Nash gives a case of acute mania, cured with *Stramonium*. " A lady about 30, overheated in the sun, on an excursion. A member of a Presbyterian church, but she imagined herself lost, and called me in six mornings in succession to see her die. Lost, lost, lost, eternally lost, was her theme, begging minister, doctor, everybody, to pray for and with her. Talked day and night about it. I had to shut her up in her room alone, for she would not sleep a wink or let anyone else.

" She imagined her head was as big as a bushel, and had me examine her legs, which she insisted were as large as a church. After treating her for several weeks with *Glon., Lach., Nat. carb.* and other remedies on the *cause* as the basis of the prescription, without the least amelioration of her condition, I gave her *Stramonium*, which covered her *symptoms*, and in twenty-four hours every vestige of that mania was gone. She was to have been sent to the Utica Asylum." (Nash gave her the sixth potency.)

SULPHUR

Sulphur is one of the greatest of " polycrests " (drugs of many uses),—is Hahnemann's Prince of " antipsorics " (remedies of non-venereal chronic diseases),—and is one of the constituents of protoplasm, thus not only occurring, but evoking and curing, symptoms in every tissue and organ of the body. Its great and wide range in homœopathic prescribing, is evidenced by the fact that Allen's *Encyclopedia* gives no fewer than 1,040-odd symptoms, each with reference that tells not only the authority but the dose responsible.

Hahnemann says of *Sulphur* : " The homœopathic physician (who alone acts in conformity with natural laws) will meet many important morbid states for which he will discover and may expect much assistance in the symptoms of *Sulphur* and *Hepar Sulphuris.*"

He points out the similarity of the eruptions produced by *Sulphur* with those of itch :—the characteristic itching eruption which *Sulphur* can excite, " in which is revealed an affection, similar (homœopathic) to but not identical with the itch   .   .   . and tells us that Homœopathy requires medicines that produce diseases only similar to those they should be administered for in order to cure them.   .   .   .   Homœopathy has never pretended to produce an identical disease with medicines, but has always enjoined the selection of a medicine for the cure, that produces only a similar affection.   .   .   .   Canova's statue of the captive of St. Helena may be very like, but it is not NAPOLEON !   .   .   . Do not our stupid opponents understand that ? Are they unable to comprehend the difference between *identical* (same) and *similar* ? or do they not wish to comprehend it ? " And he gives the difference between " true itch and the very-like pimples and vesicles of the itch of workers in wool."

In *Materia Medica Pura* he scorns the idea of employing diseases for the cure of disease : but later on, in his *Chronic Diseases*, and indeed in the *Organon* (possibly in its later editions) he discusses the fact that by preparation and potentization disease products become " so changed as to be no longer *idem* but *simillimum* " ; and it was Hahnemann himself who prepared and potentized the contents of the itch pustule, and proved it (the proving is to be found in Stapf's *Archives*) ; and showed thereby its great similarity of symptoms to those of *Sulphur*—and its great differences : thus teaching us when to prescribe the one, and when the other.

But it is believed that Hahnemann later on partly proved and used some other disease products : though he did not give us a lead to their use, since they were not sufficiently proved to be capable of scientific employment. (See an interesting article on this subject, HOMŒOPATHY, vol. I, p. 462.)

Anyway *Sulphur* is one of our great skin medicines, but only in such skin conditions as it can produce, or in typical *Sulphur-patients*. It has BOILS (*Anthrac., Tarent. cub., Arn., Bellis* and a host of others, each in its place) : crops of boils, which succeed one another. Itching, extreme ; " voluptuous " itching, relieved by scratching, then burning ; worse from heat of bed (*Merc.*). " Dry, rough, scaly or itching skin, disposed to break out or fester and won't heal " (*Hep., Sil.*) : even pustular eruptions.

And *Sulphur* eruptions may alternate with other complaints, such as asthma (*Ars.*, etc.).

When we were children a precious Riddle Book had it, "*Sulphur* comes from volcanoes and is good for eruptions," and *Sulphur* is associated in ideas with the Lake of Fire, and Everlasting Burnings ; and *Sulphur* indeed *causes* BURNINGS ; burning pain in eyes, lips, tongue ; in nostrils, face, throat ; in fauces and pharynx ; in stomach and abdomen ; in anus ; in hæmorrhoids, etc. ; between scapulæ (*Lyc., Phos.*) ; in fingers, palms (PHOS.), knees, feet, especially *at night ;* in soles, in corns, in chilblains, in skin of whole body, in parts on which he lies. The eruptions of *Sulphur* BURN. And with all its burning there may be burnings in parts—patchy or local burnings with *coldness* elsewhere, as feet cold with burning head or face ; in the same way that *Nat. mur.* may have irregular distribution of the fluids of the body, as diarrhœa with a dry mouth and tongue, or " dryness of mucous membranes with watery secretions elsewhere ".

" *Sulphur reddens orifices* in a way common to no other remedy "—lips (*Tub.*), eyelids (*Graph.*), nostrils, red, dirty, discharging (*Aurum*) ANUS, with itching ; and excoriating stools, often ; and here it is a great remedy for hæmorrhoids. One has seen low-potency *Sulphur* produce them in someone who never had them before or since. The old " low-potency " men had a trick of curing piles with *Sulphur* alternately with *Nux* (they are complementary remedies). In those days they would have held it a disgrace to have piles " operated " or injected.

Sulphur goes through the body from vertex to soles. In the former its pressure-symptoms remind one of LACH., BELL., GLON. and others, while it burns the soles so much that the feet must be thrust out of bed (PULS., MED., CHAM.).

Sulphur is, of course, a great remedy of stomach and intestinal conditions. The *Sulphur* stomach feels empty and " sinking ", especially about 11 a.m. (or noon, or an hour before the mid-day meal), but then a *Sulphur* patient will often tell you that she wants no breakfast, but starves at the later hour. And the typical *Sulphur* diarrhœa (often chronic) torments its victim with hurried early morning stools or diarrhœa, leaving them safe for the rest of the day.

It would be impossible to give all the black letter symptoms of *Sulphur*—i.e. the symptoms again and again produced and again and again cured by that drug—they are far too numerous for the space at our command ; but we will delve a little into Kent, and glean from that great prescriber his experiences derived from a very large and successful practice and from years of teaching Materia Medica. The more one goes to Kent, the more one needs to go. He, more than anyone, probably, has imbibed the spirit of Hahnemann, and expounded and perpetuated his doctrines.

KENT says, " *Sulphur* is such a full remedy that it is difficult to tell where to begin. It seems to contain a likeness of all sickness, and a beginner reading over the provings of *Sulphur* might naturally think that there was no need of any other remedy, as the image of all sickness seems to be contained in it." Yet, he says, " it will not cure all the sicknesses of man, and must not be used indiscriminately. . . It seems that the less a physician knows of Materia Medica the oftener he gives *Sulphur* ; but it is very frequently given by good prescribers, so that the line between physicians' knowledge and ignorance cannot be drawn from the frequency of their use of *Sulphur*.

" The *Sulphur* patient is lean, lank, hungry, dyspeptic with stoop-shoulders ; yet many times it must be given to fat, rotund, well-fed people."

" The *Sulphur* state may be brought on by being housed up in meditation—philosophical inquiry, taking no exercise : must eat only the simplest foods and not enough to nourish them, and end up by going into a philosophical mania. . . . Another class, dirty-looking, shrivelled, red-faced. If a child, may be often washed, but looks as if perfunctorily washed. . . . The *Sulphur* scholar—inventor—works day and night in threadbare clothes and battered hat ; has uncut hair and a dirty face ; his study is uncleanly—untidy, books piled indiscriminately, no order. *Sulphur* seems to produce this state of disorder, uncleanliness, ' don't care how things go,' and a state of selfishness. He becomes a *false philosopher*—disappointed because the world

does not consider him the greatest man on earth. . . . .
He has on a shirt that he has worn many weeks : if he had not a
wife, he would wear his shirt till it fell off him." (One has seen
with triumph how a dose or two of *Sulphur*, in such a patient, has
produced a clean shirt !) " Cleanliness is not a great idea with a
Sulphur patient," says Kent. " *Sulphur* is seldom indicated in
cleanly people, but it is commonly indicated in *those who are not
disturbed by uncleanliness.* . . . The *Sulphur* child is subject
to catarrhal discharges from nose and eyes, etc., and mothers
will tell you that the child will eat the discharges from the nose.
. . . That is peculiar, because the *Sulphur* patient is *over-
sensitive to filthy odours ;* but the filthy substances themselves
he will eat and swallow. Has filthy odours, and they nauseate
him. Imagines he smells things. . . . Discharges not only
offensive but excoriating. Stools, nasal discharge, excoriating,
burn and make raw the parts. Boils—suppurations—abscesses—
eruptions, but always with *burning.* Burning runs through
Sulphur. Burning soles : palms : vertex. Worse warm in
bed. Nightly complaints are a feature." And so on for many
pages.

　　Sulphur has some weird sensations, perhaps not often met
with, but helpful where they occur. A band tightly bound round
forehead ; as if bed too small to hold him : as if swinging, or
standing on wavering ground. Pressure vertex, as if brain
beating against skull : as if head would burst. As if scalp were
loose ; as if eyes had been punctured ; as if sounds came not
through ears but forehead ; as of a lump or hair in throat ;
intestines in knots ; as if bowels too weak to retain their contents ;
as if a lump of ice in chest ; as if chest would fly to pieces when
coughing or breathing deeply ; as of a mouse running up arms
and back. (See *Calc.*) And many others. As of a rivet through
upper third left lung to scapula . . . .

　　Sulphur has also some weird mentalities. As GUERNSEY puts
it, " fantastic illusions of the intellect, especially if one turns
everything into beauty, as an old rag or stick looks to be a beautiful
piece of workmanship—everything looks pretty which the patient
takes a fancy to. Wishing to touch something " . . . one
has had this symptom in children, and failed to find it !

　　Sulphur is one of the remedies that has *periodicity.* Pains
in head, for instance, every seven days, every fourteen days ;
" an intermittent, periodic neuralgia with aggravation every
24 hours, generally at mid-day or mid-night." Diarrhœa at 5 a.m.

　　The *Sulphur* patient hates, or is the worse for a bath : and
though a " warm patient " is worse for wet, or cold wet weather.

Sulphur has a big reputation for clearing up acute conditions that hang fire : pneumonias—exudations into serous sacs, following inflammations (as pleural effusions—we have seen this). Complaints that are continually relapsing (*Tub.*). But, in a "*Sulphur* patient".

By the way, *Sulphur* has, in poisoning, produced convulsions, and it is one of the first things one thinks of for epilepsy—in a *Sulphur* patient, or when the patient has had a *Sulphur*-like eruption.

When first one started "working out" one's cases, it seemed as if *Sulphur* must always come through, such a constant appearance does it present in the various rubrics, but that is by no means the case. Its symptoms are very definite and very striking : it has its own place and does its own work ; and often comes in, as we said, to clear up difficult conditions, and those that hang fire—in a *Sulphur* patient.

To do rapid and at all creditable out-patient work, where the patients crowd in as they do with us, and where they have to be considered as individuals, and not as this or that disease, and treated accordingly, one must have the various drug-pictures of *Sulphur*—*Sepia*—*Lycopodium* and a dozen other common remedies of common complaints at one's finger-tips. And when you get one or two of the little *Sulphur* drug-pictures by heart, and prescribe *Sulphur* correctly, it is surprising how long it will hold your patient—i.e. a chronic patient. Many of these return only after many months to ask for " the medicine you give me, which always puts me right ". *Sepia* is another of these medicines of very definite symptoms, easy to recognize ; and when one turns to the patient's page, and sees *Sepia* inscribed thereon, one nearly always knows that the patient will say, " *Much* better ! " and that the call for repetition will be long-delayed.

One must be pardoned for dragging in " out-patients " so often ; but continuous heavy out-patient work for at least thirty years has impressed some things on one's consciousness.

A few years ago we gave a Paper to the British Homœopathic Society on " DRUG-PICTURES " which still persists in pamphlet form. That little paper was so much appreciated, and one was urged so often to go on with such pictures, that it has led to the present efforts in the same direction. And the little *Sulphur*-pictures in that paper—they only ran to a page—are so concise and to the point that we are minded to reproduce them here.

Sulphur has been called the " ragged philosopher ".

An argumentative, stoop-shouldered person, who is always on the look-out for a chair to drop into.

26

Untidy—unkempt.

Coarse, lustreless hair, which takes its own rebellious way, like its owner ; not amenable to conventions.

Famished before meals : famished at 11 a.m.

Eats anything.

Craves fat.   (*Sulphur* is the only WARM drug that craves fat.)

Intolerant of clothing—of flannel on the skin.

Morning diarrhœa ; but, after that, safe for the rest of the day.

One curious aspect of the *Sulphur* mentality is the admiration for what is not admirable.   Rags may seem beautiful.   Ecstacies over things in which normal persons can see nothing to admire.

Sulphur exists in every tissue of the body : there is nothing that *Sulphur* cannot help, IN A SULPHUR PATIENT.

It is the greatest of polycrests.

Again, *elderly women with flushes.*

Throw off the bedclothes.

Starving at 11 a.m.

Put their burning soles out at night to cool.   (CHAM., MED., PULS., and one or two others do this also.}

Again,—Warm, hungry babies.   Kick off the bedclothes—impossible to keep them covered at night.

Very obstreperous hair—(?) sandy—harsh and lustreless—grows every way.

Dirty-nosed children : sore discharging nostrils.   (*Aur.*)

Orifices brilliant red ; anus, nostrils, eyelids, lips.

Itching at anus.

NASH says, " Every true homœopath knows the value of these and many more symptoms of this remedy.   No one else appreciates them.   Again, none but those who use potentized *Sulphur* can ever know what it is capable of curing."

BLACK LETTER SYMPTOMS

Foolish happiness and pride, thinks himself in possession of beautiful things ; even rags seem beautiful.

Indisposed to everything, work, pleasure, talking or motion ; indolence of mind and body.

Melancholy mood ; dwelling on religious or philosophic speculations ; anxiety about soul's salvation ; indifference about lot of others.

Too lazy to rouse himself up, and too unhappy to live.

Hypochondriasis after suppression of eruption.

Dread of being washed (in children).

Heat on crown of HEAD *; cold feet ; frequent flushing.*

Brain affections in children who do not like to be washed, have pimples, boils and other eruptions on head, face and everywhere, pick at nose, have red lips, crave sour things, feel faint in forenoon, may have diarrhœa early in morning ; sleep restless, start when falling asleep, cry out during sleep, or murmur, whine, moan or snore ; feet cold in morning, hot in evening ; they run about but do not like to stand, sit hunched and walk stooping.

Severe itching on forehead and scalp.

Itching pimples on forehead ; inflamed, painful to touch.

Inflamed and suppurating pimples on hairy scalp.

Humid, offensive eruption on top of head, filled with pus, drying up into honey-like scabs.

Dry, offensive, easily bleeding, burning eruption, begins on back of head and behind ears ; pains and cracks ; > from scratching.

Humid, offensive eruption, with thick pus, yellow crusts, bleeding and burning.

Dimness of vision ; as of a veil or gauze before EYES *; as from a fog ; with headache ; as if cornea had lost its transparency ; sudden paroxysms of nyctalopia ; while reading ; objects seem more distant ; for near and distant objects ; with weakness of eyes, blindness, cataract, glaucoma ; with innumerable, confused, dark spots floating before eyes.*

Keratitis parenchymatosa in a scrofulous subject, cornea like ground glass, photophobia, lids swollen and bleed easily.

Burning heat in eyes ; painful smarting.

Lachrymation ; in morning, followed by dryness ; and burning in morning ; profuse and burning from acrid, excoriating tears ; in open air, dry in room ; itching and biting in eyes.

DEAFNESS *; preceded by oversensitiveness of hearing ; especially for human voice ; from disposition to catarrhs ; < after eating, or blowing nose.*

Otitis ; in psoric patients with tendency to skin eruptions, coryzas, and cerebral congestion ; from a furuncle in meatus ; in children who suddenly cry out in pain, while they appear listless and unobservant, and where it seems doubtful whether irritation is in brain or in intestinal canal ; in complication with meningitis or eruptive fevers ; lancinating, stinging, tearing in ear, extending to head and throat, < by disturbance, musical sounds, and all noises, and human voice is heard imperfectly ; chronic with a purulent discharge.

Smell before nose as of an old catarrh ; as of old offensive mucus.
Frequent sneezing.
Swelling and inflammation in nose ; red nose.

FACE : *Painful eruptions about chin.*
Bright redness of lips, particularly with children, complexion
sallow.
Lips dry, rough and cracked.

TOOTHACHE : *coming on in open air ; from least draught, at night*
in bed ; from washing with cold water ; with congestion to head, or
stitches in ear.
Stomacace ; aphthæ.

Dryness of THROAT *; exciting cough ; at night ; constant desire*
to swallow saliva in order to moisten affected parts.
Stitches in throat on swallowing ; painful contraction.
Swelling of palate and tonsils, elongation of palate.

APPETITE : *excessive ; canine ; ravenous, obliged to eat fre-*
quently, if he does not he has a headache and great lassitude,
and has to lie down ; feeling of faintness with strong craving for food
at 11 *a.m. ; voracious children put everything they see into mouth,*
swallow everything, watch everyone eating.
Drinks much, but eats little.
Desire for sweets ; diseases from eating sweet things, candy, etc.
Desire to imbibe alcholic drinks, from morning until night.
Drinks much, eats but little.
Weak, empty, gone or faint feeling in stomach about 11 *a.m.*
Heaviness in stomach ; feeling of weight.

Inflation of ABDOMEN *with wind ; rumbling and gurgling in*
bowels.
Emission of flatus ; especially in evening and night ; having
odour of bad eggs, or sulphuretted hydrogen ; inodorous.
Rumbling and gurgling in bowels ; painless diarrhœa, driving
patient out of bed at 5 *a.m.*
Big belly and emaciated limbs ; children disliked to be washed.

Portal stasis ; hæmorrhoidal congestions ; with indigestion,
constipation, etc.
Sudden call to STOOL *on waking in morning.*
Desire to stool, with colic, awakes him about 5 *a.m.*
Thin stool every morning, with cutting in lower abdomen.
Diarrhœa after midnight ; painless, driving out of bed early in
morning ; as if bowels were too weak to retain their contents.

Dysentery ; child was faint regularly at 11 *a.m. ; early morning aggravation.*

Cholera Asiatica ; as a prophylactic, a pinch of the powdered milk of sulphur worn in stockings in contact with soles of feet ; diarrhœa commences between midnight and morning, with or without pain, with or without vomiting, ineffectual desire to evacuate; diarrhœa and vomiting at same time ; numbness of limbs ; cramps in soles of feet and calves ; blueness under eyes ; coldness of skin ; indifference of mind ; during convalescence, red spots, furuncles, etc. ; susceptibility to temperature, warm things feel hot ; nerve symptoms.

Burning and pressure in rectum.

Itching in rectum.

Increased congestion of hæmorrhoidal vessels.

Hæmorrhoids, moist, blind, or flowing dark blood, with violent bearing-down pains from small of back toward anus.

Suppressed hæmorrhoids, with colic, palpitation, congestion to lungs, back feels stiff as if bruised.

Large hæmorrhoids, violent burning and sticking in anus ; pressing in rectum during and after stool ; it feels full.

Burning in anus ; after sitting a while ; after soft stools in evening.

Constant bearing down towards anus ; forcing down after sitting.

Itching in anus. Bleeding from anus.

Excoriation about anus.

Burning in URETHRA.

Itching in urethra.

Both flow of urine and discharge of fæces are painful to parts over which they pass.

Involuntary discharge of semen, with burning in urethra.

Testicles relaxed, hanging down ; soreness and moisture of scrotum, or offensive sweat of genitals.

Itching on glans penis.

Discharge of prostatic fluid after micturition and stool.

Soreness and moisture of scrotum ; soreness between thighs when walking.

Fetid perspiration on genital organs, with soreness and excoriation destroying most of hair, painful in walking, with thickening and induration of scrotum.

Hot flushes at climacteric period, with hot head, hands and feet, and a great goneness in stomach.

Burning in vagina, scarcely able to keep still.

Troublesome itching of vulva, with pimples.

Feels hungry and FAINT *about* 11 *a.m. ; cannot wait for dinner.*

Shortness of breath ; and oppression on bending arms backward ; from talking too much ; when walking in open air ; in evening in bed.

Feels suffocated ; wants doors and windows wide open ; particularly in night.

Oppression, heaviness and pressure in CHEST.

Burning in chest, rising to face.

Shooting in left side of chest through to back.

Stitches through chest, extending in to left scapula ; < lying on back and during least motion.

Congestion of blood to chest.

Pleurisy : (after ACON.*) acute, plastic form.*

Rush of blood to HEART.

Palpitation : anxious ; in evening in bed ; and fluttering of heart ; without anxiety, at any time of day ; during stool ; violent at night, on turning in bed ; violent and rapid on falling asleep ; when going upstairs or when climbing a hill ; visible.

Sensation as if heart were enlarged.

Sharp stitches in præcordial region.

Sharp pain at heart going through chest, to between shoulders ; especially with dyspeptic symptoms.

Great orgasm of blood, with violent burning in hands.

Pain in small of BACK *; could not walk erect, was obliged to walk bent over ; violent only on stooping, tensive as if everything were too short ; on rising from a seat ; gnawing ; after heavy lifting and taking cold at same time ; violent, as if bruised, also in coccyx ; tiresome feeling as if bruised ; stitches.*

Curvature of spine, vertebræ softened.

Rheumatic pains in SHOULDER, *especially in left.*

Perspiration in armpits, smelling like garlic ; offensive to patient.

Tremulous sensation in HANDS *when writing ; cold trembling hands.*

Burning of hands.

Rhagades on hands, especially between fingers, on finger joints and in palms.

Stiffness in KNEES *and cracking.*

Cramps in calves and soles, particularly at night ; looseness of bowels.

Stiffness of ankle joints.

Burning in feet, wants to find a cool place for them ; puts them out of bed to cool them off.

Burning in soles ; on stepping after sitting a long time ; and itching, especially on walking ; wishes to find a cool place for them, puts them out of bed ; wants them uncovered.

Weak, fainting spells frequently during day ; feels very faint and weak, with a strong craving for food, from 11 *to* 12 *every morning.*

Excessively sensitive to open air and will not be washed ; very much inclined to take cold.

Chorea ; in chronic diseases, particularly after suppressed eruptions ; frequent spasmodic jerking of whole body ; tremor of hands ; unsteady walk ; peevish, irritable, obstinate ; faint and hungry spells at 10 *a.m. ; soles of feet burn.*

Irresistible drowsiness in day time, wakefulness at night.
Wakes up at 3, 4 *or* 5 *a.m., and cannot* SLEEP *again.*
Heavy, unrefreshing sleep.
Finds himself at night lying on his back.
Nightmare.
Dreams : vivid, anxious, as if pursued by wild beasts ; vivid, comic, with loud laughter, continued for some time after waking ; vivid, believing she sits on chamber causes her to wet bed ; horrible, with great palpitation, that he has been bitten by a dog ; that he is falling.

Wants doors and windows open.
Orgasm of blood ; frequent flushes of HEAT.
Flushing heat in face, with febrile shivering over whole body.
Heat in head ; prevents falling asleep ; in morning ; in evening with cold feet.
Hot flushes, with spells of faintness, or passing off with a little moisture, faintness or debility.

Complaints continually relapsing. Alternate : pale and red cheeks; diarrhœa and constipation ; asthma, or gout, and skin eruptions.

Offensive odour of body despite frequent washing ; averse to washing.

Does not walk erect ; stoops or bends over forward in walking or sitting ; standing is most disagreeable position.

Scrofulous chronic diseases that result from SUPPRESSED ERUP-
TIONS.

DISCHARGES *in every outlet of body acrid, excoriating skin wherever they come in contact.*

CONGESTION *to single parts ; eyes, nose, chest, abdomen, arms, legs, etc.*

Complaints are continually RELAPSING *; seems to get almost well when disease returns.*

ITCHING *: all over body ; spots painful after scratching ; itching spots bleed and bite after scratching ; in various parts, disappearing after scratching ; at times followed by sticking or burning ; over whole body, recurring every night in bed ; and biting on nates ; violent on thighs and legs, at night ; about knees ; on toes ; of toes that had been frozen ; at night, in heat of bed, now in one place, now in another, especially on nape of neck ; in palms of hands, sometimes sticking, burning ; is obliged to rub them, after which they burn ; on backs of hands ; in eyebrows ; on abdomen, at night ; in scrotum ; on inside of thighs ; in axillæ and hollows of knees ; as if she were alive beneath skin ; as if vermin were running about ; < at night, and in morning, in bed, after waking ; above left eyebrow ; in ears externally ; of nose externally ; about chin ; on neck ; on chest ; of old tetter, is obliged to scratch until it bleeds.*
BURNING *in skin of whole body.*
FORMICATION *of skin over whole body.*
Voluptuous itching ; scratching relieves after it ; burning ; sometimes little vesicles.
After violent scratching aching, numbness of skin, swelling of skin, even ulceration.
Nettlerash ; with fever ; on face, arms, neck, and lower extremities ; on back of hand.
Itching hives over whole body, hands and feet.
Boils.
Skin rough, scaly, scabby.
Soreness in folds of skin.
Comedones ; black pores of skin, particularly in face.

Lean, stoop-shouldered persons who walk and sit stooped ; standing is the most uncomfortable position.

Persons of nervous temperament, quick-motioned, quick-tempered, plethoric, skin excessively sensitive to atmospheric changes.
Dirty, filthy people, prone to skin affections.
Children : cannot bear to be washed or bathed ; emaciated, big-bellied ; restless, hot, kick off clothes at night ; have worms.
Adapted to persons of scrofulous diathesis, subject to venous congestions, especially of portal system.

SYMPHYTUM

ONE of the invaluable remedies of " smashed and bruised humanity " is *Symphytum*—Comfrey : " Bone-set,"—" Healing herb."

For accidents, extravasations and bruises, we have quite a number of priceless remedies ; and, while any one on the list will be helpful in any and every case, whether in dilute tincture form, or freshly culled and infused, especially at its own season of perfection of growth and intensity of healing virtue, yet each one differs from all the rest in its relation to the several injured tissues.

It may be useful to set forth the marked features of a few of the most common of these God-gifts for pain and disability.

Arnica montana, whose very name emphasizes its habitat and functions. It is the " Fall-krout " of the mountains : and especially valuable for the repair of " soft parts ".

Its great action is on blood, and blood vessels.

It is invaluable for combating the effects of shock, mental as well as physical, and jar ; besides those of over-exertion and strain, and sprains.

Arnica is so sore all over and so tender to touch, as to be in terror of approach.

It is used internally, always ; also externally, provided the skin is not broken ; in which case it has acquired an evil reputation for provoking inflammation of an erysipelatous nature. Here it is safer to employ, externally, any one of the others.

Calendula. Marigold, which, in addition to its ample vulnerary qualities, stimulates life mechanisms to the prevention or cure of *Sepsis*. Greatly esteemed in the surgery, and in the midwifery of homœopaths.

Bellis perennis. The common daisy ; our indigenous *Arnica*.

A grand remedy for injuries and sprains, which are like those of *Arnica*, very tender to touch.

Again, like *Arnica*, *Bellis* affects blood vessels ; and, like *Hypericum*, nerves.

It is also precious for its effects on the mammæ, when indurations persist after blows.

Hypericum. Our marvellous remedy for the comfort and relief of pierced, torn, or injured parts rich in nerves ; such as lips (we have seen a torn lip with some loss of tissue, heal in a few hours by *Hypericum*). Finger-tips also whose fine nerve-endings are wound round little hard " touch corpuscles ", in order that the slightest impact shall be registered.

Hypericum relieves nerve pain, often excruciating. It is useful in injuries to spine, even of long ago, and to coccyx, as in a recent case of persistent coccygeal pain, when later enquiry evoked the answer, " Oh ! that's gone ! "

Ruta. Has elicited, in provings, bruised sensation all over, as from a fall or blow ; with soreness of parts on which he lies (*Arnica*).

A great remedy of bruises and injuries to bones and periosteum ; of sprains ; and of periostitis and pains in consequence of external injuries with erysipelatous inflammation.

Bone lesions and fractures (*Symph.*).

Ruta is also a great eye remedy (*Symph.*). Eyestrain, and loss of power in eye muscles.

Symphytum. Specific for injuries caused, not by sharp stabbing instruments, but by blows from blunt masses that damage, but fail to penetrate.

Especially useful for blows on the eyeball.

Symphytum is our very great remedy of fractures, and of fractures that fail to unite. It has a special mission in regard to periosteum (*Ruta*) and bone.

In the case of fractures, ensure position and immobility, and *Symphytum* will take charge.

Urtica urens, the common stinging Nettle, with its marvellous properties in regard to burns, especially the more or less superficial, and therefore the most painful. The manner in which pain is instantly banished and healing starts forthwith, needs to be seen to be realized.

From a thankful heart one is constrained to repeat Hahnemann's acknowledgment : " God's great gift, HOMŒOPATHY ! "

But, you will say, there is a sameness about the indications for all these bruise worts. Happily ! because it may be possible to get one or other, but not always the one that appeals to us as the most likely curative agent.

Dr. Robert Cooper, in his *Cases of Serious Disease Saved from Operation*, gives several of the triumphs of Comfrey (*Symphytum*). One of these we are minded to reproduce *in extenso*, being of special interest, as vouched for by the then President of the Royal College of Surgeons in Ireland—an unsympathetic and incredulous witness.

SARCOMATOUS TUMOUR INFILTRATING THE BONY TISSUE OF THE UPPER JAW

Dr. William Thompson, President of the Royal College of Surgeons in Ireland, delivered an address in Dublin on November 13th, 1896, entitled " Some Surprises and Mistakes ", in which the following very important case was narrated :

" In the early part of this year I saw a man who was suffering from a growth in the nose. I recommended him to see Dr. Woods, and I saw him later with Sir Thornley Stoker and Dr. Woods. We came to the conclusion that he was suffering from a malignant tumour of the antrum which had extended to the nose. We recommended an exploratory operation, and if our opinion was confirmed, that the jaw should be at once removed. He refused the larger operation. The exploration was made by Dr. Woods. We found that the tumour did extend from the antrum, into which I could bore my finger easily. Dr. O'Sullivan, Professor of Pathology of Trinity College, declared the growth to be a round-celled sarcoma. Of that there is no doubt. The tumour returned in a couple of months, and the patient then saw Dr. Semon in London, who advised immediate removal of the jaw. He returned home, and after a further delay he asked to have the operation performed. I did this in May last by the usual method. I found the tumour occupying the whole of the antrum. The base of the skull was everywhere infiltrated. The tumour had passed into the right nose and perforated the septum so as to extend into the left. It adhered to the septum around the site of perforation. This was all removed, leaving a hole in the septum about the size of a florin. He went home within a fortnight. In a month the growth showed signs of return. It bulged through the incision and protruded upon the face. Dr. Woods saw him afterwards, as I had declared by letter that a further operation would be of no avail. The tumour had now almost closed the right eye. It was blue, tense, firm and lobulated, but it did not break. Dr. Woods reported the result of this visit to me and we agreed as to the prognosis. Early in October the patient walked into my study after a visit to Dr. Woods. He looked better in health than I had ever seen him. The tumour had completely disappeared from the face and I could not identify any trace of it in the mouth. He said he had no pain of any kind. He could speak well when the opening remaining after the removal of the hard palate was plugged, and he was in town to have an obturator made. He has since gone home apparently well. He told me he had applied poultices of comfrey root, and that the swelling had gradually disappeared. Now this was a case of which none of us had any doubt at all, and our first view was confirmed by the distinguished pathologist whom I have mentioned, and by our own observation at the time of the major operation. Here, then, was another surprise. I am satisfied as I can be of anything that the growth was malignant and of a bad type. Of course we know in the history of some tumours that growth is delayed, and that in the sarcomata recurrence is often late. But this is a case in which the recurrence occurred twice—the second time to an extreme degree, and yet this recurrent tumour had vanished. What has produced this atrophy and disappearance ? I do not know. I know nothing of the effects of comfrey root, but I do not believe that it can remove a sarcomatous tumour. Of course the time that has so far elapsed is very short ; but the fact that this big recurrent tumour no longer exists—that it has not ulcerated or sloughed away, but simply with unbroken covering disappeared —is to me one of the greatest surprises and puzzles that I have met with."

Dr. Cooper adds : Dr. Thompson's common sense leads him into direct opposition to his own observation ; were inquiries in other departments of human knowledge to act similarly, there would be little human knowledge worth having. The appeal to common sense is too often evidence of its dethronement.

Dr. Cooper gives us one more instructive *Symphytum* case ; this also recorded by Old School incredulity. . . .

He says, " A hundred and twenty years before Dr. Thompson wrote on this subject, we find the then great master of the surgical art, Mr. Percivall Pott, referring in an equally sceptical tone to the action of comfrey root, in his celebrated article on ' The palsey of the Lower Limbs ', in connection with curvature of the spine. The case was one in which Mr. Pott had diagnosed bony disease of the spine, and had applied a seton. Some weeks afterwards he met the patient walking along the street perfectly well. The patient had taken comfrey root and isinglass which, in his innocence, he supposed had cured him, but Mr. Pott would have nothing of it. It could have been the seton, and only the seton ! "

BLACK LETTER, AND OTHER MARKED INDICATIONS
PAIN IN EYES AFTER A KNOCK OR CONTUSION OF AN OBTUSE
BODY

Cured cases (Hering). More than a year ago, fell and struck knee on a stone, wound healed and left scarcely any trace, but there remained an acute stitching pain, felt when clothing touched part, or when knee was bent.

Man suffering a spontaneous laxation of thigh since childhood, fell and fractured affected thigh. After two months fragments were quite movable, an apparatus was made which allowed him to sit on a chair during the day. *Symphytum* 4, every six hours, brought about complete union in twenty days.

Inflammation of bones. Diseased spinous processes.

Psoas abscess.

Facilitates union of fractured bones, and lessens peculiar pricking pain."

Favours production of callus.

Mechanical injuries, bad effects from blows, bruises, thrusts on eye.

Peculiar pain in periosteum after wounds have healed.

Irritability of bone at point of fracture.

Gunshot wounds.

*   *   *

Dr. Oscar Hanson, in his *Therapeutics of Rare Homœopathic Remedies*, gives those of *Symphytum*, thus :

Injuries to bones. Non-union of fractures (*Calc. phos.*). Irritable stump after operation. Irritability of bone at the point of fracture. Psoas abscess from diseases of the vertebrae. Inflammation of the inferior maxillary bone. Traumatic periostitis. Wounds penetrating in periosteum and bones.

TARENTULA HISPANIA AND CUBENSIS

(Spider Poisons)

FROM scanty and rather scattered data we have tried to picture *Tarentula cubensis*—the rotten specimen of the Cuban tarentula, which is such a marvellous remedy in a number of septic conditions : but we do not seem to have attacked the better known *Tarentula* of our Materia Medica. It is a very interesting and very unique remedy, suggested in most difficult conditions—nervous and mental especially ; and like all the other drugs of Homœopathy, priceless *where it fits*.

Tarentula suggests violence and torment. Without specific power to damage parts or organs after the manner of many of our remedies, it can violently torment both body and mind in a manner utterly subversive to decency and behaviour as regards the unhappy victim, and perplexing and alarming to friends and attendants. *Tarentula*, therefore, becomes a powerful remedy in spasms, and in hysteria with its " protean manifestations ", as Clarke puts it.

After this spider bite, the victim sings and dances, with extravagant behaviour and complete loss of control, and is only to be cured, and cured again and again in its annual recurrence of symptoms, by music and dancing—so we are told.

And not only is this drug amazingly sensitive to music, but it can be even physically affected *by colour :* " an unpleasant colour may cause anguish of heart ".

Tarentula has the sudden changes of mood of *Crocus*, but its gaiety and laughter turn to sudden spitefulness ; to a paroxysm of insanity, in which she will strike herself and others, tear and rend and destroy. Sudden violent, or sly destructive movements are absolutely characteristic, and unique to this drug—so far as our knowledge goes. And then the patient may be sorry and apologize : " Couldn't help it ! "

She " feigns sick " as the Repertory has it ; feigns paroxysms ; feigns fainting and insensibility ; yet looks furtively round to see that she is being observed, and to note the effect she is producing. Incredible quickness : jumps out of bed and smashes something before she can be prevented.

Tormented, again, with frightful restlessness : especially of arms and legs.

Then, *Fear :* indefinite fears ; fears of something going to happen ; of danger from something that does not exist ; sees terrible things that are not there.

The urinary symptoms suggest *Cantharis*. The skin, its septic troubles—abscess, anthrax, etc., remind one of *Tarent. cub.*

*   *   *

Many of our most consulted Materia Medicas have shirked *Tarentula* ; but CLARKE has much that is interesting to say about the drug.

To condense, he says, *inter alia* " Tarantism " is a dancing mania, set up in persons bitten by the *Tarentula*, or who imagine themselves bitten. The cure is music and dancing. And he gives striking cases of such cures, which bring out the cardinal features of *Tarentula : Dark red, or purplish* swelling of skin and tissue. *Choreic movements ; restlessness ; apparent imminent choking :* relief by *music*, which first excites, then relieves ; *periodicity— return of symptoms annually* on the date of the bite.

The restlessness is particularly noticed in lower extremities, with desire to cry ; must keep moving, though walking aggravates all the symptoms. . . . Many of the mental symptoms, " which almost exhaust the protean range of hysteria," were in connection with sexual disorders.

*   *   *

NASH says, This spider poison has like other spider poisons very positive nervous symptoms. It acts on uterus and ovaries, and on the female sexual organs generally. " In cases of hyper-æsthesia or congestion of these organs, which set up a general hysterical condition, states simulating spinal neuræsthenia, sensitive and painful back, excessive restlessness, and impressibility to excitements, music especially. . . . Twitching or jerking of muscles in conjunction with other troubles, should always call to mind this remedy." " This remedy is not as thoroughly understood as it should be."

*   *   *

FARRINGTON says : The bitten part becomes swollen and discoloured, lymphatic glands enlarged. By conveyance of the poison to the neck, the cellular tissue there is affected, giving rise to a swelling of a dark red or purplish hue. Choking seems eminent, when epistaxis appears, with dark clots, and relieves the symptoms. Evidence of cerebral congestion is given by the violently throbbing carotid arteries ; but with all this there is a a pale, earthy hue to the face. . . . Nervous symptoms are present in all the spider poisons, but *Tarentula* applies, more than other members of the group, to hysteria. . . . Music starts her acting like one crazy ; when there are no observers she has no hysterical attacks. As soon as attention is directed to her, she begins to twitch. . . .

Has a reputation for cancer of tongue, etc., and for " fibrous tumours, abdominal, with discharge of pale blood from uterus ".

Desire to eat with intense thirst : constant desire for large quantities of cold water. Or loss of appetite.

Desire for raw articles.

Disgust for bread, for roasted meats.

Inextinguishable thirst.

Muscular contractions of epigastrium.

Many of the digestive symptoms are peculiar, because of the sympathetic pains, neuralgic or congestive, which accompany them, or arise, on sides of head, face, ears, teeth, malar bones.

BLACK LETTER SYMPTOM
HYSTERIA.

NOTEWORTHY, DIAGNOSTIC, OR ITALICIZED SYMPTOMS

Great excitement caused by music ; one hour after it, general and copious perspiration.

Paroxysms of insanity ; strikes head, pulls hair ; complains ; threatens, scratches herself ; restlessness ; her clothes annoy her ; restless legs ; threatening words of destruction and death : comes out of attack with severe headache ; eyes wide and staring.

Sees small figures hovering before her eyes.

Hysteria with bitter belchings.

They sing, dance, cry ; extreme gaiety.

Ludicrous and lascivious hysteria ; had to be restrained by force.

Visions of monsters, animals, frighten him ; of different things not present, faces, insects, ghosts.

Feigned paroxysms ; feigns fainting and insensibility ; looks sideways to observe the effect on those around her.

Taciturn, irritable ; desire to strike himself and others.

Extreme disposition to laugh and joke.

Laughs, runs, dances, gesticulates ; sings till hoarse and exhausted.

Sadness, grief, moral depression are not only the almost constant symptoms of the sting, but are present, in a striking manner, during different provings of the medicine.

Fear which could not be stopped ; tried to find a cause and leaves others to think there is one ; really there was none.

Constant fear that something would happen to prevent my finishing a thing ; would start and hastily change my position, through fear that something would fall on me ; walking, would stop and throw head to one side, through fear of striking against some imaginary object suspended a few inches above my head.

Great desire to be alone, with fear of being alone.

Changeable mood ; from gaiety to sadness ; from fixed ideas to uneasiness of mind.

Does not understand questions ; does not know the persons she sees every day ; cannot say her prayers.

Fits of nervous laughter ; desire to joke, play, laugh.

Extreme gaiety.

Great excitement caused by music ; later general, copious sweat.

Sudden fox-like destructive efforts, requiring utmost vigilance to prevent damage ; followed by laughter and apologies.

Threatening words of destruction and death.

Suddenly sprang away from attendants, swept ornaments from mantelpiece ; said she was sorry but could not help it.

Very mischievous and destructive, amusing and cheerful.

Attacks of hystero-mania daily about the same hour : first quarrelsome and despondent, suddenly a state of great exhaltation, hits and abuses everyone, destroys whatever she can lay hold of, tears her clothes, laughs and sings ; mocks aged people with their age ; if restrained becomes violent ; attacks end in a comatose sleep.

Jumps from bed, destroying whatever she could get hold of ; so quickly that she could not be prevented.

Headache as if a quantity of cold water were poured on head and body.

Intense headache, as if thousands of needles were pricking brain.

Pain in occiput, as if struck by a hammer, extends to temples.

Burning, scorching heat in occiput.

Pain in right maxillary nerve, with tickling sensation in stomach.

It seems as if a living body were moving or tingling in the stomach, with tendency to ascend to throat.

Diabetes—constant craving for raw articles. Disgust for meat ; polyuria.

Involuntary micturition when coughing, laughing, making any effort.

Precordial anxiety, tumultuous beating of heart.

Pain, shooting pain in heart and arteries of left chest, extending to left arm ; the contact with dress is very painful.

Tumours about the vertebral column.

Strange fancies in regard to colours.

Anguish of heart if they see an unpleasant colour.

Angina pectoris.

Precordial anxiety ; tumultuous beating of heart ; trembling and thumping, as if from a fright.

Precordial anguish ; movement of heart not felt. Constant want of air. Heart ceases to beat and patient fears to die.

Right pupil much dilated, left contracted. Loss of visions in right eye, till dilated pupil contracted.

Face expressed terror.

Face pale earthy, contrasting with nearly purple neck.

Burning and sweat in palms of hands.

Pain in lower jaw as if all the teeth were going to fall out.

Onanism ; violent nymphomania.

Intense, unbearable pruritis vulvæ.

Terrible pruritis, as of insects creeping and crawling.

Outer parts, as if worms or insects were boring and crawling.

Itching, burning, formication, ecchymosed spots. Painful vesicular and especially pustular eruptions.

KENT who has no lecture on *Tarentula*, gives a case exemplifying one phase of its action : " *Rolling from side to side to relieve the distress* is a characteristic of *Tarentula*. A man with inveterate constipation, who had used physics till they would no longer serve, was encouraged by his daughter to wait for further action until the proper remedy could be recognized, as advised by the doctor. In his distress he rolled from side to side, on the bed, wailing, ' Oh dear me '. *Tarentula* quieted him. Two days later he had a normal stool, and thereafter had no difficulty."

New Remedies, etc.

*   *   *

A couple of years ago a patient in the Children's Ward of our London Hospital, suffering from chorea, was making little or no progress. During the doctor's rounds this girl appeared shy and demure : but the Ward Sister said that she was " very foxy ". When she thought no one was looking she would suddenly start tearing up books and destroying such toys as lay within her reach.

Further observation led to the discovery that she was unusually sensitive to music : when the wireless was turned on, she would jump about and dance. *Tarentula* was given with success.

The following case from *The Homœopathician* for October 1913 illustrates the potentialities of *Tarentula hispania*, where symptoms, especially the marked mental symptoms match.

INSANITY—*TARENTULA HISPANIA*

By A. W. McDONOUGH, M.D., U.S.A.

1912. March 14th. Miss P., a rather delicate girl of 18 years, tall and slender, with a sort of sallow complexion, called for treatment two months prior to her high-school graduation ; had evidently been overworking. Headache intense for past week ; frontal and occipital ; increases after study ; walking. Pain behind eyes. Toward evening feels worse all over. Sensitive to cold. Very irritable. Coughs frequently; increases when quiet. Better in warm room. Desires sweet things. Perspiration scant. After carefully working out the case with a repertory gave *Sepia* 200. Result was splendid. She had no further trouble until October, when in a runaway with a horse, though not hurt, she was badly frightened.

December 12th. Amenorrhœa. Loss of appetite. Constipation. Very chilly, but feels increase in a close room. Cross and difficult to get along with : increases with heat ; increases with cold ; decreases when quiet. Headache when awakening. Desires cold. Stomach sensation of a load after eating. Because *Sepia* had formerly done good gave *Sepia*. As the remedy did not work to the satisfaction of the family, she did not return for a second prescription, but went to an old school doctor. With the aid of an osteopath he treated her for amenorrhœa until the middle of February 1913. Under the osteopathic and allopathic treatment she had become very nervous, pale, and restless, and had emaciated from 103 lb. to 78 lb. The allopath advised her to go west for her health. The osteopath said she was almost insane. She was taken to Iowa City to a nerve specialist. He pronounced her in fair condition, but said she must eat to get some strength. From the first she had refused to eat. He gave her strong stomach stimulants, similar to those she had been taking, but on the fourth day of his treatment she became so unmanageable that I was again summoned. I accepted the case only on condition that I might ask the aid of Dr. W. G. Allen, of Barnes City, whom I knew to be an accurate prescriber, homœopathically, and with whom I felt assured of ability to cure the girl. Uncontrollable. The family could do nothing with her. Exalted ; restless. Wanted everything to be in motion. Chased the cat from under the stove ; " Oh, I can't bear to see the lazy thing "

Ordered her step-father to chase himself around the house and not sit around all day. She was determined to do all the work, but everyone must move, and move rapidly. Insisted on serving at table ; loaded the dishes full, but would eat nothing herself ; feared she would get fat. Hurries ; walks rapidly ; must be active every minute ; took up her school books and began to work on physics and geometry; forced her music teacher to give her lessons; practised for hours at the piano. Cross, hateful ; appeared " possessed of the very old Nick ". Sleep impossible ; would not go to bed before midnight ; didn't want to take time to go to bed. Never tired ; feels " strung up " constantly. Cannot relax. Aversion to odour of heat. Chilly ; sensitive to cold. Weeping inclination constant ; weeps much. Craves salt ; heaps it on any small bite of food she eats. Craves and eats much chocolate candy. Would take the raw juice of lemon " to keep down the fat ". Nose bleed ; bright red from the right nostril. Skin sallow. " Strawberry tongue." Albumen in abundance in urine. Pulse 67, temperature 96·8, when standing ; as soon as sits pulse drops to 60. From our study of the case with the repertory, choice appeared to be between *Natrum mur.* and *Sulph.*, but choice was difficult.

Sulph. 200 was selected. It did but little for her ; it appeared merely to check the downward progress, but she made no improvement. As Dr. Allen was called to Rochester, I dreaded his departure, but he was glad to escape. After a few days gave *Natrum mur.* 200, as *Sulph.* appeared to be almost useless. The case remained unchanged. She continued to " run things high " from early morn to midnight. Refused to eat. Was terrible to live with. Fearful of getting fat, though she weighed only 67 lb. and was dreadful to behold. Again studying the case, beginning with the rubric REFUSES TO EAT, *Ars. alb.* was in all the symptoms. Gave *Ars.* 200. It dispelled her restlessness, warmed her, and helped. After a few days she became worse again. Reporting the case to Dr. Kent, his telegram soon came : " Give the patient *Tarentula hisp.* 10m." It suited exactly, and I hadn't seen the picture, plainly as it had presented !

Tarent. hisp. Three hours later her condition was completely changed. Instead of driving her mother from the room, not allowing her to touch her, she wanted to be with her mother every minute, as would almost any sick child. Thoroughly relaxed, she was quite a different person. Gradual improvement from the dose of *Tarent.* Hands and feet became very dry and scaly about four weeks after beginning *Tarentula.* After five weeks Dr. Kent advised *Tarent. hisp.* 50m. About four weeks after the skin scaled and became natural, fine fuzzy hair three-quarters of an inch long appeared on the entire body except the palms and soles, but at present writing the face has cleared, the hair having entirely disappeared. She now appears perfectly well, but strength and flesh not fully restored.

This is a rare case, such as will not frequently be observed in private practice. It again illustrates the wonderful power of the potentized remedy when the exact similimum is used. But for *Tarentula hispania* this patient must have died in an asylum.

TARENTULA CUBENSIS

Tarentula cubensis is a remedy that has stared and beckoned for many years : because it was one of the 144 precious " *cm* "s, " grafts from his pocket case ", sent to us by DR. NASH, after his visit to this country. If so high in the estimation of such a pre-scriber as to have a place in his pocket case, and to be one of his " 144 ", surely it was worth trying for the septic conditions for which he advocates it in his Leaders (?) as follows :

" *Tarentula cubensis*, or the hairy spider. It is one of the most efficacious remedies for boils, abscesses, felons, or swellings of any kind where the tissues put on a bluish colour, and there are intense burning pains.

"We used to think that we had two great remedies in *Arsenicum* and *Anthracinum* ; but *Tarentula cubensis* is simply wonderful. I have seen felons which had kept patients awake night after night walking the floor in agony from the terrible pains so relieved in a very short time that they could sleep in perfect comfort until the swellings spontaneously discharged and progressed to a rapid cure. This remedy should receive a thorough proving. It is a gem."

One may say, that many experiences with this remedy have more than confirmed its worth.

* * *

KENT, *New Remedies*, gives a case showing the powerful action of *Tarentula cubensis* in Carbuncle on the back of neck.

A lady, age about 30, suffered greatly from a carbuncle on the back of her neck. She had applied many domestic remedies and obtained no relief. The tumefaction seemed destined to sup-purate. It was *mottled bluish* and the pain was *intense, knife-cutting* and *burning*. She was sick at the stomach to vomiting, and at night she was delirious. Her eyes were staring and there was some fever ; the tongue was foul and the breath fetid. There was great *tension in the scalp and muscles of the face.*   She begged for morphine to " stop that *burning* and *cutting* ".   *Tarentula cubensis* 12x, one dose, produced quiet immediately and the angry-looking tumefaction failed to complete its work : it did not suppurate.   The discoloration was gone in two days, and the hardness soon disappeared also.   She regained her normal state very rapidly, and she said to me a short time ago that she had never had her old headache since that swelling left her, showing how deeply the medicine affected her whole system.

If a part is mottled (*Lach.*), bluish, growing dark, with those symptoms, *Tarentula cubensis* must be the most appropriate remedy.

*   *   *

In regard to *Tarentula cubensis*, Dr. Oscar Hansen, of Copenhagen, in his *Textbook of Rare Homœopathic Remedies*, writes : " Therapeutics.   Gangrene.   Carbuncle, even sloughing, with great prostration and diarrhœa, intermittent fever of evening exacerbation.   Acts magically in the most terrible burning, stinging pains here.   A purplish hue with the above pains is characteristic.   (Compare *Lachesis, Anthracinum, Silica*.)   Recommended in the last stage of tuberculosis pulmonum.   Diphtheria, malignant type, deposit dark-coloured, fetid breath, septic fever.   Typhoid fever, fetid dark stool, great prostration."

Our Materia Medica textbooks have so little to say about the *Tarentula*—either the *Spanish* or *Cuban*, that it may be helpful to quote a discussion in America, on a paper entitled "*Tarentula* in Meningitis " by Dr. Neiswandler (Ohio) which appeared some time ago in the *Homœopathic Recorder*.   Here we learn a great deal about *Tarentula cubensis*, for knowledge of which we are greedy, since it is such a very potent remedy, especially in septic conditions, and since so little is to be learnt about it in our textbooks.

By the way, Dr. Neiswandler's " *Tarentula* in Meningitis " was the *Hispania*.   But what Dr. Roberts has to say regarding the origin of the *cubensis*, is of the greatest interest.   He tells us that we have here not only the *Cuban Tarentula*, but *a rotten Cuban Tarentula ;* which gives us, he suggests, not only the temperament and mental symptoms of *Tarentula*, but *the septic element of the decomposed spider.*   Sounds nasty ? but it works.   And it comes into line, to some extent, with *Pyrogen*, " gotten " as they say " across the ditch ", from rotten meat.   These have powers of combating similar conditions of sepsis, and are drugs of the greatest importance and value.   We will reproduce from the discussion on the two drugs.

DR. MACFARLAN : I don't know anything about *Tarentula hispania*, but I know that *Tarentula cubensis* is a wonderful remedy. I made that proving about ten years ago. I also made a good cure with it in a terrible case of cough, something like whooping cough, that seemed to tear the patient to bits. *Tarentula* does tear them to bits, and I gave it with a marvellous response from the start.

Tarentula cubensis produces great drowsiness, I think it is more useful in whooping cough than *Ipecac.* or *Castanea vesca* or any other remedy I know ; it is marvellous.

DR. BENTHACK : I have never before heard of its use in meningitis, but *Tarentula cubensis* is my standby in any abscess where there is severe pain. I formerly thought I had a wonderful remedy for such conditions in *Arsenicum* and *Anthracinum*, but I have found *Tarentula cubensis* in the 30th potency does much better.

DR. ROBERTS : *Tarentula* is one of the most interesting of the spider poisons. I think we get a better concept of it if we study its habits. *Tarentula hispania*, as you know, is found in the western part of this country, and I have been told that before the rainy season they migrate in herds, travelling in leaps and bounds. It makes its nest in the ground, a burrow lined with web, and turning a sharp angle after going down a few inches. Here the spider sits to watch for its prey.

It does its work by violence, one sharp pounce on the neck of its victim, severing the ganglia. It strikes and retreats, never holding on. It is a perfect coward when away from home. It is in these things you get the characteristics, for you find this sudden violence all through the remedy—the sudden impulse to do harm.

One *Tarentula* patient whom I knew seemed to be quiet and peaceable ; the nurse left the room and instantly the patient jumped from bed, swept everything from the shelf and was back in bed before the nurse could get back. That is *Tarentula* : violence of onslaught, fear to face real opposition or when they are away from home—just as the spider does in its natural setting.

In regard to *Tarentula cubensis*, while it is not mentioned in this paper, it is much like *Tarentula hispania* ; it is the same spider or closely related, only coming from Cuba. Dr. T. F. Allen told me the history of this remedy. The *Tarentula cubensis* was being shipped to this country in a container with alcohol to preserve it. The container broke on the way up, the alcohol ran out and the specimen decomposed. However, a potency was made, and it is the pyogenic effect of the decomposition that is the greatest differentiation between *Tarentula hispania* and the *Tarentula cubensis*, for all our higher potencies were made from that stock. It is worth consideration, because there you get the mentality of *Tarentula hispania* and the septic conditions of *Tarentula cubensis*.

DR. FARRINGTON : It would be interesting to re-prove a fresh specimen of *Tarentula cubensis*. That is one deficiency, you might say, in our materia medica and its provings, that we have evidently not got the real symptoms of *Tarentula cubensis*. Perhaps it would result in a reproduction of what we get from *Tarentula hispania*.

DR. FARRINGTON : Probably the accident gave us a new remedy which we would not have had before, much as an accident gave us *Causticum*, because that is a compound subject, Hahnemann's *tinctura acris kali*, which cannot be found in any pharmacopœia except the Homœopathic. . . .

A number of years ago I reported a case to this society, of a young fellow of eighteen who was supposed to have had dementia præcox cured with *Tarentula*, and his symptoms and his general behaviour were just as Dr. Roberts has described. He would fly into a rage over something and throw whatever was in his hand, whatever he could reach. He nearly killed his mother with a big pitcher. She objected to something he had done or said, and he threw it at her and just missed her, and smashed an enormous mirror to smithereens.

Another interesting symptom of *Tarentula* is the heart. A number of you know those heart symptoms, sudden and violent, and in some of our materia medicas the condition *Tarentula* produces and cures is called St. Vitus' Dance of the heart.

Several years ago I was called in the middle of the night to South Bend, Indiana, and found a man of forty-five years of age, pale as death, frightened. His heart was beating rapidly and he thought he was going to die ; in fact, the physician who examined him told him that he had a serious heart trouble and did not have long to live.

I examined his heart very carefully and found no lesions whatsoever, but every now and then he would start to jump, and then it would go like that, up and down, and then settle down ; and he had a previous history of diarrhœa and digestive symptoms, referable especially to the colon, and I have to add, though I asked him a few questions, I could get very few symptoms besides the objective ones. I think what I said to him did him almost as much good as the medicine. I told him he was suffering from auto-intoxication and had no heart disease at all, and I gave him a dose of *Tarentula*. Two weeks later he was up to see me, apparently a well man.

DR. GREEN : I have had a chance to watch *Tarentula* fairly closely and I want to add to what Dr. Roberts said about the sudden sly, destructive tendency, a tendency to change one's disposition altogether from a sweet, wholesome, rational person, to someone who is so terribly self-centred and selfish, and who wants nothing but to have everyone standing around waiting on him, and even to interfere with the nurse going on or off duty, because of some imaginary ailment like feigning a swoon, or something to oblige that person to stay near.

DR. BENTHACK said that before he knew *Tarentula* was used in ulcers, he used to depend on *Arsenic* for burning ulcers. " That reminds me to say that I have learned that *Tarentula* and *Arsenicum* are complementary remedies in such chronic cases."

TEREBINTHINA
(Oil of Turpentine)

ON reading through the provings and poisoning by *Terebinth.* in the *Cyclopædia of Drug Pathogenesy*, one is struck by several points. One has always read in Materia Medica that with *Terebinth.* the "urine smells of violets " : this curious fact occurs again and again —even in the poisoning of animals by turpentine. The urine may be clear, bloody, sooty, black, but it apparently smells of violets : or, as it is once or twice expressed, it smells sweet.

Again, one notes the sleepiness and stupor so frequently produced.

Again, the character of the pains,—BURNING : burnings in gums ; in mouth ; in tongue, like fire ; in throat ; stomach ; hypochondria ; in rectum and anus ; in kidneys ; in bladder ; in umbilicus ; in urethra ; in small of back ; in testicle ; in uterus ; in air passages ; in chest ; along sternum. Burning pressure in hypochondrium.

But the opposites so often obtain, in drug action :—perhaps action and reaction : and while *Terebinth.* has " burning in umbilicus ", it has also the curious symptom, " umbilical region seems retracted, cold, just as though a cold round plate were pressed against it ".

Then one realizes its extremely hæmorrhagic nature, causing ecchymoses—" fresh ecchymoses in great numbers from day to day " ; ecchymoses in mouth and at angles of lips, which bleed ; bleeding from stomach—" burning in stomach with nausea and vomiting of mucus, bile or blood—copious hæmorrhages " ; " sooty stools like coffee grounds " ; entero-colitis, with hæmorrhages and ulceration of bowels ; hæmorrhage from anus, and bleeding piles ; " albuminuria, when blood and albumen abound ", urine, violet odour, fetid, albuminous, scanty, dark, *cloudy and smoky*, bloody ; bloody, offensive leucorrhœa ; expectoration of blood-stained sputum ; bloody expectoration. Here it vies with the snake poisons, *Crotalus hor.*, etc.

It has the credit of inducing stupefaction and deep sleep ; inability to think or work ; weariness of life. Two cases of " suicide by hanging are recorded, from persons washing lace in oil of turpentine and alcohol " : and the fumes of turpentine have been very poisonous to many people. " Comatose, can be only roused by shaking out of apparent stupor, but falls immediately into it again." Or again, it has an intoxicating effect : " slightly drunk for several hours " ; staggering gait, as if drunk : stands with feet far apart ; cannot balance body ; to insensibility of extremities, especially the lower : to, no control over hand and arm when attempting to write : weakness and prostration : tired and unable to walk, staggered and fell : "muscles feel stiff, he walks slowly and bent over like an old man": the limbs being raised fell heavily back by their own weight. Or, on the other hand, occasionally subsultus ; tetanic spasms ; lockjaw ; chorea and epilepsy, as, when at intervals of ten to fifteen minutes, there were violent convulsive paroxysms, producing the most frightful opisthotonos. Uræmic spasms.

We published last month a most interesting *Terebinth.* case : but it is wanted here, so we will venture to repeat it. It shows how the potentized drug antidotes the same crude drug : provided, of course, there has been no irremediable destruction of tissue.

A child of four years, falling in short spells of unconsciousness ; unable to control the flow of urine day or night, was absolutely cured by one dose of *Terebinthina* 1m. The history of the case was that the child had drunk a lot of turpentine when 18 months old and had gone from bad to worse ever since. She never had another fit after that dose, and gradually but quickly got over the enuresis. She got nothing but a *Placebo* from then on.—Dr. Chas. C. Bowes, U.S.A. *Recorder*, March 1931.

Terebinth. is quite an interesting remedy, but its chief use, and its chief malignity (as seen from the black letter symptoms) is centered on the urinary organs :—kidneys, bladder, and urethra.

Black Letter Symptoms

Tongue remains dry, with abdominal tension ; after cleansing becomes dry again with increase of tympanitis.

Tongue does not clean gradually but rapidly and in large flakes, first from middle, leaving tongue smooth and glossy.

Distension of abdomen : feeling of, as from flatus.
Meteorism ; excessive tympanitis, abdomen sensitive.
Hæmorrhage from bowels, with ulceration ; epithelial degeneration passive.

Violent drawing pains in the region of kidneys.
Albuminuria ; early stages when blood and albumen abound more than casts and epithelium.
Sensitiveness of hypogastrium, tenesmus of bladder.
Violent burning and cutting in bladder, alternating with a similar pain in umbilicus ; < at resi ; > when walking in open air.
Urine scanty and bloody. Burning in urethra.

Strangury ; spasmodic retention of urine.

Frequent urination at night, with intense burning and pain in small of back.

Urine cloudy and smoky, bloody ; clear, watery, profuse.

Hæmaturia.

Urine black, with coffee-ground sediment.

After scarlatina ; passes small quantities of dark, sweet-smelling urine, turbid and having a sediment like coffee-grounds ; sometimes mind dull, or patient drowsy, even in a stupor ; dropsy ; urine though rich in albumen and blood, contains few if any casts.

Metritis and peritonitis puerperalis, with tendency to mortification ; lochia checked, terrible burning in uterus, abdomen fuller than usual ; headache with thirst ; brown dry tongue, nausea and vomiting ; distended abdomen, sore to touch ; pulse small, frequent.

Bronchial catarrh and pneumonia in typhus.

Hæmorrhage from lungs.

Malarial and African fevers.

Prostration.

Purpura hæmorrhagica.

Congestion and inflammation of viscera ; kidneys, bladder, lungs, intestines and uterus.

Ascites with anasarca.

Scarlatina, especially when kidneys are involved, with stupor ; bloody, smoky urine.

Other Marked, Italicized, or Curious Symptoms

" Supposed to be dying, but found to be intoxicated by turpentine."

Pupils " violently contracted ".

Coryza without usual accompanying symptoms, and without premonition, of watery liquid from one or both nostrils.

As if he had swallowed a small ball, which remained in the pit of stomach.

As if intestines were being drawn towards spine (*Pb., Plat.*).

Terebinth. is said to prevent and dissolve renal calculi.

Constant colic of whole abdomen, extending into legs.

Movement in inguinal region, as if a hernia would protrude.

Feeling as if the pubes were suddenly forced asunder.

Burning and crawling in anus, as if worms were creeping out : (has caused the discharge of round worms and tape-worm).

A transient movement in region of bladder, during stool, as if bladder were suddenly distended and bent forward.

" Most distressing strangury, the most violent I had ever before witnessed, and attended with a greater loss of blood."

Urine very scanty and red, or else very copious and light-coloured, but in both cases smelling of violets.

" Has the so-called odour of violets in a high degree."

Whole body feels sick, with vertigo and dullness of head.

Very drowsy : difficult to keep awake.

Cold and clammy perspiration all over body.

Profuse sweat on legs, evenings in bed.

Staggering gait as if drunk.

Boger gives " Pains excite urination ".

* * *

NASH gives, as his chief indications for the use of this drug, burning and smarting on passing urine ; urine red, brown, black or *smoky* in appearance.

Tongue smooth, glossy, red, with excessive tympanites (Typhoid).

Hæmorrhages from all outlets, especially with urinary or kidney troubles.

He says, that, like *Berberis*, it has much pain in the back with kidney and bladder trouble. Painters working in the smell of turpentine are often seriously affected by it : even unable to work in it.

For burning and smarting on passing urine, Turpentine stands nearer to *Canth.* or *Cannabis sat.* than it does to *Berb.* . . . is one of our best anti-hæmorrhagic remedies. In hæmaturia, hæmoptysis, and hæmorrhage from bowels, especially in typhoid, and even in purpura hæmorrhagica it may do splendid work.

One of the chief characteristics for its use is the smooth glossy red tongue (*Crot., Pyrog.*) another is excessive tympanites. These two symptoms are often found in typhoids, and then *Terebinth.* is the remedy. . . ."

* * *

FARRINGTON says, *Terebinthina*, or turpentine, is a drug that has been much abused by old school physicians ; therefore it has been greatly neglected by homœopaths. In the revulsion from the misconception of the old school physicians, we often avoid the drug altogether. Its main action is on the kidneys and bladder. *When you find metritis, peritonitis, typhoid fever or scarlatina*, or in fact, *any serious disease of low type, with the following renal symptoms Terebinthina comes in as your remedy.* .

Dull pains in the region of the kidneys, burning in the kidneys, pains extending from the kidneys down through the ureters, burning during micturition, strangury, albuminous urine, and very characteristically the urine is dark, cloudy and smoky-looking, as though it contained decomposed blood, which it really does.

The real pathological condition of the kidneys in this case is not one of acute Bright's disease, nor one of croupous formation in the kidneys, but one of renal congestion, with oozing of blood into the pelvis of the kidney. When the above urinary symptoms are present, you may give *Terebinthina* with confidence, no matter what the patient's disease may be.

Terebinthina often acts powerfully on mucous membranes. It produces burning in the air passages, with thin expectoration very difficult of detachment.

* * *

A Proving of *Terebinth*

A woman had made her feet sore by walking and applied turpentine to them. This was followed by a state like hydrophobia : she had spasms whenever she saw water or heard it poured, or saw a bright object ; and also whenever she attempted to urinate. CLARKE. (Comp. *Lyssin.*, *Belladonna*, *Stramonium*.)

THERIDION

(Orange Spider)

THE venom of a small, very poisonous spider : found upon orange trees in the West Indies. In addition to its habitat, it has orange coloured spots on the posterior part of the body, and a large square yellow spot on the belly. The alcoholic tincture is prepared from the live spider, crushed.

This remedy was introduced and proved by Hering in 1832. It is interesting because of some very peculiar symptoms.

It has been found useful in vertigo : affections of the head : cough : spinal irritation : hysteria : and scrofulous conditions.

The spider poisons are especially virulent, and are found curative in the difficult states known as hysteria, with extraordinary and perverted sensitiveness to external impressions. We have already discussed that very important drug, *Tarentula*, with its intense reaction to *music*, and its *violence* and *suddenness*.

Theridion reacts more especially to *noise*. Its keynote is, " Every sound seems to penetrate through the whole body, causing nausea and vertigo : every shrill sound penetrates the teeth."

It is one of the remedies to be thought of in Ménière's disease (*Salicylic acid*). Here, as in sea-sickness, its peculiar indications are : Vertigo *on closing the eyes* : or, " when they close their eyes to get rid of the ship's motion, they grow deathly sick ".

This spider poison has extreme nervous sensitiveness.

We will give extracts from provings, of some of its RARE, PECULIAR AND NOTEWORTHY SYMPTOMS, leading to its successful employment where symptoms correspond.

WHENEVER SHE CLOSES HER EYES *she is afflicted with nausea and vertigo ; worse by noise, motion, stooping.*

It feels so thick in her HEAD *as if it were another strange head.*

Nausea and vomiting on least movement, particularly on closing the eyes.

VERTIGO *with nausea even to vomiting ; worse stooping ; from least movement ; from every noise and sound ; with cold sweat.*

Wakes at 11 p.m. with slow pulse.

Vertigo with blindness caused by pain in eyes.

Violent frontal HEADACHE, *with throbbing extending to occiput ; or with heavy pressure behind eyes.*

Headache on beginning to move.

For days feeling as if vertex did not belong to her : it felt as if separated from the rest of head ; as if she could lift it off ; felt she would like to remove it.

Headache deep in eyes, or behind eyes, worse left.

A remedy for sunstroke.

Head feels like another strange head, or as if she had something else upon it.

Headache like a pressing band in root of nose and over and round ears.

Head internally hot and oppressed and heavy, at the same time joyousness and singing.

Owing to pains deep in brain she must sit or walk : it is impossible to lie.

Headaches with nausea and vomiting like seasickness, and shaking chills.

Flickering before EYES *in frequent paroxysms.   Like a veil before eyes.   Must lie down.*

Things look double : through this fluttering, nausea is created : cold hands.   Long afterwards she dares not stoop.

Dizziness and confusion of vision : everything went together and became indistinct.

Worse from the least NOISE *: every shrill sound and reverberation penetrates her whole body, especially teeth : makes vertigo worse and causes nausea.*

Rushing, roaring in both EARS *: itching behind ears, would like to scratch them off.*

Coryza and ozæna.   Chronic, offensive discharge thick, yellow, or greenish yellow.

NOSE *dry as if too much air passed in : itching : violent sneezing.*

At times, and on waking, lower jaw is immovable.   (Has been used in tetanus.)

Cold water affects TEETH *: every shrill sound penetrates teeth.*

MOUTH *benumbed ; salty taste, and salty mucus.*

CRAVES *oranges and bananas ; wine, brandy, tobacco, and acid fruits and drinks.*

SENSATION *as if a child were bounding in body (Croc., Thuja).*

Anxiety about HEART : *sharp pains radiate to arm and left shoulder.*

Slow pulse with vertigo.

SPINAL *irritation ; great sensitiveness between vertebræ ; sits sideways in chair to avoid pressure against spine.*

Spinal irritation : could not bear least noise : jar of foot on floor was so aggravating that it made her cry out.

Pains in BONES *as if broken, as if they were about to fall asunder.*

After every exertion, fainting.

During sleep bites tip of tongue.

It has been found useful in Angina pectoris.

Also in spinal irritation ; rickets ; caries ; necrosis ; phthisis florida ; infantile atrophy with enlargement of glands.

*   *   *

Of *Theridion* Clarke says (*Dictionary of Materia Medica*) : It is very poisonous. It produces a highly sensitive, nervous condition with weakness, trembling, coldness, anxiety, faintness, and easily excited cold sweat.

There are two well-marked keynotes, one or other of which will be found in most cases calling for *Therid.* (1) *extreme sensitiveness to noise :* worse by least noise : sounds penetrate the teeth. The sensitiveness extends to vibrations of any kind, jar of a step, riding in a carriage or in a boat. The symptom also shows the relation *Therid.* has to bony structures as well as the nervous organs they enclose ; it meets cases of spinal irritation ; and also cases of disease of the spinal and other bones. Caries, necrosis and scrofulous disease of bones have all been cured with it. . . . (2) *Worse closing eyes.* This applies to vertigo and symptoms of the head and stomach, and this forms the indication in many cases of seasickness, or sickness of pregnancy. . . . but though there is worse closing eyes, there is also intolerance of light. . . . A species of intoxication, hilarity, talkativeness. . . .

*   *   *

BOERICKE says : " . . . has an affinity for the tubercular diathesis. . . . noises seem to strike on painful spots over

27

the body.　Restless : finds pleasure in nothing.　Time passes too quickly.　Stinging thrusts everywhere.　. . ."

He suggests the 30th potency.

* 　 　 * 　 　 *

Theridion is worse for NOISE ; touch ; CLOSING EYES ; least motion.　Better for rest and warmth.

* 　 　 * 　 　 *

NASH writes of *Theridion* : There is one peculiar and characteristic symptom under this remedy, which has been verified by myself and others. " *Vertigo with nausea especially on closing the eyes.*" Allen puts it—vertigo *on closing the eyes* (*Lach., Thuja*), on opening them (*Tabacum*), on looking upwards (*Puls., Sil.*), *from any, even least noise* ; aural or labyrinthine (Ménière's disease).

Again, " *Every sound seems to penetrate through the whole body, causing nausea and vertigo.*" *Asarum* has a similar symptom which is worth remembering, " *Oversensitiveness of nerves, scratching of linen or silk*, crackling of paper is unbearable." (*Ferr., Tarax.*)

The vertigo occurs in different affections of the head or stomach, and cures the whole trouble when it is present.　. . .

Another symptom which seems to be very valuable in chest affections is, " pain runs through upper left chest to shoulder." (Phthisis florida has been cured on this symptom for a guide, if given early.)　This is like *Myrtus communis*, with which I have helped many cases having that peculiar local symptom. (*Sulphur, Pix liquida* and *Anisum stellatum* also have it.)

THUJA OCCIDENTALIS

(" Arbor Vitæ ")

Arbor vitæ !—indeed a " Tree of Life, for the healing of the nations ! " as we shall see.

Hahnemann says that no serious medical employment was made of this plant " before now ".

He says " the pure effects of this uncommonly powerful medicinal substance will be regarded by the homœopathic practitioner as a great addition to his medicinal treasury in some of the most serious diseases of mankind, for which hitherto there has been no remedy." He specifies it as " the only efficacious remedy " for fig-warts and gonorrhœa. He used the 30th potency, and then found that in the 60th potency, " it had not sunk to complete powerlessness,* but on the contrary had rather become even more intensely charged with the medicinal virtue of *Thuja* ".

Thuja produces intense headaches and neuralgias. It affects especially the left temple. Its characteristic pain is " sensation of a nail being driven into head ".

It affects the kidneys, with frequent urination and all sorts of pathological urine including sugar ; also urine like water (*Ign.*). It has great action on anus and genitalia :—anus fissured, painful to touch, often with warts, " sometimes immense numbers of flat, moist, mucous tubercles or condylomata around anus, especially in sycotic subjects." Sweat about genitalia ; offensive. Warty and cauliflower excrescences about anus and genitalia. It has the severe backache of small-pox, for which it has proved a most useful remedy, being one of the drugs that produces and cures pustular eruptions.

That *Thuja* can produce warts, we had a curious proof years ago. One of our horses had a few warts, and scars where warts, probably, had been cauterized at some time or other. The coachman was given a small bottle of *Thuja* φ, with instructions to put some of this into water, to bathe the warts. He misunderstood, and put the lot into the horse's drinking water, and presently there was a most extraordinary exemplification of the *Thuja* warts, their character, and their most typical situations.

*. Hahnemann began with strong tinctures and only as experience led the way, worked gradually up to " Potentization " : when he found, as here, that drugs in extreme sub-division, instead of becoming powerless, became more intensely charged with their healing virtue.—ED.

One of Hahnemann's black letter symptoms is, " On exposure of the body to warm air, shivering all over. Rigor with much yawning, the warm air feels cold to him, and the sun seems to have no power to warm him."

Thuja has peculiar sweats, oily, sweetish, fetid : and a unique condition of "*profuse sweat only on uncovered parts*". This has suggested the curative use of *Thuja* in diverse diseases and conditions, reported from time to time in our literature.

It was the determining symptom in a case of myositis ossificans : where it made an extraordinary change in the case and started de-ossification.

Mentally, *Thuja* makes mistakes in reading and writing. Speaks slowly, as if at a loss for the words : has " prolonged thoughtfulness about the merest trifles ". Has fixed ideas, as if the body were brittle and would easily break ; when walking, as if legs were made of wood ; as if a live animal were in abdomen (*Croc.*) ; as if under the influence of a superior power. Uneasy sleep with dreams :—of falling from a height—of dead people, etc.

KENT describes the typical *Thuja* patient, sickly-looking, with waxy face, that looks as if smeared over with grease.

The perspiration is peculiar, sweetish—strong—pungent.

He says that *Arsenic* is often the acute, and *Thuja* the chronic remedy, as in asthma : here cases in which *Arsenic* would seem to be the remedy, but it only palliates, *Thuja* or *Natrum sulph.* will take up the work and cure. And here they may do so by bringing back a primitive manifestation that has been suppressed.

He describes the *Thuja* wart-like excrescences, soft and pulpy and very sensitive : burn, itch and bleed easily when rubbed by the clothing. Cauliflower excrescences in vagina, on cervix uteri, about anus and mucous membranes generally.

" Herpes everywhere, with excessive neuralgic pains. . . . " *Thuja* leads all medicines for symptoms coming from suppressed fig-warts.

" It is a pre-eminently strong medicine for cases where you have in the history snake-bite, small-pox, vaccination."

But to Dr. James Compton BURNETT with his theory of " Vaccinosis " belongs the honour of having brought *Thuja* within the range of practical politics as regards our everyday needs. He used to say that *Thuja* was worth £200 a year to him.

CLARKE also acknowledges its very wide usefulness : " People are all vaccinated and drink tea," he used to say, " and *Thuja* is the great antidote to tea and vaccination."

Burnett, in the preface to his brilliant and epoch-making little monograph, *Vaccinosis and Homœoprophylaxis*, writes, " Truth is not Truth save only to the Infinite ; to the mind of mortal man Truth is not necessarily Truth, but only that which *appears* to be true. Hence that which is a glorious truth to one man is inglorious nonsense to another, and both individuals may be equally honest of purpose and of like earnestness in their search after Truth. . · . . The idea of using *Thuja occidentalis* as here recommended is not new, nor is it peculiar to the writer, though it is but very little known in this country, and still less acted upon, and hence it is hoped that the publication of these pages may help to establish *vaccinosis as a form of disease, and* Thuja *as one of its chief remedies.*"

Burnett concedes that vaccination *does* protect, to a very large extent, from small-pox ; he is no anti-vaccinator : his aim is " to show (1) that there exists a diseased state of the constitution which is engendered by the vaccinial virus (the so-called lymph), which he proposes to call VACCINOSIS, or the Vaccinial state ; and (2) that there exists also in nature a notable remedy for said Vaccinosis, viz. the *Thuja occidentalis* ; and (3) that *Thuja* is a remedy for Vaccinosis by reason of its homœopathicity thereto ; and (4) that the law of similars also applies to the prevention of disease."

" Vaccinosis," for Burnett, does not mean the acute reaction to vaccination, the febrile state, with local phenomena at the point where the pus was inserted—not even a general varioloid eruption following vaccination.

He says, " all this is included in his term vaccinosis, but not merely this :—but also the profound and often long-lasting morbid constitutional state engendered by the vaccine virus :—*Lymph., of course, it is not, but pus.* . . . The protective power of vaccination is due to a diseased state of the body.

" One suffering from vaccinosis may not be ill in the ordinary sense. But he must be in a subdued morbid state, he has been blighted, or he is no vaccinate" . . . and he says that some of his worst cases of vaccinosis were those in whom the vaccination did not " take ". He has noticed that " not a few persons date their ill-health from a so-called unsuccessful vaccination." And he claims that " ' taking ' is the constitutional reaction whereby the organism frees itself more or less from the inserted virus. Whereas if the person does not take *and the virus has been absorbed*, the taking becomes a chronic process—paresis, neuralgia, cephalalgia, pimples, acne, etc."

Burnett's little book is full of wonderful cases that bear out this theory : and we who follow-on, have delightful experiences of our own to relate, which further prove his proposition.

Here are, in brief, some of his cases . . . *A dying baby*, ghastly, collapsed : suddenly taken ill only a few hours previously. It was found that the (new) wet-nurse had a recently vaccinated arm which was " a little painful ". Burnett pondered the strange case, and gave *Thuja* 6 to both babe and nurse.   Result, the baby next morning was still pale, but practically well, and the vaccinial vesicles on the nurse's arm had withered : they proceeded to dry up completely, and never became pustular.   The baby continued well.

[We once saw a case of very severe illness after vaccination in a baby; high temperature, eruption all over body, while the area of vaccination was in the vesicle stage. *Thuja* promptly cured the infant—it was practically well next day : and there was no pustulation, and no scarring.   So, *Thuja* IS AN ANTIDOTE TO VACCINATION in its early, acute stage.]

Among Burnett's cases are . . .   Middle-aged man : *eczema for* 20 *years with a pustular eruption on leg.*   The eczema dated from a re-vaccination twenty years before. *Thuja* 30x cured.   The pustules at once began to wither, and patient, " too busy to come himself ", sent word later that his skin was well.

Young lady, after re-vaccination got an *eruption on chin involving lower lip.*   She had to wear a dense veil to hide the repulsive disfiguration. *Thuja* 30x cured in a fortnight, leaving no thickening of skin and no scar.

Post-orbital neuralgia of twenty years' standing :—even good homœopathy had failed to touch it.   Her " existence was one life-long crucifixion ".   She came " in utter despair ".   Burnett found that she had been vaccinated five or six times, and he gave *Thuja* 30x—which cured. The neuralgia disappeared slowly. About six weeks later he was able to record " The eyes are well ". A year later she wrote him, that she had been in very much better health, " and except one or two *attempts* at a return of the enemy, I have been quite free from suffering".

Chronic headache of nine years' duration.   Head attacks once or twice a week.   Very severe, constricting and bursting headaches.   He gave first *Graphites* : when a red tender patch appeared over right eye, with two or three white-headed pustules.   Then discovering that she had been vaccinated at three months, revaccinated at seven and fourteen years, and had had small-pox about ten years ago he gave *Thuja*.   She started improving ; then became acutely ill with fever, nausea and perspiration. Then pimples broke out on face and in different parts of the body, which filled with pus, and died away.   The symptoms were said to resemble those of her attack of small-pox.   The headaches were well before this bout came on, and a couple of years later Burnett learned that the cure held good. No more headaches.

He gives cases of *glands—hairless patches,—habitual influenza with ill-health and headaches*, where the patient had been successfully vaccinated four times—of *acne*, face and nose, nasal dermatitis, after unsuccessful re-vaccination—*neuralgia* of right eye in a man who, when asked *re* vaccination seemed frightened, " I should not like to be vaccinated again ! " because his last vaccination had made him so ill for a month—of *diseased finger nails* —of *paresis* (vaccinated six or seven times, when it never took),— of *spinal irritation*, a severe case with sickness and disability, had been vaccinated four times and a fifth unsuccessfully—of *arrested development and hemiparesis*—and a number of others showing the wide range of *Thuja*, and its amazing curative powers ; the indications being less the present actual symptoms, for which *Thuja* might or might not be thought of, but the symptoms of the original malady, now latent and chronic, the *fons et origo*.

Burnett's " Vaccinosis " is rendered easily comprehensible by going back to Hahnemann. Even Burnett never seems to have grasped the true inwardness of the matter :—i.e. that vaccination can, to a certain extent, protect from, or modify small-pox *because the vaccinate has been endowed with a similar chronic parasitic disease, which renders him, more or less, immune from that " like " disease, small-pox.*

Hahnemann tells us that, two similar diseases cannot *repel* one another ; nor can they, like dissimilar diseases, *suspend* one another ; nor can two similar diseases *exist together* in the same organism, to form a *double*, complex disease.

No—two diseases (different in kind, but very similar in symptoms and effects) will annihilate one another when they meet in the organism ; the new, stronger morbific power, because of its similitude, will take possession of precisely the parts affected by the weaker, which is consequently annihilated—when vital force remains affected only—temporarily—by the new morbific influence.

Probably the modern explanation would be that the chronic disease, to be kept in abeyance, must call forth the protective mechanisms of the body, which are therefore on tap for the repulse of a " similar " foe.

The manner of infection, and the after-history of the vaccinate, answers Hahnemann's postulates regarding his chronic parasitic diseases :—

Infection takes place in a moment.

Then follows a quiescent period, till the whole organism, being infected, reacts vigorously, and endeavours to throw out the disease on to the skin :—at the place of entry of infection.

Then, after a more or less violent reaction, the body ceases to struggle, and accommodates itself to a kind of latent toleration, in which, though no longer infectious, the organism lives on, scotched, not killed, to influence adversely the whole life-history of its host, together with his reactions to diseases and drugs :— in such way that the latter, even when homœopathically indicated, having helped at first, help less and less, and finally fail to cure, —*because not corresponding to the underlying cause of the patient's continued ill-health.*

Burnett's Vaccinosis—a state of indefinite, chronic ill-health, takes different forms in different individuals according to their personal make-up : one becoming asthmatic—another epileptic— while others develop stomach or joint conditions—and others, again, neuralgias, or life-long headaches. Such cases are puzzling and baffling—terribly resistant to treatment—and never to be unlocked without the key that fits—*Thuja* . . . THUJA, that wonderful antidote to vaccination, alike in its acute and chronic forms; in those *much vaccinated,* or *who have been excessively affected by vaccination,* or again, *those who have failed to " take ",* i.e. to react acutely to the implanted virus. These last, as we have shown, being, in Burnett's experience, the worst cases.

Hahnemann gives us only 634 symptoms of *Thuja,* but the drug has been extensively proved since his day—often in the potencies, and Allen's *Encyclopedia* gives no less than 3,370 symptoms (with, as usual, authorities for each symptom).

In these later careful re-provings on one hundred persons of both sexes, we find that *Thuja* has caused, in sensitive persons, such serious conditions as asthma, epileptic convulsions, lumps in the breast : so it not only does, but *should* cure these things, with or without Burnett's " vaccinosis " thrown in to give the casting vote. *Thuja* is also responsible for the most terrific headaches—for skin troubles,—and has determined, reproduced and cured urethral and other discharges. Some of these things you cannot touch without *Thuja.*

Then gonorrhœal rheumatism. One has seen a case of rheumatoid arthritis (? gonorrhœal in origin), where *Thuja* did wonders in loosening up the joints, and restoring locomotion and power, when other, seemingly-indicated, remedies had failed.

Clarke has a striking article on *Thuja* in his Dictionary, well worth reading. He gives the gist of Burnett's little book, with many observations of his own.

Hering's *Guiding Symptoms* also gives interesting *Thuja* cases, some after vaccination.

But where I imagine that I am " going one better " than the lot, is by trying to put forward the theory that *why* vaccinosis is what it is, and why it can do what it can do in the way of vitiating health, is because it is one of Hahnemann's CHRONIC PARASITIC DISEASES. Nothing else will completely account for its course—or its cure.

And now for a few recent cases, in one's own ken, which still further widen one's knowledge of the curative virtues of *Thuja* ; prescribed on the basis of Burnett's Vaccinosis and its great remedy *Thuja*, and on *Hahnemann's conception of the parasitic nature of chronic diseases* ; passed with merely a shrug of the shoulders, and regarded as a stumbling-block and rock of offence, till Science took the matter in hand to demonstrate its truth. These cases will be found detailed in my pamphlet *Hahnemann's Conception of Chronic Diseases as caused by Parasitic Micro-Organisms*. We will only give them briefly as quoted in a letter to one of the big medical journals, which roused the interest of the Editor, but not sufficiently to secure its insertion.

This letter pointed out :

" In regard to Professor Maitland's Presidential address to the Pathological Society of Manchester (to which you refer in your issue of October 29th, 1932), and his suggestion that resistance to vaccination after recovery from infection might depend on the PERSISTENCE OF THE LIVING VIRUS in the tissues :—it is interesting to note that a similar suggestion was made by Hahnemann one hundred years ago—*in regard to all Chronic Diseases :*—and that homœopathic practice, based on that theory, is producing results which appear to confirm it.

" Our great antidote to vaccination is *Thuja occidentalis*, which will abort vaccination, as we have seen, and which proves powerfully curative in chronic conditions of persons who have been repeatedly vaccinated, often without result, or have been made very ill by vaccination and ' never been well since '.

" Here are a few cases . . . Small girl, ever since vaccination, *pustules* on legs, or alternately, when these disappeared, epileptic fits. *Thuja* quickly cured.

" Small boy, *purulent onychia*, very intractable. Nail removed and thumb healed. Then abscesses in different parts of the body, till it was discovered that he had been eight times vaccinated by a persistent and conscientious G.P. *Thuja* promptly ended the trouble.

" Woman of twenty-nine, *epileptic fits* at least once a week, with (for Aura) a *Thuja* symptom, ' *Before attacks ears feel*

27*

numbed'. She had other *Thuja* symptoms, *worse for onions, which provoke an attack next morning: drops in sleep*. Twice vaccinated, the last took badly. After the first dose of *Thuja*, in ' high ' homœopathic potency, the fits entirely stopped for the ten months she was under observation. She said, ' I don't have them now.'

" Woman of sixty. *Blinding headaches all her life*. Vaccinated three times, last took very badly : ' laid up with it, and delirious.' She was given *Thuja*. A month later,' only one headache, and not a bad one ; putting on weight '. But ' breathless, as when vaccinated, and bones have been aching, as when vaccinated '. The return of old symptoms, on the road to extinction, proves the remedy. Patient had lost headaches, had put on 8 lb., and was returning to work when last heard of five months later. She had, what most of these *Thuja* patients have, sensations rousing her from sleep, of dropping into a bottomless pit.

" A nurse, thirty-nine. Severe attacks of *asthma* for two years : they last three to four days, when she can hardly breathe. Vaccinated five times, the last did not take. She got *Thuja*, in high potency. Result : no asthma at all for three and a half years : then a return, and again *Thuja*. That was nine months ago, and not heard of since.

" Girl of nineteen. Discharge between, or instead of periods. Vague symptoms, but *quite unlike herself in behaviour*. Vaccinated once eighteen months ago and had very high temperature and ill for fourteen days, the arm only being red for one day. It was said to have ' taken internally '. She got *Thuja*. A month later, the doctor who sent her up wrote : ' Miss H. is cured ': and her mother wrote : ' She is quite well and jolly. She had been so unlike herself in her behaviour to me that I had wondered if it were the vaccination.'

" Woman, fifty-nine, *boils* on and off for six years. Worse about vulva and anus. Began with a carbuncle. Inoculations for typhoid. Vaccinated four or five times, ' doesn't take as a rule'. Was given *Thuja*. Under observation for nine months, and still ' No further trouble. Hope they are things of the past.'

" Woman with grown-up children. *Eruption* between toes, then wrists, then palms : now also on soles and sides of feet : very irritable, especially feet at night. A touch starts the itching. Vaccinated three times. *Thuja*. Her daughter, a doctor, wrote six days later, ' No trouble at all since taking the first powder, so grateful. Eruption all fading away, no new ones coming.' *Thuja* had ended it.

" Years of incapacitating *headaches* in the mother of a very noisy family of young children. Much vaccinated. Was given *Thuja*. This was some thirty years ago. Seen recently. ' Never had a recurrence of those headaches.'

" *Woman of forty-seven*. Gassed during the war, *asthma* same night and again in 1921. Now (1931), asthma every two months, or more often. Remedies losing effect. Drops in sleep. Vaccinated lots of times, never seems to take. *Thuja*. No attack for four months, her longest spell without asthma. Now, with a cold, a bad attack and *Thuja* repeated. In this case it was ten years of asthma at least every two months, practically well for eighteen months ('only one real attack after four months, and two slight threatenings').

" *Miss X*. *Asthma* for seven years, *hay fever* for fifteen years. Mother has asthma : father had asthma. T.B. history, mother's side. Asthma started after a very bad vaccination seven years previously. Had been treated by injections. *Thuja*. The happy condition of ' no asthma ' thereupon lasted a whole year, and the medicine did not need to be repeated. For the whole Summer, no asthma and no hay fever. Then, thirteen months later, for a slight return, *Thuja* was repeated, since when she has remained ' extraordinarily fit '.

" Wee boy of three. Comes as *mentally deficient*. Very dirty : incontinence of stool and urine by night. Ate a dog's fæces. At the children's hospital the mother was told ' You can't replace brains : he will never be normal.' Was vaccinated and did not take : done again at nine months. Mother had also, before his birth, a filthy discharge (? gonorrhœal), another indication for *Thuja*. He was given *Thuja*, with almost miraculous results. Already, four weeks later, ' Wonderfully better. Wonderfully different. Understands what you say, talks : getting fatter. Sleeps better. Very observant, asks " What's that ?—What's that ? " Had a birthday party four days ago, and was as normal as anybody.' Mother says, ' The Great Ormond Street doctor said, " You cannot replace brains"—*but you have !* ' Another month ; plays about the room and chatters. When his mother calls him to have his coat on says, ' Just a minute, Mummie ! ' But of course this was not a real case of mental deficiency, merely arrested development—no longer arrested, thanks to Hahnemann, Burnett and *Thuja*.

" But a word of warning. If any one desires to repeat these experiments, he must remember that he is using a homœopathic remedy, whose preparation and posology are absolutely different from the remedies he is in the habit of using. If you desire to produce an effect on a patient, to make him sleep, sweat, vomit, or to dull pain, you must give the dose that will to that extent do violence to his organism. But the remedy of ' like symptoms ' is merely *a vital stimulus, to start in the patient curative reaction,* and requires to be given only in the minimal infrequent dose that has been established by 100 years of experience as being the most suitable for the purpose. You are using cell-poisons : and here, according to the Arndt-Schulz law, large doses may be lethal, smaller doses inhibit, while smallest doses stimulate."

And now a word of warning to homœopaths in regard to *Thuja*. It is not a safe drug in careless or ignorant hands. The " *Thuja-disease* ", where the remedy is persisted in, may also become chronic, according to Kent. We will quote . . .

He says, in regard to *Thuja* : " If you repeat again and again, you will have that which will remain a lifetime. . . . Crude drugs do not impress the vital force so lastingly: but an individual who is thoroughly sensitive and properly sensitive, as sensitive as contagion, then if you undertake to prove (in potency) by giving it night and morning, you will rivet upon him a lifelong miasm."

Always, *the greater the power the greater its capabilities for good and evil, and the more the knowledge needed for its employment.* And I think we have proved that *Thuja* is, as Hahnemann says, " an uncommonly powerful medicinal substance . . . useful in some of the most serious diseases of mankind, for which hitherto there has been no remedy."

Black Letter Symptoms

Nervous, sycotic or syphilitic headaches.
White, scaly dandruff ; hair dry and falling out.

Ophthalmia neonatorum.

Condylomata at ANUS.
Anus fissured, painful to touch, often with warts, sometimes immense numbers of flat, moist, mucous tubercles or condylomata surround anus, especially in syphilitic subjects.
Prostatic affections from suppressed or badly treated gonorrhœa.
Gonorrhœa ; scalding when urinating, urethra swollen ; urinal stream forked ; discharge yellow, green, watery ; with warts , red erosions on glans ; subacute and chronic cases, especially when injections have been used and prostate is involved.

Condylomata, mucous tubercles, sycotic cauliflower excrescences ; fig-warts, smelling like old cheese or herring brine.
Warts, condylomata and other excrescences about vulva.
Condylomata moist, suppurating, stinging and bleeding.

SLEEPLESSNESS ; *sees apparitions on closing eyes ; parts lain on painful ; from heat and restlessness ; from mental depression ; after re-vaccination.*

Wart-like excrescences on back of hand, on chin and on other places.
Warts and condylomata, large, seedy and pedunculated ; sometimes oozing moisture and bleeding readily.

QUEER SYMPTOMS

Body feels very thin and delicate : frail, easily broken : as if made of glass.
As if a living animal were in abdomen.
" Nail " sensations, driven into, or out from parts of brain.
As if abdominal muscles were pushed out by arm of a child.
As if boiling lead were passing through rectum.
As if anus would fly to pieces during stool.
As if moisture, or a drop were running through urethra.
As if legs were made of wood : or elongated.
Stinging and stitching pains, in various parts of body.
Coldness through length of spine : in arms.
Burning; scalp, eyes, lids, small of back to between scapulæ, etc.
" A surplus of producing life ; nearly unlimited proliferation of pathological vegetations, condylomata, warty sycotic excrescences, spongy tumours . . . All morbid manifestations are excessive, but appear quietly, so that beginning of diseased state is scarcely known."
Rheumatism : flesh feels beaten off bones.
Bad effects from vaccination.
Luxuriant growth of hair on parts otherwise not covered by hair.
Skin looks dirty : cannot be washed clean. (*Psor.*)
Warts, condylomata, large, seedy, pedunculated, sometimes ooze moisture and bleed readily.
Eruptions only on covered parts, burn violently after scratching.
Sweat only on uncovered parts, while covered parts were dry and hot.

TUBERCULIN NOSODES

Bacillinum (Burnett); Tuberculinum (Kent)
Tuberculinum (Koch); Tuberculinum bovinum

Bacillinum (originally called *Tuberculinum*) was the earlier production ; and, glancing through Burnett's epoch-making *New Cure of Consumption*, in the light of one's large experience in the use of, chiefly, *Tuberculinum bovinum*, probably the infinitely more potent for good of the two.

There have been many preparations from different manifestations of tubercle, and they all act. It is a " nosode " which, in one form or another, one would be sorry to be without. Human nature is strange, and interesting. When Burnett brought out his book, and one started using the " phthisic virus " on his lines, one of our doctors expressed disgust at the very idea of employing such loathsome material for curative purposes. " He would not take it himself, and certainly would not give it to his patients . . ." and then, not very much later, inspired by Koch, he was *injecting it !* Imagine !—too loathsome in potency, killed and sterile and triturated and, in the 30th potency, merely one part in a decillion, in alcoholic tincture ; and of that, only sufficient used to medicate a few tiniest pellets of milk-sugar. Can one *imagine* anything more disgusting ? But, *by the methods of Hahnemann*, the most terrible poisons and disease-products can be so tamed and roped-in as to affect curatively the strong man, who needs them and is therefore hyper-sensitive to their action, and yet perfectly innocuous " to a healthy infant a day old ". It is a question, perhaps, of making contact ? Neither is the delicate preparation, *per se*, a power, nor is the sick man sensitive all round : but it is only " like to like " that makes contact—and then things happen.

And as to any objections to its use, founded on its unpleasant origin, Burnett says, " If phthisis can be cured by bread and butter or *attar of roses*, well and good : but if not, then let us have something that will cure it."

These are some of the preparations of the tubercle disease-poison. Dr. H. C. Allen, who did so much in furthering the use of the nosodes, says in his *Keynotes*, " The potencies of Fincke and Swan were prepared from a drop of pus obtained from a pulmonary tubercular abscess, or sputa. Those of Heath from a tuberculous lung in which the *bacillus tuberculosis* had been found microscopically ; hence the former was called *Tuberculinum* and the latter *Bacillinum*. Both preparations are reliable and effective."

BURNETT, who introduced the nosode into practical politics by the brilliant little monograph above mentioned, used Heath's preparation, "made especially for him". Burnett tells us that the Homœopaths, ever in the van were, years earlier, using the virus of consumption to cure consumption itself but " the leaders of the dominant sect of the medical profession raised a hue and cry against those of the homœopaths who were so unspeakable as to use the virus of consumption against the disease itself ; and for fear of an unbearable amount of opposition and ignorant prejudice, the practice was discountenanced and almost discontinued—a few only publishing here and there a striking case of the cure of consumption by the virus of the process itself ".

Burnett had been steadily using his preparation for five years in his daily practice, when Dr. Koch " breaks in with his great epoch-making discovery of a new cure for consumption and which turns out to be none other than our old homœopathically-administered virus, against which the hue and cry was long ago raised by the very men who now lie prone at Dr. Koch's feet in abject adoration."

Burnett says the difference between our old friend *Tuberculinum* (which I have ventured to call " *Bacillinum* " as the bacilli were proved to be in the preparation) and that of Koch lies in the way it is obtained: ours is the virus of the natural disease itself, while Koch's is the same virus artificially obtained in an incubator from colonies of bacilli thriving in beef jelly : ours is the chick hatched under the hen, Koch's is the chick hatched in an incubator. The artificial hatching is Koch's discovery, not " the remedy itself or its use as a cure for consumption ". . . . But " There is one other difference, i.e. the mode of administering it to the patient. I use the remedy in high potency, which is not fraught with the palpable dangers of Koch's method of injecting material quantities under the skin, or, in other words, straight into the blood. . . ."

A year later, in a second Preface to a new edition, Burnett wrote of Koch's remedy, " Almost universally voted ' useless as a cure, and terribly dangerous ', Koch and his world-famed remedy have come and—gone ! But they will return anon and . . . remain ! only the dose will get smaller and smaller, until the long-contemned homœopathic dilutions will acquire rights of citizenship in the universities and hospitals of the world. What now bars the way to the further progress of Kochism is the awful admission that will have to be made of the therapeutic efficacy of the infinitesimally small : the *little* dose is the *great* barrier to its onward march. . . ."

" Homœopathy," says Burnett, " is the winning horse at the Medical Derby of the world, and will presently be hurried past the winning post by Orthodoxy itself as her rider."

So much for Burnett's preparation ; now for Kent's preparation of *Tuberculin* :—" a little different from that generally found on the market. This preparation I procured through a Professor of Veterinary Surgery. In Pennsylvania a handsome herd of cattle had to be slaughtered because of tuberculosis. Through the Veterinary Surgeon of the Pennsylvania University I secured some of the tubercular glands from these slaughtered cattle. I examined and selected the most likely specimen. This was potentized by Boericke & Tafel as far as the 6th, and has since been prepared carefully on the Skinner machine—the 30th, 200th, 1,000th, and the higher potencies. This preparation I have been using for ten years."

All the preparations do good work, but one has found them of more use, I think, for " consumptiveness " ; for the ill-health, or the failure of normal recovery from acute disease of persons with an (even distant) " T.B." family history, or who may themselves have long ago had tuberculous activities, apparently recovered from. But Burnett's work seems to go further, and his *Bacillinum* seems to be able to deal magnificently with pulmonary and cerebral tuberculosis : and he found it of more use in suitable cases of rheumatoid arthritis than we seem to do. It will be interesting, provided that his preparations are still available—one must enquire into this—to test them, and observe whether one gets even better, or wider results, than from our usual preparations of " *Tuberculinum* ", or " *Tuberculinum bov.*"

Clarke, in his *Dictionary*, uses the term " *Tuberculinum* " for Koch's preparation, of which we have potencies ; and *Bacillinum* for Burnett's, prepared by Heath, which, as said, was originally called *Tuberculinum*. The preparation of Swan, probably the originator of the virus as a remedy, was also called *Tuberculinum*. It is a pity that there should be this confusion, and one should know what one is using.

Besides all these, there are " *Bacillinum testium* ", and " *Aviare* " from bird tubercle : and Dr. Nebel, who was for years at Davos Platz, prepared quite a number of different tubercle remedies. He sent over a whole selection : but I am afraid they were allowed to dry up.

Thus far, as regards the origin and preparation of the remedy, now for its uses, and the indications for its use.

Remedies must be proved on the healthy—and this is of the

essence of Homœopathy, in order that they may be used with scientific assurance on the sick.   But, as Swan contends, " *Morbillinum, Scarlatinum, Variolinum* " (and the rest) " are the fullest proved poisons in existence : they have been proving for hundreds of years by tens of thousands of persons, old and young, male and female. . . . Here we have the provings ready made by nature for us on healthy persons. Collate the symptoms . . . and you have the pathogenetic effect of that poison, and when you have found such in the sick, administer the potentized " (whichever it may be), " and you will cure the effects of that poison."

Burnett was in the habit of proving likely remedies on himself, and this is his experience with his *Bacillinum.*

" A severe headache, worse the day after taking the poison, and lasting on till the third day.   This headache I felt every time I took it ; I fancied the headache from the 30th was much worse than from the 100th.   The headache I could only describe as far in, and compelling quiet fixedness.   The headaches recurred from time to time for many weeks.

" The next constant effect upon me was expectoration of non-viscid, very easily detached, thick phlegm from the air-passages, followed after a day or two by very clear ring of the voice.

" The third effect was not quite so constant, viz. windy dyspepsia and pinching pains under the ribs of the right side in the mammary line.

" And, finally, disturbed sleep—distressful."   Then he says, he began to use the virus with, not more confidence exactly, but with more familiarity.   He also notes " very slight cough, only just enough to raise the phlegm, which came so easily that one might almost say it came of itself."

*   *   *

Dr. Clarke was asked by Burnett for his experience with the new remedy, and his answer, with a small proving, appears in the third edition of Burnett's book. . . .

Clarke wrote, " I began to use *Bacillin*, and at the same time I proved it on myself, in the 30th and afterwards the 100th potency," with the following result.

1.   Pain in glands of neck, worse turning head or stretching neck.   Right side more affected.

2.   Pain deep in head, worse on shaking the head.

3.   Aching in teeth, especially lower incisors (all sound). This was felt at the roots, especially on raising lower lip : the

symptoms persisted many months, and I occasionally feel it now. Teeth very sensitive to cold air.

4. Sharp pains of short duration in chest and various parts of body.

5. Pain in left knee whilst walking one evening : passed off after persevering in walking for a short distance.

6. Nasal catarrh. Pricking in throat (larynx) then sudden cough. Single cough on rising from bed in the morning. Cough waking me in the night. Easy expectoration. Sharp pain in precordial region, arresting breathing. Very sharp pain in left scapula, worse lying down in bed at night, relieved by warmth.

7. An indolent angry pimple on left cheek. This persisted many weeks, and I began to fear it was something worse. After it had healed it broke out several times at long intervals, and even still a slight indentation can be felt at the spot.

Then he gives cases treated by the nosode. Several of these are *inflammatory conditions of the eyelids*, in which doses of *Bacillinum* acted very promptly and curatively. (And we have found it almost specific for ulceration of cornea in children.—M.L.T.)

*   *   *

Burnett gives other partial provings of *Bacillinum*, one by Dr. Boocock (U.S.A.), published in the *Homœopathic Recorder*. Dr. Boocock, not having the 100th potency but only the 30th and 200th potencies, and engaged in further potentizing the 30th, grew tired of shaking, put down the vial, and dried his fingers on his tongue. Soon after experienced " a flush, some perspiration, and a severe headache, deep in." . . . Later, finished his potentizing, and foolishly did the same thing—" dried my finger on my tongue. Headache increased all over, mostly in temples and occiput. Stinging, stitch-like pains through my piles, and a stitching, creeping pain through left lung and a tickling cough. I felt very weak. I had no cough before, and yet now I had a tickling in my fauces and must cough ; the headache continued, and weakness, and feeling in and under left breast, deep in. . . .

" If this dilution, 2 drops or so, can make one in health feel as I did, I am sure there is a power in dynamization. A very restless feeling, not able to read with profit, so went to bed early ; very restless, slept well, had to rise to urinate three times, urine clear, but of a very bad smell ; putrid. Awoke at daybreak and could not sleep, feeling very tired " . . . and the proving symptoms are recounted for ten more days. Like Burnett and Clarke, he found that it had power to set up a very severe headache, *deep in*; that it irritated the throat; the *left* lung, especially,

and also inflated the bowels with gas (see Burnett's proving);
caused a soft, dark-green mushy stool, and affected the anus,
relieving a troublesome eczematous condition there.

We make no apologies for reproducing these slender provings
of *Bacillinum*. Most of our common remedies have been magnificently proved, and have received a thousandfold confirmation
in the treatment of the sick : but with some of these scantily-
proved remedies of great significance, we need all the light that
can be thrown upon them by those who have actually experienced,
on their state of health, the effect of the subversive—i.e. curative
agent ; together with the localities or organs primarily hit, and in
exactly what manner. Little, actual pictures of drug-action, by
keen and competent observers, are invaluable. Even Allen in his
Keynotes, where he gives so many of the guiding symptoms of
Tuberculinum, does not notice the headache, " deep in ", recorded
by these three doctors.

Dr. H. C. Allen, in his larger *Materia Medica of the Nosodes*,
gives a long Schema of *Tuberculinum* : but, curiously, he does not
tell us there on what authorities, or how provings were made.
Nash quotes Allen's smaller *Keynotes* (which gives many invaluable
indications for the use of the drug) ; and gives cases, to prove its
great value.

* * *

And now, let us take NASH's little list of indications. . . .

" Cosmopolitan : never satisfied to remain in one place long :
wants to travel.

" Wandering pains in limbs and joints : stiff when beginning
to move : < standing : > continued motion.

" Longs for open air, wants doors and windows open, or to ride
in a strong wind.

" Takes cold on least exposure, can't get rid of one before
another comes.

" Emaciation, even while eating well : so hungry must get
up nights to eat.

" Pain through left upper lung to back. Tubercular deposits
begin there.

" Persons with a history of tuberculosis in the family.

" Symptoms ever changing, begin suddenly, ceasing suddenly."

* * *

HERING, *Guiding Symptoms*, says that fragmentary provings
were made by Swan : and he quotes, *inter alia*, Burnett's *New
Cure of Consumption*.

KENT gives many of his personal observations, " recorded in his interleaved copy of Hering's *Guiding Symptoms* " ; these " now guide me in the use of *Tuberculinum* ", and on these he drew for his Lecture. We will extract and condense.

" I do not use *Tuberc.* merely because it is a nosode, or with the idea that generally prevails of using nosodes—that is, a product of the disease for the disease, and the results of the disease . . . that is not the better idea of Homœopathy. It belongs to a hysterical homœopathy that prevails in this century. Yet much good has come out of it. It is to be hoped that provings may be made, so that we may be able to prescribe it just as we would use any other drug.

" It is deep-acting, constitutionally deep. . . . When our deepest remedies act only a few weeks, and they have to be changed, this medicine comes in as one of the remedies—when the symptoms agree.

" One of its most prominent uses is in intermittent fever : stubborn cases that relapse and continue relapsing. . . . When the well-selected remedy has acted, and the constitution shows a tendency to break down, and the well-selected remedy does not hold because of vital weakness and deep-seated tendencies ; then it is that this remedy sometimes comes in.

" Burnett dropped an idea that has been confirmed many times —patients who have inherited phthisis, whose parents have died of phthisis are often of feeble vitality. They are always tired : take on sicknesses easily : are anæmic, nervous, waxy or pale. Burnett evidently used this medicine in a sort of routine way for this kind of constitution, which he called ' Consumptiveness '.

" The mental symptoms that have given way when the patient was under treatment, the mental symptoms I have seen crop out under the provings, and the mental symptoms that I have so often seen associated when the patient is poisoned by the tubercular toxins are such as belong to many complaints and are cured by *Tuberculinum*. Hopeless : aversion to mental work : anxiety evening till midnight : anxiety during fever : loquacity during fever : weary of life ; cosmopolitan : thoughts intrude and crowd upon one another during the night. A person running down, never finding the right remedy, or relief only momentarily, has a constant desire to change, to travel, to go somewhere and do something different. That cosmopolitan condition of mind belongs so strongly to the one who needs *Tuberculinum*. Persons on the borderland of insanity : and phthisis and insanity are convertible conditions, the one falls into the other.

" The most violent and the most chronic periodical sick

headaches, periodical nervous headaches. *Tuberc.* breaks up the tendency to periodical headache, when the symptoms agree.

" Sore, bruised feeling. Aching of bones. Sore, bruised eye-balls, sensitive to touch, and on turning the eyes sideways.

" Face red to purple. Aversion to all food. Aversion to meat—impossible to eat it. Desire for large quantities of cold water during chill and heat. Craving for cold milk. Emptiness, faint feeling ; all-gone, hungry feeling that drives him to eat.

" Emaciation : gradually losing flesh : a growing weakness : growing fatigue.

" Constipation is a strong feature of *Tuberculinum.* Stool large and hard, then diarrhœa. Excessive sweat in chronic diarrhœa. Driven out of bed with a diarrhœa, or diarrhœa worse in the morning. (*Aloe, Sulph.*)

" Menses too early, too profuse, long-lasting : amenorrhœa, dysmenorrhœa.

" Desire for deep-breathing. Longs for open air.

" Especially when the tubercular deposits begin in apex of left lung : an indication verified by a number of observers.

" Perspiration from mental exertion : stains linen yellow. Nightsweats. Sensitive to changes in the weather ; to cold damp, or warm damp weather : to rainy weather. Worse before a storm : sensitive to every electric change in the weather."

*   *   *

In regard to one's own personal experiences—well !—their name is legion. It is a drug that comes continually into use in out-patient work, in cases that hang fire and that give a T.B. family history. " Any consumption ?—father, mother, brothers, sisters, uncles, aunts ? " is one of the first questions one puts to a new patient, with questions as to vaccinations, and previous illnesses. The answers may save much work. Used as a powerful inter-current, where cases, *with that history*, hang fire, one has often felt, after tardily prescribing the drug, " If I'd only *started* with it, how much quicker we should have got on ! "—such a big difference has it made to the patient.

When a pneumonia hangs fire, and refuses to clear up, and a T.B. history is elicited, and *Tub. bov.* (generally 200 for preference) is given, there is apt to be a rise of temperature for a few hours, then it drops and does not rise again, while the patient makes the desired recovery. It may help, in the same way, an acute rheu-matism, where carefully prescribed remedies have failed to benefit.

It appears to be complementary to *Dros.* and *Silica* ; these drugs seem to play into each other's hands, so to speak, especially in cases of T.B. bones and glands : also in some cases of mental deficiency with that taint.   One could tell wonderful tales of T.B. glands and bone cases, treated in our children's clinic.   One should probably add *Calc.* and *Sil.*—but with less of remembered personal experience.

Again, *Tuberculinum* comes in specially to regulate menstrual activities—in persons with the family history, or with tell-tale scars in the neck, etc.   One thinks of it when menses are late to appear, or are too profuse, or even painful, or scanty.   One has seen Burnett's suggestion in regard to its use in *arrested development*, mental or physical, bear fruit.   In the case of one young woman, who had never succeeded in getting anything like her full complement of teeth through and who, after a dose of *Tub.* produced (to her surprise also)—I think it was eight in a couple of weeks.

*   *   *

One began with Burnett and his wonderful little book : we will now end with it : remembering that it was his *Bacillinum*, made direct from active, advanced tuberculosis, that he used. He details over fifty cases in his first edition, and a number more in the two succeeding editions, which are bound together to form one volume.

He gives many cases of children with brain troubles ; for instance—Child about 20 months old, with, for days, high fever, restlessness and constant screaming : in a " fallen in and collapsing state ".   A peculiarly fetid smell about the child, and a strong family history of consumption.   After a dose of *Bacc.*, in high potency, the child fell asleep within ten minutes and screamed no more.   Made a rapid and complete recovery.   He needed two more doses later on : and his head, in course of time, became quite shapely, and he " a gifted boy ".

Many of the cases recounted of phthisis, etc., had been vaccinated, and received benefit from *Thuja* also : and many of the cases during somewhat lengthy treatment, required other constitutional remedies.   In regard to this Burnett writes :

" As to the use of the other remedies, I would especially insist on the fact that the phthisic virus only acts *within its own sphere*, and that this sphere is very *sharply defined* as to time, and what it does not do soon, and promptly, it does not do at all.   Its action is, if I may so express myself, *acute* : its chronic equivalent in *Psorinum.*"   But he explains in a footnote, " When I say soon, I mean that the action *begins* at once ; only, of course, as phthisic processes are generally chronic, the treatment must also be the same, i.e. chronic."

In cases of miserable, ailing, hopeless-seeming children, Burnett says, " Having grown wiser, and fully recognizing that the stop-spot of such remedies as *Aconite, Chamomilla, Pulsatilla,*" which had helped, " was a long way on the hither side of a cure ", he said to himself . . . " ' This sort of remedy only goes *up* to the tubercle, and the tubercle-sphere is their stop-points. . . . But it is the tubercles that kill ! ' I therefore began with the phthisic virus."

He tells us, he used the *Bacillic virus* " Always in very infrequent dose : this is to be understood in all his cases, so he need not restate this *all-important* fact." His potencies were the 30th, 100th, and 200th.

Case XXIII is interesting. An author of eminence, with terrible pain in the head, almost absolute sleeplessness and profound adynamia : had had phthisis, with blood-spitting for years, with a solid right lung, but who had " grown out " of his consumptiveness. His brothers and sisters had died of water on the brain. He was being " shadowed " on advice, as he was thought to be on the verge of insanity. The pain in his head is " as if he had a tight hoop of iron round it ; and he has a distressing sensation of damp clothes on his spine. It sounds hardly credible, but in less than a month after beginning with the virus the pain in the head had gone, the sensation of damp clothes had gone, and his sleep was fairly good. He got a few more doses at long intervals, then needed no further treatment. Continued in good health, hard at work finishing his forthcoming publication."

Many cases of consumption are here cured—the earlier cases : but Burnett gives a case " which is quite in accordance with my previous experience ; *when the consumptive process is in full blaze the virus is unavailing.*" (This is of course what is called galloping consumption. And such is, I believe, the general experience. In fact one has come to think that *Tuberculinum* is more useful in " consumptiveness ", and in cases where structures other than lungs are affected.)

Burnett gives several cases of phthisis, less rapid, which yielded to occasional doses of *Bacillinum*, intercurrently with other homœopathic remedies, as demanded by symptoms ; or, where a double chronic affection, such as " tuberculosis " plus " vaccinosis " co-existed, with occasional doses of first *Thuja* then *Bacillinum.*

Of course Burnett was looked upon as an innovator and sharply criticised by some of his homœopathic confrères ; indeed he was a person about whom some of them could not " speak comfortably ". But in all this he was only following Hahnemann, whom they also professed to follow—more or less—and who, sixty years earlier had pointed out, in regard to his (then) three chronic miasms, that two or more might co-exist in a chronic patient, interfering with his normal reactions to indicated remedies, and that these miasms would require to be " annihilated " one by one. " Their different remedies," he said, " are to be alternately employed, if necessary, until the cure is completed." But—he warns us— *" Leave to each medicine the necessary time to complete its action."*

Sixty odd years earlier, then, Hahnemann had already reached the " stop-spot " of the obvious remedies of present symptoms in chronic disease : but not the " stop-spot " of his deductive genius. Utterly refusing to acknowledge the failure of Homœopathy in these cases of apparent failure, he realized that it was just a question of further extension of the principle, and of digging deeper into causes. Therefore he set to work, " day and night, for ten years," to elucidate the matter, and arrived at the *parasitic nature of chronic disease*, and at the fact that remedies homœopathic to their primary manifestations must be employed—in turn, where more than one such disease was in question—if real progress towards cure were to be achieved . . . and all this years before the microscope began to confirm him in regard to their real parasitic nature.

Burnett, in his turn, came up against the stop-spot of the remedies of present conditions and symptoms " on the hither-side of a cure ", where one of the " chronic miasms ", tubercle, was in question. Such remedies as *Aconite, Pulsatilla, Chamomilla* and their like, " only go up to tubercle : the tubercle-sphere is their stop-spot " ; so he began to interpose doses of the tubercle-virus.

But, in the same way—and this one must take to heart !—he found the stop-spot of the T.B. virus, *which acts within its own sphere only*. Other remedies, he says, " are needed for the non-consumptive part of the case ".

It is thought, by inferences from his writings, that Hahnemann was already working with other disease-products as remedies, besides the one (*Psorinum*) which he proved and gave to the world. He designated certain drugs, as needed intercurrently when treating chronic cases—notably " *The best preparation of Mercury* " on the one hand and *Thuja* or *Nitric acid* on the other, where the chronicity was based on one or other of the venereal diseases. But here, within their limits, the most potent of all are the disease-products themselves. Hahnemann's " isopathic remedies " changed, as he contends, by preparation, till no longer " *idem* ", the same, but "simillimum "—" like" or " homœopathic ", are by far the closest " like ", and of that there can be no question.

For Hahnemann, incessant toil ceased after eighty years ; and Burnett obtained his release unexpectedly, alone, in a hotel room one evening ; and now it devolves on us to carry on, and extend the wonderful work for humanity. *Homœopathy has not necessarily failed where we fail to deal with*—for instance—cancer ; that is a lesson we may learn from Hahnemann and Burnett. Hahnemann refused, so he tells us, the plausible excuse for failure, in the too few proved drugs ; and, instead, delved deeper than the superficial symptoms of the moment, into CAUSE ; and thus attained still wider success.   As Burnett wrote :

" *Mach's nach, aber mach's besser,*" " get on with it, but go one better."

Burnett ends his first edition with the following: " Now, little book, go forth and tell to all concerned that, thanks to the labours of Paracelsus, Fludd, Lux, Hahnemann, Hering, Pasteur, Swan, Berridge, Skinner, Koch, and many others, phthisis and the tubercular diseases generally have definitely entered the list of medicable diseases.   But finally, and for the last time, the remedy must *not* be administered by injection : it must be given in high, higher, and highest potencies, and the doses must be FAR APART.

To those who can only use low dilutions I solemnly say— Hands off ! "

*   *   *

In his second edition he says, further : " Of course, it is not suggested that *Bacillinum* is a specific for all cases of phthisis, and necessarily it will not avail in the many cases that do not come for treatment till very late on : something that will cure *every* case of any malady bearing a given name is, of course, non-existent.

" Still, Bacillary phthisis taken early, and complicated with nothing else, is curable by *Bacillinum*, and this I say after eight years' experience at the bedside and in the consulting room. Anything even approaching it in therapeutic efficacy is thus far absolutely unknown.

" Where, for instance, vaccinosis is also present, the vaccinosis must be first cured, or the phthisis remains uncured, do what you will.

" Where there is a primary spleen affection that led up to the phthisis, such a case must be approached from the spleen as a starting point, or the treatment fails.   When a liver disease underlies the whole maladive state, and phthisis only co-exists with it, the liver malady must first be cured.

" When this state arises from an hereditary syphilitic *taint* (I say *taint*, not the disease proper) the specific nosode may be required first.

" When the phthisis arises from a cancerous parentage, *Bacillinum* will not always suffice, until other remedies have prepared the way.

" When the constitution has been damaged by typhoid, by malarialism, by alcoholism, by cinchonism, and so on, all these must be therapeutically reckoned with, or success will not reward our efforts. Wherever, in fact, phthisis co-exists with other diseases or taints of diseases, the *Bacillinum touches the bacillary part of the case* ONLY.

" When phthisis supervenes upon over-crowding . . . bad food, foul air, chronic sewage poisonings, wounded pride, . . . it will be vain to expect the simple administration of a remedy of any kind to cure unaidedly if the active cause still remains present and operative. . . . It is simple uncomplicated phthisis taken early that can be cured right off the reel by its pathologic simillimum. . . .

" To my brother practitioners I would say, Shake off the shackles of prejudice and try for yourselves whether, and how far, I may be personally carried away on the wings of enthusiasm for my subject. But, mind, only high dilutions and *no* Kochian injections – and moreover, if you give the doses too often you will *fail*, as I formerly did before I learned the lesson that the pathologic simillimums of a disease must be administered in high potency and infrequently. Moreover, the worse the case the higher the potency, as a rule."

*   *   *

Again, we make no apology for these long and interesting quotations. Dr. Burnett was a great and original thinker, and a most charming writer, and it is not everybody who can get at his booklets to be charmed and instructed.

URTICA URENS

In the country it is difficult to get away from *stinging nettles*. We call them *weeds* : we belabour them with sticks : we cut them down with bill-hooks : we dig them up : and in spite of the old saw,

> " Cut them in June
> And they come again soon,
> Cut them in July,
> You cut them down tru-ly "

they are always with us.

WHY ? Is it perhaps because they are invaluable, and must be at hand for emergencies ? Test them ! *Make an infusion by pouring boiling water on stinging nettles, and cover the burn with clean linen steeped therein, and see !*

The dictionary calls them " neglected weeds witn stinging hairs". And yet, no home in town or country should be without stinging-nettle tincture, *Urtica urens*, if only because of its magic power over

BURNS,

for almost instant relief of pain, and rapid healing. (This applies, of course, to fairly superficial burns—" burns of the first and second degrees ".)

Someone, doing a chemical experiment, exploded a small tube of boiling sulphuric acid (oil of vitriol) into face and eyes. It was quickly washed away, but there were extensive superficial burns, and a corneal ulcer. Good old RUDDOCK, in his *Domestic Homœopathy*, advised : . . . and soft rag, moistened with a few drops of *Urtica* in water quickly wiped the pain out, and healed in a couple of days—so far as the skin was concerned.

One remembers a hotel-boy, hurried into hospital, having severely scalded his face. He had to be admitted on account of shock, and *Urtica* was quickly applied. Next morning it was difficult to see where the scalds had been, except on edges of lips, etc., which had not been well covered. Otherwise there was no vesication, and no inflammation.

A doctor who could not believe the fairy tales told him regarding this power of *Urtica*, was advised to " burn his finger and try". He did accidentally burn it a few hours later, and was convinced. The pain went in a few minutes, and it soon healed.

One could multiply, indefinitely, instances of the soothing and healing power of *stinging nettles* in burns.

One remembers with a shiver the burnt and scalded children of student days ; and their shrieks, day after day, when we were instructed to get the dressings off—stuck to intensely painful wounds. But when one uses *Urtica* (*pace asepsis* !) there is no need by removing the dressings, to constantly interfere with healing. Be glad that they do " stick " : and merely water them well, from time to time, with *Urtica* lotion, to cleanse and keep them moist. They will drop off, as healing takes place. I have seen a small ulcer with a surface of pus, heal quickly *under the little scab of pus*, when kept moistened with *Urtica*.

Old burns, also ! that have never healed. One small boy came up with terrible scars and contractions on thigh, and with considerable areas still ulcerated. These began to heal rapidly when compresses of *Urtica* were applied. And a cottage woman, one remembers, where an old burn just above the wrist had refused to heal, *did* heal promptly under the magic touch of a stinging nettle compress.

But . . . There is always a " but " ! Remember, what a remedy can cure, it can cause. And if you use *Urtica* externally too long, or too strong, you will be surprised to find fresh vesicles, matching those of the burn, outside the burn-area—proving Homœopathicity. And then ?—why, a little soap and water finishes that.

But, one grows curious ! Evidently a powerful medicinal herb !—what else is it good for ?

It has long been in domestic use for " gravel, and urinary affections, provoking, as DIOSCORIDES says, urine, and expelling stones out of the kidneys ".

CULPEPPER, who lived from 1615 to 1654, praises it as a remedy for chest troubles ; " to provoke urine and expel the gravel and stone " ; to wash " old, rotten or stinking sores, etc." and for GOUT (more of this anon) ; also for " joint aches in any part—found an admirable help thereunto ".

But we want to know more than that. We want to know the mischief a drug can do to a sensitive, in order to KNOW *what it is capable of curing in a sensitive : a sensitive being a person suffering from " like " symptoms.*

NETTLE-RASH.

Burnett says, " It seems to me that if any honest enquirer is really desirous of putting the truth of Homœopathy roughly to the test, he need only handle a few nice nettles with gloveless hands, when he will find that nettles *do* produce nettle-rash ; and then if he will treat a few cases of nettle-rash with nettle-tea or tincture, he will find that the nettle really does cure the disease nettle-rash . . . and if that is not homœopathy, pray what *is* it ? "

Urtica has not been well proved ; and has never been proved, for finer symptoms, in the potencies. But several provings are recorded. One, a most dramatic one, in " a woman who drank two cupfuls of a hot infusion of two ounces of the herb ".

The result was a most intense urticaria, " with burning, itching, numbness, swelling, œdema and vesication. Face, arms, chest and shoulders were affected—the whole upper part of the body down to the navel. The itching was so intense that the vesicles were scratched off, and exuded a large amount of serum. The look of the patient was monstrous : eyelids completely closed ; upper lip, nose and ears frightfully swollen". But the most astonishing thing was that "in this woman, who had had no children for 3 years, and who had nursed none of her children, the breasts swelled up and discharged, first serum, then perfect milk ; and a very copious secretion of milk lasted for eight days ".

Other provers got nettle-rash " especially on fingers and hands ". (See Allen's *Encyclopedia*, etc.)

We will quote two cases of nettle-rash, showing, *inter alia*, that the *potency* is of less importance than the *remedy*.

The first. After a prolonged course of Camembert cheese, there came occasional urticarial swellings of palms ; but only when hot with walking. Camembert was suspected and let alone. Again Camembert, as a test, with the same result. Then Camembert was let finally alone. (This was in the early days of the Boer War, about 1900.)

Years later (some years after the *Great* War) in a strange place in the country one afternoon, a cup of tea with goat's milk was drunk. A few hours later, after getting home, terrific irritation began, first in one place, then in another, then everywhere, till the victim was obliged to retire and tear off her clothes, in agonies of itching from scalp to heels, and she was forced to rub, till black and blue. She had been inclined to laugh at nettle-rash—*till then* ! Happily *Urtica* was remembered, and a few drops of the strong tincture in water, sipped, brought speedy relief, and it was all gone by night, *never to return since*, i.e. in some ten years.

A second case. " She looked as if she had fallen, stripped, into a bed of nettles : not an inch free from weals. *She got Urtica Urens* 10m., one dose, and was clear next morning."

* * *

LACTATION.

Urtica has been used to promote the secretion of milk, and also to suppress it, in women who are weaning. In a case quoted in Clarke's *Dictionary*, a woman with a lump in her breast was seen six weeks after childbirth, with stinging pains in the lump and in various parts of the body, and with entire absence of milk. Nothing helped till *Urtica* was given, " when in three days the breasts filled with milk, and the pains were relieved. The breasts had now to be supported on account of their fullness ".

DELTOID RHEUMATISM.

Another notable feature of the provings of *Urtica* was *a very severe right deltoid rheumatism*, and *Urtica* has proved curative in this distressing condition.

*   *   *

Dr. Compton Burnett, who had a perfect genius for spotting, roughly proving, and making play with rather unusual remedies, tells us a great deal about *Urtica urens* in his brilliant little monograph on GOUT. It is to him that we owe much of our knowledge of this despised but supremely-useful weed.

AGUE—MALARIA.

In a charming and characteristic little story, he gives an account of his " first acquaintance with the nettle as a medicine ".

" Twenty years ago I was treating a lady for intermittent fever of the mild English type, when one day my patient came tripping somewhat jauntily into my consulting room and informed me that she was quite cured of her fever, and wished to consult me in regard to another matter. I at once turned to my notes of her case, and inquired more closely into the matter of the cure, in order to duly credit my prescribed remedy with the cure, and the more so as ague is not always easily disposed of therapeutically. ' Oh! ' said the lady, ' I did not take your medicine at all, for when I got home I had such a severe attack of fever that my charwoman begged me to allow her to make me some nettle-tea, as that was a sure cure of fever. I consented, and she at once went into our garden, where there are plenty of nettles growing in a heap of rubbish and brickbats, and got some nettles, of which she made me a tea, and I drank it. It made me very hot. The fever left me, and I have not had it since.' "

Burnett adds, " Honour to the charwoman of nettle-tea fame! "

Burnett continues, " The thing escaped my mind for years, but one day being in difficulty about a case of ague, I treated it with a tincture of nettles and cured it straight away, and my next case also, and my next, and almost every case ever since, with very nearly uniform success. Some of my cases of ague cured with nettle tincture were most severe ones, invalided home from India and Burmah. And quite lately a patient in Siam, to whom I had sent a big bottle of nettle tincture, wrote me, ' The tincture you sent us has very greatly mitigated the fever we get here. Please order us another bottle.' ''

" I say *almost* every case has yielded to *Urtica urens* ; every case, of course, has not."

This use is also homœopathic, for Burnett says, " *Urtica urens, in my hands, has produced fever over and over again*." One sensitive to whom he gave rather large doses of the φ reported, " I cannot go on with this medicine, it sets all my pulses beating, makes me terribly giddy as if I were going to topple forwards in my bed, and then a bad headache comes on ; and when I take it at night it makes me very feverish."

In an Indian officer, suffering from Scinde boils (? of malarial origin), to whom Burnett gave *Urtica*, this " was followed by a furious outburst of fever, so severe that his condition caused his friends considerable anxiety ". But " he made a quick and complete recovery ".

In another such case, followed by very severe fever with unusually long stages, the patient recovered under *Nat. mur.*

Burnett says, " It is distinctly curious to note the remarkable effects of *Natrum muriaticum* and *Urtica urens* in gout as well as in ague and malarialism."

Gout.

Urtica urens was one of Burnett's great remedies, not only for *malaria* and *ague-cake* (he found in it a powerful " *splenic* ", but also " *for its gravel-expelling power* " and for *gout*.

He says, " Patients under the influence of small material doses of *Urtica* will often pass quantities of gravel " ; (one of his patients " used to point to a spot under her spleen as her gravel-pit ") and he says, " when I observed others who, being under the influence of *Urtica urens*, passed grit and gravel pretty freely for the first time in their lives, I came to the conclusion that *Urtica* possesses the power of eliminating urates from the economy. And it slowly became clear to my mind that *Urtica* might be the very remedy I had long been in quest of, viz., a quickly-acting, easily-obtained homœopathic remedy for the ATTACKS of gout, or some of them ; for of course we, of experience, never expect uniform results, any more than we expect all the trees of the forest to be of the same height ".

He says, " I have no faith in gout cures unless they thicken the urine." And he says, " *in acute gout, it cuts short the attack in a safe manner, viz., vy ridding the economy of the disease product, its actual suffering-producing material.*"

His usual way was to give five drops of the mother tincture in a wineglassful of quite warm water, say every two or three hours : and a few hours later he would hear, " Oh ! the pain is gone, and I have passed a lot of gravel."

Acute gout was more common in his day, than with us : but I remember one case in a lady, whose foot was red and swollen and intensely painful, and who was in the habit of getting gouty attacks. *Urtica urens* φ cured very promptly.

For his success in curing acute gout, Dr. Burnett came to be known as " Dr. URTICA " in London West-end Clubland.

Then again, for suppression of urine, and uræmia. One remembers a small boy, dying of tubercular meningitis, where the urine was suppressed, and the body had a highly urinous odour. A few drops of the strong tincture of stinging nettles caused the passage of urine, and the odour disappeared, and life was, *pro tem.*, prolonged. The same restoration of the urinary function was seen in a case of uræmia in the hospital a few years ago.

Burnett's little book is crowded with brilliant cases, told in his inimitable style ; we are here giving only the results of his experiences.

As said, he used *Urtica* " in small material doses ", repeated pretty frequently (since they were acute illnesses) for some days.

In the course of his so using the remedy he got, as we have seen, some pretty severe provings in some of his patients, which show the homœopathicity of the drug : as able to *cause*, as well as to *cure*.

It was in exactly this way that Hahnemann started, originally, when administering his " similars ". Then he had to dilute, to avoid severe aggravations ; this especially where poisonous drugs were concerned. Then, going further and further in attenuation— as it seemed !—he discovered that Dilutions became Potencies.

Poor old Culpepper ! how surprised he would have been to learn that he was advocating Homœopathy an odd hundred years before its time !—just as Molière's *Bourgeois Gentilhomme* was enchanted with the wonderful news that he had been speaking prose all his life ! But Culpepper only tells what he knew had *cured*. While we know, that *what will cure, will also cause.*

* * *

By the way, if you are being stung by a mosquito, don't smack it dead on your face, thus expressing its maximum poison : but flick it off lightly.   In the same way, if you have the misfortune to be badly stung by nettles, don't " rub it in " but pass a sharp knife lightly over the painful places, after the manner of shaving, and so extract those little terrors, the poison hairs.

After all this, I think we shall all GRASP THE NETTLE ; remembering that it is only out of sufferings that we can ever extract CURE.

*   *   *

The strong tincture of *Arnica* applied to a *wasp* sting, prevents the pain and swelling, and in a couple of hours the sting is forgotten.

Urtica is said to do likewise for bee stings.

And *Cantharis* 200, given internally, quickly cures the inflamed and horrible swellings that may follow gnat bites.

VERATRUM ALBUM

(White hellebore)

EVERYBODY knows *Veratrum alb.* as one of the great remedies of collapse : collapse with icy coldness ; with profuse cold sweat, especially on the forehead : with profuse evacuations : with great thirst. But far from everybody knows *Veratrum alb.* as a notable *pain* remedy : or in its *mental* aspects—as Hahnemann knew it and left it for us, and as Hahnemann's most faithful followers have experienced and taught it.

It is an old folly to substitute opinions for facts. Hahnemann gave us facts, results of actual experiments carefully conducted, and the experience of one of the most astute observers who ever put pen to paper. But since his day some of the teachers of Homœopathy, wise in their own conceits, have crippled knowledge and therefore usefulness, by substituting their opinions for facts. Perhaps the worst of these was Hughes, whose " *Pharmaco-dynamics* " was dubbed by his contemporaries " Homœopathic milk for Allopathic babes", and who, always ready to go one better than Hahnemann, by his dicta and omissions has robbed us of, or belittled much of Hahnemann's experience. He threw doubt, for instance, on Hahnemann's observation that " a single dose of *Drosera* 30 is quite sufficient for the homœopathic cure of epidemic whooping cough according to the indications of symptoms " (which he enumerates) : " the cure taking place with certainty in from seven to nine days, under a non-medicinal diet " (See HOMŒOPATHY, Vol. III, p. 24). This was not the Homœopathy of Hughes, who favoured repeated doses of low potency, from which, according to his own showing, he got very inferior results : but Hughes was obliged to print a footnote in later editions of his work, to the effect that this observation of Hahnemann had been confirmed by other doctors. And one may say that, recently, one doctor after another has volunteered with great joy results from following Hahnemann's directions in regard to whooping cough.

Later writers again, have robbed us of a " lead " to good work, by ignoring Hahnemann's black type *Drosera* symptoms in regard to bones and joints, as if its true, and indeed only sphere was whooping cough and laryngitis. Thus certain cases of even

rheumatoid arthritis, where *Drosera* might have helped, have
been left uncured.

Again in regard to *Veratrum alb.* Hughes, from his lofty assumption of critic is pleased to say that " the marked symptoms of
insanity which stand at the head of Hahnemann's list " (of mental
symptoms) " were observed upon insane patients taking the drug,
and are worse than useless ".   Imagine that ! worse than useless !
—in Dr. Hughes's *opinion*.   And in Allen's *Encyclopædia*, where
one of the " contributors" was Dr. Richard Hughes, a footnote
is to the following effect : " All symptoms of the mind and
disposition occurring in the first two classes, and all the spasmodic
phenomena manifested by the third, have been bracketed, *as the
doses administered were too small to induce them.*"—HUGHES.

Again, Opinion *versus* Fact ! One cannot help wondering
how much of Hahnemann has been deleted or slurred by Hughes !
One only discovers these things gradually. Hering's *Guiding
Symptoms* has no hint of such follies ; and Kent, a far greater
teacher and prescriber than Hughes—or so one gathers—realizes
the great importance of *Veratrum alb.* in insanity ; as we shall see.

Meanwhile, hear Hahnemann on the subject : " . . . It is
quite false that patients affected with emotional and mental
diseases require and bear enormous doses of medicine, as physicians still imagine. . . . In such cases ", he says, " health is often
but little affected and the patients are often very robust . . .
the malady has settled in the fine invisible organs of the mental
and emotional spheres undiscoverable by anatomy . . ."
and, in his experience, " patients suffering from mental and
emotional diseases soon regained a healthy state of their mental
and emotional organs, i.e. perfect recovery of health and reason,
by doses as small as those that suffice for other non-psychical
maladies, but only of the appropriate and perfectly homœopathic medicine ".   One may say here, by the way, that in the
provings of drugs, to ascertain their powers of sick-making,
mental and physical, in order to use them to neutralize a like
sickness, the mental symptoms are best elicited by provings with
the higher potencies.

But Hahnemann knew what he was talking about in the
matter of insanity. He describes (*Lesser Writings*) how (having
been for several years much occupied with the treatment of
diseases of the most tedious and desperate character, including
hypochondriasis and insanity in particular) with the assistance
of the reigning duke he established a convalescent asylum for
patients affected with such disorders, in Georgenthal, near Gotha.
Here he treated and cured, " the Privy Secretary of the Chancery,

one Klockenbring of Hanover : a man who, when in health, "attracted the admiration of Germany by his practical talents for business and his profound sagacity, as also by his knowledge of ancient and modern lore and his acquirements in various branches of science ". " His almost superhuman labours in the department of state police, for which he had a great talent, his constant sedentary life, combined with a too nutritious diet " had gradually deranged him : " possibly also his copious indulgence in strong wines contributed ". Anyway, the last straw was some horrible lampoon which completed his mental catastrophy.

Hahnemann describes in detail his wild maniacal condition ; now quoting from different authors in different languages ; now throwing himself, in an agony of sobbing at the feet of his amazed attendants ; now hacking and tearing to pieces his attire and his bed ; now running about naked, bellowing : demanding foods or drinks which were spilt and fouled.

At first Hahnemann merely watched him, while he treated him and causing him to be treated with the greatest kindness and consideration, so earning his confidence. Then gradually, with remedies—no doubt at all, *Veratrum* among them, the big man's reason was gradually restored—indeed so perfectly restored that a governmental post—but less arduous, was found for him.

And, out of his experiences, this is what Hahnemann has to tell us in regard to *Veratrum alb.*

" *Physicians have no notion of the power possessed by this drug to promote a cure of almost one-third of the insane in lunatic asylums* (*at all events as a homœopathic intermediate remedy*) *because they know not the peculiar kind of insanity in which to employ it, nor the dose in which it should be administered in order to be efficacious and yet not injurious.*"

In his treatment of mental patients Hahnemann entirely departed from the treatment customary at that time, which was brutal in the extreme. His absolutely new methods, he thus describes.

" I never allow any insane person to be punished by blows or other painful bodily chastisement, because there can be no punishment for involuntary actions, and because these patients are always made worse and not better by such rough treatment. He (Klockenbring) used often to show me with tears the remains of the marks of the ropes which his former guardians had employed in order to restrain him. The physician in charge of such unhappy people must indeed have at his command an attitude which inspires respect but also creates confidence ; he will never feel insulted by them, because a being that cannot reason is incapable of insulting anyone. Their outbreaks of unreasonable anger only arouse his sympathy for their pitiful state, and call forth his charity to relieve their sad condition."

And again, in the *Organon*, he deals with the treatment of mental aberration. . . . Raving madness to be met by calm fearlessness and firmness : plaintive melancholy soothed by silent compassion by gesture and expression : silly loquacity listened to in silence, with attention ; indecent behaviour and obscene language treated with indifference : destruction and injury of objects prevented by placing them out of reach, without reproaching the patient : corporal punishment or torture to be absolutely avoided. Even the administration of medicines need not require coercion : the smallness of the dose, and the taste-lessness of homœopathic medicines allows them to be mixed with the patient's drink, obviating any kind of compulsion, and not exciting his suspicion. . . . He adds, " *there is nothing that embitters the insane and augments their diseases so much as expressions of contempt, and ill-disguised deception. Physician and attendants should always treat such patients as if they regarded them as rational beings* ".

BLACK LETTER SYMPTOMS (*Hahnemann, Allen, and Hering*).

Persistent raging.

Inconsolable over a fancied misfortune, runs about the room howling and screaming, looking upon the ground ; or sits brooding in a corner, wailing and weeping in an inconsolable manner.

Taciturnity.

Crossness, when cause given.

Attacks of pain with delirium, driving to madness.

Mania with desire to cut and tear everything, especially clothes ; with lewdness and lascivious talk : religious or amorous.

Delusions of grandeur.

Cold sweat on forehead with anguish and fear of death.

Despair of salvation with suppressed catamenia.

His consciousness is as if in a dream.

Flat-pressing headache, vertex : which became throbbing when moving.

Sensation of a lump of ice in vertex.

Cold sweat on forehead.

Pale face : sunken : with anxious expression.

He became pale in the face with frequent stools.

He cannot speak.
Saliva runs incessantly out of mouth like waterbrash.
Tasteless saliva   want of taste in mouth.
Taste and coolness in mouth, as from peppermint.
Pungent peppermint taste in throat : sensation of heat rises into the mouth.

Thirst for coldest drinks.   Craves ice : fruit.
Violent hunger.   Excessive thirst during perspiration.
Great thirst with hunger.
Great nausea before vomiting.
Violent vomiting of slimy, acid liquid, with food.
Forcible, excessive vomiting.
Vomiting and diarrhœa as many as ten times, with pale sunken face, covered with cold sweat.
Vomiting of green mucus.
Gastric catarrh, great weakness : cold, sudden sinking.

Colic, as if intestines twisted into a knot.
Cold feeling in abdomen.
Colic with burning, as if intestines twisted into a knot, with cold sweat.
Cutting pains : flatulent colic, which attacks the lower bowels here and there and the whole abdomen : the longer the flatus is retained, the more difficult it is to be expelled.

Diarrhœa with profuse perspiration.
Frequent and violent diarrhœa : very profuse and painful.
Excessive evacuations : copious evacuations.
Constipation on account of the hardness and size of the evacuations.
Cholera morbus : worse at night : cold sweat on forehead ; vomiting and purging at the same time, after fruits : profuse brownish discharges : thirst : cramps : prostration : cold sweats : great weakness after stool.
Asiatic cholera . . . violent evacuations upwards and downwards : icy coldness of body : cramps in calves : vomiting with constant desire for cold drinks : face colourless or bluish : blue margins round eyes : deathly anguish in features : cold tongue and breath : . . . great oppressive anguish in chest, with desire to escape from bed : violent colic, especially about umbilicus, as if abdomen would be torn open : sensitive to contact : drawing and cramps, fingers : wrinkled skin in palms : retention of urine.

Palpitation of heart with great anxiety and quickened audible respiration.

Excessive anxiety that takes away the breath.
Spasmodic constriction of larynx with contracted pupils.
Suffocative attacks of constriction in larynx.
Deep hollow cough in three or four shocks.
Seems in danger of suffocation, the respiration is so restricted.
Cold breath (in cholera).

Hands icy cold, blue. Blue nails.
Rheumatic pain, felt when moving. . . .
Very great difficulty of walking, like paralysis, first right then left hip-joint.
Pain under knee, as if bone had been broken and was not quite firm.
Heavy pain of legs, as from fatigue. . . .

Prostration and weakness of the whole body : extreme weakness.
Syncope. Yawning. Paralytic sinking of strength.
Whole body and face pale.

Chill and shivering with frequent stools.
Febrile chill with coldness and thirst.
Creeping coldness through whole body.
Cold skin.
Creeping coldness over head, especially vertex. " Lump of ice " sensation, vertex.
Face cold, collapsed.
Coldness back : extremities cold. Great coldness of hands.
Cold sweat. Cold sweat on forehead. Profuse perspiration on forehead with the evacuation.
Cold perspiration over whole body.
Typhoid forms of fever when vital forces sink : cold sweat : coma.
Vomiting and watery diarrhœa : bluish face : pointed nose : wrinkled skin.
Internal chill ran through him from head to toes of feet with thirst.
Hahnemann gives also, heat and redness of face.

Among the peculiar sensations of *Verat. alb.* we find :
As if pregnant, or in throes of childbirth.
As if he had a bad conscience and had committed a crime.
As if a lump of ice on vertex.
As if tongue too heavy.
As if peppermint—coolness—in mouth and throat.

As if something alive were rising from stomach into throat.

As if knives cutting bowels : hot coals in abdomen : pinching as with pincers in abdomen : intestines twisted into a knot.

Cold water running through veins.

Bones pressed or broken. As if a heavy stone were tied to feet and knees.

As if she would have to fly away.

Veratrum, then, has mania, insanity, delirium, all of great violence. KENT condenses these far more tellingly than one can hope to do, so we will quote. He says :

" The mental symptoms are marked by violence and destructiveness : he wants to destroy, to tear something ; he tears the clothes from his body. Always wants to be busy, to carry on his daily work. A cooper who was suffering from the *Veratrum* insanity would pile up chairs on top of one another : when asked what he was doing, he replied that he was piling up staves. When not occupied with this he was tearing his clothes, or praying " (*Stram.*) " for hours on his knees, and so loud that he could be heard blocks away.

" Excited state of religious frenzy : believes he is the risen Christ : screams and screeches until he is blue in the face : head cold as ice, cold sweat, reaches out and exhorts to repentance.

" Exhorts to repent, preaches, howls, sings obscene songs, exposes the person " (*Hyos.*). " Fear and the effects of fear : fear of death and of being damned : imagines the world is on fire.

" Mania with desire to cut and tear everything especially the clothes. . . . puerperal mania and convulsions with violent cerebral congestion ; bluish and bloated face ; protruding eyes ; wild shrieks, with disposition to bite and tear. . . . Alternate states of brooding, screaming and screeching. A few such remedies would empty our insane asylums, especially of recent cases. Insanity is curable if there are no incurable results of disease."

Kent says again, " *Veratrum* is a remedy that would keep many women out of the insane asylum, especially those with uterine trouble. . . . During menses, cold as death, lips blue, extremities cold and blue, dreadful pains, sinking sensations, mania to kiss everybody " (*Crocus*) ; " hysteria with a coldness at the menstrual period, copious sweat, vomiting and diarrhœa . . ."

Kent remembers a farmer, one summer, who had a strange sensation when he drank water, as if it ran down the outside and did not go down the œsophagus—so marked that he requested his friends to see if it did not run down the outside. *Veratrum 2m* cured him. " No remedy has produced that sensation, but I figured it out by analogy," says Kent. *Verat.* has also a sensation of cold water running in the veins.

In regard to the symptom, " head feels as if packed in ice ; as if ice lay on the vertex ", one remembers a hospital patient, a sturdy, elderly woman, full of common sense and cheery to the last degree, who developed terrific pains in the head, and was admitted, almost insane with the suffering. Face distorted with its anguish. Remedy after remedy failed to touch her, till one day it turned out that she had a sensation of a block of ice lying on vertex : this suggested *Veratrum*, as did the symptom, " attacks of pain with delirium, driving to madness "—it was almost as bad as that ! and *Veratrum* quickly changed the picture, and her old self re-emerged. One will never forget *Veratrum* for terrific, unbearable pains in the head that change the face, almost induce insanity, with that *icy sensation on vertex.*

And in regard to PAIN, Hahnemann says, " Paroxysms of pains, similar to those the white hellebore root can itself produce, and which always brought the patient for a short time into a sort of delirium and mania, often yielded to the smallest dose of the above solution " (the quadrillionth of a grain of the root).

The cry for *Veratrum* then, consists of excessive coldness ; excessive cold sweat ; extreme thirst ; extreme violence of evacuations ; extreme copiousness of vomiting, purging and sweat ; collapse ; paralytic weakness and loss of power : with violence of reactions to pain and mania.

The remedies that probably come nearest to it are *Arsenicum* and *Carbo veg.* But *Arsenicum* has extreme anxiety and restlessness, " the *Veratrum* patient is quiet " ; and *Carbo veg.* lacks the profuseness of evacuations and sweat. The excessive evacuations also distinguish it from *Camphor* and *Cuprum* (in cholera).

Homœopathy scored its laurels in CHOLERA, with its three principle remedies designated by Hahnemann, who had never seen the disease, but had studied its symptoms and wrote pamphlet after pamphlet to help. Early stages, with collapse, coldness and sudden prostration, *Camphor* : with excessive cramps, not only in abdomen, but in, and beginning in, fingers and toes, *Cuprum* : with excessive cold sweat, and excessive vomiting and purging, *Veratrum alb.* (See HOMŒOPATHY, Vol. I, 126 ; Vol. III, 338).

VERATRUM VIRIDE

Variously named *American white hellebore : American green hellebore : Poke weed. (Veratrum alb.* is a different plant of different symptoms and uses : it grows in Europe and Asia.)

Veratrum viride " grows in swamps ; wet meadows ; along mountain creeks from Canada to the Carolinas ".

Veratrum viride has produced and cured pneumonia : it is, in fact, one of Homœopathy's greatest pneumonia medicines, symptoms agreeing. One has seen astonishing cases, in the hands of one of our doctors especially, who knows exactiy when to prescribe the drug. These are his indications : " The case looks very like a *Phos.* case. The face is red, flushed ; with profuse sweat. *Red streak down centre of tongue.* High temperature ; bounding pulse : perhaps delirium. Thirst. The patient has an aversion to sweets, and may complain that water tastes sweet." So we can all " go and do likewise ".

A red streak (perhaps dry) down the centre of the tongue is its most suggestive and arresting symptoms. But, like so many drugs, it may have just the opposite : for, looking down the provings, one finds that it has also produced a *white* streak down the centre of the tongue. It evidently has some action on the blood supply to the tongue.

It has, " tongue white, not coated ; looks bleached . . . Tongue white in centre, with red edges and white tip. It does not look like a coated tongue, but as if the blood were pressed out . . . Tongue feels scalded WITH RED STREAK IN CENTRE." And this last is the classical appeal of *Veratrum viride* for employment not only in pneumonia but in any of the conditions it can so greatly benefit.

Glancing down the provings, as given in the *Cyclopædia of Drug Pàthogenesy,* one is struck by several of its other peculiarities. For instance, nearly all the provers promptly developed *hiccough.* And again, the astonishing effect it had—quickly— on pulse-rate. Pulses dropped, sometimes to 40, 34, or lower. Or, in other cases, perhaps better observed, the pulse would rise at once, and *then* fall. Pulse generally very small and weak ; often hardly perceptible.

*　　　*　　　*

NASH says this remedy had once a great reputation in the first, or congestive stage of inflammatory diseases . . . for a time the journals fairly bristled with reported cures of pneumonia ; and its curative action was attributed to the influence of the remedy to control the action of the heart and pulse . . . I was a young physician and thought I had found a prize in this remedy. " But one day," he says, he " left a patient relieved by *Verat. vir.*, and returning later found him dead." He watched others treated by this remedy, and " found every little while a patient with pneumonia dropping out suddenly when reported better. Now we do not hear so much of *Veratrum viride* as the greatest remedy for the first stage of this disease. (1) It was (like other fads) used too indiscriminately. (2) It is wrong to control or depress the pulse, regardless of all other considerations. (3) The patients who had weak hearts were killed by this powerful heart-depressant. A quickened circulation is salutary in all inflammatory diseases, and is evidence that the Natural power to resist diseases is there, and at work."

One presumes that as Nash is alluding to his early experiences ; that the dosage " to bring down the pulse " was, as it would have to be, a physiological dose. In homœopathic prescribing, the drug is used, like any other, in accordance with symptoms, not to do something subversive, perhaps dangerous, but to stimulate the patient to do something curative : a very different proposition. As a matter of fact one would think of *Veratrum viride* where the pulse is *slow*.

Nash gives, as his chief indications for the remedy, " A narrow, well-developed red streak right through the middle of the tongue : intense fever, with twitching, and tendency to spasms."

* * *

CLARKE (*Dictionary*) gives an instructive case, which we will quote—a nearly fatal accidental proving of the drug. He says, " Burt made a heroic proving of the liquid extract ; and his infant daughter (twenty-one months) very nearly died from taking a few drops of the tincture from a phial. In two minutes she began vomiting. Coffee and camphor were given as antidotes. In five minutes her jaws were rigid ; pupils widely dilated ; face blue ; hands and feet cold ; no pulse at wrist. Abdomen and back were rubbed with camphor, when she went into spasms with violent shrieks. These spasms were frequently repeated, a hot bath being most effective in relaxing the muscles. Vomiting ropy mucus kept up for three hours. Pulseless ; hands and feet shrivelled. After three and a half hours she slept quietly and soundly and next morning was well but a little weak."

* * *

Glancing down the provings, one thing one notices is the rapid recovery from the drug, especially after sleep. " Slept well, and awoke without any trace of trouble." " Next morning felt well."

In some cases, the prover " dreamt much, especially of water ". Again, a cup of hot, strong coffee did more good than anything else.

In one case " clothes would not fit him, seemed as if they were scratching him somewhere : constant twitchings of different parts of the body."

In a case of severe poisoning, with excessive and prolonged vomiting; cold surface ; clammy sweat ; pulse feeble and irregular, forty-four beats to the minute ; a couch in front of a warm fire, and brandy repeated at short intervals restored warmth to the surface and improved the pulse, and after about an hour he fell asleep, slept for fifteen minutes, and woke saying, " I'm all right now ", as he appeared to be. Next day there was only soreness of muscles from retching.

*　　　*　　　*

H. C. ALLEN (*Keynotes*) says, for full-blooded, plethoric persons.

Congestions, especially to *base of brain, chest, spine and stomach*.

Inflammation with violent pains.

Acute rheumatism, with high fever . . .

Cerebral congestion ; intense, almost apoplectic, with violent nausea and vomiting.

Congestive apoplexy, hot head, bloodshot eyes, thick speech, *slow full pulse, hard as iron*.

Child on the verge of convulsions, continued jerking or nodding of head.

Cerebro-spinal disease (compare *Cicuta*) : spasms : dilated pupils : tetanic convulsions : opisthotonos: *cold clammy perspiration*.

Sunstroke (see *Gels., Glon., Bell.*).

Pulse suddenly increases and gradually decreases below normal : *slow, soft, weak*.

And then the characteristic tongue : (here we need not repeat).

He also says, " *Veratrum viride* should not be given simply ' to bring down the pulse or control the heart's action ' but like any other remedy, for the totality of the symptoms."

*　　　*　　　*

BOGER (*Synoptic Key*), with later experience (?), has quite a lot to say about *Verat. vir.* " SUDDEN VIOLENT CONGESTIONS

(brain, chest, etc.) with nausea and vomiting.   Muscle prostration.
. . . Head thrown back : nodding or rolling motions . . .
Vision of red spots, purple on closing eyes.   LIVID, TURGID FACE,
BUT BECOMES FAINT ON SITTING UP.   Red or dry streak down
centre of tongue.   Violent vomiting without nausea . . .   Slow,
heavy breathing . . . Full, large, soft pulse, or slow, with
strong or violent heart-beat.   Violent cough from the very
start.   Hyperpyrexia, or rapidly oscillating temperature . . .
Cerebo-spinal fever . . .''

BLACK LETTER SYMPTOMS

Quarrelsome and delirious.
Dilated pupils.
Face flushed.   Dry mouth, and lips, dry all day.
Tongue somewhat red in centre.
Tongue (? coated yellow) with red streak in centre.
Tongue : white or yellow, with red streak down middle ; dry
or moist, with white or yellow coating, or no coating on either side.
Feels scalded.

Vomiting.
Menstrual colic, with dysmenorrhœa : much nausea and vomiting ;
plethora ;   cerebral congestion.
Suppressed menses, with cerebral congestion.

Pneumonia, pulse hard, strong, quick ;   engorgement of lungs,
with faint feeling in stomach, nausea, vomiting :—or slow, or
intermittent pulse.

Congestions, especially to base of brain, chest, spine and stomach.
Pain and soreness just above the pelvis.

OTHER MARKED, OR CURIOUS SYMPTOMS

Immense green circles appear round candle, which, as vertigo
comes on, turn to red.
Hiccough : almost constant : painful, with spasms upper
end of oesophagus.
Vomiting, long-continued, of glairy mucus, after food ; painful empty retching, with inflammatory and cerebral diseases ;
smallest quantity of food or drink is immediately rejected ;
with collapse, very slow pulse and cold sweat.
Puerperal convulsions ; furious delirium ; arterial excitement ;
cold clammy sweat.   Hands and feet shrivelled.
Convulsions with mania.

Breathing : laboured, must sit up, cold sweat on face ; difficult, convulsive, almost to suffocation ; sensation of a heavy load on chest.

Pleurisy : holds side : " can't breathe " stitching pain.   (*Bry.*)

Bathed in cold perspiration.   (Compare *Verat. alb.*)

Chorea : twitchings and contortions of body, *unaffected by sleep*.   (Reverse of *Agar.*)

Head jerking or continually nodding, is peculiar here.

Makes faces : bobs head : face livid and covered with cold sweat.

When rising makes a series of springs, apparently from impossibility of raising one foot from the ground without lifting the other.

Sensations : as if head would burst : as if stomach tightly drawn against spine (compare *Plumb.*, *Plat.*).

As if damp clothing on arms and legs (*Sepia*).

Tongue as if scalded : a load on chest.

Excruciating pain lower part stomach.

As if boiling water were poured over parts.

Dreams of water.

VIBURNUM OPULUS
Cramp Bark ; High Cranberry Bush

(Clarke says, " Our Guelder Rose, is the cultivated and sterile variety.")

Provings by H. C. Allen, with eleven provers, male and female. The ϕ and the first and thirtieth strengths were used.

and VIBURNUM PRUNIFOLIUM
Black Haw

ONE learns most about the *Viburnums* from HALE'S *Materia Medica of the New Remedies* (1880 Edition).

He says : " The physician who shall find a remedy for *painful menstruation* will have the blessings of thousands of suffering women."

That VIBURNUM OPULUS, for the treatment of dysmenorrhœa, is traditional in this country (U.S.A.). That the aborigines so used it, and handed the secret down to the white people ; . . . that it has been successfully used as a domestic remedy for more than a century. Hale says that he first realized its value, from observation of its domestic uses. He used a weak infusion ; or drop doses of the ϕ, finally dilutions up to the 3*x*. It appears to have been used most in the lower potencies.

He says that it is specifically indicated in *spasmodic dysmenorrhœa* : for " *false labour pains*, which may render a woman's life a torture for weeks " ; for " *after-pains*—a dose after every pain ". He says that " *cramps in the abdomen and legs* of pregnant women are controlled very quickly by it."—" It will prevent *miscarriage*, if given before the membranes are injured, and when pains are spasmodic or threatening." He predicts that it will prove useful in spasmodic conditions of all *hollow muscular organs*. He says he has used *Viburnum* in many cases of neuralgia and spasmodic dysmenorrhœa, " and has yet to meet a single case where it has failed to cure." . . . So much so, that he had taken pains to look up old cases, dismissed as incurable years ago, and " in every instance, so far, it has cured these old, obstinate cases."

He tells of corroboration from physicians who have written him since his first accounts of the value of *Viburnum*. One reports a cure of a membraneous dysmenorrhœa :—" if this should be

verified, we have now four remedies for that painful condition—
Borax, Guaiacum, Ustilago and *Viburnum.*

" I shall not be surprised," he says, " if it is found useful in
heart cramp, which is the real condition, in angina pectoris ; also
perhaps in *spasmodia laryngitis.*"

[Why not, also, in *Asthma* ?]

In regard to the VIBURNUM PRUNIFOLIUM, he writes : This
species seems to possess some of the properties of the *Viburnum op.*
But is probably not identical in its powers.   He had used the
tincture in *threatened premature labour* or *miscarriage, dysmenorrhœa*
and spasmodic uterine pains, with good results.

He quotes a Dr. Phares of Alabama (Allopath), who says : " It
is particularly valuable in preventing abortion and miscarriage,
whether habitual or otherwise ;   whether threatened from
accidental causes, or criminal drugging. . . . It completely
neutralizes the action of *Gossypium* (used for purposes of abortion)
and compels the delinquent mother, however unwilling, to carry
the fœtus to full term.   Some farmers on whose plantations I have
used this medicine and who have seen much of its effects on negro
women who always managed to miscarry, declare their belief that
no woman can possibly abort if compelled to use the Viburnum."   He
says, that " it has certainly prevented abortion in every case in
which I have ordered it for the purpose, . . . that miscarriage
has never taken place, so he is informed, in any case where this
medicine has been used as a preventive."   He gives a number
of interesting cases.

*   *   *

One may say, that one has given *Viburnum prun.* in the ϕ to
a certain number of cases of threatened abortion, with, so far as
one can remember, success.

That VIBURNUM is absolutely homœopathic to the conditions,
which, by long native and domestic practice it traditionally cures,
will be gathered from the following provings—some made with the
30th potency.   It would, therefore, probably work as well—
possibly better, needing less frequent repetition, in the higher
potencies.   Of these we have no personal experience—*yet !*

BLACK LETTER SYMPTOMS, AND ITALICS (*Viburnum opulus*)

Dull frontal headache.

She has cramping colic pains in lower abdomen, almost unbearable.
Pains come suddenly and with terrible severity.
Cramp-like colic pains in lower abdomen (during menstruation).

Before menses : severe bearing down ; drawing in anterior muscles of thigh : heavy aching in sacral region and over pubes ; occasional sharp, shooting pains in ovaries ; they make her so nervous that she cannot sit still. Excruciating, cramping, colicky pains in lower abdomen and through womb. Pains begin in back and go around, ending in cramps in uterus.

During menses : nausea ; cramping pain and great nervous restlessness : flow ceases for several hours, then returns in clots.

Menstrual flow scanty, thin, light-coloured, with sensation of lightness of head, faint when trying to sit up. Spasmodic, or membraneous dysmenorrhœa.

Leucorrhœa, thin, yellow-white or colourless, except with stool, when it is thick, white, blood-streaked.

NEURALGIC AND SPASMODIC DYSMENORRHŒA.

Pain beginning in back and going round to loins and across pubic bone like labour pains.

Irritable ovaries, with dysmenorrhœa.

Cramp-like pains and spasms of stomach, bowels, bladder or other organs, when reflex from uterine irritation.

Cramps in abdomen and legs of pregnant women.

Will prevent miscarriage if given before the membranes are injured, and when the pains are spasmodic and threatening.

Hysterical convulsions from uterine irritation.

General irritation of nervous system.

Cramps and contractions of extremities, especially during pregnancy.

Among peculiar sensations are also :

Opening and shutting in left parietal region (in occiput *Cocc.* Compare also *Cann. ind.*).

Stabbed with a knife in eyes and ears.

Ears pinned to head.

As if she could not live : sick feeling in stomach.

Pelvic organs turning upside down.

As if she would collapse, from waist to lower pelvis.

As if breath would leave body and heart would cease beating.

Clutching and cramping pains in heart.

Excruciating, cramping pain in heart.

Oppression over whole chest : dyspnœa, as if chest muscles failed to act.

As if hands would burst.

In sleep, sensation of falling, wakes with a start. (Compare *Thuja.*)

Dr. Boger, writing later, stresses a few more points.

Violent nervous, or spasmodic effects *in females.* Can't keep still.

CRAMPING.

Hæmorrhage.

Frequent profuse urination : during headache, menses, hæmorrhage, etc.

Heavy ache, or EXCRUCIATING CRAMPS IN PELVIS : > menses.

Dysmenorrhœa ; with flatulency, loud eructations and nervousness.

MISCARRIAGE. False labour pains.

UTERINE HÆMORRHAGE.

SUFFOCATION : at night ; worse cold damp.

Infantile asthma.

Pains in back, end in CRAMP IN UTERUS, OR GO DOWN ANTERIOR SURFACE OF THIGHS.

VISCUM ALBUM

Mistletoe

ONE of our little-known remedies, and not too well proved, one gathers. But a remedy for chorea and epilepsy is not to be lightly set aside.

It was one of the late Dr. Robert Cooper's cases that brought the drug to mind, and we will try to do it justice and make it available for us all.

BOGER (*Synoptic Key*) gives it only a few lines, but says it is related to *Bufo*. One of his points is, " Vertigo persists after epileptic attacks ". A late edition of BOERICKE gives many symptoms ; and CLARKE has a great deal to say about it in his *Dictionary*.

Clarke, Burnett and Cooper—it is difficult to talk of them in the past tense ; since they, being dead, still speak convincingly. They were a wonderful trio of geniuses in their several ways. Each seems always to supplement the others.

Actually the mistletoe is a very ancient remedy—for epilepsy, for chorea, for disorders of the spleen and for " imposthumes " (abscesses) according to old Culpepper, some three hundred years ago. We shall see how far he is followed, in our day. He speaks not only of the mistletoe, but of the virtues of bird-lime made from the berries of the mistletoe, " to ripen and draw forth thick and thin humours from remote parts of the body, digesting and separating them ; to mollify the hardness of the spleen ; to help old ulcers and sores, and mixed with sanderick and orpiment, it helps to draw off foul nails. Mistletoe, made into powder and given to drink, is good for falling sickness (epilepsy). The fresh wood bruised and the juice extracted and dropped into the ears is effectual in curing the imposthumes in them. Mistletoe is a cephalic and nervine medicine, useful for convulsive fits, palsy and vertigo."

These ancient uses still obtain.

Viscum alb. has been proved. In one of the provings symptoms were those of aura epileptica and petit mal, which recurred frequently for two years.

Clarke has much of most interest to say in regard to the mistletoe. It cured a fine breed of horses which became epileptic at four years of age. It has cured chorea ; ear troubles ; spleen ;

uterine diseases. A number of cases " of catarrhal deafness with noises in the ears " are also recorded as cured.

He gives some curious mental and physical symptoms : Feels as if going to do something dreadful while the tremblings are on. Wakes in the night thinking of most horrible things. Trembling limbs. Teeth chatter ; jerkings. He says it has cured whooping cough in two days. There is a sensation on dorsum of left hand as if a large spider were crawling over it, then the same on dorsum of right hand. Another queer sensation, as if something dragging her down from the waist, and directly afterwards as if upper part of body were floating in air.

In fatal cases of poisoning, all muscles of body were paralysed except those of eyes. The victims could neither speak nor swallow and died on the eighth or ninth day.

This is what Dr. Robert Cooper has to say in regard to a case he cured :

" As to my reasons for prescribing *Viscum alb.*—they are, firstly, its well-known effects over choreic symptoms. Here we had a trembling heart, twitching of the limbs at night, and severe shaking fits with a cataleptoid state of insensibility for hours. The prescription of *Viscum* was amply justified by the Hahne-mannian principle that the symptoms, and not the names merely of diseases, are to correspond to the remedy . . ." He also quotes a writer who expresses his opinion that the *Viscum* is far superior, in labour cases, to all remedies he had hitherto tried.